# 2013
## YEAR BOOK OF
# PEDIATRICS®

# The 2013 Year Book Series

**Year Book of Anesthesiology and Pain Management™:** Drs Chestnut, Abram, Black, Gravlee, Lien, Mathru, and Roizen

**Year Book of Cardiology®:** Drs Gersh, Cheitlin, Elliott, Gold, Graham, and Thourani

**Year Book of Critical Care Medicine®:** Drs Dries, Zanotti-Cavazzoni, Latenser, Martinez, Rincon, and Zwank

**Year Book of Dermatology and Dermatologic Surgery™:** Dr Del Rosso

**Year Book of Diagnostic Radiology®:** Drs Elster, Abbara, Oestreich, Offiah, Rosado de Christenson, Stephens, and Strickland

**Year Book of Emergency Medicine®:** Drs Hamilton, Bruno, Handly, Minczak, Mullin, Quintana, and Ramoska

**Year Book of Endocrinology®:** Drs Schott, Apovian, Clarke, Eugster, Meikle, Oetgen, Ovalle, Schteingart, and Toth

**Year Book of Hand and Upper Limb Surgery®:** Drs Yao, Adams, Isaacs, Lee, and Rizzo

**Year Book of Medicine®:** Drs Barker, Garrick, Gersh, Khardori, LeRoith, Panush, Talley, and Thigpen

**Year Book of Neonatal and Perinatal Medicine®:** Drs Fanaroff, Benitz, Donn, Neu, Papile, and Van Marter

**Year Book of Neurology and Neurosurgery®:** Drs Klimo, Minagar, Gandhi, House, Kevill, Liu, Mazia, Panagariya, Ragel, Riesenburger, Robottom, Schwendimann, Shafazand, Uhm, and Yang

**Year Book of Obstetrics, Gynecology, and Women's Health®:** Drs Dungan and Shulman

**Year Book of Oncology®:** Drs Arceci, Bauer, Chiorean, Gordon, Lawton, Murphy, Thigpen, and Tsao

**Year Book of Ophthalmology®:** Drs Rapuano, Cohen, Flanders, Hammersmith, Milman, Myers, Nagra, Nelson, Penne, Pyfer, Sergott, Shields, Talekar, and Vander

**Year Book of Orthopedics®:** Drs Morrey, Huddleston, Rose, Swiontkowski, and Trigg

**Year Book of Otolaryngology-Head and Neck Surgery®:** Drs Sindwani, Balough, Franco, Gapany, and Mitchell

**Year Book of Pathology and Laboratory Medicine®:** Drs Raab and Bissell

**Year Book of Pediatrics®:** Dr Stockman

**Year Book of Plastic and Aesthetic Surgery™:** Drs Miller, Gosman, Gurtner, Gutowski, Ruberg, Salisbury, and Smith

2013

# The Year Book of PEDIATRICS®

Editor

## James A. Stockman III, MD

*President, The American Board of Pediatrics; Clinical Professor of Pediatrics, University of North Carolina Medical School at Chapel Hill, and Duke University Medical Center, Durham, North Carolina*

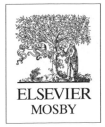

ELSEVIER
MOSBY

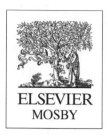

**ELSEVIER**
MOSBY

*Vice President, Continuity:* Kimberly Murphy
*Editor:* Kerry Holland
*Production Supervisor, Electronic Year Books:* Donna M. Skelton
*Electronic Article Manager:* Emily Ogle
*Illustrations and Permissions Coordinator:* Dawn Vohsen

**2013 EDITION**

Printed in the United States of America
Composition by TNQ Books and Journals Pvt Ltd, India

Editorial Office:
Elsevier
Suite 1800
1600 John F. Kennedy Blvd.
Philadelphia, PA 19103-2899

International Standard Serial Number: 0084-3954
International Standard Book Number: 978-1-4557-7286-5

Transferred to Digital Printing, 2012

# Table of Contents

# Journals Represented

Journals represented in this YEAR BOOK are listed below.

Acta Paediatrica
Annals of Internal Medicine
Archives of Disease in Childhood
Archives of Pediatrics & Adolescent Medicine
Blood
British Medical Journal
Clinical Pediatrics
Journal of Adolescent Health
Journal of Developmental and Behavioral Pediatrics
Journal of Pediatric Gastroenterology and Nutrition
Journal of Pediatric Hematology/Oncology
Journal of Pediatric Ophthalmology and Strabismus
Journal of Pediatric Orthopedics
Journal of Pediatric Surgery
Journal of Pediatrics
Journal of the American Academy of Child & Adolescent Psychiatry
Journal of the American Medical Association
Lancet
Nature Medicine
New England Journal of Medicine
Pediatric Cardiology
Pediatric Emergency Care
Pediatric Infectious Disease Journal
Pediatrics
Science

---

## STANDARD ABBREVIATIONS

The following terms are abbreviated in this edition: acquired immunodeficiency syndrome (AIDS), cardiopulmonary resuscitation (CPR), central nervous system (CNS), cerebrospinal fluid (CSF), computed tomography (CT), deoxyribonucleic acid (DNA), electrocardiography (ECG), health maintenance organization (HMO), human immunodeficiency virus (HIV), intensive care unit (ICU), intramuscular (IM), intravenous (IV), magnetic resonance (MR) imaging (MRI), ribonucleic acid (RNA), ultrasound (US), and ultraviolet (UV).

---

## NOTE

The YEAR BOOK OF PEDIATRICS® is a literature survey service providing abstracts of articles published in the professional literature. Every effort is made to assure the accuracy of the information presented in these pages. Neither the editors nor the publisher of the YEAR BOOK OF PEDIATRICS® can be responsible for errors in the original materials. The editors' comments are their own opinions. Mention of specific products within this publication does not constitute endorsement.

To facilitate the use of the YEAR BOOK OF PEDIATRICS® as a reference tool, all illustrations and tables included in this publication are now identified as they appear in the original article. This change is meant to help the reader recognize that any illustration or table appearing in the YEAR BOOK OF PEDIATRICS® may be only one of many in the original article. For this reason, figure and table numbers will often appear to be out of sequence within the YEAR BOOK OF PEDIATRICS.®

# Introduction

*"However beautiful the strategy, you should occasionally look at results."*
- **Winston Churchill**

The YEAR BOOK OF PEDIATRICS stands proud in the history of medical education, an instrument that for over a century has assisted those providing care to children. The YEAR BOOK exists in hard copy book format, a "traditional" transfer of knowledge available to humans since the written word first went from appearing on rocks then onto papyrus. The same YEAR BOOK material exists in an electronic format available to be read on computers, Kindle Fires, iPads and other electronic media. No matter how well one is doing with the transfer of knowledge, however, one should occasionally look at the results, as Sir Winston suggests. It is interesting to note how medical education and its results have evolved over time.

It was in 1910 that the revolutionary Flexner Report changed the face of medical education in the United States. Commissioned by the Carnegie Foundation for the Advancement of Teaching at the request of the American Medical Association's Council on Medical Education, Abraham Flexner collected information about the current state of medical education in the United States and Canada by visiting all 155 medical schools in North America. His report highlighted several university-based programs that had already adopted a system firmly rooted in scientific inquiry and concomitantly called for extensive reform and standardization of our medical education system. Many substandard medical schools were closed, state licensing systems improved, and methods to certify specialists established.

A century later we are again seeing the status quo in medical education and the methods for the transfer of knowledge undergoing a transition, a second revolution of sorts. Changes in this regard are occurring at a pace impossible to imagine 100 years ago. Take for example, the Medical College Admission Test (MCAT), which has been formatted exactly the same way for decades and has consisted of four sessions looking at the physical sciences, verbal reasoning, a writing sample, and the biological sciences. Beginning in 2015, the test will now include a section on behavioral and social sciences and a section on critical analysis and reading that will replace the writing sample.[1] This reflects the recognition that behavioral and social factors not only now claim major roles in health and illness, but also interact with biological factors to influence health outcomes. Once in medical school, students are experiencing a very different curriculum from students a generation ago. Curriculum has evolved in ways Flexner could not have predicted. For example Stanford School of Medicine has initiated the concept of lecture halls without lectures.[2] This is a flipped-classroom model in which students absorb an instructor's lecture in digital format as homework, freeing up "lecture hall" time for a focus on applications, mind-expanding exercises, and discussions of case-based, problem-based, and team-based activities that call for retrieval and integration of prior knowledge.

The variability that exists in graduate medical education is undergoing a different revolution. The Accreditation Council for Graduate Medical Education, the entity that accredits the environment of residency learning in the United States, has entered into a new era called "The Next Accreditation System (NAS)." With a phase starting in 2013, NAS allows training programs to be more innovative and to evaluate trainees based on measurements and reporting of outcomes through the creation of educational milestones, a natural progression of the work on the six general competencies introduced more than a decade ago.[3] The aim is to facilitate a logical trajectory of professional development permitting the essential elements of competency to be evaluated based not on time in training but on the achievement of relevant educational and performance milestones.

The continuing education and assessment of the practicing physician is clearly undergoing an even more fundamental series of dramatic changes. The question has even been asked whether traditional continuing medical education (CME) delivered through medical conferences will remain viable or of importance in assisting physicians of all types in keeping up to date.[4] It has been estimated that there may be more than 100 000 medical meetings held annually in the United States. In an electronic age in which information can be shared around the world instantly, the contribution of large medical conferences in the dissemination of knowledge is unclear. The Internet and other social media technologies have enabled new experiments, including open-access journals, that have shifted the costs of journal production to authors so that research results may be freely shared globally.[5] Blogs, listservs, Twitter feeds, etc, permit everyone an authorial voice and increasingly influence what counts as relevant medical information. There are few if any creditable journals not available for reading on iPads or other electronic media. The iPad soon may be adapted to become a portable ultrasound machine, an example of how technology used to acquire knowledge can serve a dual function as a diagnostic tool.[6] There is also a race to replace hard copy textbooks with electronic versions, although the majority of students still seem to prefer traditional print books when offered the choice. It appears that reading electronic textbooks (as opposed to leisure reading of ebooks) takes longer, on average, than reading hard copy print and may elicit a higher level of reader fatigue.[7] Nonetheless, the cognitive consequences of having information at our fingertips and being continuously "wired" are inestimable. This "Google effect" on learning and recall has opened a whole new era of educational research that shows that the experience of losing our Internet connection becomes more and more like losing a friend. We must remain plugged in to know what Google knows; it is our contemporary "Hal" of Space Odyssey 2001.

This introduction closes with the observation that the YEAR BOOK OF PEDIATRICS will continuously evolve to meet our readers' needs and interests. It will, however, remain anchored to the belief that most advances in medicine come from inquisitive minds underpinned by current knowledge.

In this regard, we suggest you read an editorial in *Science* that highlights these concepts by Alphonso Joseph D'Abruzzo, also known as Alan Alda, the actor.[8] Alda notes that when he was 11, he was a curious creature and had been thinking for days about the flame at the end of a candle. He finally took the problem to his teacher. "What's a flame?" he asked. The only answer he got was "It's oxidation." Deflated, he knew there needed to be more to the mystery of a flame than just giving the mystery another name. In his editorial, Alda suggested a playful experiment and asked the journal reader to have a go at writing one's own explanation of what a flame is—one that an 11-year-old would find intelligible and maybe even fun. The intent would be to ignite people's curiosity, to seek out knowledge, and to pass this knowledge on to the next generation.

What Mr Alda suggests is in some ways quite similar to what the YEAR BOOK OF PEDIATRICS is about. If you are innately curious, this book will provide knowledge and hopefully some fun at times. It is up to you, however, to ask the probing questions, to integrate the knowledge you acquire, and just as importantly, to pass it on to the next generation of learners. There is more to the educational process than just the Google effect.

This introduction to the 2013 YEAR BOOK OF PEDIATRICS has been longer than in the past. It is always a challenge to decide how long is long enough and how long is perhaps too long. In that regard:

*"Writing should end not when there is nothing more to add, rather, when there is nothing more to take away."*

- **Anonymous**

Additionally, if you want to read about the flame challenge and the challenge to the readers of *Science*, go to: http://flamechallenge.com.[8]

**J. A. Stockman III, MD**

*References*

1. Kaplan RM, Satterfield JM, Kington RS. Building a better physician—the case for the new MCAT. *N Engl J Med*. 2012;366:1265-1268.
2. Prober CG, Heath C. Lecture halls without lectures—a proposal for medical education. *N Engl J Med*. 2012;366:1657-1659.
3. Nasca TJ, Philibert I, Brigham T, Flynn TC. The next GME accreditation system—rationale and benefits. *N Engl J Med*. 2012;366:1051-1056.
4. Ioannidis JP. Are medical conferences useful? And for whom? *JAMA*. 2012;307:1257-1258.
5. Podolsky SH, Greene JA, Jones DS. The evolving roles of the medical journal. *N Engl J Med*. 2012;366:1457-1461.
6. Spence D. Medical heresy: ditch the eponyms. *BMJ*. 2012;344:e2503.
7. National Association of College Stores. Update: electronic book and ereader device report: March 2011. *NCAS OnCampus Research*. Feb 2011. http://www.nacs.org/LinkClick.aspx?fileticket=ulf2NoXApKQ%3d&tabid=2471&mid=3210. Accessed August 27, 2012.
8. Alda A. The flame challenge. *Science*. 2012;335:1019.

# 1 Adolescent Medicine

## Celebrity Worship and Incidence of Elective Cosmetic Surgery: Evidence of a Link Among Young Adults

Maltby J, Day L (Univ of Leicester, UK; Sheffield Hallam Univ, UK)
*J Adolesc Health* 49.483-489, 2011

*Purpose.*—The purpose of the current study was to explore among young adults whether celebrity worship predicted the incidence of elective cosmetic surgery within the period of 8 months after controlling for several known predictors of elective cosmetic surgery.

*Methods.* A total of 137 young adults completed questionnaire measures of attitudes toward a celebrity whose body image they admired, previous and vicarious experience of elective cosmetic surgery, attitudes toward cosmetic surgery, and a range of psychological and demographic measures at time 1. Participants were then asked to report whether they had undergone elective cosmetic surgery 8 months later.

*Results.*—After controlling for several known predictors of elective cosmetic surgery, intense-personal celebrity worship of a celebrity whose body shape was admired by the participant predicted the incidence of elective cosmetic surgery within an 8-month period.

*Conclusions.*—The current findings suggest that the type of para-social relationship that young adults form with celebrities, particularly with those whose body shape is admired, may need to be considered by those when speaking to, and educating, young people about their choices around elective cosmetic surgery.

▶ Cosmetic procedures have become pervasive in our society and are being advertised in the mass media. Teens are exposed continuously to TV programs emphasizing "natural" beauty. The American Society of Aesthetic Plastic Surgery estimates that the number of children younger than 18 years undergoing cosmetic surgery procedures by members of the organization has increased from 33 000 to 65 000 procedures annually over the last decade, with nonsurgical cosmetic procedures increasing from 91 000 to 190 000 per year. We should all be asking ourselves whether the increase in cosmetic surgery among teens raises health concerns. While surgery to correct deformities such as cleft lip and palate have clear benefits, procedures such as liposuction and breast augmentation or reduction in adolescence are much more controversial. Indeed, there is no scientific evidence that surgery improves self-esteem or confidence in the long term.

Maltby et al undertook a study to examine whether celebrity worship in any way predicts the incidence of elective cosmetic surgery among young adults. In a study carried out in Great Britain, 137 young adults (mean age, 19.74 years; range, 18 to 23 years) in 2 cities completed questionnaires regarding attitudes toward celebrities whose body image they admired, previous experiences regarding cosmetic surgery, and a host of psychological and demographic measures, such as measures of body shape, self-esteem, life satisfaction, and self-rated attractiveness. These young adults were followed up within a year to also determine whether they had undergone any elective cosmetic surgical procedures. The most frequent procedures reported by the subjects were Botox, soft tissue fillers, breast augmentation, breast lift, laser skin resurfacing, and nose reshaping. After controlling for known predictors of cosmetic surgery, such as body-image preoccupation, self-esteem, sex, and previous cosmetic surgery, the researchers found that celebrity worship of an individual whose body was admired predicted the likelihood of cosmetic surgery.

The results from the Maltby et al study shed light on celebrity worship as a potential risk factor for undergoing elective cosmetic surgery in late adolescence and early adulthood. Given that there are very few "ugly" or "untrim" individuals in *People Magazine* or *Teen Magazine*, you can see the problem. The data provided by Maltby et al show there is much we need to address regarding cosmetic surgery in adolescents.

As preteens and teenagers growing up, some of us had role models such as Fats Domino and Aretha Franklin. There was little desire to want to remake one's image in a similar body composition in those days.

This commentary closes with an observation about a problem that affects a number of adolescents. In case you are not aware, *phthisis nervosa* and *apepsia hysterica* were names used to describe "modern day" anorexia nervosa as far back as 1689 and 1868, respectively. Both describe the phenomenon of extreme emaciation without apparent organic cause. The term *anorexia nervosa*, however, was first coined in 1874. In France—although not apparently elsewhere—anorexia was considered to be a visual manifestation of the malignant effects of the self-pollution of masturbation. The role of family dynamics was probably first recognized by Alfred Taylor Schofield (1846-1929), who was a writer on religious matters as well as a physician and police surgeon.

**J. A. Stockman III, MD**

---

**Prevalence and Characteristics of Youth Sexting: A National Study**
Mitchell KJ, Finkelhor D, Jones LM, et al (Univ of New Hampshire, Durham)
*Pediatrics* 129:13-20, 2012

---

*Objectives.*—To obtain national estimates of youth involved in sexting in the past year (the transmission via cell phone, the Internet, and other electronic media of sexual images), as well as provide details of the youth involved and the nature of the sexual images.

*Methods.*—The study was based on a cross-sectional national telephone survey of 1560 youth Internet users, ages 10 through 17.

*Results.*—Estimates varied considerably depending on the nature of the images or videos and the role of the youth involved. Two and one-half percent of youth had appeared in or created nude or nearly nude pictures or videos. However, this percentage is reduced to 1.0% when the definition is restricted to only include images that were sexually explicit (ie, showed naked breasts, genitals, or bottoms). Of the youth who participated in the survey, 7.1% said they had received nude or nearly nude images of others; 5.9% of youth reported receiving sexually explicit images. Few youth distributed these images.

*Conclusions.*—Because policy debates on youth sexting behavior focus on concerns about the production and possession of illegal child pornography, it is important to have research that collects details about the nature of the sexual images rather than using ambiguous screening questions without follow-ups. The rate of youth exposure to sexting highlights a need to provide them with information about legal consequences of sexting and advice about what to do if they receive a sexting image. However, the data suggest that appearing in, creating, or receiving sexual images is far from being a normative behavior for youth.

▶ Teens and even preteens are engaging in activities that were essentially unimaginable just a decade or more ago, including *sexting*, a word many parents still have never heard of. *Sexting* generally refers to sending sexual images and sometimes sexual texts via cell phone or other electronic devices. Youngsters may not know it, but in doing so they may be creating illegal child pornography, exposing themselves possibly to serious legal sanctions. That aside, such youngsters may be jeopardizing their future by putting compromising ineradicable images online that could become available to potential employers, academic institutions, and family members. It is not inconceivable that youth can be charged with serious sex crimes and placed on sex offender registries for what some might call impulsive teenage indiscretions. Thus, the topic of sexting is a critical one for parents and care providers to understand and understand thoroughly.

Mitchell et al have assessed in detail the range of youth sexting behaviors, including the content of images that a youth receives, distributes, and creates. The body of information they have generated allows parents, policy makers, and professionals to understand the entire scope of sexting. The information was collected from a survey of more than 1500 youths who were independently contacted by a national survey research firm. The eligible participants were youths ages 10 years to 17 years who had used the Internet at least once a month for the past 6 months. Parents and children provided informed consent, and the interviews were carried out anonymously. Interviewers assured youths that answers would be confidential and they could skip any question and end the interview at any time. Screeners asked the following questions:

1. Has anyone ever sent you nude or nearly nude pictures or videos of kids who were under the age of 18 that someone else took?
2. Have you ever forwarded or posted any nude or nearly nude pictures or videos of other kids who were under the age of 18 that someone else took?
3. Have you ever taken nude or nearly nude pictures or videos of yourself?
4. Has someone else ever taken nude or nearly nude pictures or videos of you?

5. Have you taken nude or nearly nude pictures or videos of other kids who were under the age of 18?

Each of these questions had follow-up questions if the answer was yes.

The results from this survey showed that 10% of youths reported appearing in or creating nude or nearly nude images or receiving such images in the past year. Assuming the results of this report are accurate, one could view the results as the cup is half full versus half empty, meaning that 10% could be considered a high number by some and 10% could be considered a low number by others.

Whether you consider a 10% prevalence of sexting among our youth high or low, it certainly can get youngsters into trouble. Recently, Wolak et al surveyed 2712 law enforcement agencies to ask whether they had handled sexting cases from 2008 to 2009.[1] The investigators undertook detailed telephone interviews to determine the scope of the trouble kids get themselves into. The study results suggested that production of sexual images by teens, or what has come to be called *sexting*, is a pervasive phenomenon that can result in serious criminal activity, such as adults interacting sexually with underage youths, young people engaging in blackmail or other criminal or malicious behavior, or youths just recklessly circulating nude images. About one-third of police reports involving sexting were found to have no malicious elements, probably best characterized as experimental romantic and sexual attention-seeking among adolescents. The estimate is that the total number of cases coming to police attention was 3477 in 2008 and 2009 or about 1750 per year. One can guess that this is a number that is simply the tip of the iceberg. In most cases, law enforcement officers were fairly restrained in terms of how they deal with youth sexting. Most youths were not arrested and, of the few youths who were subject to sex offender registration laws, most had committed additional sex crimes, such as sexual assault. Many cases in this series involved criminal, malicious, or reckless behavior. Although such cases are probably overrepresented in police data and not frequent among the general population of adolescents, these are the most concerning that should be targeted for intervention by clinicians.

The report of Wolak is important for all of us to read. It contains an extensive appendix showing examples of cases of sexting that have come to police attention and how they were handled. As pediatric care providers, you can be certain that parents will come to you with questions about their children's sexting. Learning about this problem is imperative.

This commentary closes with an observation having to do with marriage during adolescence. It has been estimated that worldwide some 60 million or more women were married as children (before the age of 18 years). More than half of such marriages occur in South Asia. Child marriage is recognized as a violation of human rights and is associated with severe limitation of educational and work opportunities; early, frequent, and unplanned pregnancies; and increased maternal and infant morbidity and mortality. In India since 1978, marriages for girls under the age of 18 years has been illegal, but a 1998 to 1999 survey showed that 50% of women aged 20 years to 24 years had married as children. More recent studies show that such child marriages still remain quite common particularly in India. Among 2807 Indian women age 20 years to 24 years, 45% were married before the age of 18, 23% before the age of 16, and 3% before the age of 13 years. Child marriage in India is associated with lack of contraceptive use, high fertility, short time between child births (less than 24 months), multiple unwanted pregnancies, pregnancy termination, and female sterilization. Recent data for the United States for comparative purposes are not available.[2]

**J. A. Stockman III, MD**

*References*

1. Wolak J, Finkelhor D, Mitchell KJ. How often are teens arrested for sexting? Data from a national sample of police cases. *Pediatrics*. 2012;129:4-12.
2. Editorial comment. Teen marriages. *Arch Dis Child*. 2009;94:822.

---

**Comparison of rates of adverse events in adolescent and adult women undergoing medical abortion: population register based study**
Niinimäki M, Suhonen S, Mentula M, et al (Univ Hosp of Oulu, Finland; City of Helsinki Health Centre, Finland; Helsinki Univ Central Hosp, Finland; et al)
*BMJ* 342:d2111, 2011

---

*Objective.*—To determine the risks of short term adverse events in adolescent and older women undergoing medical abortion.

*Design.*—Population based retrospective cohort study.

*Setting.*—Finnish abortion register 2000-6.

*Participants.*—All women (n = 27 030) undergoing medical abortion during 2000-6, with only the first induced abortion analysed for each woman.

*Main Outcome Measures.*—Incidence of adverse events (haemorrhage, infection, incomplete abortion, surgical evacuation, psychiatric morbidity, injury, thromboembolic disease, and death) among adolescent (< 18 years) and older (≥ 18 years) women through record linkage of Finnish registries and genital *Chlamydia trachomatis* infections detected concomitantly with abortion and linked with data from the abortion register for 2004-6.

*Results.*—During 2000-6, 3024 adolescents and 24 006 adults underwent at least one medical abortion. The rate of chlamydia infections was higher in the adolescent cohort (5.7% v 3.7%, P < 0.001). The incidence of adverse events among adolescents was similar or lower than that among the adults. The risks of haemorrhage (adjusted odds ratio 0.87, 95% confidence interval 0.77 to 0.99), incomplete abortion (0.69, 0.59 to 0.82), and surgical evacuation (0.78, 0.67 to 0.90) were lower in the adolescent cohort. In subgroup analysis of primigravid women, the risks of incomplete abortion (0.68, 0.56 to 0.81) and surgical evacuation (0.75, 0.64 to 0.88) were lower in the adolescent cohort. In logistic regression, duration of gestation was the most important risk factor for infection, incomplete abortion, and surgical evacuation.

*Conclusions.*—The incidence of adverse events after medical abortion was similar or lower among adolescents than among older women.

Thus, medical abortion seems to be at least as safe in adolescents as it is in adults.

▶ A few studies have specifically assessed the risks of medical abortion in adolescents. In the linked retrospective cohort study, Niinimäki et al assess the outcomes in 3024 adolescent females and 24006 adults who underwent medical abortion between 2000 and 2006. The study was reported from Helsinki, Finland. The development of "modern" methods for medical abortion began in the 1970s. Initial approaches used prostaglandins alone. When given at any point in pregnancy, prostaglandins induce uterine contractions that can lead to expulsion of the embryo or fetus. However, the effectiveness of medical abortion with early generation prostaglandin compounds alone was not uniformly effective for the purpose of inducing an abortion. Side effects were common, particularly gastrointestinal ones.

The early situation with medical abortion changed with the development of mifepristone. Early in pregnancy, this antiprogestin causes the trophoblast to detach from the uterine wall and softens the cervix. Mifepristone also increases endogenous prostaglandin release while sensitizing the uterus to the uterotonic prostaglandin effects. When this agent is combined with a prostaglandin, an abortion will be induced in between 92% and 99% of women treated with this combination during the first trimester. Generally, the way this is done is with a single oral dose of mifepristone, 200 mg, followed in 1 to 2 days by the administration of misoprostol, a prostaglandin E1 derivative. The latter drug is usually swallowed or placed in the vagina, under the tongue, or against the cheek. In typical clinical use (not in research studies), only about 2 women per 1000 experience a complication requiring inpatient or outpatient hospital treatment when such a combination of drugs is used to induce abortion. The most common complication is heavy bleeding. The risk of mortality is similar to that with surgical abortion, about 1 in 100000.

So what did Niinimäki et al find? They noted that serious adverse events (thromboembolic disease, surgical interventions, death) were rare in adolescents undergoing medical abortion. The actual incidence of adverse events among adolescents was similar or lower than in adults, including the risk of hemorrhage, incomplete abortion, and the need for surgical evacuation. The risk of infection did not differ between the cohorts. As might be expected, risks increased the longer pregnancy had been in place.

Whether one is pro-life or pro-choice, the information from this report is useful in that it provides objective data on the risks of medical abortion that inform all of us. The investigators obviously took no opinion other than to state the facts.

This commentary closes with an observation having to do with teenage fatherhood. It is clear that becoming a father in one's teens has both educational and economic consequences according to a journal report.[1] Teenage fatherhood is a topic far less researched than teenage motherhood, but this study found that teenage fatherhood significantly reduces the chances of graduating from high school but increases the chance of full-time employment by 6 percentage points and military employment by 6 percentage points after a birth. Teenage fatherhood also leads to an increased likelihood of early marriage and cohabitation. This must be a difficult way to grow up fast given the responsibilities associated with becoming a father at a young age.

**J. A. Stockman III, MD**

*Reference*

1. Fletcher JM, Wolfe BL. The effects of teenage fatherhood on young adult outcomes. *Economic Inquiry.* 2011; http://dx.doi.org/10.1111/j.1465-7295.2011.00372.x.

## The Association of Religion and Virginity Status Among Brazilian Adolescents

Ogland CP, Xu X, Bartkowski JP, et al (Univ of Texas at San Antonio)
*J Adolesc Health* 48:651-653, 2011

This study examines the association between religious factors and the virginity status of unmarried Brazilian female adolescents aged 15–19 years. The analysis draws on data from the Brazilian National Demographic and Health Survey (2006) using a sub-sample of unmarried Brazilian female adolescents aged 15–19 years (N = 2,364). Multinomial logistic regression is used to test the association between denominational affiliation, worship service participation, and self-reported virginity status. The findings reveal that adolescents affiliated with Protestant faiths, particularly Pentecostalism, and those who attend worship services often have significantly higher odds of remaining a virgin because of a commitment to not have sex until marriage. This premarital chastity rationale for virginity is most strongly evidenced among frequently attending teens who are affiliated with Protestant and Pentecostal faiths. Similar to patterns observed in the United States, teen involvement with Protestant faiths, particularly strict traditions, such as Pentecostalism, is associated with a commitment to virginity in Brazil.

▶ Brazil is no different than many other countries. It is Latin America's most populous nation, and sexual behavior has changed there significantly in recent years. In keeping with similar trends across Latin America, Brazilian adolescents are increasingly likely to become sexually active during their teen years. A study in 1986 found that 94% of never-married female teens reported being abstinent, but by 2006, this percentage had declined to 52%.[1] The intersection of religion and sexual behavior has become of significant interest to investigators who look at Brazilian youth.

Ogland et al have documented that teens who show significant degrees of religiosity are much more likely to report virginity in comparison with teens who have no religious affiliation. This was true of teens who were Catholic, Protestant, or Pentecostal. Interestingly, the most robust data showing the relationship between religion and virginity were for those teens who practiced Protestantism and Pentecostalism. These findings suggest that Pentecostalism and other Protestant (likely non-Pentecostal Evangelical) faiths sacralize marriage in Brazil as they do in the United States. As part of this broader sacralization of marriage, sexual behavior is defined as an activity that is morally appropriate only within the confines of marriage. What is a tad unusual is that those professing Catholicism, which also has similar definitions, do not, in general, maintain the same level of virginity.

While on the topic of sexuality, a new study has come up with 41 definitions of what "having sex" means. A major survey of sexual behavior among Americans has shown that among men who said they had an orgasm during their last sexual encounter, 85% believed that their partner also had an orgasm, yet only 64% of women indicated they had experienced an orgasm. The study of nearly 6000 men and women age 14 to 94 also found that penetrative sex was most common among men 25 to 39 years and women 20 to 29 years and declined progressively among older age groups. However, between 20% and 30% of men and women remained sexually active well into their 80s.[2] Over time, both in teens and older adults, oral and anal sex appear to have become much more common. The study indicated that some people consider sex to be only vaginal intercourse, while some people consider anal sex or oral sex to be sex. The study found there were a total of 41 combinations of what constitutes "sex."

This study was funded by a church group and the Dwight Company, the maker of Trojan condoms. The investigators noted in their report that scientific integrity was maintained throughout their research. For more on this topic, see the comment by Tanne.[3] Last, this commentary closes with some additional insights, having to do with adolescent fatherhood. It appears that adolescent fatherhood is "catching"—or at least there seems to be an intergenerational cycle of adolescent fatherhood. Data from nearly 1500 young men who were interviewed annually for the US National Longitudinal Survey of Youth 1997 show that sons of adolescent fathers are 1.8 times more likely to become adolescent fathers themselves than are sons of older fathers. Other factors that independently predict adolescent fatherhood are delinquency, maternal education, and early adolescent dating. The authors recommend that interventional programs tackle all these risk factors.[4]

**J. A. Stockman III, MD**

*References*

1. Brazil Ministry of Health, 2006. *Brazil National Demographic and Health Survey Data (Online)*. http://bvsms.saude.gov.br/bvs/pnds/index.php. Accessed January 1, 2010.
2. Reece M, Herbenick D, Fortenberry JD, Dodge B, Sanders SA, Schick V. National survey of sexual health and behavior (NSSHB): Center for sexual health promotion. http://www.nationalsexstudy.indiana.edu. Accessed November 8, 2011.
3. Tanne JH. Study comes up with 41 definitions of what "having sex" means. *BMJ*. 2010;341:752.
4. Sipsma H, Biello KB, Cole-Lewis H, Kershaw T. Like father, like son: the intergenerational cycle of adolescent fatherhood. *Amer J Public Health*. 2010;100: 517-524.

## Sexual Abuse in Childhood and Adolescence and the Risk of Early Pregnancy Among Women Ages 18–22

Young M-ED, Deardorff J, Ozer E, et al (Univ of California, Berkeley)
*J Adolesc Health* 49:287-293, 2011

*Purpose.*—This clinic- and community-based study of young women investigated the relationship between previous sexual abuse and early pregnancy, examining the effect of the developmental period in which sexual abuse occurred and type of sexual abuse, while also providing methodological advances in the assessment of distinctive sexual abuse and its sequelae.

*Methods.*—Secondary data analysis using Cox proportional hazards models was conducted to determine the association between sexual abuse in childhood, in adolescence, or both, and risk of early pregnancy among 1,790 young women. In addition, this study examined the type of sexual abuse that occurred during each period.

*Results.*—As compared with women with no history of sexual abuse, women who experienced sexual abuse only in childhood had a 20% greater hazard of pregnancy; women who experienced sexual abuse only in adolescence had a 30% greater hazard of pregnancy; and women who experienced sexual abuse in both childhood and adolescence had an 80% greater hazard of pregnancy. Across these periods, attempted rape and rape were associated with an increased hazard of pregnancy. The association between sexual abuse and pregnancy was mediated by age at first intercourse and moderated by a woman's education level.

*Conclusion.*—This study provides evidence that both the developmental timing and the type of sexual abuse contributes to an increased risk for early pregnancy. The study findings indicate that sexual abuse leads to an earlier age of first sexual intercourse, which in turn increases the likelihood of an early pregnancy. Women with higher educational attainment are less likely to experience early pregnancy as a result of abuse.

▶ This is an important study. There have been no previous studies that have examined whether sexual abuse during adolescence affects the risk of early preg nancy. The authors of this report studied the association between sexual abuse and early pregnancy based on the age when sexual abuse occurred and the most severe types of sexual abuse involving molestation, coercion, attempted rape, or rape. More than 2000 women age 18 to 22 years were interviewed for this study.

The study documented that most women who experienced sexual abuse exclusively in childhood experienced episodes of molestation, consistent with data from previous studies. By comparison, the majority who were revictimized in adolescence experienced rape. Women who were abused only in adolescence reported all types of abuse. Survivors of sexual abuse exclusively in childhood may be more likely to experience the abuse within the context of family relationships compared with survivors of sexual abuse in adolescence, who may be more likely to be victimized by an acquaintance or romantic or sexual partner. Research has suggested that forced sex is most likely to be perpetrated by a non—family member, whereas molestation is more likely to be perpetrated by a family member. Women who experience sexual abuse in both childhood and adolescence were at the highest risk for early pregnancy. The study clearly emphasizes the importance of sexual abuse prevention to reduce pregnancy risk among adolescent women.

It should also be noted that a recent report in the *American Journal of Psychiatry* documents that adults who were maltreated as children are 43% more likely to have episodes of severe depression.[1] This finding was true irrespective of gender and age at which the maltreatment had started. The findings were based on a combined meta-analysis of 16 studies and 10 clinical trials with maltreatment being defined as physical or sexual abuse, neglect, or family conflict or violence.

This commentary closes with some findings reported in *Pediatrics* a couple of years back that are quite disturbing. The report shows that repeated penile-genital penetration may leave no definitive evidence in children who are sexually abused.[2] In a study of 506 girls age 10 years or older, definitive hymenal evidence was absent in most of those who reported repetitive penetration. Analysis of data found no association between the number of reported penetrative events and definitive genital findings. The results were similar for children who claimed repetitive assaults over long periods of time and for those with a history of consensual sex. Child abuse experts: take note.

**J. A. Stockman III, MD**

*References*

1. Nanni V, Uher R, Danese A. Childhood maltreatment predicts unfavorable course of illness and treatment outcome in depression: a meta-analysis. *Am J Psychiatry.* 2011 Aug 14 [Epub ahead of print].
2. Anderst J, Kellogg N, Jung I. Reports of repetitive penile-genital penetration often have no evidence of penetration. *Pediatrics.* 2009;124:e403-e409.

---

**Prevalence of Oral HPV Infection in the United States, 2009-2010**
Gillison ML, Broutian T, Pickard RKL, et al (Ohio State Univ Comprehensive Cancer Ctr, Columbus; et al)
*JAMA* 307:693-703, 2012

---

*Context.*—Human papillomavirus (HPV) infection is the principal cause of a distinct form of oropharyngeal squamous cell carcinoma that is increasing in incidence among men in the United States. However, little is known about the epidemiology of oral HPV infection.

*Objective.*—To determine the prevalence of oral HPV infection in the United States.

*Design, Setting, and Participants.*—A cross-sectional study was conducted as part of the National Health and Nutrition Examination Survey (NHANES) 2009-2010, a statistically representative sample of the civilian noninstitutionalized US population. Men and women aged 14 to 69 years examined at mobile examination centers were eligible. Participants (N = 5579) provided a 30-second oral rinse and gargle with mouthwash. For detection of HPV types, DNA purified from oral exfoliated cells was evaluated by polymerase chain reaction and type-specific hybridization. Demographic and behavioral data were obtained by standardized interview. Statistical analyses used NHANES sample weights to provide weighted prevalence estimates for the US population.

*Main Outcome Measures.*—Prevalence of oral HPV infection.

*Results.*—The prevalence of oral HPV infection among men and women aged 14 to 69 years was 6.9% (95% CI, 5.7%-8.3%) and of HPV type 16 was 1.0% (95% CI, 0.7%-1.3%). Oral HPV infection followed a bimodal pattern with respect to age, with peak prevalence among individuals aged 30 to 34 years (7.3%; 95% CI, 4.6%-11.4%) and 60 to 64 years (11.4%; 95% CI, 8.5%-15.1%). Men had a significantly higher prevalence than women for any oral HPV infection (10.1% [95% CI, 8.3%-12.3%] vs 3.6% [95% CI, 2.6%-5.0%], P < .001; unadjusted prevalence ratio [PR], 2.80 [95% CI, 2.02-3.88]). Infection was less common among those without vs those with a history of any type of sexual contact (0.9% [95% CI, 0.4%-1.8%] vs 7.5% [95% CI, 6.1%-9.1%], P < .001; PR, 8.69 [95% CI, 3.91-19.31]) and increased with number of sexual partners (P < .001 for trend) and cigarettes smoked per day (P < .001 for trend). Associations with age, sex, number of sexual partners, and current number of cigarettes smoked per day were independently associated with oral HPV infection in multivariable models.

*Conclusion.*—Among men and women aged 14 to 69 years in the United States, the overall prevalence of oral HPV infection was 6.9%, and the prevalence was higher among men than among women.

▶ When I was a medical student, human papillomavirus (HPV) was simply thought to be a cause of the common skin wart, the anogenital wart, or perhaps a rare skin cancer. It was only in the late 1970s and early 1980s that HPV infection was linked to cervical cancer. The work documenting this link was awarded a Nobel Prize. In the interim period of time, research has linked HPV infection to most squamous cell cancers of the vagina and anus, many cancers of the vulva and penis, and more recently, oropharyngeal cancers. In fact, more oropharyngeal cancers are caused by HPV infection than by tobacco or alcohol.

The report abstracted tells us about the first major prevalence study of oral HPV infection for the United States population through analysis of the National Health and Nutrition Examination Survey. The investigators studied 5579 participants aged 14 to 69 years who provided a 30-second oral rinse for HPV DNA analysis. The study found an overall prevalence of oral HPV infection of 6.9%. This prevalence peaked at 30 to 34 years and again at 60 to 64 years. Men had a higher overall HPV prevalence than women (10.1% vs 3.6%, respectively). A history of sexual activity versus none, smoking, and a higher number of lifetime sexual partners correlated with oral HPV infection. This study reports an overall HPV-16 oral prevalence of 1.0%, which is important because 85% of HPV-related oropharyngeal cancers are positive for this subtype.

The prevalence of oral HPV infection is much lower than that seen in other body sites. The prevalence of cervical-vaginal HPV infection runs 42% in women aged 14 to 59 years. Penile/scrotal HPV prevalence in this age group ranges from 14% to 50% depending on what study one is reading. The study of Gillison et al also showed that current smoking is independently associated with oral HPV infection rates. Curiously, this effect was stronger among women than men. These findings are consistent with the known immunosuppressive effects of smoking.

The data from this study have important research as well as public health in implications. The Centers for Disease Control and Prevention currently recommends routine HPV vaccination for females aged 9 to 26 years and males aged 9 to 21 years for prevention of genital warts and anogenital cancers based on demonstrated efficacy in randomized trials. The vaccine efficacy against oral HPV infection is unknown, and therefore vaccination cannot currently be recommended for the primary prevention of oral pharyngeal cancer. An analysis of US cancer registry data recently projected that the number of HPV-positive oropharyngeal cancers diagnosed each year will surpass that of invasive cervical cancers by 2020. Given these numbers, vaccine trials do seem warranted to prevent this problem.

This commentary closes with an observation related to sexual activity. Recently noted in the literature was the fact that an estimated 1.35 million defective condoms were distributed free of charge in South Africa. The condoms had been distributed to hotels, restaurants, and bars as part of the African National Congress centenary celebrations in January 2012. Unfortunately, most of these condoms were found to be highly porous![1] Also, a recent report tells us just how prevalent human papilloma virus is in men and strengthens the case for vaccinating men and boys against this virus.[2] Starting in 2005, a team of investigators from Tampa, Florida, recruited more than 4000 men living in Brazil, Mexico, and Florida for a study of the human papilloma virus. The average age of these men was 32 years. None had been vaccinated against this virus. Swabs of the penis and genital area of each man revealed that 50% were infected with at least one strain of human papilloma virus upon enrollment in the study. Over a median of 28 months, the group acquired 1572 new human papilloma virus infections. Once a new infection was acquired, it took a median of 7.5 months to clear the infection. Clearance times did not vary substantially among the countries involved in the study but did vary among human papilloma virus types. Some cases lingered as long as 20 months. The investigators of this report noted that male circumcision and the use of condoms showed little protection against human papilloma virus infection.

**J. A. Stockman III, MD**

*References*

1. Editorial comment. Free condoms "porous." *Lancet*. 2012;379:222.
2. Seppa N. Half of adult males may carry the human papilloma virus: Sexually transmitted virus can linger for months. *Science News*. March 26, 2011:12.

### Risk of venous thromboembolism in users of oral contraceptives containing drospirenone or levonorgestrel: Nested case-control study based on UK General Practice Research Database

Parkin L, Sharples K, Hernandez RK, et al (Univ of Otago, Dunedin, New Zealand; Boston Univ School of Medicine, Lexington, MA)
*BMJ* 342:d2139, 2011

*Objective.*—To examine the risk of non-fatal idiopathic venous thromboembolism in current users of a combined oral contraceptive containing drospirenone, relative to current users of preparations containing levonorgestrel.

*Design.*—Nested case-control study.

*Setting.*—UK General Practice Research Database.

*Participants.*—Women aged 15-44 years without major risk factors for venous thromboembolism who started a new episode of use of an oral contraceptive containing 30 µg oestrogen in combination with either drospirenone or levonorgestrel between May 2002 and September 2009. Cases were women with a first diagnosis of venous thromboembolism; up to four controls, matched by age, duration of recorded information, and general practice, were randomly selected for each case.

*Main Outcome Measures.*—Odds ratios and 95% confidence intervals estimated with conditional logistic regression; age adjusted incidence rate ratio estimated with Poisson regression.

*Results.*—61 cases of idiopathic venous thromboembolism and 215 matched controls were identified. In the case-control analysis, current use of the drospirenone contraceptive was associated with a threefold higher risk of non-fatal idiopathic venous thromboembolism compared with levonorgestrel use; the odds ratio adjusted for body mass index was 3.3 (95% confidence interval 1.4 to 7.6). Subanalyses suggested that referral, diagnostic, first time user, duration of use, and switching biases were unlikely explanations for this finding. The crude incidence rate was 23.0 (95% confidence interval 13.4 to 36.9) per 100 000 woman years in current users of drospirenone and 9.1 (6.6 to 12.2) per 100 000 woman years in current users of levonorgestrel oral contraceptives. The age adjusted incidence rate ratio was 2.7 (1.5 to 4.7).

*Conclusions.*—These findings contribute to emerging evidence that the combined oral contraceptive containing drospirenone carries a higher risk of venous thromboembolism than do formulations containing levonorgestrel.

▶ This report is 1 of 2 case-controlled studies appearing in the same issue of the *British Medical Journal* addressing the risk of nonfatal venous thromboembolism in women taking oral contraceptives that contain drospirenone versus those containing levonorgestrel. One report was from the United States,[1] and the other, that of Parkin et al, was from Great Britain. Both analyses found an increased risk associated with drospirenone compared with levonorgestrel, about double in the US study and triple in the UK study.

The report by Parkin et al and by Jick et al (from the United States) represent what are known as observational studies. The British study had comparatively low numbers (61 cases and 215 controls). There were 27 cases of deep venous thrombosis and 34 cases of pulmonary embolism (a case mix that does not reflect clinical practice given the relatively higher percentage of pulmonary emboli). There are no data presented regarding other risk factors in these patients, including rates of obesity, smoking, etc. In the US study, data on obesity were incomplete; height and weight measurements were not available.[1]

So why would anyone want to use drospirenone contraceptives? The latter are said to improve acne, but there is actually little evidence to support their superiority over low-dose oral contraceptives. It seems sensible to prescribe an oral contraceptive with a well-known favorable safety profile (one that contains levonorgestrel) unless there is a persistent reason to use the other type. While these observational studies are not perfect, they are consistent with enough concern about oral contraceptives containing drospirenone to suggest that these contraceptives should not be used, even though the overall risk of thromboembolism is low.

While on the topic of sexual activity, this commentary closes with the observation that nothing compares in humans to what happens to certain spiders when they copulate. The spider *Nephilengys malabararensis* is into rough sex. Like many species of spiders, the male is devoured by the female during copulation, giving new meaning to the term rough sex. In order to avoid demise, the male spider will often voluntarily break off his whole sex organ, or palp, while it still lodged in the female's abdomen, rather than risk being eaten alive by her. Now a group of researchers think they know why evolution has allowed dead-end dads to survive. Investigators collected 25 pairs of spiders and introduced them to one another. After each pair had mated and the male's palp was left in the female, the researchers dissected the female's abdomen and counted the sperm in her abdomen and also the amount remaining in the embedded palp. It appears that the palp will continue to transfer sperm into the female long after the male has fled or has been consumed. The longer it's embedded, the more sperm is transferred, and it is even more efficient when the male breaks himself away to run off rather than letting the female eat him. To read more about all this interesting but odd activity, see article that appeared recently in the journal *Science*.[2]

**J. A. Stockman III, MD**

*References*

1. Jick SS, Hernandez RK. Risk of non-fatal venous thromboembolism in women using oral contraceptives containing drospirenone compared with women using oral contraceptives containing levonorgestrel: case-control study using United States claims data. *BMJ*. 2011;342:d2151.
2. Editorial comment. Spider can inseminate female from afar. *Science*. 2012;335:509.

## Reciprocal Relations Between Objectively Measured Sleep Patterns and Diurnal Cortisol Rhythms in Late Adolescence

Zeiders KH, Doane LD, Adam EK (Arizona State Univ, Tempe; Northwestern Univ, Evanston, IL)

*J Adolesc Health* 48:566-571, 2011

*Purpose.*—To examine how hours of sleep and wake times relate to between-person differences and day-to-day changes in diurnal cortisol rhythms in late adolescence.

*Methods.*—Older adolescents (N = 119) provided six cortisol samples (wakeup, +30 minutes, +2 hours, +8 hours, +12 hours, and bedtime) on each of three consecutive days while wearing an actigraph. We examined how average (across 3 days) and day-to-day changes in hours of sleep and wake times related to diurnal cortisol patterns.

*Results.*—On average, more hours of sleep related to steeper decline in cortisol across the days. Day-to-day analyses revealed that the hours of sleep of the previous night predicted steeper diurnal slopes the next day, whereas greater waking cortisol levels and steeper slopes predicted more hours of sleep and a later wake time the next day.

*Conclusion.* Our results suggest a bidirectional relationship between sleep and hypothalamic-pituitary-adrenal axis activity.

▶ More than 10 years ago, it was noted that approximately two-thirds of college students were reporting sleep problems, a sharp increase from the 25% figure found in 1982.[1] It has been suggested that the average college student is deprived of anywhere from between 1 and 1.5 hours of sleep consistently each night.

Zeiders et al have examined the relationship between sleep duration and diurnal cortisol rhythms in late adolescence. The findings from the report suggest that across individuals, average hours of sleep are related to a steeper diurnal decline in cortisol across the day, even after accounting for adolescents' average awake times. These findings are consistent with those seen in adults, suggesting that individuals who sleep more have diurnal cortisol rhythms characterized by a steeper decline across the day and align with health findings suggesting that such patterns are considered quite normal and healthy. The findings suggest that choices made about sleep have substantive consequences for hormonal physiology.

The National Sleep Foundation suggests that adults need 7 to 9 hours of sleep per night. Both shorter and longer sleep durations have been associated with increased morbidity and mortality. Studies reported from the Centers for Disease Control and Prevention have shown that young and older adults who report sleeping less than 7 hours on weekdays or workdays are more likely to have difficulties with daily activities than adults who reported getting 7 to 9 hours of sleep.[2]

The message here is tell your patients to get a good night's sleep. As an aside, not getting enough sleep, at least in boys and men, can affect one's testosterone levels. A study carried out by the University of Chicago in which adult men were studied after a week of 8-hour bedtimes, followed by a period of 3 nights of 10-hour bedtimes, followed by 8 nights of 5-hour bedtimes documented that daytime testosterone levels decrease anywhere from 10% to 15% in these young healthy men who underwent the period of sleep restriction. The testosterone decline was associated with lower vigor scores and symptoms of androgen deficiency including low energy, reduced libido, poor concentration, and increased sleepiness, all of which may be produced by sleep deprivation. To read more about this report, see the research letter that appeared recently in *JAMA*.[3] Sleep deprivation is a tough way to exercise birth control, but it may well work for this purpose if for nothing else.

**J. A. Stockman III, MD**

*References*

1. Hicks RA, Fernandez C, Pellegrini RJ. Self-reported sleep durations of college students: normative data for 1978-79, 1988-89, and 2000-01. *Percept Mot Skills*. 2001;93:139-140.
2. Editorial comment Effect of short sleep duration on daily activities—United States, 2005—2008. *MMWR Morb Mortal Wkly Rep*. 2011;60:239-242.
3. Leproult R, Van Cauter E. Effect of 1 week of sleep restriction on testosterone levels in young healthy men. *JAMA*. 2011;305:2173-2174.

---

**Profanity in Media Associated With Attitudes and Behavior Regarding Profanity Use and Aggression**
Coyne SM, Stockdale LA, Nelson DA, et al (Brigham Young Univ, Provo, UT)
*Pediatrics* 128:867-872, 2011

---

*Objective.*—We hypothesized that exposure to profanity in media would be directly related to beliefs and behavior regarding profanity and indirectly to aggressive behavior.

*Methods.*—We examined these associations among 223 adolescents attending a large Midwestern middle school. Participants completed a number of questionnaires examining their exposure to media, attitudes and behavior regarding profanity, and aggressive behavior.

*Results.*—Results revealed a positive association between exposure to profanity in multiple forms of media and beliefs about profanity, profanity use, and engagement in physical and relational aggression. Specifically, attitudes toward profanity use mediated the relationship between exposure to profanity in media and subsequent behavior involving profanity use and aggression.

*Conclusions.*—The main hypothesis was confirmed, and implications for the rating industry and research field are discussed.

▶ This interesting little report shows how impressionable youth are—perhaps not that different from adults when it comes to mimicking what we see in the media. The Motion Picture Association of America rates films on 4 main criteria: profanity use, violence, sexual behavior, and substance abuse. Hundreds of studies have shown links between exposure to violence, sexual behavior, and substance abuse in the media and subsequent behavior. The authors of this report, however, reviewed the literature and did not find a single study examining the effects of exposure to profanity in media and subsequent profanity use.

Coyne et al designed a study intended to provide an initial examination of the relationship between exposure to profanity in the media and behavior. They examined exposure to profanity in multiple types of media, including television and video games. Some 223 middle school children ranging in age from 11 to 15 years completed a series of questionnaires based on their viewing of their 3 favorite television programs and video games, rating each with respect to what they perceived to be the amount of profanity that each contained. Participants in the study were asked about their beliefs regarding profanity use, their own use of profanity, and the number hours a day they spent playing video games and watching TV on average. Participants also rated their favorite TV programs and video games with respect to physical and relational aggression. An analysis of the information provided showed that exposure to profanity in all types of media was positively associated with attitudes toward profanity, profanity use, and physical and relational aggression.

This is the first study to examine the link between exposure to profanity in media and attitudes and behavior regarding profanity among adolescents. The most interesting aspect of this report is that exposure to profanity ultimately turns out to be associated with both physical and relational aggression. Although this study had some limitations related to the fact that it represented survey information, it does add greatly to the literature on profanity and media as the first study to reveal that exposure to profanity in the media is associated with harmful outcomes for adolescents.

While on the topic of imprinting from exposure to media, the Centers for Disease Control and Prevention (CDC) recently reported a study on smoking in top-grossing movies in the United States.[1] Data show that by 2010, the number of onscreen tobacco scenes in youth-rated (G, PG, or PG-13) movies had decreased 71.6% from 2005. This rate of decline, however, varied substantially by motion picture company. Three major film companies with published policies designed to reduce tobacco use in their movies had an average decrease in tobacco incidences of 95.8% compared with an average of 41.7% among the 3 major motion picture companies and independents without such policies. It should be noted that in 2010, 55% of 137 top-grossing films had no tobacco scene compared with 33% of 147 films in 2005. Among R-rated films, 29.2% of 48 such films had no tobacco scene in 2010 compared with 4.7% of 43 in 2005. From 2005 to 2010, the total number of tobacco scenes in top-grossing films decreased 56% from 4152 to 1825. These findings indicate continuing progress toward the US Department of Health and Human Services goal of reducing youth exposure to onscreen smoking. It is hard to say whether this decreased presence of onscreen smoking might have contributed to the documented decline in cigarette use among middle school and high school students in that same 2005 to 2010 period.

Until I read the CDC report, I did not realize that almost all states offer movie producers subsidies in the form of tax credits or cash rebates to attract movie production to their states. Financially, this contributes about $1 billion annually to the movie industry. The 15 states subsidizing top-grossing movies with tobacco incidence spent more on these productions in 2010 ($280 million) than they budgeted for their own state tobacco control programs in 2011. What irony!

**J. A. Stockman III, MD**

*Reference*

1. Editorial comment. Smoking in top-grossing movies—United States, 2010. *MMWR Morb Mortal Wkly Rep.* 2011;60:909-913.

## Underdiagnosed Menorrhagia in Adolescents is Associated with Underdiagnosed Anemia

Revel-Vilk S, Paltiel O, Lipschuetz M, et al (Hadassah Hebrew-Univ Hosp, Jerusalem, Israel)

*J Pediatr* 160:468-472, 2012

*Objective.*—To test the hypothesis that adolescent girls with menorrhagia rarely seek medical attention.

*Study Design.*—A total of 705 adolescent girls attended a lecture on menorrhagia, completed an initial anonymous questionnaire, and were asked to participate in a more comprehensive study comprising a detailed bleeding questionnaire, a pictorial blood loss assessment chart, and blood tests.

*Results.*—A total of 105 adolescents (15%) reported they had heavy periods on the initial questionnaire. Among the 94 girls who completed the full questionnaire, 34 reported menorrhagia (36%; 95% CI, 26.5%-46.7%). Almost one-third (11 of 34) of these girls did not perceive having menorrhagia according to their response to the initial questionnaire. Menorrhagia was not related to age, years since menarche, or family history of menorrhagia. Among the 62 girls who consented to blood testing, 6 had anemia (9.6%; 95% CI, 3.6%-19.6%), all of whom had bleeding symptoms.

*Conclusion.*—Using standardized questionnaires, we were able to identify adolescents with menorrhagia associated with anemia. Importantly, some of these adolescents were not aware of having menorrhagia and/or anemia. Screening programs for menorrhagia in schools could result in better detection of menorrhagia among adolescents and consequent appropriate referral for medical consultation.

▶ This interesting report from Jerusalem studied over 700 adolescent girls to determine the prevalence of menorrhagia. The technical definition of menorrhagia is "excessive menstrual blood loss of greater than 80 mL per cycle or menstrual periods lasting longer than 7 days."[1] Unfortunately the term is frequently used to mean blood loss perceived as excessive by the patient. There is a gold standard for determining whether an individual has menorrhagia. This involves quantification of alkaline hematin, a very complicated and time-consuming technique. An alternative approach to quantifying menstrual blood loss is with a pictorial blood loss assessment chart, which is based on the fraction of blood soiling of sanitary products, as well as the total number of pads or tampons used. A score greater than 100 is equivalent to a blood loss of greater than 80 mL. The latter method is simple, inexpensive, and reasonably accurate for assessing menstrual blood loss with greater than 80% specificity and sensitivity. It is the latter method that the authors used to determine the presence or absence of menorrhagia in the adolescent girls studied in this report. These young girls were attending school in grades 10 through 12. All were asked: "Do you think you have heavy periods?" The girls were then given the pictorial survey to answer the question that would determine whether they really had or did not have menorrhagia. Just 15% reported that they had heavy periods, but when assessed using the pictorial blood loss assessment chart, it turns out that 36% had menorrhagia. Approximately one-third of these girls did not perceive themselves as having menorrhagia, according to the response based on the initial question. The prevalence of anemia in this population was 9.6%, seen exclusively in those with menorrhagia.

It is clear that teenagers do not necessarily recognize when they have menorrhagia. At the same time, some thought they had menorrhagia when they did not. This study was not designed to assess why some adolescents with menorrhagia are not aware of the problem. One can speculate that this lack of awareness is related in part to not sharing their menstrual experience with others. Those who do share their experience with female family members may find falsely reassuring responses, because family members frequently have similar menstrual patterns that they consider "normal." For these reasons and since menorrhagia in adolescents is so relatively frequent, it is reasonable to suggest that teenage girls should be screened with both a bleeding history as well as a pictorial blood loss assessment, looking for a score of over 100. Given the high prevalence of anemia in teenage girls, they also should be screened for anemia at the time of routine examinations.

**J. A. Stockman III, MD**

*Reference*

1. Hallberg L, Högdahl AM, Nilsson L, Rybo G. Menstrual blood loss a population study. Variation at different ages and attempts to define normality. *Acta Obstet Gynecol Scand.* 1966;45:320-351.

---

## Prospective Study of Sunburn and Sun Behavior Patterns During Adolescence

Dusza SW, Halpern AC, Satagopan JM, et al (Memorial Sloan-Kettering Cancer Ctr, NY; et al)
*Pediatrics* 129:309-317, 2012

---

*Objectives.*—Early childhood UV light radiation (UVR) exposures have been shown to be associated with melanoma development later in life. The objective of this study was to assess sunburn and changes in sunburn and sun behaviors during periadolescence.

*Methods.*—A prospective, population-based study was conducted in fifth-grade children ( ~ 10 years of age) from Framingham, Massachusetts. Surveys were administered at baseline (September–October 2004) and again 3 years later (September–October 2007). Surveys were analyzed to assess prevalence of reported sunburn and sun behaviors and to examine changes in response over the follow-up period.

*Results.*—Data were analyzed from 360 participants who had complete information regarding sunburn at both time points. In 2004, ~ 53% of the students reported having at least 1 sunburn during the previous summer, and this proportion did not significantly change by 2007 (55%, $P = .79$), whereas liking a tan and spending time outside to get a tan significantly increased ($P < .001$). In 2004, 50% of students reported "often or always" use of sunscreen when outside for at least 6 hours in the summer; this proportion dropped to 25% at the follow-up evaluation ($P < .001$).

*Conclusions.*—With at least 50% of children experiencing sunburns before age 11 and again 3 years later, targeting children in pediatric offices and community settings regarding unprotected UV exposure may be a practical approach. Because periadolescence is a time of volatility with regard to sun behaviors, learning more about children who receive sunburns versus those who avoid them is a critical research task.

▶ The incidence of melanoma has increased dramatically in the past 30 years. In 2006, a total of 55 034 new cases of melanoma were diagnosed in the United States. Long-term exposure to ultraviolet radiation and a history of sunburn during childhood and adolescence are significant risk factors for both malignant and nonmalignant skin cancer. Having ever had a sunburn during childhood essentially doubles the risk for the development of cutaneous melanoma in adulthood. During the past decade, there have been numerous public health efforts to increase the use of sun protection at a multitude of sites, including beaches, schools, pediatrician offices, pools, and ski slopes. Despite these efforts, reported prevalence of recent sunburn in children and adolescents remains high.

The authors of this report tell about nevi in children, a prospective population-based study exploring the natural history of nevi in adolescence. The investigators report the results of questionnaires summarizing sun exposure experience with some behaviors and attitudes relevant to sun exposure during this important time of life. A total of 366 high school students were evaluated over a 3-year period of time. At the beginning of the study, 53% of students had already reported having at least 1 sunburn during the summer and more than half reported liking a suntan. This proportion increased to 66% 3 years later. A higher proportion of students reported spending time in the sun to get a tan at the follow-up evaluation compared with baseline (39.8% vs 21.8%). Students with very fair to fair skin were 40% more likely to report 2 or more sunburns over the 3-year period of time, whereas those students with light olive or black skin were 70% less likely to report 2 or more sunburns at follow-up.

Sunburn is an observable response to a high dose of ultraviolet radiation and is implicated in the chain of causation leading to skin cancer. Thus, a high priority for skin cancer prevention programs should be to understand the factors needed to reduce the occurrence of sunburn, in particular, frequent sunburns that are strongly implicated in the development of cancer, especially melanoma. Unfortunately, sunscreen use is not the sole answer to this problem. A report showed that over a recent 10-year period, the percentage of white students who never or rarely wore sunscreen when outside on a sunny day had increased, as did the percentage among Hispanic students. This increase in no sunscreen use was most pronounced in white female students.[1] The finding that sunscreen use is diminishing in our adolescent population suggests need for renewed public health efforts among clinical, school, and community health professionals to warn our youth about the risks of skin cancer later in life. It is easier, safer, and less time-consuming to get a tan out of a bottle of artificial tanning solution than it is to go out into the sun or to hop into a tanning booth.

**J. A. Stockman III, MD**

*Reference*

1. Jones SE, Saraiya M, Miyamoto J, Berkowitz Z. Trends in sunscreen use among U.S. high school students: 1999–2009. *J Adolescent Health*. 2012;50:304-307.

## Sickle Cell Trait Screening in Athletes: Pediatricians' Attitudes and Concerns

Koopmans J, Cox LA, Benjamin H, et al (Univ of Chicago, IL; Cook County Public Defender Service, Chicago, IL; et al)
*Pediatrics* 128:477-483, 2011

*Background.*—As part of a legal settlement in 2010, the National Collegiate Athletic Association (NCAA) adopted a recommendation that all Division I athletes be screened for sickle cell trait (SCT) or sign an exemption waiver. Pediatricians' attitudes about this policy are unknown.

*Objective.*—We queried 3 specialty sections of the American Academy of Pediatrics (AAP)—the Section on Adolescent Health, the Council on Sports Medicine and Fitness (COSMF), and the Section on Bioethics—to determine attitudes about and knowledge of SCT testing of athletes.

*Methods.*—Three e-mail surveys were sent to 600 members of the AAP chosen equally from the Section on Bioethics, the Section on Adolescent Health, and the COSMF. The survey queried respondents about their awareness of the NCAA policy and whether they supported universal or targeted screening based on gender, race/ethnicity, level of play, and type of sport.

*Results.*—Usable responses from 254 of 574 eligible respondents (44%) were received. Respondents were 54% male and 84% white. Almost half were aware of the NCAA policy, with highest awareness in members of COSMF ($P < .001$). Only 40% supported universal screening, whereas 70% supported targeted screening of athletes in all NCAA divisions and would focus on black student-athletes more than on Hispanic or white-Mediterranean student-athletes (no differences among AAP sections/council). More than 75% of all respondents support allowing athletes or their parents to waive screening. A majority expressed some concern that athletes with SCT might experience discrimination in sports participation and/or insurance. Members of COSMF were least concerned about discrimination.

*Conclusions.*—The NCAA policy to universally screen Division I athletes is not uniformly supported by pediatricians, who prefer targeted screening based on race/ethnicity and sport in all NCAA divisions. We found little difference in policy considerations between members of the different AAP sections/council except that members of the COSMF were least concerned about discrimination.

▶ Most are familiar with the background that led to the National Collegiate Athletic Association (NCAA) adoption of a recommendation that all Division I athletes be screened for sickle cell trait or sign an exemption waiver. It was in 2006 that Dale Lloyd II, a freshman at Rice University, died during football practice. The autopsy report showed that Dale died of "exertional rhabdomyolysis associated with sickle cell trait." Dale's family brought a lawsuit against the NCAA. In June 2009, as part of a legal settlement with the Lloyd family, the NCAA recommended its member colleges and universities test student-athletes to confirm sickle cell trait status if that information was not already known. In April 2010, this policy was revised by the NCAA District I Legislative Council, which approved a measure that requires only District I athletes to be screened for the sickle cell trait unless they can show results of a prior test or they sign a release to decline testing. In October 2010, the District I Legislative Council announced that it will ask the Board of Directors of that district to enter a proposal eliminating the ability of incoming student-athletes to decline the test for sickle cell trait into the 2010–2011 legislative cycle. As of April 2011, no action had been taken on this legislation.

It should be noted that Dale Lloyd's death was not the first associated with sickle cell trait and exertional rhabdomyolysis. Sickle cell trait had been linked to exertional rhabdomyolysis and fatal exertional heat illness after strenuous exercise in college sports, the difference being that although exertional heat illness is related to heat and humidity, exertional rhabdomyolysis is not. Both exertional rhabdomyolysis and exertional heat illness can occur in players with and without sickle cell trait, and neither is uniformly fatal as evidenced by the hospitalization for exertional rhabdomyolysis of 13 University of Iowa football players after a very rigorous weightlifting practice following a winter break.[1] The first association between sickle cell trait and fatal exercise heat illness was described during military basic training back in 1970, a finding confirmed in several larger military studies. Some branches of the military responded to this finding by excluding those individuals with sickle cell trait from service. The interesting observation, however, in the military was that one could remarkably reduce the likelihood of exertional heat illness and exercise-related rhabdomyolysis simply by altering training programs. This has raised the question of whether universal screening to identify all athletes with sickle cell trait is necessary or whether all college sports programs should modify training to reduce the risk of these disorders.

The literature has raised several issues with respect to the screening of athletes for sickle cell trait. One issue is whether all athletes need to be screened or rather those at highest risk for having sickle cell trait, such as black athletes. To screen only black athletes, however, is to ignore the diverse populations in which sickle hemoglobin is found. Also, to screen only Division I athletes ignores the fact that sickle cell trait has been found in players of all divisions. Another ethical issue relates to cost. More than 90% of individuals born in or after 1992 have had hemoglobin screening as a part of universal newborn screening. Many do not know their results and will undergo repeat screening. Because of cost, many NCAA Division I teams elect to use the Sickledex test, which costs less than $10 per student-athlete in contrast with hemoglobin electrophoresis, which costs in excess of $100 per student-athlete. This raises moral economic and medical trade-off issues with using the Sickledex test because it is known to have false-positive and false-negative results and cannot distinguish between sickle cell trait and sickle cell disease. It also does not capture other hemoglobin abnormalities. A third ethical issue is the student's right to consent or waive out of screening. A waiver, of course, respects the right to refuse genetic testing and addresses the concerns of stigma and discrimination that some student-athletes may fear.

The authors of this report surveyed 3 specialty sections of the American Academy of Pediatrics to get a sense of what pediatricians feel about the need and method of screening for sickle cell trait in athletes. They queried the Section on Adolescent Health, the Council on Sports Medicine and Fitness and the Section on Bioethics. The surveyors theorized that the Council on Sports Medicine and Fitness would be the most supportive of the 3 sections for universal screening and the most tolerant of using the Sickledex screening modality. They also theorized that members of the Section on Bioethics would be the least supportive of targeted testing, especially one based on race/ethnicity; the most supportive of modifying practice for all athletes; and the most concerned about the potential for discrimination. Of those surveyed and those who were aware of the NCAA policy, only 40% supported universal screening, whereas 70% supported targeted screening of athletes in all NCAA divisions, focusing on black student-athletes. There were no differences in the 3 academy sections on this point. The majority (75%) of those responding supported allowing athletes and their parents to waive sickle cell trait screening, and the majority also expressed some concern that athletes with sickle cell trait might experience discrimination, the latter either in sports participation or from insurance companies. Members of the Council on Sports Medicine and Fitness were the least concerned about discrimination. The slight majority of respondents preferred the Sickledex test to hemoglobin electrophoresis for the detection of sickle cell trait.

It is fairly obvious that pediatricians do not uniformly accept the NCAA policy to universally screen for sickle cell trait among Division I athletes. Although pediatricians in general would prefer targeted screening based on race/ethnicity and the particular sport involved in the athletic activity, the NCAA policy differs. It is hard to say whether pediatricians in any way can or will influence the policies that are currently in place.

**J. A. Stockman III, MD**

*Reference*

1. Report of the Special presidential commission to investigate the January 2011 hospitalization of university of Iowa football players. http://www.regents.iowa. gov/news/emailcommunications/2011/suireport032211.pdf. Accessed November 3, 2011.

---

### Graduated Driver Licensing and Fatal Crashes Involving 16- to 19-Year-Old Drivers

Masten SV, Foss RD, Marshall SW (Res and Development Branch, Sacramento, CA; Univ of North Carolina, Chapel Hill)
*JAMA* 306:1098-1103, 2011

---

*Context.*—In the United States, graduated driver licensing (GDL) systems allow full, unrestricted licensure for drivers younger than 18 years only after an initial period of supervised driving and an intermediate period of unsupervised driving that limits driving at night, transporting multiple young passengers, or both.

*Objective.*—To estimate the association of GDL programs with involvement in fatal crashes among 16- to 19-year-old drivers.

*Design, Setting, and Participants.*—Pooled cross-sectional time series analysis of quarterly 1986-2007 incidence of fatal crashes involving drivers aged 16 to 19 years for all 50 states and the District of Columbia combined.

*Main Outcome Measures.*—Population-based rates of fatal crash involvement for 16-, 17-, 18-, and 19-year-old drivers. Rate ratios and 95% CIs comparing statequarters with stronger (restrictions on both nighttime driving and allowed passengers) or weaker (restrictions on either nighttime driving or allowed passengers) GDL programs with state-quarters without GDL.

*Results.*—Fatal crash incidence among teen drivers increased with age, from 28.2 per 100 000 person-years (16-year-old drivers) to 36.9 per 100 000 (17-year-olds), before reaching a plateau of 46.2 per 100 000 (18-year-olds) and 44.0 per 100 000 (19-year-olds). After adjusting for potential confounders, stronger GDL programs were associated with lower incidence of fatal crashes for 16-year-old drivers, compared with programs having none of the key GDL elements (rate ratio, 0.74 [95% CI, 0.65-0.84]). However, stronger GDL programs were associated with higher fatal crash incidence for 18-year-old drivers (rate ratio, 1.12 [95% CI, 1.01-1.23]). Rate ratios for 17-year-olds (0.91 [95% CI, 0.83-1.01]), 19-year-olds (1.05 [95% CI, 0.98-1.13]), and 16- to 19-year-olds combined (0.97 [95% CI, 0.92-1.03]) were not statistically different from the null.

*Conclusions.*—In the United States, stronger GDL programs with restrictions on nighttime driving as well as allowed passengers, relative to programs with none of the key GDL elements, were associated with substantially lower fatal crash incidence for 16-year-old drivers but somewhat higher fatal crash incidence for 18-year-old drivers. Future studies should seek to determine what accounts for the increase among 18-year-old drivers and whether refinements in GDL programs can reduce this association.

▶ Currently, all states and the District of Columbia have enacted some form of graduated driver licensing. Florida is credited with having enacted the first graduated driver licensing program in the United States. That was in 1996. It should be noted, however, that the benefits of delayed licensure and the restriction of nighttime driving were demonstrated as early as the 1980s.[1] The data have been in for some time documenting how graduated driver licensing has reduced rates of fatal crashes among teenage drivers. Between 1996 and 2009, for example, large declines occurred in such crashes. The decline for 15-year-olds was 69%, for 16-year-olds 68%, and for 17-year-olds 53%.[2] In jurisdictions that have adopted elements of graduated driver licensing, overall crash rates among young teenagers have declined on average 20% to 40%.

The study by Masten et al shows a 26% lower per capita rate of fatal crash incidence for 16-year-olds associated with stronger than less strong graduated driver licensing programs. Masten et al report a 12% higher rate of fatal crash incidence for 18-year-olds and a nonsignificant, slightly lower rate for 16- to 19-year-olds combined. This report, along with others, supports the benefits of graduated driver licensing for the youngest drivers. In the United States, depending on state law, graduated driver licensing programs have been directed primarily at 16-year-olds and, to a lesser extent, 15- and 17-year-olds. Most evaluations have focused on just these age groups. A relatively small number of states have graduated licensing programs for all license applicants who are younger than 21 years of age. If all states were to adopt this provision, younger teenagers would be unable to avoid graduated driver licensing by waiting until age 18 (the age at which new drivers are not subject to graduated driver licensing restrictions in most states). New Jersey is a prime example of a state that has the strictest requirements and has shown significant reduction in crashes for 18- to 20-year-olds who are applying for licenses for the first time.

When I was a teenager, getting a driver's license as soon as possible was a rite of passage, for both girls and boys. Nowadays, we are seeing more and more teens taking a pass on getting a driver's license as soon as they are eligible to do so. This social change seems to be progressing. It is not at all uncommon to see many college students without driver's licenses these days. Should all who apply for a driver's license, at any age, be subjected to a graduated licensing program? Food for thought or a mindless edible?

This commentary closes with a "whodunit." You are seeing a teenager in your office who has a history of substance abuse. Physical examination shows patches of blackened, dying skin on the ears, face, trunk, and extremities. It is obvious that these represent small areas of skin necrosis. What do think is the etiology of the problem? If your answer is adulterated cocaine use, you would be right. Recently patients began showing up in emergency rooms with this problem. The cause of the outbreak appears to be a veterinary medication that has become the most common ingredient used to dilute or cut cocaine coming into the United States from South America. The drug, levamisole, was once approved for cancer treatment but was later pulled because of its side effects. Three-quarters of the cocaine bricks seized by the US Drug Enforcement Agency in 2011 were shown to contain levamisole. Equally of concern is another side effect of this drug, a sometimes fatal lowering of the white blood cell count. To read more about this, see the report by Chung et al.[3]

**J. A. Stockman III, MD**

*References*

1. Preusser DF, Williams AF, Zador PL, et al. The effect of curfew laws on motor vehicle crashes. *Law Policy.* 1994;6:115-128.
2. Fatality analysis reporting system, 1996—2009. National Highway Safety Administration Web Site. Ftt.nhtsa.dot.gov/FARS/. Accessed October 7, 2010.
3. Chung C, Tumeh PC, Birnbaum R. Characteristic purpura of the ears, vasculitis, and neutropenia—a potential public health epidemic associated with levamisole-adulterated cocaine. *J Amer Acad Dermatol.* 2011;65:722-725.

# 2 Allergy and Dermatology

**Recognising haemorrhagic rash in children with fever: a survey of parents' knowledge**
Aurel M, Dubos F, Motte B, et al (Univ of Lille Nord de France, Lille)
*Arch Dis Child* 96:697-698, 2011

*Background.*—Early recognition and treatment of meningococcal disease improves its outcome. Haemorrhagic rash is one of the most specific signs that parents can learn to recognise.

*Objective.*—To determine the percentage of parents able to recognise a haemorrhagic rash and perform the tumbler test.

*Methods.*—123 parents of children consulting for mild injuries were interviewed about the significance and recognition of haemorrhagic rash in febrile children.

*Results.*—Although 88% of parents undressed their children when they were febrile, it was never to look specifically for a skin rash. Only 7% (95% CI 3% to 12%) were able to recognise a petechial rash and knew the tumbler test.

*Conclusion.*—Information campaigns about the significance of haemorrhagic rash and about the tumbler test are needed.

▶ Meningococcal disease remains a major cause of morbidity and mortality in both children and adults. Obviously one of the early signs of infection with meningococcus is the development of a nonblanching skin rash. The authors of this report demonstrate that parents can be taught how to recognize the significance of petechial rashes. Without instruction, only a low percentage of parents are able to recognize a petechial rash, and few are aware of what is known as the tumbler test. One can say with some assurance that many physicians are not aware of the latter test either, thus the importance of this report. In Great Britain, the "tumbler" or "glass" test has been promoted in national guidelines as a way to address the detection of serious petechial rashes. Parents are taught to "press a glass tumbler firmly against the rash — if you see the spots through the glass and they do not fade, seek medical advice immediately."[1]

Use of the tumbler test is not well known in the United States. Perhaps it should be. Last, this commentary closes with a "whodunit." You are seeing a 14-year-old boy who presents with an asymptomatic bruiselike lesion on his left thigh. Examination reveals a solitary reticular area of pigmentary abnormality consistent with erythema ab igne. The patient strongly denies any regular exposure to heat in this area, but on more careful questioning admits to one other activity. What is that activity? If you answer that this youngster frequently has his laptop computer resting on his left thigh, you would be right. This phenomenon of erythema ab igne has been documented to be at times related to the heat produced by laptop computers. In the case of the 14-year-old, the diagnosis was made by ruling out any underlying vascular abnormalities by the performance of a skin biopsy.[2] Erythema ab igne is also commonly called "hot water bottle rash," "toasted skin syndrome," and "laptop thigh."

**J. A. Stockman III, MD**

*References*

1. National Institute for Health and Clinical Excellence. Fever in children younger than five years. http://www.nice.org/UK/nicemedia/lide/11010/30526/30526.pdf. Accessed August 31, 2010.
2. Simpson RC, Burd R. Skin rash secondary to a laptop computer. *BMJ*. 2010;340: 322.

---

**Delayed Acyclovir and Outcomes of Children Hospitalized With Eczema Herpeticum**

Aronson PL, Yan AC, Mittal MK, et al (Children's Hosp of Philadelphia, PA; Univ of Pennsylvania School of Medicine, Philadelphia)
*Pediatrics* 128:1161-1167, 2011

*Objective.*—To describe the epidemiology and outcomes of children hospitalized with eczema herpeticum and to determine the association with delayed acyclovir on outcomes.

*Patients and Methods.*—This was a multicenter retrospective cohort study conducted between January 1, 2001, and March 31, 2010, of 1331 children aged 2 months to 17 years with eczema herpeticum from 42 tertiary care children's hospitals in the Pediatric Health Information System database. Multivariable linear regression models determined the association between delayed acyclovir therapy and the main outcome measure: hospital length of stay (LOS).

*Results.*—There were no deaths during the study period. *Staphylococcus aureus* infection was diagnosed in 30.3% of the patients; 3.9% of the patients had a bloodstream infection. Fifty-one patients (3.8%) required ICU admission. There were 893 patients (67.1%) who received acyclovir on the first day of admission. The median LOS increased with each day delay in acyclovir initiation. In multivariable analysis, delay of acyclovir initiation by 1 day was associated with an 11% increased LOS (95% confidence interval [CI]: 3%−20%; $P = .008$), and LOS increased by 41% when acyclovir was started on day 3 (95% CI: 19%−67%; $P < .001$) and by 98% when started on day 4 to 7 (95% CI: 60%−145%; $P < .001$). Use of topical corticosteroids on day 1 of hospitalization was not associated with LOS.

*Conclusions.*—Delay of acyclovir initiation is associated with increased LOS in hospitalized children with eczema herpeticum. Use of topical corticosteroids on admission is not associated with increased LOS. The mortality rate of hospitalized children with eczema herpeticum is low.

▶ Eczema herpeticum is a rare problem affecting only a subset of patients with atopic dermatitis who seem to have a predisposition to herpes simplex virus (HSV) infection because of defects in specific proteins critical for skin barrier function and innate immunity. There are several things that increase the risk of eczema herpeticum. These include early onset of atopic dermatitis, more extensive skin involvement, eczematous lesions located on the head and neck, and higher IgE levels. Given the infrequency of the problem, it is easy to understand why there has been so little in the way of information about its management and the benefits of the antiviral agent acyclovir. Prior to the use of acyclovir, mortality rates reported in the literature ranged from 10% to 50%. The current mortality rate of eczema herpeticum with moderate antiviral therapy has not been reported. The study of Aronson et al describes the epidemiology of eczema herpeticum in hospitalized patients and explores the effect of delayed acyclovir on outcomes in this patient population. Using a multicenter retrospective analysis, some 1300 children 2 months to 17 years of age with eczema herpeticum were evaluated. There were no deaths reported. One-third of patients developed a *Staphylococcus aureus* infection. Delay of acyclovir initiation by day 1 was associated with an 11% increased length of stay. Length of stay increased by 41% when acyclovir was delayed until day 3 of hospitalization. Length of stay increased by 98% when started on days 4 to 7.

There is no question, based on the data from this report, that even if one merely suspects a child with eczema as having developed eczema herpeticum, one should immediately institute oral acyclovir therapy. Every day of delaying such therapy increases the likelihood of complications and extended hospital stays. Fortunately, this report also shows that topical steroid use early in hospitalization (which is generally considered a no-no) was not associated with an increased length of stay, although additional investigation into the safety of topical steroid use in the context of eczema herpeticum does seem warranted.

**J. A. Stockman III, MD**

---

**2-cm versus 4-cm surgical excision margins for primary cutaneous melanoma thicker than 2 mm: a randomised, multicentre trial**
Gillgren P, Drzewiecki KT, Niin M, et al (Karolinska Institutet, Stockholm, Sweden; Univ Hosp Rigshospitalet, Copenhagen, Denmark; North Estonian Regional Hosp, Tallin, Estonia; et al)
*Lancet* 378:1635-1642, 2011

---

*Background.*—Optimum surgical resection margins for patients with clinical stage IIA—C cutaneous melanoma thicker than 2 mm are controversial.

The aim of the study was to test whether survival was different for a wide local excision margin of 2 cm compared with a 4-cm excision margin.

*Methods.*—We undertook a randomised controlled trial in nine European centres. Patients with cutaneous melanoma thicker than 2 mm, at clinical stage IIA—C, were allocated to have either a 2-cm or a 4-cm surgical resection margin. Patients were randomised in a 1:1 allocation to one of the two groups and stratified by geographic region. Randomisation was done by sealed envelope or by computer generated lists with permuted blocks. Our primary endpoint was overall survival. The trial was not masked at any stage. Analyses were by intention to treat. Adverse events were not systematically recorded. The study is registered with ClinicalTrials.gov, number NCT01183936.

*Findings.*—936 patients were enrolled from Jan 22, 1992, to May 19, 2004; 465 were randomly allocated to treatment with a 2-cm resection margin, and 471 to receive treatment with a 4-cm resection margin. One patient in each group was lost to follow-up but included in the analysis. After a median follow-up of 6·7 years (IQR 4·3—9·5) 181 patients in the 2-cm margin group and 177 in the 4-cm group had died (hazard ratio 1·05, 95 CI 0·85—1·29; $p = 0.64$). 5-year overall survival was 65 (95 CI 60—69) in the 2-cm group and 65 (40—70) in the 4-cm group ($p = 0.69$).

*Interpretation.*—Our findings suggest that a 2-cm resection margin is sufficient and safe for patients with cutaneous melanoma thicker than 2 mm. Swedish Cancer Society and Stockholm Cancer Society.

▶ Despite more than a century of debate, the optimum excision margins for cutaneous melanoma in both children and adults are still unclear. This question is of great importance. A wider excision margin might be oncologically safer, but the closure method needed for such incision is more often a skin graft or a complex flap-plastic surgical procedure, resulting in greater morbidity and increased cost compared with a more narrow margin. About half of patients treated with 4-cm margins will require a skin graft. A distinct minority requires such grafts with just a 2-cm margin. One hundred years ago, a 5-cm radial margin was recommended for all patients with melanoma in the hope of reducing local recurrence and improving overall survival. Over the past 100 years, however, surgeons have begun to selectively use narrower margins and still have reported low local recurrence rates and no apparent reduction in overall survival. It is clear that when a melanoma is less than 1 mm thick, narrower margins can be used.

The clinical trial of Gillgren et al is quite welcome. Nine hundred thirty-six patients with melanomas thicker than 2 mm were randomly assigned to either a 2-cm or a 4-cm resection margin. The authors report no significant difference in overall survival rates (65% in both groups) or recurrence-free survival (56% in both groups) for the 2 treatment groups at 5-year follow-up. One hundred thirty-four patients died of melanoma (2-cm resection margin group), compared with 138 deaths (4-cm group) giving a hazard ratio of just 0.99. There were 109 before recurrences in the 2-cm group compared with 200 recurrences in the 4-cm group for a hazard ratio of 0.98. The authors conclude that a 2-cm margin is sufficient for patients with melanomas that are 2-mm or thicker. These conclusions need to be tempered with the knowledge that the originally planned trial had a target accrual of 2000 patients, yet fewer than 1000 were enrolled. Thus, the statistical power required for an equivalence trial was lacking, and the study should be classified as an unplanned, noninferiority trial, which shows that a 2-cm margin is not inferior to a 4-cm margin.

It should be noted that a previous trial comparing outcomes for a 3-cm versus a 1-cm margin excision of melanomas also showed no significant overall survival benefit from a wide margin.[1] The next study that needs to be designed should determine whether a 2-cm margin is preferable to a 1-cm margin. Morbidity and health care costs could be remarkably decreased if a 1-cm margin is equivalent or noninferior to a 2-cm margin. It appears that a proposal for such a large-scale multicenter trial is underway.

Recent data from the Centers for Disease Control and Prevention have documented that the annual percentage change in the incidence of melanoma has increased in the past 10 years in both sexes and all age groups. The annual percentage change in mortality rate has generally decreased in those younger than 65 but has increased in older individuals. Melanoma awareness in people younger than 65 years probably leads to earlier detection and therefore treatment. The melanoma mortality rate per 100 000 people during the period 2004 to 2006 was highest in non-Hispanic white individuals compared with black people and Asian or Pacific Islanders (3.31 vs 0.44 vs 3.37, respectively). To read more about skin cancer in the United States, including the statistics about melanoma, see the editorial that appeared recently in *The Lancet*.[2]

**J. A. Stockman III, MD**

*References*

1. Thomas JM, Newton-Bishop J, A'Hern R, et al. Excision margins in high-risk malignant melanoma. *N Engl J Med*. 2004;350:757-766.
2. Melanoma surveillance in the United States (Centers for Disease Control and Prevention). Skin cancer in the USA. *Lancet*. 2011;378:1528.

---

## gp100 Peptide Vaccine and Interleukin-2 in Patients with Advanced Melanoma

Schwartzentruber DJ, Lawson DH, Richards JM, et al (Indiana Univ Health Goshen Ctr for Cancer Care; Emory Univ, Atlanta, GA; Oncology Specialists, Park Ridge, IL; et al)
*N Engl J Med* 364:2119-2127, 2011

---

*Background.*—Stimulating an immune response against cancer with the use of vaccines remains a challenge. We hypothesized that combining a melanoma vaccine with interleukin-2, an immune activating agent, could improve outcomes. In a previous phase 2 study, patients with metastatic melanoma receiving high-dose interleukin-2 plus the gp100:209-217 (210M) peptide vaccine had a higher rate of response than the rate that is expected among patients who are treated with interleukin-2 alone.

*Methods.*—We conducted a randomized, phase 3 trial involving 185 patients at 21 centers. Eligibility criteria included stage IV or locally advanced stage III cutaneous melanoma, expression of HLA*A0201, an absence of brain metastases, and suitability for high-dose interleukin-2 therapy. Patients were randomly assigned to receive interleukin-2 alone (720,000 IU per kilogram of body weight per dose) or gp100:209-217 (210M) plus incomplete Freund's adjuvant (Montanide ISA-51) once per cycle, followed by interleukin-2. The primary end point was clinical response. Secondary end points included toxic effects and progression-free survival.

*Results.*—The treatment groups were well balanced with respect to baseline characteristics and received a similar amount of interleukin-2 per cycle. The toxic effects were consistent with those expected with interleukin-2 therapy. The vaccine—interleukin-2 group, as compared with the interleukin-2—only group, had a significant improvement in centrally verified overall clinical response (16% vs. 6%, $P = 0.03$), as well as longer progression-free survival (2.2 months; 95% confidence interval [CI], 1.7 to 3.9 vs. 1.6 months; 95% CI, 1.5 to 1.8; $P = 0.008$). The median overall survival was also longer in the vaccine—interleukin-2 group than in the interleukin-2—only group (17.8 months; 95% CI, 11.9 to 25.8 vs. 11.1 months; 95% CI, 8.7 to 16.3; $P = 0.06$).

*Conclusions.*—In patients with advanced melanoma, the response rate was higher and progression-free survival longer with vaccine and interleukin-2 than with interleukin-2 alone. (Funded by the National Cancer Institute and others; ClinicalTrials.gov number, NCT00019682.)

▶ The past few years have been banner ones with respect to innovative and somewhat effective new therapies for the management of patients with melanoma. The report of Schwartzentruber et al tells us about immunotherapy as part of the management of melanoma.

Melanoma, a tumor that may be innately immunogenic in humans, is an important model for the study of tumor immunity. Although the early stages of melanoma can be cured by surgery, the prognosis for patients with metastatic melanoma has remained grim, with a 5-year survival rate of less than 10%. To date, only 3 agents have been approved for the treatment of metastatic melanoma, but these agents have low response rates. Interleukin-2, a cytokine that induces T-cell activation and proliferation, is associated with an overall response rate of 13% to 16%, and up to 6% of patients have a complete response that can be reasonably durable. A variety of agents have been combined with interleukin-2 in an effort to improve its efficacy, including chemotherapy and other cytokines. Vaccination with the gp100:209-217 (210M) peptide has resulted in very high levels of circulating T cells that are capable of recognizing and killing melanoma cells at least in the laboratory, leading to the theory that activation of these T cells with cytokines such as interleukin-2 could be synergistic.

Schwartzentruber et al looked at the combination of interleukin-2 plus vaccination with this peptide as a novel way to manage patients with metastatic melanoma. These investigators conducted a randomized trial of almost 200 patients with stage IV or locally advanced stage III cutaneous melanoma. These patients were assigned to receive either interleukin-2 alone or the gp100:209-217 (210M) vaccine plus interleukin-2. The primary objective of this study was to determine whether the addition of the peptide vaccine to high-dose interleukin-2 would result in a higher rate of clinical response than that with interleukin-2 alone. This randomized study showed the clinical benefit of the vaccine in the treatment of patients with metastatic melanoma. Patients receiving the peptide vaccine with interleukin-2 were more than twice as likely to have a clinical response compared with those receiving interleukin-2 alone. The response rate with the combined approach was 16% versus 6%. These studies did not include an interleukin-2 only control group, and consequently, conclusions about the efficacy of vaccine itself could not be drawn.

As an aside, the first drug to extend overall survival for people with metastatic melanoma won approval from the US Food and Drug Administration in March 2011. A monoclonal antibody marketed under the brand name Yervoy by Bristol-Meyers-Squibb increased life span significantly more than either chemotherapy or an experimental vaccine.[1] Last, an investigational new drug has seen a remarkably high response rate (81%) in patients with metastatic melanoma. The drug, labeled PLX4032, inhibits B-RAF kinase, an enzyme that regulates signaling pathways in cells to control cell division and differentiation. B-RAF kinase is the most frequently mutated protein kinase in cancer cells. The drug blocks a particular pathway in cells with mutations of B-RAF gene, known to be associated with the development of cancer. Phase I clinical data revealed the very high response rate in metastatic melanoma patients treated with an oral dose of 960 mg twice daily. These data demonstrate that B-RAF-mutant melanomas are very dependant on this specific kinase.[2] The achievement of complete or partial regression of tumors in this group of patients with a single agent is unprecedented.

**J. A. Stockman III, MD**

*References*

1. Editorial comment. Melanoma milestone. *Science Med.* 2011;17:527.
2. Mayor S. Researchers describe how melanoma drug blocks key cancer pathway. *BMJ.* 2010;341:628.

---

**Cryotherapy versus salicylic acid for the treatment of plantar warts (verrucae): a randomised controlled trial**

Cockayne S, on behalf of the EVerT Team (Univ of York, UK; et al)
*BMJ* 342:d3271, 2011

*Objective.*—To compare the clinical effectiveness of cryotherapy versus salicylic acid for the treatment of plantar warts.

*Design.*—A multicentre, open, two arm randomised controlled trial.

*Setting.*—University podiatry school clinics, NHS podiatry clinics, and primary care in England, Scotland, and Ireland.

*Participants.*—240 patients aged 12 years and over, with a plantar wart that in the opinion of the healthcare professional was suitable for treatment with both cryotherapy and salicylic acid.

*Interventions.*—Cryotherapy with liquid nitrogen delivered by a health-care professional, up to four treatments two to three weeks apart. Patient self treatment with 50% salicylic acid (Verrugon) daily up to a maximum of eight weeks.

*Main Outcome Measures.*—Complete clearance of all plantar warts at 12 weeks. Secondary outcomes were (*a*) complete clearance of all plantar warts at 12 weeks controlling for age, whether the wart had been treated previously, and type of wart, (*b*) patient self reported clearance of plantar warts at six months, (*c*) time to clearance of plantar wart, (*d*) number of plantar warts at 12 weeks, and (*e*) patient satisfaction with the treatment.

*Results.*—There was no evidence of a difference between the salicylic acid and cryotherapy groups in the proportions of participants with complete clearance of all plantar warts at 12 weeks (17/119 (14%) *v* 15/110 (14%), difference 0.65% (95% CI −8.33 to 9.63), $P = 0.89$). The results did not change when the analysis was repeated but with adjustment for age, whether the wart had been treated previously, and type of plantar wart or for patients' preferences at baseline. There was no evidence of a difference between the salicylic acid and cryotherapy groups in self reported clearance of plantar warts at six months (29/95 (31%) *v* 33/98 (34%), difference −3.15% (−16.31 to 10.02), $P = 0.64$) or in time to clearance (hazard ratio 0.80 (95% CI 0.51 to 1.25), $P = 0.33$). There was also no evidence of a difference in the number of plantar warts at 12 weeks (incident rate ratio 1.08 (0.81 to 1.43), $P = 0.62$).

*Conclusions.*—Salicylic acid and the cryotherapy were equally effective for clearance of plantar warts.

*Trial Registration.*—Current Controlled Trials ISRCTN18994246, National Research Register N0484189151.

▶ Everyone knows that warts are common. Everyone knows they are benign. Not everyone is totally confident, however, about how to best manage cutaneous warts. These present in various forms and sizes and are caused by infection with human papillomavirus (HPV). They usually present as common warts (verrucae vulgaris), which occur most often on the hands or as plantar warts (verrucae plantares), usually found on the soles of the feet. Somewhere between 10% and 30% of young school-age children will have cutaneous warts and most of these resolve quite spontaneously.

Treatment of cutaneous warts has been based on destruction (cryotherapy, photodynamic treatment, pulsed dye laser), keratolysis (salicylic acid), immunostimulation (dinitrochlorobenzene, interferons), or the effects of antimitotics (bleomycin, fluorouracil). The rub is that the literature does not seem to be clear on which form of therapy is ideal.

Cockayne et al studied 240 patients aged 12 years or older with plantar warts to determine the effectiveness of various forms of therapy. In 1 group of patients, professionals delivered cryotherapy using liquid nitrogen 2 to 3 weeks apart for a maximum of 4 treatments. This was compared with daily self-treatment with 50% salicylic acid for a maximum of 8 weeks. The trial found no significant differences in the proportion of study subjects who had complete clearance of all plantar warts at 12 weeks. Thus, salicylic acid and cryotherapy were equally effective (14.3% vs 13.6% clearance). Although no group was allocated to a wait-and-see approach, the cure rates after intervention were probably not higher than without intervention, a finding seen in previous studies.

It is clear that less is probably more when it comes to plantar warts, but it should be noted that it is easier to treat plantar warts in those under 12 years of age because these warts tend to be less persistent than those seen in adolescents and young adults. Some cases may warrant treatment, such as those associated with considerable social stigma, particularly when lesions are on the face and hands. Warts can cause pain, particularly some on the soles of the feet or close to nails. These may also require treatment.

To read more about treatment for common plantar warts, see the excellent review of this topic by Bavinck et al [1] We are reminded that there are a number of HPV types and we know little about the epidemiology and prevalence of these various types as causes of common and plantar warts. It might be possible using simple DNA-related assays to determine which type of HPV is more susceptible to one form of therapy or another. Such a study might seem a bit over the top, but having warts is no laughing matter. Plantar warts, in particular, are not something on which to tread lightly (pardon the pun).

This commentary closes with some information provided from Denmark on nickel allergy. Over the 20th century, the prevalence of nickel allergy increased in Western Europe and the United States. This increase has been attributed to increased skin exposure to nickel in buttons, zippers, and other objects, earrings in particular. Nickel allergy may lead to nickel dermatitis at the site of contact and is a risk factor for the development of hand eczema. Our colleagues in Denmark have attempted to address this problem in a headlong way, unlike in the United States. In 1990, the Danish government began regulating the release of nickel from consumer products including jewelry. Investigators have recently reported the benefits of such regulation.[2] Investigators had baseline data prior to 1990 on the prevalence of nickel allergy and nickel dermatitis. It was clear that both the prevalence of nickel allergy and the presence of nickel dermatitis were significantly lower among women who have had their ears pierced after the start of nickel regulation in 1990 than among women who had had their ears pierced before that year. Specifically, the prevalence of nickel allergy declined from 15.6% to 6.9% and the prevalence of dermatitis dropped from 44% to 30.5%. The investigators commented that the drop probably would have been greater except for the fact that jewelry is jewelry and, like herpes, is around forever. Even after 1990 women may have had access to older jewelry in addition to jewelry from other countries which lack such regulation. By the way, the prevalence of nickel allergy among men was not significantly higher among those whose ears were pierced before 1990 than those whose ears were pierced between 1990 and 2006. Obviously men are a hardier breed, particularly those who are of the sufficient psychological fortitude to have their ears pierced.

**J. A. Stockman III, MD**

*References*

1. Bavinck JNB, Eekhof JAH, Bruggink SC. Treatments for common and plantar warts. *BMJ.* 2011;342:d3119.
2. Thyssen JP, Johansen JD, Menne T, Nielsen NH, Linneberg A. Nickel allergy in Danish women before and after nickel regulation. *N Engl J Med.* 2009;360: 2259-2260.

---

**The Association of Psoriasis and Elevated Blood Lipids in Overweight and Obese Children**
Koebnick C, Black MH, Smith N, et al (Kaiser Permanente Southern California, Pasadena; et al)
*J Pediatr* 159:577-583, 2011

---

*Objective.*—To investigate whether obesity and cardiovascular risk factors are associated with psoriasis in children and adolescents.

*Study Design.*—For this population-based, cross-sectional study, measured weight and height, laboratory data, and psoriasis diagnoses were extracted from electronic medical records of 710 949 patients age 2 to 19 years enrolled in an integrated health plan. Weight class was assigned on the basis of body mass index—for—age.

*Results.*—The OR for psoriasis was 0.68, 1.00, 1.31, 1.39, and 1.78 (95% CI, 1.49 to 2.14) for underweight, normal-weight, overweight, moderately obese, and extremely obese children, respectively (*P* for trend < .001). The OR for psoriasis treated with systemic therapy or phototherapy as an indicator of severe or widespread psoriasis was 0.00, 1.00, 2.78, 2.93, and 4.19 (95% CI, 1.81 to 9.68) for underweight, normal-weight, overweight, moderately obese, and extremely obese children, respectively (*P* for trend < .003). In adolescents, mean total cholesterol, low-density lipoprotein cholesterol, triglycerides, and alanine aminotransferase were significantly higher in children with psoriasis compared with children without psoriasis after adjustment for body mass index.

*Conclusion.*—Overweight and obesity are associated with higher odds of psoriasis in youths. Independent of body weight, adolescent patients with psoriasis have higher blood lipids. These data suggest that pediatricians and dermatologists should screen youths with psoriasis for cardiovascular disease risk factors.

▶ An association between obesity and psoriasis has been documented in adults.[1] One study has also examined a potential association in children.[2] This study found obesity to be 1.7 times higher in frequency in children with psoriasis compared with those without. This same study also noted a higher prevalence of dyslipidemia and hypertension in obese children who had developed psoriasis.

The report of Koebnick et al used the power of numbers to determine the potential association between obesity and psoriasis. Specifically, the authors undertook a cross-sectional study of more than 700 000 racially and ethnically diverse children who were being cared for within the Kaiser Permanente health care system. They evaluated the association of psoriasis and cardiovascular risk factors such as cholesterol, low-density lipoprotein, high-density lipoprotein, triglycerides, alanine aminotransferase levels, and body mass index. They identified 1350 patients with psoriasis. The odds ratios for developing psoriasis were 0.62, 1.00, 1.38, 1.33, and 1.86 for underweight, normal weight, overweight, moderately obese, and extremely obese children, respectively. Among the overweight to extremely obese adolescents in this report, those with psoriasis had significantly higher total cholesterol, low-density lipid cholesterol, triglycerides, and alanine aminotransferase levels compared with those without psoriasis. The mean high-density lipid cholesterol was not significantly different between patients with and without psoriasis.

There are a number of other interesting findings in this report. The severity (not just incidence) of psoriasis was associated with high body weight. The use of systemic therapy or phototherapy, indicating severe or widespread psoriasis, was almost 3 times as likely to occur in moderately obese children and more than 4 times as likely to occur in extremely obese children compared with normal-weight children. Also, although the absolute differences in cholesterol and other lipid levels were small, they are of clinical significance. These differences compared with a reference group show that kids with psoriasis have lipid levels roughly in the 70th percentile for total cholesterol. This finding is consistent with adult studies showing a link between psoriasis and the development of metabolic syndrome.

The obvious question that arises from this report is, what the link is between obesity and the development of psoriasis? There is no question that obesity is associated with an inflammatory state in and of itself. Psoriasis is known to be an inflammatory condition of unknown origin. Given that remission of psoriasis has been reported after bariatric surgery, it seems reasonable to believe there is a genuine link between the 2 entities. If there is a lesson to be learned from this report, it is that if you are caring for a patient with psoriasis and that patient is overweight, treat the obesity and the psoriasis may just go away.

This commentary closes with a relatively unimportant historical observation and that is that the oldest human hair that has been discovered was found a few years ago in the feces of a 200 000-year-old hyena.[3] Researchers have found fossils of early humans and their evolutionary forbearers in many South African caves. Some think the hominins either died or were buried there, but others think it more likely that wild animals dragged their bones or bodies into the caves. Along with the bones, fossilized hyena feces or coprolites have been found. These were discovered in the Galdysvale Cave north of Johannesburg, where Australopithecine teeth and a hominin head bone were found in the 1990s. A paleontologist at the University of Witwatersrand in Johannesburg teased 40 hairs from a coprolite and examined half of them with a scanning electron microscope. Comparing their microscopic structure with that of other animal hairs, this individual found that five of the hairs were highly likely to be human. They are the oldest known hairs—20 times as old as the previous record holder, hair from a 9000-year-old mummy found in Chile. Needless to say it is obvious that a hyena ate at least part of a hominin, our ancestors from Africa.

**J. A. Stockman III, MD**

*References*

1. Neimann AL, Shin DB, Wang X, Margolis DJ, Troxel AB, Gelfand JM. Prevalence of cardiovascular risk factors in patients with psoriasis. *J Am Acad Dermatol.* 2006;55:829-835.
2. Augustin M, Glaeske G, Radtke MA, Christophers E, Reich K, Schäfer I. Epidemiology and comorbidity of psoriasis in children. *Br J Dermatol.* 2010;12:633-636.
3. Editorial comment. Oldest human hair found? *Science.* 2009;323:1651.

---

**Recognition of Tuberous Sclerosis in Adult Women: Delayed Presentation With Life-Threatening Consequences**

Seibert D, Hong C-H, Takeuchi F, et al (Uniformed Services Univ of the Health Sciences, Bethesda, MD; Kaohsiung Veterans General Hosp, Taiwan)

*Ann Intern Med* 154:806-813, 2011

---

*Background.*—Tuberous sclerosis complex (TSC) is associated with tumor development in the brain, retina, kidney, skin, heart, and lung. Seizures, intellectual disability, and characteristic skin lesions commonly manifest in early childhood, but some findings, notably renal angiomyolipomas and pulmonary lymphangioleiomyomatosis (LAM), emerge later, placing adults with undiagnosed TSC at increased risk for morbidity and mortality.

*Objective.*—To describe the clinical presentation and severity of TSC in adult women.

*Design.*—Retrospective cohort study.

*Setting.*—National Institutes of Health Clinical Center, Bethesda, Maryland, 1995 to 2010.

*Patients.*—79 women aged 18 years or older who were enrolled in an observational cohort study of TSC to evaluate disease manifestations.

*Measurements.*—History, physical examination, pulmonary function testing, chest radiography, abdominal computed tomography, high-resolution chest computed tomography, and brain magnetic resonance imaging were used to evaluate patients.

*Results.*—Among the 45 patients who received a diagnosis of TSC in adulthood, 21 presented with symptoms due to LAM, 19 with renal angiomyolipomas, and 10 with seizures. Of the 45 patients, 30 met clinical criteria for TSC in childhood that remained undiagnosed for a median of 21.5 years and 15 were older than 18 years before meeting the clinical criteria for TSC. Patients diagnosed in adulthood and those diagnosed in childhood had similar occurrences of pneumothorax, shortness of breath, hemoptysis, nephrectomy, and death.

*Limitation.*—No men were included in the study, and selection was biased toward patients having pulmonary LAM.

*Conclusion.*—Women who received a TSC diagnosis in adulthood had minimal morbidity during childhood but were still at risk for life-threatening pulmonary and renal manifestations.

▶ Most of us think of tuberous sclerosis as a disease of children. Indeed, it is because it is an autosomal dominant disorder and therefore is present from birth. The rub is that many get through childhood without being adequately diagnosed or diagnosed at all with the disorder and that is what the report of Seibert et al is all about. Siebert et al looked at 79 women, age 18 years or older who were first diagnosed as having tuberous sclerosis as adults. Approximately two-thirds of the women, in fact, reported problems during childhood that were consistent with the disease but were not recognized at the time. In the remaining women, some features of tuberous sclerosis may have been present earlier in life but were not sufficient to make a diagnosis.

So how does tuberous sclerosis present in the young or even more mature adult? Among patients who received a diagnosis of tuberous sclerosis in adulthood, about half presented with symptoms related to renal angiolipomas or pulmonary lymphangioleiomyomatosis. About 1 in 4 presented with seizures. Two-thirds of adults met clinical criteria for tuberous sclerosis in childhood if the disorder had been properly diagnosed on the basis of history or physical examination.

As an autosomal dominant disorder, tuberous sclerosis is characterized by the development of hamartomatous tumors in many organs, most notably the brain, retina, kidney, skin, heart and lung. While the condition may present early in life with a classic triad of seizures, intellectual disability, and cutaneous angiofibromas, fewer than 30% of affected individuals will have all 3 characteristic findings and 6% have none. If left undiagnosed, the disorder will eventually catch up with an individual in adulthood, often presenting as a pneumothorax, shortness of breath, or hemoptysis, leading to respiratory failure and death. Once diagnosed, those with tuberous sclerosis can be treated with a surveillance program that looks for all of the complications that can be managed at an early stage of development. Fig 2 in the original article shows the clinical characteristics of tuberous sclerosis complex with early or late penetrance. Fig 1 in the original article shows many of the anatomic findings that should be a tipoff to the diagnosis.

Tuberous sclerosis has many skin findings so this commentary closes with an observation about the skin. It turns out that skin hosts more bacteria than previously thought. Researchers at the National Institute of Health Human Microbiome Project sequenced genes from skin samples from healthy volunteers and found bacteria that hailed from 19 different phyla and 205 genera and that possessed more than 112 000 individual gene sequences. Previous studies of skin cultures supposed that only one type of bacteria, Staphylococcus, was the main resident of skin. The researchers' purpose in carrying out this investigation was to establish a bacteriological baseline so as to better treat skin diseases, such as acne and eczema, where bacterial populations might be out of balance and contributing to the underlying skin disorder.[1]

**J. A. Stockman III, MD**

Reference

1. Harmon K. Skin so bacterial. *Scientific American.* August 2009:26.

## Leukotriene Antagonists as First-Line or Add-on Asthma-Controller Therapy

Price D, Musgrave SD, Shepstone L, et al (Univ of Aberdeen, UK; Univ of East Anglia, Norwich, UK; et al)

*N Engl J Med* 364:1695-1707, 2011

*Background.*—Most randomized trials of treatment for asthma study highly selected patients under idealized conditions.

*Methods.*—We conducted two parallel, multicenter, pragmatic trials to evaluate the real-world effectiveness of a leukotriene-receptor antagonist (LTRA) as compared with either an inhaled glucocorticoid for first-line asthma-controller therapy or a long-acting beta$_2$-agonist (LABA) as add-on therapy in patients already receiving inhaled glucocorticoid therapy. Eligible primary care patients 12 to 80 years of age had impaired asthma-related quality of life (Mini Asthma Quality of Life Questionnaire [MiniAQLQ] score $\leq 6$) or inadequate asthma control (Asthma Control Questionnaire [ACQ] score $\geq 1$). We randomly assigned patients to 2 years of open-label therapy, under the care of their usual physician, with LTRA (148 patients) or an inhaled glucocorticoid (158 patients) in the first-line controller therapy trial and LTRA (170 patients) or LABA (182 patients) added to an inhaled glucocorticoid in the add-on therapy trial.

*Results.*—Mean MiniAQLQ scores increased by 0.8 to 1.0 point over a period of 2 years in both trials. At 2 months, differences in the MiniAQLQ scores between the two treatment groups met our definition of equivalence (95% confidence interval [CI] for an adjusted mean difference, $-0.3$ to $0.3$). At 2 years, mean MiniAQLQ scores approached equivalence, with an adjusted mean difference between treatment groups of $-0.11$ (95% CI, $-0.35$ to $0.13$) in the first-line controller therapy trial and of $-0.11$ (95% CI, $-0.32$ to $0.11$) in the add-on therapy trial. Exacerbation rates and ACQ scores did not differ significantly between the two groups.

*Conclusions.*—Study results at 2 months suggest that LTRA was equivalent to an inhaled glucocorticoid as first-line controller therapy and to LABA as add-on therapy for diverse primary care patients. Equivalence was not proved at 2 years. The interpretation of results of pragmatic research may be limited by the crossover between treatment groups and lack of a placebo group. (Funded by the National Coordinating Centre for Health Technology Assessment U.K. and others; Controlled Clinical Trials number, ISRCTN99132811.)

▶ This report introduces the concept to many readers of what is known as pragmatic clinical trials. Generally speaking, guidelines for treating asthma are built on results from randomized, tightly controlled trials. Patients enrolled in these trials make up a small and selected fraction of the real-world population with asthma. This is because so many exclusions exist in such trials that few patients with the disease can be enrolled. It is estimated that 95% or so of asthmatics are never eligible to enter such randomized tightly controlled trials because of variables that exclude them. What Price et al have done is to report on 2 "pragmatic" trials in which a much larger fraction of patients with asthma are able to be enrolled than the case in randomized, controlled trials. Their results challenge current guidelines. Asthma treatment guidelines generally recommend glucocorticoids as the first-line controller medication for asthma in patients with mild persistent asthma. These agents have little effect on the formation or action of cysteinyl leukotrienes, inflammatory mediators in asthma. Leukotriene-receptor antagonists (LTRAs) have proved to be beneficial in double-blind, randomized, placebo-controlled trials. Results of prior comparisons of LTRA and inhaled glucocorticoids (mostly double-blind, randomized, controlled trials) have been mixed, with some suggesting that LTRAs are less efficacious than inhaled glucocorticoids for patients with mild persistent asthma, and others reporting similar overall asthma control and proportions of patients meeting asthma-controlled criteria. For patients whose symptoms are not controlled with low-dose inhaled glucocorticoids, step-up therapy consists of an increased dose or the addition of LTRA or an inhaled long acting beta2 agonist (LABA).

Price et al describe 2 real life community studies of patients with asthma. In the first trial, patients whose asthma required first-line controller therapy were treated with an inhaled glucocorticoid or an LTRA. In the second trial, patients were receiving an inhaled glucocorticoid as first-line controller therapy but needed additional therapy to control their asthma; the second study compared adding either LTRA or a long-acting inhaled beta2 agonist. In each trial, the LTRA was essentially equivalent in efficacy to either the inhaled glucocorticoid as first-line controller therapy or to the LABA as add-on therapy. In both trials the patients were followed for 2 years, making the results relevant to ordinary clinical practice.

Much has been written about the strengths and weaknesses of pragmatic trials, but in the real-world setting, the results of this study seem quite reasonable. It is far easier to take a pill once or twice a day than to use an inhaler. The data from the 2 studies of Price et al support this view because the rates of adherence to the oral LTRA were 65% and 74% in the first-line controller and add-on therapy trials, respectively, compared with only 41% and 46% for the inhaled glucocorticoid. Antileukotrienes may have other advantages in clinical practice. The cost of this treatment will most likely become competitive since montelukast and zafirlukast are expected to be available soon as generic medications. Also, many patients with asthma have rhinitis or other coexisting conditions in which leukotrienes only contribute to the symptoms. Antileukotrienes have a very good safety profile unlike inhaled glucocorticoids that may have some measurable systemic effects, including inhibition of bone growth in children.

This report is worth reading in some detail. It certainly changes one's thinking about the potential management of asthma. It will be interesting to see how national treatment guidelines for children evolve with this new information.

To read more about asthma treatment guidelines, see the editorial by Dahlén et al.[1]

**J. A. Stockman III, MD**

*Reference*

1. Dahlén S-E, Dahlén B, Drazen JM. Asthma treatment guidelines meet the real world [Editorials]. *N Engl J Med.* 2011;364:1769-1770.

**Feather bedding and childhood asthma associated with house dust mite sensitisation: a randomised controlled trial**
Glasgow NJ, Ponsonby A-L, Kemp A, et al (The Australian Natl Univ, Acton, Australia; Univ of Sydney, New South Wales, Australia; et al)
*Arch Dis Child* 96:541-547, 2011

*Introduction.*—Observational studies report inverse associations between the use of feather upper bedding (pillow and/or quilt) and asthma symptoms but there is no randomised controlled trial (RCT) evidence assessing the role of feather upper bedding as a secondary prevention measure.

*Objective.*—To determine whether, among children not using feather upper bedding, a new feather pillow and feather quilt reduces asthma severity among house dust mite (HDM) sensitised children with asthma over a 1-year period compared with standard dust mite avoidance advice, and giving children a new mite-occlusive mattress cover.

*Design.*—RCT.

*Setting.*—The Calvary Hospital in the Australian Capital Territory and the Children's Hospital at Westmead, Sydney, New South Wales.

*Patients.*—197 children with HDM sensitisation and moderate to severe asthma.

*Intervention.*—New upper bedding duck feather pillow and quilt and a mite-occlusive mattress cover (feather) versus standard care and a mite-occlusive mattress cover (standard).

*Main Outcome Measures.*—The proportion of children reporting four or more episodes of wheeze in the past year; an episode of speech-limiting wheeze; or one or more episodes of sleep disturbance caused by wheezing; and spirometry with challenge testing. Statistical analysis included multiple logistic and linear regression.

*Results.*—No differences between groups were found for primary end points — frequent wheeze (OR 1.51, 95% CI 0.83 to 2.76, $p = 0.17$), speech-limiting wheeze (OR 0.70, 95% CI 0.32 to 1.48, $p = 0.35$), sleep disturbed because of wheezing (OR 1.17, 95% CI 0.64 to 2.13, $p = 0.61$) or for any secondary end points. Secondary analyses indicated the intervention reduced the risk of sleep being disturbed because of wheezing and severe wheeze to a greater extent for children who slept supine.

*Conclusion.*—No differences in respiratory symptoms or lung function were observed 1 year after children with moderate—severe asthma and

HDM sensitisation were given a mite-occlusive mattress cover and then received either feather upper bedding (pillow and quilt) or standard bedding care.

▶ It is interesting that over the last 20 years or so, various studies have reported an inverse association between feather upper bedding and asthma symptoms. Feather upper bedding refers to feather pillows as opposed to synthetic pillows. It has been suggested that synthetic bedding may be more problematic than feather bedding because synthetic bedding may have higher levels of dust mite allergens, proinflammatory fungal-related products, volatile organic compounds, and lower levels of bacterial endotoxins, the latter having been inversely correlated with asthma prevalence if a child is exposed early. The authors of this report attempted to determine whether among children not using feather pillows, a new feather pillow and feather quilt would reduce asthma severity. All study subjects received a new mite-occlusive mattress cover and instructions about how to avoid dust mite exposure, to the extent possible.

The findings of this report show no overall differences in respiratory symptoms, lung function, or quality of life 1 year after children with moderate to severe asthma and house dust mite sensitization were given a mite-occlusive mattress cover along with receiving either feather upper bedding (pillow and quilt) or standard bedding materials. Interestingly, this study did find that children's sleep position influences bedding—wheeze associations. There was a protective effect of feather bedding observed in children who slept in the supine but not prone position. The overall findings do not provide support for previous recommendations that feather bedding should be avoided for children with asthma. Child sleep position should be considered in the design phase of any future studies.

While on the topic of exposure to various things that can trigger asthma, children who live on farms have been documented to have less asthma and atopy than children who grow up in other settings. Even indoors, such children are exposed to a greater variety of bacteria and fungi. This seems to explain a large part of the association with asthma but not with atopy. These findings come from 2 large observational studies with many thousands of children in rural areas of Austria, South Germany, and Switzerland. It may be that exposure to a wide range of microbes prevents colonization of lower airways with harmful bacteria, stopping them from contributing to the development of asthma. The mechanism supporting such a belief remains unknown. Unfortunately, there is a long way to go before the health benefits of growing up on a farm can translate into anything preventative in a practical sense.[1]

**J. A. Stockman III, MD**

*Reference*

1. Ege MJ, Mayer M, Normand A-C, et al. Exposure to environmental microorganisms and childhood asthma. *N Engl J Med*. 2011;364:701-709.

## Sex-specific trends in prevalence of childhood asthma over 30 years in Patras, Greece

Anthracopoulos MB, Pandiora A, Fouzas S, et al (Univ Hosp of Patras, Greece; et al)

*Acta Paediatr* 100:1000-1005, 2011

*Aim.*—According to four surveys conducted during 1978–2003, the prevalence of childhood asthma and wheezing has risen in the city of Patras, Greece, albeit at a decelerating rate. We examined sex-specific wheeze and asthma prevalence in the same urban environment in 2008.

*Methods.*—A cross-sectional parental questionnaire survey was performed in 2008 among third and fourth grade schoolchildren (8–9 year old), which was identical to previously conducted surveys in 1978 (n = 3003), 1991 (n = 2417), 1998 (n = 3076) and 2003 (n = 2725).

*Results.*—The prevalence of current wheeze and asthma in 1978, 1991, 1998, 2003 and 2008 (n = 2688) was 1.5%, 4.6%, 6.0%, 6.9% and 6.9%, respectively ($p$ for trend < 0.001). Respective values for lifetime (ever had) wheeze and asthma in the 1991–2008 surveys were 8.0%, 9.6%, 12.4% and 12.6% ($p$ for trend < 0.001). The male:female ratio of current and lifetime wheeze and asthma increased during the 30-year surveillance period ($p$ for trend < 0.001). Irrespective of sex, diagnosed asthma declined among current wheezers by 17% ($p < 0.001$), but not among non-current ones (6.7%, $p = 0.16$) during 2003–2008.

*Conclusions.*—Childhood wheeze and asthma have reached a plateau in an urban environment in Greece, while the male:female ratio increased. Asthma diagnosis declined among schoolage but not preschool wheezers during 2003–2008.

▶ Everyone knows that in the last 50 years there has been an explosion in the prevalence of asthma, at least in western societies. More recent reports, however, suggest that this asthma epidemic may have reached its plateau in countries that have experienced rapid increases. This is indicated by the results of several studies of the prevalence of asthma in children and adolescents, including the International Study of Asthma and Allergies in Childhood Phase III (ISAAC Phase III).[1] The study reported by Anthracopoulos from Patras, Greece, adds valuable information to support the view that the prevalence of asthma is no longer increasing.

Patras is the regional capital of Western Greece. It is located about 200 km west of Athens and has a population of about 250 000. Asthma studies have been conducted there over the last 40 years. The prevalence of asthma in children for the periods 1978, 1991, 1998, and 2003 were 1.5%, 4.6%, 6.0%, and 6.9%, respectively. In this study, based on data in 2008, there has been no increase in prevalence of asthma for more than a half decade. The prevalence sits at 6.9%. At least in this area of the world, asthma prevalence has reached a plateau.

It is interesting to note that similar findings on the prevalence of asthma are now being observed in adults. Why this prevalence has reached a plateau is unknown. It has been suggested that the progressive induction of asthma in genetically predisposed children is a self-limiting process with an upper limit that has now been reached, that is, the leveling off reflects a saturation effect. Another contributing factor could be the decreased frequency of smoking in the general population, including the decreased exposure of pregnant women to secondary smoke. This explanation may not be particularly applicable in Greece, where the maternal smoking rate is still very high.

The results of the study from Greece, as well as several others, support the notion that the increase in asthma prevalence seen starting in the 1950s has now reached a plateau, at least in many parts of the western world.

**J. A. Stockman III, MD**

*Reference*

1. Zilmer M, Steen N, Zachariassen G, Duus T, Kristiansen B, Halken S. Prevalence of asthma and bronchial hyperreactivity in Danish school children: no change over 10 years. *Acta Paediatr.* 2011;100:385-389.

**Antibiotic Prescribing During Pediatric Ambulatory Care Visits for Asthma**
Paul IM, Maselli JH, Hersh AL, et al (Penn State College of Medicine, Hershey, PA; Univ of California at San Francisco; Univ of Utah School of Medicine, Salt Lake City)
*Pediatrics* 127:1014-1021, 2011

*Objective.*—National guidelines do not recommend antibiotics as an asthma therapy. We sought to examine the frequency of inappropriate antibiotic prescribing during US ambulatory care pediatric asthma visits as well as the patient, provider, and systemic variables associated with such practice.

*Patients and Methods.*—Data from the National Ambulatory Medical Care Surveys and National Hospital Ambulatory Medical Care Survey were examined to assess office and emergency-department asthma visits made by children (aged <18 years) for frequencies of antibiotic prescription. *International Classification of Diseases, Ninth Revision* (ICD-9) codes were used to assess the presence of coexisting conditions warranting antibiotics. Multivariable logistic regression models assessed associations with the prescription of antibiotics.

*Results.*—From 1998 to 2007, an estimated 60.4 million visits occurred for asthma without another ICD-9 code justifying antibiotic prescription. Antibiotics were prescribed during 16% of these visits, most commonly macrolides (48.8%). In multivariate analysis, controlling for patient age, gender, race, insurance type, region, and controller medication use, systemic corticosteroid prescription (odds ratio [OR]: 2.69 [95% confidence interval (CI): 1.68—4.30]) and treatment during the winter (OR: 1.92 [95% CI: 1.05—3.52]) were associated with an increased likelihood of antibiotic prescription, whereas treatment in an emergency department was associated with decreased likelihood (OR: 0.48 [95% CI: 0.26—0.89]). A second multivariate analysis of only office-based visits demonstrated that asthma education during the visits was associated with reduced antibiotic prescriptions (OR: 0.46 [95% CI: 0.24–0.86]).

*Conclusions.*—Antibiotics are prescribed during nearly 1 in 6 US pediatric ambulatory care visits for asthma, ~1 million prescriptions annually, when antibiotic need is undocumented. Additional education and interventions are needed to prevent unnecessary antibiotic prescribing for asthma.

▶ This report, along with one other,[1] remind us all too vividly that many who care for children with asthma write prescriptions for antibiotics that are not likely to be indicated as part of the management of the presenting problem. A study by De Boeck et al[1] used health insurance database information that encompassed the records of almost 1 million Belgian children seen in 1 year to examine antibiotic-prescribing practices. It was observed that antibiotics were dispensed to 44% of children covered by insurance. An asthmatic drug (β-adrenergic agents, inhaled corticosteroids, tiotropium, or leukotriene receptor agonist) was dispensed to 16.04% of children. An antibiotic was dispensed to 39% of children without an asthmatic drug versus 73.5% of children when an asthmatic drug was also dispensed.

The findings of Paul et al from the National Ambulatory Medical Care Survey and the National Hospital Ambulatory Medical Care Survey also demonstrate the frequency of antibiotic prescribing during office and emergency department visits for children with asthmatic symptoms. Between 1998 and 2007, just more than 60 million visits were noted for asthma in which the prescription for an antibiotic was given, but without supporting information for the use of the antibiotic. Antibiotics were prescribed in 16% of overall visits with macrolides being the most commonly prescribed antibiotic (almost 50% of the time). Children who were prescribed systemic steroids were significantly more likely to receive an antibiotic.

Obviously, prescribing for a bacterial illness when none is present is not a new phenomenon. The assumption is that physicians are likely to be treating for presumed "bacterial"-associated respiratory tract infections including sinusitis, pharyngitis, and acute otitis media, even though the clinical findings to support such antibiotic use may not be fully there.

Other studies have reminded us that asthma education at the time of a routine office visit can produce remarkable reductions in the need for antibiotic prescription writing. In a commentary that accompanied this report, Mangione-Smith and Krogstad[2] tell us that it would be terrific if a national quality improvement program could be established to address inappropriate antibiotic prescribing in the pediatric outpatient setting. This would be a worthwhile endeavor.

**J. A. Stockman III, MD**

*References*

1. De Boeck K, Vermeulen F, Meyts I, Hutsebaut L, Franckaert D, Proesmans M. Coprescription of antibiotics and asthma drugs in children. *Pediatrics.* 2011; 127:1022-1026.

2. Mangione-Smith R, Krogstad P. Antibiotic prescription with asthma medications: why is it so common? *Pediatrics*. 2011;127:1174-1176.

## Prenatal or Early-Life Exposure to Antibiotics and Risk of Childhood Asthma: A Systematic Review

Murk W, Risnes KR, Bracken MB (Yale Univ School of Public Health, New Haven, CT)
*Pediatrics* 127:1125-1138, 2011

*Context.*—The increasing prevalence of childhood asthma has been associated with low microbial exposure as described by the hygiene hypothesis.

*Objective.*—We sought to evaluate the evidence of association between antibiotic exposure during pregnancy or in the first year of life and risk of childhood asthma.

*Methods.*—PubMed was systematically searched for studies published between 1950 and July 1, 2010. Those that assessed associations between antibiotic exposure during pregnancy or in the first year of life and asthma at ages 0 to 18 years (for pregnancy exposures) or ages 3 to 18 years (for first-year-of-life exposures) were included. Validity was assessed according to study design, age at asthma diagnosis, adjustment for respiratory infections, and consultation rates.

*Results.*—For exposure in the first year of life, the pooled odds ratio (OR) for all studies ($N = 20$) was 1.52 (95% confidence interval [CI]: 1.30–1.77). Retrospective studies had the highest pooled risk estimate for asthma (OR: 2.04 [95% CI: 1.83–2.27]; $n = 8$) compared with database and prospective studies (OR: 1.25 [95% CI: 1.08–1.45]; $n = 12$). Risk estimates for studies that adjusted for respiratory infections (pooled OR: 1.16 [95% CI: 1.08–1.25]; $n = 5$) or later asthma onset (pooled OR for asthma at or after 2 years: OR: 1.16 [95% CI: 1.06–1.25]; $n = 3$) were weaker but remained significant. For exposure during pregnancy ($n = 3$ studies), the pooled OR was 1.24 (95% CI: 1.02–1.50).

*Conclusions.*—Antibiotics seem to slightly increase the risk of childhood asthma. Reverse causality and protopathic bias seem to be possible confounders for this relationship.

▶ Here we have another report having to do with precedents that increase or decrease the long-term risk of the development of childhood asthma. This report comes from New Haven, Connecticut, and Trondheim, Norway, and represents an analysis of literature over the last 60 years examining any associations between antibiotic exposure during pregnancy or in the first year of life and the development of asthma by 18 years of age. The data indicate an excess risk of asthma as the result of early antibiotic exposure (relative risk, 1.13). Assuming a baseline childhood asthma incidence of 10% and an odds ratio of 1.13, the number needed to harm is 87. This specifically means that for every 87 children exposed to antibiotics, one child will develop asthma presumably because of his or her antibiotic exposure. If it turns out that there is a true causal relationship between antibiotics and asthma, the total number of children who develop asthma as a result of such exposure would not be insignificant, even for small-effect estimates such as those noted in this report. The authors of this study conclude that evidence does suggest that antibiotic exposure early in life or in utero will increase the risk of developing childhood asthma, albeit only very modestly for any specific child. The authors also note that this conclusion remains tentative because evidence for bias was observed in a number of the studies that formed the basis for the authors' conclusions. One will need to see studies of large prospective cohorts to really answer the question of whether there is a true relationship between early antibiotic exposure and a risk of the development of asthma, but it does seem reasonable to suspect that where there is smoke there is fire, at least in terms of the evidence that exists to date.

While on the topic of asthma, in February 2010, the US Food and Drug Administration (FDA) sought to improve the safety of long-acting beta-agonists (LABAs)—drugs that provide bronchodilation for 12 hours or longer by stimulating the beta-2 adrenergic receptor—by issuing a requirement for manufacturers of products containing LABAs to make changes in their labelling with respect to asthma treatment. This is based on the observation that LABAs have been associated with severe and serious asthma outcomes, such as asthma-related hospitalization, need for intubation, and even death in some patients.[1] On April 14, 2011, the FDA issued a requirement for all manufacturers of LABAs that are marketed for asthma treatment in the United States to conduct controlled clinical trials to assess the safety of a regimen of LABAs plus inhaled corticosteroids compared with inhaled corticosteroids alone. The FDA believes that these clinical trials will provide data in a timely fashion that will clarify the safety risk associated with LABAs when used concurrently with inhaled corticosteroids and will inform the safe use of these medications for the treatment of asthma.

To read more about assessing the safety of adding LABAs to inhaled corticosteroids for treating asthma in both children and adults, see the excellent editorial on this topic by Chowdhury et al.[2]

**J. A. Stockman III, MD**

*References*

1. Chowdhury BA, Dal Pan G. The FDA and safe use of long-acting beta-agonists in the treatment of asthma. *N Engl J Med.* 2010;362:1169-1171.
2. Chowdhury BA, Seymour SM, Levenson MS. Assessing the safety of adding LABAs to inhaled corticosteroids for treating asthma. *N Engl J Med.* 2011;364:2473-2475.

## Hospital-Level Compliance With Asthma Care Quality Measures at Children's Hospitals and Subsequent Asthma-Related Outcomes

Morse RB, Hall M, Fieldston ES, et al (Univ of Arizona College of Medicine, Phoenix; Child Health Corporation of America, Shawnee Mission, KS; Univ of Pennsylvania School of Medicine, Philadelphia; et al)

*JAMA* 306:1454-1460, 2011

*Context.*—The Children's Asthma Care (CAC) measure set evaluates whether children admitted to hospitals with asthma receive relievers (CAC-1) and systemic corticosteroids (CAC-2) and whether they are discharged with a home management plan of care (CAC-3). It is the only Joint Commission core measure applicable to evaluate the quality of care for hospitalized children.

*Objectives.*—To evaluate longitudinal trends in CAC measure compliance and to determine if an association exists between compliance and outcomes.

*Design, Setting, and Patients.*—Cross-sectional study using administrative data and CAC compliance data for 30 US children's hospitals. A total of 37 267 children admitted with asthma between January 1, 2008, and September 30, 2010, with follow-up through December 31, 2010, accounted for 45 499 hospital admissions. Hospital-level CAC measure compliance data were obtained from the National Association of Children's Hospitals and Related Institutions. Readmission and postdischarge emergency department (ED) utilization data were obtained from the Pediatric Health Information System.

*Main Outcome Measures.*—Children's Asthma Care measure compliance trends; postdischarge ED utilization and asthma-related readmission rates at 7, 30, and 90 days.

*Results.*—The minimum quarterly CAC-1 and CAC-2 measure compliance rates reported by any hospital were 97.1% and 89.5%, respectively. Individual hospital CAC-2 compliance exceeded 95% for 97.9% of the quarters. Lack of variability in CAC-1 and CAC-2 compliance precluded examination of their association with the specified outcomes. Mean CAC-3 compliance was 40.6% (95% CI, 34.1%-47.1%) and 72.9% (95% CI, 68.8%-76.9%) for the initial and final 3 quarters of the study, respectively. The mean 7-, 30-, and 90-day postdischarge ED utilization rates were 1.5% (95% CI, 1.3%-1.6%), 4.3% (95% CI, 4.0%-4.5%), and 11.1% (95% CI, 10.5%-11.7%) and the mean quarterly 7-, 30-, and 90-day readmission rates were 1.4% (95% CI, 1.2%-1.6%), 3.1% (95% CI, 2.8%-3.3%), and 7.6% (95% CI, 7.2%-8.1%). There was no significant association between overall CAC-3 compliance (odds ratio [OR] for 5% improvement in compliance) and postdischarge ED utilization rates at 7 days (OR, 1.00; 95% CI, 0.98-1.02), 30 days (OR, 0.97; 95% CI, 0.90-1.04), and 90 days (OR, 0.96; 95% CI, 0.77-1.18). In addition, there was no significant association between overall CAC-3 compliance (OR for 5% improvement in compliance) and readmission rates at

7 days (OR, 1.00; 95% CI, 0.99-1.02), 30 days (OR, 0.99; 95% CI, 0.96-1.02), and 90 days (OR, 1.01; 95% CI, 0.90-1.12).

*Conclusion.*—Among children admitted to pediatric hospitals for asthma, there was high hospital-level compliance with CAC-1 and CAC-2 quality measures and moderate compliance with the CAC-3 measure but no association between CAC-3 compliance and subsequent ED visits and asthma-related readmissions.

▶ Everyone is involved in quality improvement initiatives these days, and, if not, they should be. Measurement is the cornerstone for improving quality. Well-accepted criteria for high-quality measures include that the indicator chosen shows opportunity for improvement based on either low performance, high variability, or both and that the measure to be assessed is linked to a specific desired outcome. Morse et al tell us how well compliance occurs with the Children's Asthma Care Measures as studied in children's hospitals.

Using administrative data from 2 sources and 30 children's hospitals, the authors of this report examined rates of performance on 3 measures: use of asthma relievers, use of systemic steroids, and use of a written home asthma management plan. The authors looked at the rates of performance of these measures over time across participating hospitals and sought to correlate performance with accepted outcome measures for asthma care emergency department revisits and hospitalizations. They found that levels of performance were extremely high for the use of asthma relievers and systemic steroids, whereas performance on the third measure, a written home management plan, was lower with modest variability improving from 41%—73% over a 3-year period. However, the use of a plan was not associated with reductions in subsequent emergency department visits or rehospitalizations.

A lot of hope was placed in the early part of this decade on having a home management plan that would significantly improve long-term outcomes of children with asthma. In an editorial that accompanied this report, Homer noted how we must have been off base with some of our thinking.[1] Based on the findings of Morse et al, use of a written discharge management plan no longer meets the criteria for a high-quality measure. Even so, asthma remains the major cause of preventable hospitalizations in childhood in the United States, and children with this and similar chronic conditions overall are frequently hospitalized and readmitted.

This report raises a number of questions. Are there other measures than a home treatment plan that would be more suitable to produce better outcomes for children with asthma who have been hospitalized? Should hospitals stop providing written management plans when sending a child home with asthma? Although such written plans alone are insufficient, they certainly are capable of being integrated into a more comprehensive transition from the inpatient setting to home.

Homer notes that the study by Morse et al documents that the Joint Commissions' Children Asthma Care Measure 3, an asthma discharge plan, no longer reaches the threshold of a high-quality measure and should be retired as should the other components if the nonvariability found in this study is replicated in nonspecialty hospitals. That is a powerful statement, but that is what the data show.

While on the topic of hospitals, this commentary ends with validation of a belief that many have had, namely that there is a "weekend effect" showing poor outcomes when patients are admitted to the hospital on weekends. The belief in this weekend effect, that those admitted to the hospital during the weekend fare worse than those admitted during the week, has spread. A study was performed examining patients who were admitted to the hospital on a weekend with stroke. There was a significantly worse outcome observed at days 7, 14, and 30 days in such patients compared with those who were admitted during the week. The overall risk of dying in the hospital with a cerebral hemorrhage was 12% higher for weekend admission![2] Timing is everything in life, isn't it?

**J. A. Stockman III, MD**

*References*

1. Homer CJ. Improvement for childhood asthma. *JAMA*. 2011;306:487-488.
2. Crowley RW, Yeoh HK, Stukenborg GJ, Medel R, Kassell NF, Dumont AS. Influence of weekend hospital admission on short-term mortality after intracerebral hemorrhage. *Stroke*. 2009;40:2387-2392.

# 3  Blood

**Intravenous iron for the treatment of fatigue in nonanemic, premenopausal women with low serum ferritin concentration**
Krayenbuehl PA, Battegay E, Breymann C, et al (Univ Hosp Zurich, Switzerland; et al)
*Blood* 118:3222-3227, 2011

This is the first study to investigate the efficacy of intravenous iron in treating fatigue in nonanemic patients with low serum ferritin concentration. In a randomized, double-blinded, placebo-controlled study, 90 premenopausal women presenting with fatigue, serum ferritin $\leq 50$ ng/mL, and hemoglobin $\geq 120$ g/L were randomized to receive either 800 mg of intravenous iron (III)—hydroxide sucrose or intravenous placebo. Fatigue and serum iron status were assessed at baseline and after 6 and 12 weeks. Median fatigue at baseline was 4.5 (on a 0-10 scale). Fatigue decreased during the initial 6 weeks by 1.1 in the iron group compared with 0.7 in the placebo group ($P = .07$). Efficacy of iron was bound to depleted iron stores: In patients with baseline serum ferritin $\leq 15$ ng/mL, fatigue decreased by 1.8 in the iron group compared with 0.4 in the placebo group ($P = .005$), and 82% of iron-treated compared with 47% of placebo-treated patients reported improved fatigue ($P = .03$). Drug-associated adverse events were observed in 21% of iron-treated patients and in 7% of placebo-treated patients ($P = .05$); none of these events was serious. Intravenous administration of iron improved fatigue in iron-deficient, nonanemic women with a good safety and tolerability profile. The efficacy of intravenous iron was bound to a serum ferritin concentration $\leq 15$ ng/mL. This study was registered at the International Standard Randomized Controlled Trial Number Register (www.isrctn.org) as ISRCTN78430425.

▶ This is a very important report. Several studies have suggested that iron deficiency (sans anemia) can cause fatigue symptoms. Data from the pediatric literature also have noted an association between the status of body iron stores and aerobic adaptation during exercise as well as with cognitive function. Studies done some time ago have shown that women with normal hemoglobin concentration, but depleted or reduced bone marrow iron stores, experience some improvement in fatigue after oral iron therapy. The problem with oral iron therapy is that it is very difficult to "blind" a study to document its effectiveness given that oral iron can produce intestinal effects, including a change in color of the stool, so the individuals receiving it probably know that they are taking iron as opposed to a placebo. The report abstracted solves this investigational dilemma by studying how intravenous iron affects fatigue in nonanemic female patients with low serum ferritin concentration.

Women entered into this study had baseline fatigue scores determined and had comparable low levels of serum ferritin. Their hemoglobin levels, both in the iron and placebo group, were normal (mean, 13.3 ± 6). The iron group received 4 intravenous infusions containing 200 mg of iron, while the placebo-treated group received a comparable volume of a saline containing fluid. In women whose serum ferritin values were < 15 ng/mL, 82% had remarkable improvements in levels of fatigue compared with 47% of placebo-treated individuals. These are the first results providing evidence that intravenous supplementation of iron can improve fatigue syndrome in iron-deficient, nonanemic premenopausal women.

The results of this study are in agreement with those of previous studies indicating a beneficial effect of oral iron therapy in nonanemic, iron-deficient young women. One can assume that these data would equally apply to an adolescent population. It should be noted that improvement in fatigue after 6 weeks was reported by 40% of placebo-treated patients. This highlights the importance of the emotional component of fatigue in patients who consider themselves to be severely fatigued. It seems clear that iron deficiency has many nonhematologic effects in those who may not be anemic. It is important, therefore, to detect iron deficiency in nonanemic individuals in the pediatric population. How to best do this remains a bit of a mystery, but one has to look at more than just the hemoglobin level.

**J. A. Stockman III, MD**

---

**Tmprss6 is a genetic modifier of the *Hfe*-hemochromatosis phenotype in mice**

Finberg KE, Whittlesey RL, Andrews NC (Duke Univ School of Medicine, Durham, NC)
*Blood* 117:4590-4599, 2011

---

The hereditary hemochromatosis protein HFE promotes the expression of hepcidin, a circulating hormone produced by the liver that inhibits dietary iron absorption and macrophage iron release. *HFE* mutations are associated with impaired hepatic bone morphogenetic protein (BMP)/SMAD signaling for hepcidin production. TMPRSS6, a transmembrane serine protease mutated in iron-refractory iron deficiency anemia, inhibits hepcidin expression by dampening BMP/SMAD signaling. In the present study, we used genetic approaches in mice to examine the relationship between Hfe and Tmprss6 in the regulation of systemic iron homeostasis. Heterozygous loss of Tmprss6 in $Hfe^{-/-}$ mice reduced systemic iron overload, whereas homozygous loss caused systemic iron deficiency and elevated hepatic expression of hepcidin and other Bmp/Smad target genes. In contrast, neither genetic loss of Hfe nor hepatic Hfe overexpression modulated the hepcidin elevation and systemic iron deficiency of $Tmprss6^{-/-}$ mice. These results indicate that genetic loss of Tmprss6 increases Bmp/Smad signaling in an *Hfe*-independent manner that can restore Bmp/Smad signaling in $Hfe^{-/-}$ mice.

Furthermore, these results suggest that natural genetic variation in the human ortholog *TMPRSS6* might modify the clinical penetrance of *HFE*-associated hereditary hemochromatosis, raising the possibility that pharmacologic inhibition of TMPRSS6 could attenuate iron loading in this disorder.

▶ Most pediatricians are not all that aware of the problem of hereditary hemochromatosis. It does exist in pediatrics both in the newborn period (neonatal hemochromatosis) as well as in any age child or adolescent, as the disorder is hereditary and is present from birth. Hereditary hemochromatosis is associated with an *HFE* mutation and is a disorder of variable penetrance in which excessive absorption of dietary iron causes iron to accumulate in tissues. This can lead to organ failure. The gene mutation is characterized by insufficient expression of hepcidin, a circulating peptide hormone produced by the liver in response to several physiologic stimuli, including iron loading. Hepcidin inhibits the absorption of dietary iron and the release of iron from macrophage stores by triggering the internalization and degradation of ferroportin, a cellular iron exporter present in enterocytes and the plasma membrane of macrophages. Finberg et al describe in much greater detail than has been previously known exactly how hemochromatosis develops on a genetic basis. The report is fairly complex but well worth reading for any savant of the disorder. I included it to allow readers to keep up to date with what is going on in this important area.

2011 was the tenth anniversary of the initial publication on hepcidin.[1] In the intervening years, we have learned that hepcidin is the major link in the transfer of iron back and forth throughout the body, including absorption of iron from the gut. This iron regulator hormone controls the dietary absorption, storage, and tissue distribution of iron. Hepcidin is feedback regulated by iron concentrations in plasma and in the liver and by erythropoietic demand for iron. Genetic malfunctions affecting hepcidin ferroportin axis are a main cause of iron disorders but can also cause iron deficiency anemias. If you are not that knowledgeable about hepcidin, see the superb review of hepcidin and its role in iron regulation.[2]

**J. A. Stockman III, MD**

*References*

1. Park CH, Valore EV, Waring AJ, Ganz T. Hepcidin, a urinary antimicrobial peptide synthesized in the liver. *J Biol Chem*. 2001;276:7806-7810.
2. Ganz T. Hepcidin and iron regulation, 10 years later. *Blood*. 2011;117:4425-4433.

---

**Defective ribosome assembly in Shwachman-Diamond syndrome**
Wong CC, Traynor D, Basse N, et al (Med Res Council Laboratory of Molecular Biology, Cambridge, UK)
*Blood* 118:4305-4312, 2011

---

Shwachman-Diamond syndrome (SDS), a recessive leukemia predisposition disorder characterized by bone marrow failure, exocrine pancreatic insufficiency, skeletal abnormalities and poor growth, is caused by mutations in the highly conserved *SBDS* gene. Here, we test the hypothesis that defective ribosome biogenesis underlies the pathogenesis of SDS. We create conditional mutants in the essential SBDS ortholog of the ancient eukaryote *Dictyostelium discoideum* using temperature-sensitive, self-splicing inteins, showing that mutant cells fail to grow at the restrictive temperature because ribosomal subunit joining is markedly impaired. Remarkably, wild type human SBDS complements the growth and ribosome assembly defects in mutant *Dictyostelium* cells, but disease-associated human SBDS variants are defective. SBDS directly interacts with the GTPase elongation factor-like 1 (EFL1) on nascent 60S subunits in vivo and together they catalyze eviction of the ribosome antiassociation factor eukaryotic initiation factor 6 (eIF6), a prerequisite for the translational activation of ribosomes. Importantly, lymphoblasts from SDS patients harbor a striking defect in ribosomal subunit joining whose magnitude is inversely proportional to the level of SBDS protein. These findings in *Dictyostelium* and SDS patient cells provide compelling support for the hypothesis that SDS is a ribosomopathy caused by corruption of an essential cytoplasmic step in 60S subunit maturation.

▶ Most of us learned about the Shwachman Diamond syndrome back in medical school. This syndrome is a rare autosomal disorder characterized by exocrine pancreatic insufficiency, ineffective hematopoiesis, and an increased risk for leukemia. In roughly 90% of patients with the disease, it is caused by a mutation in the SBDS (Shwachman-Bodian-Diamond syndrome) gene. SBDS has been implicated in multiple biologic processes, including ribosome biogenesis, stabilization of the mitotic spindle, and cell motility, but the functional defect that causes the Shwachman-Diamond syndrome phenotype has not been clear at least to date. Studies in yeast cell lines and mammals have demonstrated a role for SBDS in the final stages of cellular ribosome maturation.

Wong et al have studied the SBDS gene and have produced data that strongly indicate that Shwachman-Diamond syndrome is a ribosomopathy, adding another intriguing disorder to a fascinating class of diseases only recently described. Diamond-Blackfan anemia, the first human disease to be linked to ribosome dysfunction, is characterized by a profound macrocytic anemia and a range of physical abnormalities, including craniofacial and cardiac defects. Ten different ribosomal proteins have now been described in patients with Diamond-Blackfan syndrome, and a similar pattern has been described in the 5q-syndrome, a subtype of myelodysplastic syndrome. Another disorder with convincing links to ribosomal dysfunction is Treacher Collins syndrome. Patients with Treacher Collins syndrome have craniofacial abnormalities that are similar to patients with Diamond-Blackfan anemia but do not develop bone marrow failure. Patients with Treacher Collins syndrome have a gene mutated that encodes a protein that is essential for transcription of ribosomal DNA.

We do not know how defects in ribosome biogenesis lead to divergent clinical phenotypes. Both Diamond-Blackfan anemia and Shwachman-Diamond syndrome cause bone marrow failure, but patients with the former have a more severe defect in erythropoiesis, whereas the latter tend to have worse neutropenia. Patients with Treacher Collins syndrome and some with Diamond-Blackfan anemia develop craniofacial abnormalities, but patients with Treacher Collins syndrome have normal hematopoiesis. These differences remain to be elucidated.

Despite the many unanswered questions, it is increasingly clear that genetic lesions causing specific defects in ribosome biogenesis are fundamental to the pathophysiology of human disorders. Before reports in this regard began to appear, there was little understanding that ribosomes themselves could be affected by gene mutations that cause serious human genetic defects.

In honor of Drs Diamond and Blackfan, this commentary closes with some thoughts on eponyms. The old English dictionary defines an eponym as a person...after whom a discovery, invention, institution, etc, is named or thought to be named. Eponyms are deeply rooted in medical tradition, but some have wondered whether they may have outlived their usefulness. From time to time, eponyms provide less than truthful accounts of how diseases were discovered and reflect the influence of politics, language, habit or even sheer luck rather than scientific behavior. The continued use of tainted eponyms is certainly inappropriate and not accepted by patients, families, or the public at large. Take for example the atrocities committed by Nazi doctors who still have diseases named after them. One such example is Hans Reiter, a German doctor who is remembered for his discovery of a variant of reactive arthritis. He took part in human experimentation in World War II. These revelations have resulted in decline in the use of the term "Reiter syndrome." In hindsight, the facts about Reiter escape the scientific community only because no one had bothered to investigate the person behind the eponym. The same is probably true of Friedrich Wegener, the pathologist for whom Wegener granulomatosis is named. Wegener had been an early member of the Nazi Brown Shirts and he had been the pupil of a prolific expert on "racial hygiene." He was also wanted as a war criminal for a period of time. Prompted by these revelations about Friedrich Wegener, the Vasculitis Foundation of North America has stated: "As patients and family members, we would prefer a different name be used for our disease."[1]

Not everyone believes that eponyms should be euthanized.[2] Witworth notes that some years back, filling in time between candidates as a clinical examiner, he was chatting with a colleague about eponyms. The colleague's view was the eponyms were not particularly useful and he recalled an encounter with a young woman struggling with a clinical examination. She could not find lymph nodes and seemed unfamiliar with listening to the lungs. To bolster her spirits, this fellow asked her who discovered Koch bacillus. Thinking he would get a ready answer, he did not. The young lady became even more anxious and at a loss for words. He then said "who wrote Mendelsohn's *Spring Song*?" The young examinee then burst into tears. He gave up when the examinee could not identify who designed the Eiffel Tower.

Witworth suggests that eponyms bring color to medicine and embed medical traditions and culture in our history. Yes, the use of eponyms in medicine, as in other areas, is often random, inconsistent, idiosyncratic, confused, and heavily influenced by geography and culture. Nonetheless, do we really want to say "cyanotic congenital heart disease due to ventricular septal defect, pulmonary stenosis, right ventricular hypertrophy and aortic dextroposition" rather than Tetralogy of Fallot? What about the hereditary disorder of renal tubular function with vitamin D—resistant rickets, glycosuria, amino aciduria, and hyperphosphatemia? It is easier simply to say Fanconi syndrome, isn't it? The same is true of Tourette syndrome as opposed to a syndrome consisting of violent muscular jerks of the face, shoulders, and extremities with spasmodic grunting, explosive noises, and coprolalia!

Face it; if we do away with medical eponyms, then we might as well do away with Avogadro number, Boyles Law, the Joule, the Kelvin, and the Hertz (the unit of measure, not the rental company).

**J. A. Stockman III, MD**

*References*

1. Woywod A, Matteson E. Should eponyms be abandoned? *BMJ.* 2007;335:424.
2. Witworth JA. Should eponyms be abandoned? No. *BMJ.* 2007;335:425.

**Proof of principle for transfusion of in vitro—generated red blood cells**
Giarratana M-C, Rouard H, Dumont A, et al (UPMC Paris 06, France; EFS Ile de France, Créteil, France; AP-HP Hôpital St Antoine, Paris, France; et al)
*Blood* 118:5071-5079, 2011

In vitro RBC production from stem cells could represent an alternative to classic transfusion products. Until now the clinical feasibility of this concept has not been demonstrated. We addressed the question of the capacity of cultured RBCs (cRBCs) to survive in humans. By using a culture protocol permitting erythroid differentiation from peripheral CD34+ HSC, we generated a homogeneous population of cRBC functional in terms of their deformability, enzyme content, capacity of their hemoglobin to fix/release oxygen, and expression of blood group antigens. We then demonstrated in the nonobese diabetes/severe combined immunodeficiency mouse that cRBC encountered in vivo the conditions necessary for their complete maturation. These data provided the rationale for injecting into one human a homogeneous sample of $10^{10}$ cRBCs generated under good manufacturing practice conditions and labeled with $^{51}$Cr. The level of these cells in the circulation 26 days after injection was between 41% and 63%, which compares favorably with the reported half-life of 28 ± 2 days for native RBCs. Their survival in vivo testifies globally to their quality and functionality. These data establish the proof of principle for transfusion of in vitro-generated RBCs and path the way toward new developments in transfusion medicine. This study is registered at http://www.clinicaltrials.gov as NCT0929266.

▶ This report is preliminary, but it is so intriguing that it is impossible not to comment on it. The generation of red blood cells in vitro with the use of current biotechnologies could represent an interesting alternative to transfusion of human red blood cell components. The chronic difficulty of maintaining a red blood cell supply relates to the high annual requirement of red blood cells of nearly 90 million units worldwide. It would be wonderful if there were new ways to create and design hemoglobin-containing products. Because of the disappointing results with oxygen-carrier substitutes, the production of bioengineered red blood cells is a promising alternative.

It is now possible to initiate complete maturation of red blood cell lines in vitro to the stage of enucleation, starting from hematopoietic stem cells obtained from peripheral blood, bone marrow, umbilical cord blood, and fetal liver embryonic cells. Until recently, the clinical feasibility of this concept has not been demonstrated, whatever the origin of the cells and the experimental protocol. What Giarrantana et al have done is to evaluate the in vitro functionality and the in vivo behavior in an animal model and in humans of cultured red blood cells produced by bioengineering cell techniques. The authors report the first injection of cultured red blood cells into humans that were generated under good manufacturing practice conditions. If you have any interest at all in this topic, the report details exactly how one can bioengineer red blood cells. The process takes 2 to 4 weeks. These investigators were also able to store their newly developed product at refrigerated temperatures. They showed that the survival time was quite comparable with that of normal red blood cells obtained from humans.

This study represents a significant step forward and a tribute to a long-standing international investment in the basic biology of hematopoiesis. That is the good news, but there are a lot of caveats before anyone can anticipate replacing any of the estimated 90 million-plus units transfused worldwide with cultured red blood cells. A standard unit of red blood cells contains approximately $2.5 \times 10^{12}$ red blood cells, whereas the method described in this report required 13 L of culture medium to produce $10^{10}$ cultured red blood cells. Needless to say, human scaleup remains a formidable hurdle. It is anticipated that proliferation can be improved by some 10-fold if the results of small-scale studies are useful. Current technology and state of knowledge, however, indicate that near-term prospects for preparing first-generation hematopoietic stem cell—derived cultured red blood cells in sufficient amounts to address the needs of those difficult-to-transfuse patients with rare phenotypes or multiple alloantibodies are more than an idle hope. This relatively small market already relies on red blood cell units that are difficult to acquire and extremely expensive it available.

Despite all the caveats noted, the findings of Giarrantana et al should encourage investigators and funding agencies in this field to keep persevering. In a commentary that accompanied this report, Klein noted that "after all, small volumes of reasonably safe and tasty beer were brewed from gravity-drained, wood-lined, copper vats even before microbes were discovered to be the source of fermentation. Now via scientific progress and control of the fermentation process, coupled with stainless steel tanks and automated, microprocessor-controlled operations, we have an almost limitless source of wholesome ales and lagers of predictable flavor and body. Might we aspire to no less purity and predictability in our blood supply?"[1]

Please note that the article dealing with transfusion had many authors. This commentary closes with an observation having to do with authorship in medical journals, a hot topic these days. It turns out that at least a fifth of articles published in medical journals are likely to have a guest (or honorary) author. Journals are not doing enough to tackle this problem as indicated by the results of two studies. A guest author is someone who has not contributed sufficiently to the work, but whose name is included in the list of authors. In a survey of corresponding authors of nearly 900 articles published at high-impact general medical journals in 2008, 20% of respondents admitted that their paper had at least one guest author. In addition, nearly 8% admitted that their article had at least one ghost author—someone who had written the article or otherwise contributed substantially to the work, but was not listed as an author. The percentages of ghost or guest authors differ in the 6 journals studied. Both types of authorship misconduct were higher among research articles than in review articles and editorials. Since the results of this study are based on self-reporting, they most likely underestimate the true picture. In the medical editing field, such ghost writing and honorary guest authoring are considered dishonest unless the relationship of such authors is clearly described. Much of the problem of ghost authorship relates to concerns about drug companies preparing articles without the true authorship being acknowledged.[2]

**J. A. Stockman III, MD**

*References*

1. Klein HG. Brewing blood. *Blood.* 2011;118:5069-5070.
2. Godlee F. More than 20% of medical articles have a "guest author". *BMJ.* 2009; 339:652-653.

**A randomized controlled study in patients with newly diagnosed severe aplastic anemia receiving antithymocyte globulin (ATG), cyclosporine, with or without G-CSF: a study of the SAA Working Party of the European Group for Blood and Marrow Transplantation**

Tichelli A, Schrezenmeier H, Socié G, et al (Univ Hosp Basel, Switzerland; Univ Hosp Ulm, Germany; Hematology Transplantation and Univ Paris VII, France; et al)
*Blood* 117:4434-4441, 2011

We evaluated the role of granulocyte colony-stimulating factor (G-CSF) in patients with severe aplastic anemia (SAA) treated with antithymocyte globulin (ATG) and cyclosporine (CSA). Between January 2002 and July 2008, 192 patients with newly diagnosed SAA not eligible for transplantation were entered into this multicenter, randomized study to receive ATG/CSA with or without G-CSF. Overall survival (OS) at 6 years was 76% ± 4%, and event-free survival (EFS) was 42% ± 4%. No difference in OS/EFS was seen between patients randomly assigned to receive or not to receive G-CSF, neither for the entire cohort nor in subgroups stratified by age and disease severity. Patients treated with G-CSF had fewer infectious episodes (24%) and hospitalization days (82%) compared with patients without G-CSF (36%; $P = .006$; 87%; $P = .0003$). In a post hoc analysis of patients receiving G-CSF, the lack of a neutrophil response by day 30 was associated with significantly lower response rate (56% vs 81%; $P = .048$) and survival

(65% vs 87%; $P = .031$). G-CSF added to standard ATG and CSA reduces the rate of early infectious episodes and days of hospitalization in very SAA patients and might allow early identification of nonresponders but has no effect on OS, EFS, remission, relapse rates, and mortality. This study was registered at www.clinicaltrials.gov as NCT01163942.

▶ I have not dealt with aplastic anemia in quite some time, and a lot has changed with respect to management of this difficult-to-treat disorder. Immunosuppressive therapy with antithymocyte globulin (ATG) and cyclosporin (CSA) remains the treatment of choice for patients not eligible for bone marrow transplantation. Overall, the survival at 10 years ranges between 60% and 80% for the combination of therapies that are currently available. Among these therapies, immunosuppression remains a less than optimal option that does not result in a cure. Approximately 30% of patients fail to respond, and even in those who do, bone marrow function remains less than ideal. Relapse and the development of myelodysplastic syndromes occur all too frequently. Infectious complications remain the main cause of death, and newer regimens have failed to improve survival over standard ATG plus CSA combinations.

The use of growth factors in combination with immunosuppressive therapy with ATG and CSA has not been fully investigated in patients who cannot undergo bone marrow transplant. Despite lack of evidence for preemptive use, many centers add granulocyte colony-stimulating factor (G-CSF) to ATG plus CSA, particularly in pediatric-age patients or in patients with very low neutrophil counts. The report abstracted represents a randomized controlled trial from Europe that has compared ATG and CSA with or without the addition of G-CSF. Patients as young as 2 years and as old as 81 years were included in the report. The overall survival among all patients at 6-year follow-up was 76% with an event-free survival of 42%. No difference in outcome was seen between patients randomly assigned to receive or not to receive G-CSF. Survival was better for young patients under the age of 20 and also in patients aged 20 to 40 years compared with older patients. When the patients were stratified according to age and severity of the disease, there was no difference in survival with respect to the addition or not of G-CSF.

This is the largest randomized trial examining the addition of G-CSF to standard immunosuppression with ATG/CSA, and it shows that G-CSF has no significant effect on event-free survival, overall survival remission rates, mortality and relapse rates. The only singular benefit appears to be a reduced rate of early infection episodes and reduced number of hospitalization days related to the latter. Such shorter hospitalization stays and fewer infections can have clinical implications in the daily care of patients with aplastic anemia, particularly high-risk patients.

The bottom line here is that G-CSF, an expensive therapeutic option, when added to standard immunosuppression with ATG and CSA, reduces the rate of early infection episodes and days of hospitalization but does not seem to affect the long-term outcome of patients with aplastic anemia, including pediatric patients. One can suspect that the data from this report will be interpreted in differing ways by differing groups. There is nothing wrong with fewer days of infection and hospitalization. The latter may be a goal that balances out the over-all cost of management of this serious and potentially lethal disease.

**J. A. Stockman III, MD**

---

**Late effects among pediatric patients followed for nearly 4 decades after transplantation for severe aplastic anemia**
Sanders JE, Woolfrey AE, Carpenter PA, et al (Fred Hutchinson Cancer Res Ctr, Seattle, WA)
*Blood* 118:1421-1428, 2011

---

Aplastic anemia (AA), a potentially fatal disease, may be cured with marrow transplantation. Survival in pediatric patients has been excellent early after transplantation, but only limited data are available regarding late effects. This study evaluates late effects among 152 patients followed 1-38 years (median, 21.8 years). Transplantation-preparative regimes were mostly cyclophosphamide with or without antithymocyte globulin. Survival at 30 years for the acquired AA patients is 82%, and for the Fanconi anemia patients it is 58% ($P = .01$). Multivariate analysis demonstrated that chronic GVHD ($P = .02$) and Fanconi anemia ($P = .03$) negatively impacted survival. Two Fanconi patients and 18 acquired AA patients developed a malignancy that was fatal for 4. There was an increased incidence of thyroid function test abnormalities among those who received total body irradiation. Cyclophosphamide recipients demonstrated normal growth, basically normal development, and pregnancies with mostly normal offspring. Quality-of-life studies in adult survivors of this pediatric transplantation cohort indicated that patients were comparable with control patients except for difficulty with health and life insurance. These data indicate that the majority of long-term survivors after transplantation for AA during childhood can have a normal productive life.

▶ Allogeneic hematopoietic stem cell transplantation (HSCT) is the treatment of choice for many malignant and nonmalignant hematologic disorders. Survival rates after HSCT have improved substantially over the last couple of decades. More than 40 000 HSCTs are performed yearly now worldwide. Thus, the number of long-term disease-free survivors is continuously increasing. These survivors, unfortunately, sometimes face late transplantation-associated morbidity and mortality issues. The latter include a host of malignant and nonmalignant complications that can affect general health. Awareness of the long-term effects is critical to design appropriate screening methodologies to deal with these effects in the earliest timeframe possible.

Sanders et al describe delayed effects among patients followed up for nearly 4 decades after HSCT for severe aplastic anemia. These transplants were performed at the Fred Hutchinson Cancer Research Center in Seattle. The authors report on 154 patients of whom 137 had acquired severe aplastic anemia and 15 had Fanconi anemia. Risk factors for survival largely related to the presence of chronic graft-versus-host (GVH) disease. Those with Fanconi anemia did not do as well. Late complications included thyroid abnormalities (increased in patients who received irradiation and solid tumors, particularly in patients with Fanconi anemia or those having chronic GVH disease). The staff at the Fred Hutchinson Center has developed conditioning regimens over the last several decades that have become the gold standard worldwide leading to sustained engraftment in most patients with fewer linked effects, notably preserving fertility. Unfortunately, even good survival is hardly perfect in the sense that survival in patients who have been transplanted for severe aplastic anemia does not yet match that of the general population.

For patients with Fanconi anemia, posttransplantation, the genetic defect is still present in other somatic tissues. This results in a high propensity for the development of secondary solid cancers, in particular, those of the head and neck, even if the patient is cured of their aplastic anemia by the transplant. Transplantation for Fanconi anemia, probably because of the result of GVH disease, increases the risk of head and neck cancers, and patients must be followed up throughout their entire life with careful surveillance for the latter.

**J. A. Stockman III, MD**

---

**Polymeric IgA1 controls erythroblast proliferation and accelerates erythropoiesis recovery in anemia**
Coulon S, Dussiot M, Grapton D, et al (Université Paris Descartes, France; et al)
*Nat Med* 17:1456-1465, 2011

---

Anemia because of insufficient production of and/or response to erythropoietin (Epo) is a major complication of chronic kidney disease and cancer. The mechanisms modulating the sensitivity of erythroblasts to Epo remain poorly understood. We show that, when cultured with Epo at suboptimal concentrations, the growth and clonogenic potential of erythroblasts was rescued by transferrin receptor 1 (TfR1)-bound polymeric IgA1 (pIgA1). Under homeostatic conditions, erythroblast numbers were increased in mice expressing human IgA1 compared to control mice. Hypoxic stress of these mice led to increased amounts of pIgA1 and erythroblast expansion. Expression of human IgA1 or treatment of wild-type mice with the TfR1 ligands pIgA1 or iron-loaded transferrin (Fe-Tf) accelerated recovery from acute anemia. TfR1 engagement by either pIgA1 or Fe-Tf increased cell sensitivity to Epo by inducing activation of mitogen-activated protein kinase (MAPK) and phosphatidylinositol 3-kinase (PI3K) signaling pathways. These cellular responses were mediated through the TfR1-internalization motif, YXXΦ. Our results show that pIgA1 and TfR1 are positive regulators of erythropoiesis in both physiological and pathological situations. Targeting this pathway may provide alternate approaches to the treatment of ineffective erythropoiesis and anemia.

▶ This report may not have immediate relevance to one's immediate clinical practice, but it is good sometimes to take a peek into the future to see what might be coming down the pike in terms of new therapies. For many years, recombinant human erythropoietin (Epo) has been used as a front-line therapy for anemia because it stimulates erythropoiesis in children and adults who cannot make Epo or in whom inflammation has inhibited erythropoiesis. Without question, Epo has improved the quality of life and decreased the dependence of patients on transfusions, but recent studies have identified risks associated with Epo therapy. Several studies have associated Epo therapy with an increased risk of venous thromboembolic events, especially those treatment regimens with high hemoglobin target values. This has been particularly true in those being treated with Epo for the anemia associated with chronic renal disease. Increased mortality has also been observed in patients with cancer undergoing Epo therapy, and some studies have suggested that Epo stimulation of Epo receptors on breast cancer cells can antagonize the effects of chemotherapeutic agents. Given such risks of Epo therapy, new ways of stimulating erythropoiesis are sorely needed.

It is well known that erythropoietic capacity far exceeds that necessary to maintain steady state erythrocyte numbers. With that as a given, a rational approach to identifying new targets to manage anemia would be to study the mechanisms that regulate erythroid output at times of acute or chronic stress. For example, hypoxia has long been known to stimulate erythropoiesis. Logically, drugs that activate hypoxia-inducible transcription factor should augment erythropoiesis.

Coulon et al have identified polymeric IgA1 (pIgA1) as a novel erythropoiesis-stimulating agent. IgA is one of the potential antibody subtypes generated by B cells during infection. In humans, only a small fraction of IgA is polymeric IgA, which consists of a polymer of IgA molecules that are covalently attached to their J chains. pIgA1 binds transferrin to receptor 1. Erythropoiesis requires iron. Coulon et al show that pIgA1 improves the response to suboptimal Epo stimulation. Somehow or other, pIgA1 signals cells to respond better to Epo than Epo alone can do.

It is not entirely clear how pIgA1 works. It is produced by plasma cells, and on the basis of what is known about plasma cells, there is no reason to assume a connection between pIgA1 production and a response to anemia. However, Coulon et al convincingly show that hypoxia increases pIgA1 production in mouse models and in humans with chronic hypoxic conditions. On the basis of these observations, the authors present a model, wherein anemia leads to tissue hypoxia, which increases pIgA1 concentrations, which in turn delivers more iron to boost erythroid output. The role of pIgA1 becomes more important in iron deficiency anemia, in which transferrin saturation is low, limiting the ability of transferrin-bound iron to stimulate erythropoiesis.

It may not be that far into the future where we will be hearing about a new drug, pIgA1, to treat anemia. Only time will tell whether this interesting new potential therapy plays out.

**J. A. Stockman III, MD**

## A Functional Element Necessary for Fetal Hemoglobin Silencing

Sankaran VG, Xu J, Byron R, et al (Children's Hosp Boston, MA; Fred Hutchinson Cancer Ctr, Seattle, WA; et al)
*N Engl J Med* 365:807-814, 2011

*Background.*—An improved understanding of the regulation of the fetal hemoglobin genes holds promise for the development of targeted therapeutic approaches for fetal hemoglobin induction in the β-hemoglobinopathies. Although recent studies have uncovered *trans*-acting factors necessary for this regulation, limited insight has been gained into the *cis*-regulatory elements involved.

*Methods.*—We identified three families with unusual patterns of hemoglobin expression, suggestive of deletions in the locus of the β-globin gene (β-globin locus). We performed array comparative genomic hybridization to map these deletions and confirmed breakpoints by means of polymerase-chain-reaction assays and DNA sequencing. We compared these deletions, along with previously mapped deletions, and studied the *trans*-acting factors binding to these sites in the β-globin locus by using chromatin immunoprecipitation.

*Results.*—We found a new $(\delta\beta)^0$-thalassemia deletion and a rare hereditary persistence of fetal hemoglobin deletion with identical downstream breakpoints. Comparison of the two deletions resulted in the identification of a small intergenic region required for γ-globin (fetal hemoglobin) gene silencing. We mapped a Kurdish $\beta^0$-thalassemia deletion, which retains the required intergenic region, deletes other surrounding sequences, and maintains fetal hemoglobin silencing. By comparing these deletions and other previously mapped deletions, we elucidated a 3.5-kb intergenic region near the 5′ end of the δ-globin gene that is necessary for γ-globin silencing. We found that a critical fetal hemoglobin silencing factor, BCL11A, and its partners bind within this region in the chromatin of adult erythroid cells.

*Conclusions.*—By studying three families with unusual deletions in the β-globin locus, we identified an intergenic region near the δ-globin gene that is necessary for fetal hemoglobin silencing. (Funded by the National Institutes of Health and others.)

► One has to be fairly wide awake to read this complicated report, but it is well worth the read. Regulation of the switch from fetal hemoglobin to adult hemoglobin in humans is a fascinating subject of immense interest to those trying to improve the lives of youngsters with sickle cell anemia and certain forms of thalassemia. Most of us recall from medical school that after a brief period of embryonic globin gene expression, the gamma-globin chain of fetal hemoglobin (HbF) begins to be expressed and then is replaced by the beta-globin chain of adult hemoglobin. These globin genes are clustered together on chromosome 11 and are arranged in precisely the same order that they are expressed during development with the gamma-globin genes located between the embryonic globin gene and the adult genes responsible for the production of hemoglobin A2 (that contain delta-globin) and beta-globin for hemoglobin A. It is also well known that certain inherited mutations in binding sites on this chromosome are associated with different forms of hereditary persistence of fetal hemoglobin (HPFH). Patients with HPFH have inherited mutations associated with persistence of HPF that cause high levels of uniformly distributed HbF or somewhat lower levels of HbF heterogeneously distributed among red blood cells. The latter is known as delta-beta0-thalassemia.

Sankaran et al now describe new mutations in the beta-globin gene cluster that cause either HPFH or delta-beta0-thalassemia. This report provides great insights into a critical region of the gene cluster that appears to be required for efficient gamma-globin gene suppression.

A thorough reading of this article is not for the lighthearted, nor is the associated commentary by Forget,[1] but the importance of the findings from this report is that it provides hope for the future development of targeted molecular therapies for both sickle cell disease and beta thalassemia. Imagine the day, with a rather minor bit of gene manipulation, when one can reactivate the production of gamma-globin genes and essentially cure patients with serious forms of hemoglobinopathies of their symptomatology.

**J. A. Stockman III, MD**

*Reference*

1. Forget BG. Progress in understanding the hemoglobin switch. *N Engl J Med*. 2011; 365:852-854.

---

### Iron chelation with deferasirox in adult and pediatric patients with thalassemia major: efficacy and safety during 5 years' follow-up

Cappellini MD, Bejaoui M, Agaoglu L, et al (Universitá di Milano, Italy; Centre National de Greffe de Moelle Osseuse, Tunis, Tunisia; Istanbul Univ Med Faculty, Turkey; et al)
*Blood* 118:884-893, 2011

---

Patients with β-thalassemia require lifelong iron chelation therapy from early childhood to prevent complications associated with transfusional iron overload. To evaluate long-term efficacy and safety of once-daily oral iron chelation with deferasirox, patients aged ≥2 years who completed a 1-year, phase 3, randomized trial entered a 4-year extension study, either continuing on deferasirox (deferasirox cohort) or switching from deferoxamine to deferasirox (crossover cohort). Of 555 patients who received ≥1 deferasirox dose, 66.8% completed the study; 43 patients (7.7%) discontinued because of adverse events. In patients with ≥4 years' deferasirox exposure who had liver biopsy, mean liver iron concentration significantly decreased by $7.8 \pm 11.2$ mg Fe/g dry weight (dw; n = 103; $P < .001$) and $3.1 \pm 7.9$ mg Fe/g dw (n = 68; $P < .001$) in the deferasirox and crossover cohorts, respectively. Median serum ferritin significantly decreased by 706 ng/mL (n = 196; $P < .001$) and 371 ng/mL (n = 147; $P < .001$), respectively, after ≥4 years' exposure. Investigator-assessed, drug-related adverse events, including increased blood creatinine (11.2%), abdominal pain (9.0%), and nausea (7.4%), were generally mild to moderate, transient, and reduced in frequency over time. No adverse effect was observed on pediatric growth or adolescent sexual development. This first prospective study of long-term deferasirox use in pediatric and adult patients with β-thalassemia suggests treatment for ≤5 years is generally well tolerated and effectively reduces iron burden. This trial was registered at www. clinicaltrials.gov as #NCT00171210.

▶ It is disheartening to know that while we can make the lives of children with thalassemia major essentially normal with transfusional therapy, we are causing these children's death as young to middle-age adults as a result of iron overload. Iron overload is the ultimate leading cause of morbidity and mortality in transfusion-dependent patients with thalassemia major. Although the introduction of iron chelation therapy does lead to improvement in survival, the long-term management of iron overload is less than ideal in many patients. Part of the problem is compliance associated with the parenteral chelation therapy with deferoxamine (DFO). Investigators have been exploring oral forms of iron chelators to get around the compliance problem.

Deferasirox is a once-daily oral iron chelator that has shown some effectivity in reducing iron accumulation as well as serum ferritin levels, at least in 1 study that spanned a relatively short period of time.[1] Since oral iron chelators would have to be given over a lifespan, it is critical that the long-term safety, as well as efficacy, of deferasirox be studied in both pediatric and adult patients. Cappellini et al report on a phase 3 study that initially randomly assigned patients with β-thalassemia 2 years of age and older to receive deferasirox or DFO for 1 year. Patients who completed the 1-year core study were eligible to enter a 4-year crossover, switching from DFO to deferasirox and vice versa. Efficacy and safety data for patients treated with deferasirox for 5 years were the basis of this report.

The report of Cappellini et al is the first prospective study to report long-term monitoring of the efficacy and safety of iron chelation with deferasirox in both pediatric and adult patients with β-thalassemia major. Overall, two-thirds of the patients completed the 5-year study. During the study, deferasirox became commercially available for others to use. Some of the patients who were enrolled in the study elected to go off protocol and take the commercially available deferasirox. It was clear from the data of this report that long-term deferasirox treatment did lead to a sustained reduction in the iron burden. Iron burden in the liver decreased by almost 50%, as did the fall in serum ferritin values. Renal and liver function studies were also monitored carefully. No progressive increases in serum creatinine or liver transaminase levels were observed during long-term deferasirox treatment. Deferasirox was generally well tolerated in both pediatric and adult patients. Only 1 in 7 patients discontinued the drug as a result of side effects. It should be noted that during this 5-year study, pediatric patients showed continued growth and development during deferasirox treatment, suffering none of the endocrine problems commonly seen with iron overload.

This first study to show significant reduction of liver and total body iron overload with long-term deferasirox treatment supports the potential use of this drug for more widespread use.[1] Deferasirox with dosing tailored to individual patient requirements does appear to be an effective long-term treatment for transfusional iron overload in both children and adults. It will be interesting to see how the pediatric hematology community adopts the information gleaned from the study reported by Cappellini et al.

**J. A. Stockman III, MD**

*Reference*

1. Cappellini MD, Cohen A, Piga A, et al. A phase 3 study of deferasirox (ICL670), a once-daily oral iron chelator, in patients with beta-thalassemia. *Blood*. 2006; 107:3455-3462.

---

**Hydroxycarbamide in very young children with sickle-cell anaemia: a multicentre, randomised, controlled trial (BABY HUG)**
Wang WC, for the BABY HUG investigators (St Jude Children's Res Hosp, Memphis, TN; et al)
*Lancet* 377:1663-1672, 2011

---

*Background.*—Sickle-cell anaemia is associated with substantial morbidity from acute complications and organ dysfunction beginning in the first year of life. Hydroxycarbamide substantially reduces episodes of pain and acute chest syndrome, admissions to hospital, and transfusions in adults with sickle-cell anaemia. We assessed the effect of hydroxycarbamide therapy on organ dysfunction and clinical complications, and examined laboratory findings and toxic effects.

*Methods.*—This randomised trial was undertaken in 13 centres in the USA between October, 2003, and September, 2009. Eligible participants had haemoglobin SS (HbSS) or haemoglobin $S\beta^0$thalassaemia, were aged 9—18 months at randomisation, and were not selected for clinical severity. Participants received liquid hydroxycarbamide, 20 mg/kg per day, or placebo for 2 years. Randomisation assignments were generated by the medical coordinating centre by a pre-decided schedule. Identical appearing and tasting formulations were used for hydroxycarbamide and placebo. Patients, caregivers, and coordinating centre staff were masked to treatment allocation. Primary study endpoints were splenic function (qualitative uptake on $^{99}$Tc spleen scan) and renal function (glomerular filtration rate by $^{99m}$Tc-DTPA clearance). Additional assessments included blood counts, fetal haemoglobin concentration, chemistry profiles, spleen function biomarkers, urine osmolality, neurodevelopment, transcranial Doppler ultrasonography, growth, and mutagenicity. Study visits occurred every 2—4 weeks. Analysis was by intention to treat. The trial is registered with ClinicalTrials.gov, number NCT00006400.

*Findings.*—96 patients received hydroxycarbamide and 97 placebo, of whom 83 patients in the hydroxycarbamide group and 84 in the placebo group completed the study. Significant differences were not seen between groups for the primary endpoints (19 of 70 patients with decreased spleen function at exit in the hydroxycarbamide group *vs* 28 of 74 patients in the placebo group, $p=0·21$; and a difference in the mean increase in DTPA glomerular filtration rate in the hydroxycarbamide group versus the placebo group of 2 mL/min per $1·73 \text{ m}^2$, $p=0·84$). Hydroxycarbamide significantly decreased pain (177 events in 62 patients *vs* 375 events in 75 patients in the placebo group, $p=0·002$) and dactylitis (24 events in 14 patients *vs* 123 events in 42 patients in the placebo group, $p<0·0001$), with some evidence for decreased acute chest syndrome, hospitalisation rates, and transfusion. Hydroxyurea increased haemoglobin and fetal haemoglobin, and decreased white blood-cell count. Toxicity was limited to mild-to-moderate neutropenia.

*Interpretation.*—On the basis of the safety and efficacy data from this trial, hydroxycarbamide can now be considered for all very young children with sickle-cell anaemia.

▶ If you are not familiar with hydroxycarbamide, it is an antineoplastic drug that inhibits ribonucleotide reductase. This increases fetal hemoglobin concentration in red blood cells and has other potentially beneficial effects in patients with sickle cell disease, including improved nitric oxide metabolism, reduced red cell-endothelial interaction, and decreased erythrocyte density. More than a decade and a half ago, the double-blind placebo-controlled Multi-Center Study of Hydroxyurea (MSH) in adults with severe sickle cell anemia showed that hydroxycarbamide substantially reduces episodes of pain and acute chest syndrome, admissions to hospital, and also transfusion requirements.[1] Subsequently, smaller studies have shown similar benefits and few toxic effects in school-age children and adolescents. Wang et al have now assessed the effects of hydroxycarbamide therapy on organ dysfunction and clinical complications, also examining laboratory findings and other possible toxic effects.

The study reported by Wang et al represents a clinical trial that involved 13 centers in the United States looking at patients with sickle cell anemia over a 6-year period. Data from the report show that hydroxycarbamide was safe and resulted in a decrease in common but serious adverse effects, particularly pain and dactylitis. Some laboratory parameters were improved. Several secondary measures of spleen, kidney, and central nervous system function suggested benefit, but these results were not in and of themselves conclusive. It is possible that few differences were seen because the dose of hydroxycarbamide used (20 mg/kg per day) is lower than the usual maximum tolerated dose and perhaps clinically less effective. Nonetheless, 3 secondary measures of splenic function (liver count ratios, pit count, and Howell-Jolly bodies) suggested some benefit from hydroxycarbamide when adjusted for baseline values.

The report of Wang et al is the only double-blind prospective pediatric trial to investigate the effect of hydroxycarbamide in very young children with sickle cell anemia. Patients in this trial differed from other trials in 2 important ways: they were very young and eligible irrespective of whether they had severe clinical course of disease. On the basis of safety and efficacy data from this trial, one can conclude that hydroxycarbamide should be considered for all children with sickle cell anemia, starting at an early age. It is likely that not everyone will buy into this conclusion, but it seems to be based on solid information.

**J. A. Stockman III, MD**

*Reference*

1. Charache S, Terrin ML, Moore RD, et al. Effect of hydroxyurea on the frequency of painful crises in sickle cell anemia. Investigators of the multi-center study of hydroxyurea in sickle cell anemia. *N Engl J Med.* 1995;332:1317-1322.

## Complete Resolution of Sickle Cell Chronic Pain With High Dose Vitamin D Therapy: A Case Report and Review of the Literature

Osunkwo I (Aflac Ctr for Cancer and Blood Disorders Service Comprehensive Sickle Cell Program of Children's Healthcare of Atlanta, GA)
*J Pediatr Hematol Oncol* 33:549-551, 2011

With age, individuals with sickle cell disease (SCD) experience daily chronic pain. Vitamin D deficiency (VDD) can result in chronic pain, osteoporosis, fractures, and muscle weakness. Several studies report a high prevalence of VDD in SCD; however, the clinical correlates have not been well described. We describe a case of SCD chronic pain associated with profound VDD, osteoporosis, and osteonecrosis. Treatment with high-dose vitamin D resulted in complete resolution of chronic pain symptoms and improvement in bone density. Randomized studies of vitamin D in SCD may help elucidate its role in the management of chronic pain and bone disease.

▶ In recent years, it has become obvious that low serum levels of 25 hydroxy-vitamin D (25 OHD) levels can be associated with chronic bone pain, osteoporosis, muscle weakness, and an increased predisposition to falls and fractures. The precise relationship between vitamin D and pain is not fully understood, but there are numerous case series that report a beneficial effect of vitamin D on chronic pain. For example, in a study of 33 female African asylum seekers with unexplained chronic pain, 67% of patients were found to have profound vitamin D deficiency. All experienced improvement in their pain symptoms with initiation of daily high-dose vitamin D therapy.[1] The evidence for the use of vitamin D to treat chronic pain, however, remains poor because of the lack of adequate randomized trials of high quality.

Based on their experience with a 16-year-old premenarchal young lady with homozygous sickle cell disease with a history of severe throbbing headaches and chronic pain involving her neck, lower mid back, left shoulder, and lower extremities, who was found to be vitamin D deficient and who responded to vitamin D therapy with resolution of her pain symptoms, Osunkwo speculates that some patients with sickle cell disease and musculoskeletal pain may in fact be responsive to vitamin D therapy. Patients with sickle cell disease not uncommonly develop vitamin D deficiency as a result of inadequate sun exposure and increased utilization of vitamin D for regulation of bone remodeling after recurrent sickle-related insults. Also, as is true of many patients with sickle cell disease, lactase deficiency can exacerbate the malabsorption of vitamin D. The 16-year-old in this report had significant improvement in bone mineral density with vitamin D treatment as well as complete resolution of her chronic pain and headaches. One could argue that these symptoms are simply complications of sickle cell disease rather than vitamin D deficiency, but the improvement in both the pain and bone density truly suggests a role for vitamin D in the pathogenesis of these musculoskeletal complications, findings that warrant further exploration.

It will be interesting to see if others pick up on this report by Osunkwo. We need to carefully evaluate the role of vitamin D deficiency in the pathogenesis of musculoskeletal pain in patients with sickle cell disease, perhaps with a properly designed randomized, controlled trial.

**J. A. Stockman III, MD**

*Reference*

1. de Torrenté de la Jara G, Pécoud A, Favrat B. Female asylum seekers with musculoskeletal pain: the importance of diagnosis and treatment of hypovitaminosis D. *BMC Fam Pract.* 2006;7:4.

## Growing Up With Sickle Cell Disease: A Pilot Study of a Transition Program for Adolescents With Sickle Cell Disease

Smith GM, Lewis VR, Whitworth E, et al (Duke Univ, Durham, NC; Duke Univ Med Ctr, Durham, NC)

*J Pediatr Hematol Oncol* 33:379-382, 2011

We implemented the Duke Sickle Cell Disease (SCD) Transition Program for adolescents with SCD and investigated the knowledge about SCD; concerns and emotions about transitioning; and the initial impact of the Transition Program. Thirty-three adolescents participated in the initial study. Gaps in knowledge included ethnicities affected by SCD and inheritance of SCD. Adolescents were primarily concerned about transferring to a new medical team. There was a mix of both positive and negative emotions that varied over time. Overall, we have identified educational gaps and concerns and emotions about transitioning, which we will address through the Duke SCD Transition Program.

▶ Children with sickle cell disease (SCD) are living longer and longer. This means that transition of care into adulthood is becoming increasingly more important. All too often, these kids fall between the cracks of our health care system in the late teenage or young adulthood years. A recent survey of children with special health care needs demonstrated that only 42% of those in a transitional age group discuss shifting care to an adult provider with their current pediatric provider.[1]

Smith et al have examined the impact of the Duke Sickle Cell Disease Transition Program on adolescents with SCD. The transition program was developed by a team of pediatric and adult hematologists, a child life specialist, social workers, undergraduate students, and the North Carolina Sickle Cell Consortium, an advocacy group. All adolescents with SCD aged 13 years and more are eligible to participate in the Transition Program if followed at the Duke Pediatric Sickle Cell Clinic. The program is funded by the Department of Pediatrics. A child life specialist teaches Duke undergraduates about SCD and trains them to administer the transition program through lecture and written materials. Adolescents can participate in this program until they are transitioned into the Adult Sickle Cell Clinic at 18 years of age or once they have completed high school. A transition team member accompanies the participants in the program to meet the adult staff team and schedule the first appointment in the Adult Sickle Cell Clinic. The participants are not followed up by the transition team after moving to the adult clinic. The transition program contains a thorough curriculum for patients with SCD and contains basic education about SCD and its sequelae, including disease management skills. In the aggregate, there are more than 100 specific topics covered in the reading material. Thirty-three adolescents with SCD aged 15 to 18 years have participated in this study.

This report documents that those in the transition program clearly enter the program with knowledge deficits about their SCD and voice concerns about transition of care into adulthood. The study showed that participating in a transition program will better inform patients with SCD, but future studies will need to address how participating in such a transition program ultimately benefits adolescents with SCD.

While on the topic of SCD in adolescence and young adulthood, it is worth mentioning that although myeloablative allogenic hematopoietic stem cell transplantation is increasingly being used for young children with SCD and is curative, it has been largely restricted to those who are 16 years and younger. This is because of concerns about the ability of such a procedure to be tolerated by older patients with SCD. Recently, Shieh et al[2] have reviewed the topic of allogenic hematopoietic stem cell transplantation for SCD in older-age adolescents and adults. It was noted that efforts to use nonmyeloablative transplantation strategies in adults logically followed pilot use in children but were initially met with largely disappointing results. More recently, however, data indicate that nonmyeloablative allogenic hematopoietic stem cell transplantation in adult patients with SCD can be undertaken and allows for stable mixed hematopoietic chimerism with associated full-donor red cell engraftment and normalization of blood counts and persistence in some without continued need for immunosuppression, suggesting immunologic tolerance. It is clear that efforts to build on these experiences should be undertaken to explore the use of allogenic hematopoietic stem cell transplantation in patients with SCD while minimizing morbidity and mortality.

**J. A. Stockman III, MD**

References

1. Lotstein DS, Ghandour R, Cash A, McGuire E, Strickland B, Newacheck P. Planning for health care transitions: results from the 2005—2006 national survey of children with special health care needs. *Pediatrics.* 2009;123:e145-e152.
2. Hsieh MM, Fitzhugh CD, Tisdale JF. Allogeneic hematopoietic stem cell transplantation for sickle cell disease: the time is now. *Blood.* 2011;118:1197-1207.

## Genetic predictors for stroke in children with sickle cell anemia

Flanagan JM, Frohlich DM, Howard TA, et al (St Jude Children's Res Hosp, Memphis, TN; et al)

*Blood* 117:6681-6684, 2011

Stroke is a devastating complication of sickle cell anemia (SCA), affecting 5% to 10% of patients before adulthood. Several candidate genetic polymorphisms have been proposed to affect stroke risk, but few have been validated, mainly because previous studies were hampered by relatively small sample sizes and the absence of additional patient cohorts for validation testing. To verify the accuracy of proposed genetic modifiers influencing stroke risk in SCA, we performed genotyping for 38 published single nucleotide polymorphisms (SNPs), as well as α-thalassemia, G6PD A⁻ variant deficiency, and β-globin haplotype in 2 cohorts of children with well-defined stroke phenotypes (130 stroke, 103 nonstroke). Five polymorphisms had significant influence ($P < .05$): SNPs in the *ANXA2*, *TGFBR3*, and *TEK* genes were associated with increased stroke risk, whereas α-thalassemia and a SNP in the *ADCY9* gene were linked with decreased stroke risk. Further investigation at these genetic regions may help define mutations that confer stroke risk or protection in children with SCA.

▶ Currently, the only useful prognostic tool available for primary stroke prevention of patients who have sickle cell anemia (SCA) is periodic screening of time-averaged mean velocities (TAMVs) in the distal internal carotid arteries and middle cerebral arteries using transcranial Doppler (TCD) ultrasonography. Stroke remains a catastrophic complication in SCA patients, affecting somewhere between 5% and 10% of pediatric age-affected individuals. Currently, if a patient has an abnormal TAMV, the youngster can be offered intervention consisting of blood transfusions. Transfusional therapy will lower the risk of stroke by more than 90%. Unfortunately, TCD is not available at all institutions that provide care to patients with SCA, and the test itself is hardly perfect. The limitations of TCD to accurately identify all SCA patients who will develop cerebrovascular complications as well as the reluctance for care providers and families to commit to an indefinite chronic transfusion program expose the need for a more sensitive and specific set of predictors for stroke. The latter is what Flanagan et al have attempted to do. They have looked at specific genetic modifiers that could influence the development of cerebrovascular disease in patients with SCA.

Flanagan et al looked at a variety of genotype characteristics (some 38 single nucleotide polymorphisms [SNPs], as well as alpha-thalassemia, G6PD A-variant deficiency, and beta-globin haplotype in patients with SCA who have and who have not had a stroke). Four of the 38 SNPs were found to be significantly associated with stroke risk. Some decreased the risk by more than half and others increased the risk by as much as almost 3-fold. As suspected, the presence of alpha-thalassemia is associated with a decreased risk of stroke as well.

The objective of this study was to corroborate published genetic modifiers that might aid prediction of stroke in children with SCA. One of the genes that modified the risk of stroke has been shown to help prevent and recover from stroke events. It will be interesting to see if this panel of genetic modifiers enters the clinical arena to assist care providers in following more closely those who are at the greatest risk of the development of stroke.

While on the topic of SCA, the gene mutation that causes the disorder is a double-edged sword. Individuals who carry 1 copy of the mutant hemoglobin allele do not develop sickle cell disease (simply the trait) but show a greater resistance to malaria. This may be because despite not developing full-blown disease, their blood still carries some consequences of the mutated allele. Investigators have developed a strain of mice that have the sickle cell trait. These mice are less likely to develop malaria than normal mice despite similar exposures to the malaria parasite. The protective effect was documented to be caused by heme oxygenase-1, which metabolizes free heme, generating carbon monoxide as one of the derivatives. For whatever reason, this makes the host mouse intolerant to malaria infection. The studies were carried out by Ferreira et al.[1] Needless to say, investigators are now hot on the trail of agents that might stimulate heme oxygenase activity or carbon monoxide production to block the rapid progression of the spread of the malaria organism throughout the body. To read more about this, see the excellent editorial by Rosenthal.[2]

**J. A. Stockman III, MD**

*References*

1. Ferreira A, Marguti I, Bechmann I, et al. Sickle hemoglobin confers tolerance to Plasmodium infection. *Cell*. 2011;145:398 409.
2. Rosenthal PJ. Lessons from sickle cell disease in the treatment and control of malaria. *N Engl J Med*. 2011;364:2549-2551.

---

**Discontinuing prophylactic transfusions increases the risk of silent brain infarction in children with sickle cell disease: data from STOP II**

Abboud MR, for the STOP II Study Investigators (American Univ of Beirut Med Ctr, Lebanon)
*Blood* 118:894-898, 2011

---

In the STOP II trial, discontinuation of prophylactic transfusions in high risk children with sickle cell disease (SCD) resulted in a high rate of reversion to abnormal blood-flow velocities on transcranial Doppler (TCD) ultrasonography and strokes. We analyzed data from STOP II to determine the effect of discontinuing transfusions on the development or progression of silent brain infarcts on magnetic resonance imaging (MRI). At study entry, 21 of 79 (27%) patients had evidence of silent infarcts. There were no statistically significant differences in baseline characteristics between patients with normal brain MRI or silent infarcts at study entry. At study end, 3 of 37 (8.1%) patients in the continued-transfusion group developed new brain MRI lesions compared with 11 of 40 (27.5%) in the transfusion-halted group ($P = .03$). The total number of lesions remained essentially unchanged decreasing from 25 to 24 in the continued-transfusion group while increasing from 27 to 45 in transfusion-halted patients. Thus, discontinuation of transfusions in children with SCD and abnormal TCD who revert to low-risk increases the risk of silent brain infarction. Together with data from STOP, these findings demonstrate that transfusions prevent the development of silent infarcts in patients with SCD and abnormal TCD but normal MRA.

▶ Silent brain infarcts are quite common in children with sickle cell disease. Estimates of the prevalence of this problem range from 17% to 35%.[1] Even though these infarcts are silent, they are problematic in that they can portend overt stroke and are associated with neurocognitive deficits in school-age children. The only significant therapy that has been available for the prevention of stroke or its recurrence is transfusion therapy. Hematologists are now routinely using transcranial Doppler ultrasonography to identify youngsters with sickle cell disease who have diminished brain flow and who, therefore, are at high risk for the development of a stroke. These children are placed on transfusion therapy. This will result in a reduced risk of silent strokes. There is concern, however, about the adverse effects of chronic transfusion therapy, especially iron overload. Many will therefore stop transfusion therapy after a period of time. Abboud et al have attempted to determine the effect of discontinuing transfusions on the development or progression of silent brain infarcts as determined by magnetic resonance imaging.

The study of Abboud et al is called STOP II. Data from this report show that in patients who have had silent strokes and their transfusions stopped, the risk of recurrent silent strokes increases by more than 3-fold. Not good news. Thus, for the time being, most care providers will keep patients who have had strokes (overt or silent) on transfusions indefinitely.

While on the topic of sickle cell disease, elsewhere noted is the high prevalence of pulmonary hypertension in many affected individuals. In adults with pulmonary hypertension (individuals without sickle cell disease) sildenafil has been shown to improve exercise capacity. The effect of sildenafil has now been studied in sickle cell disease patients. Unfortunately, sickle cell disease patients treated with sildenafil appear to have a much higher than expected occurrence of painful crises. One trial of sildenafil had to be stopped because of this complication.[2] As good as sildenafil may be for the management for erectile dysfunction, it does little or nothing for patients with sickle cell disease who have pulmonary hypertension.

**J. A. Stockman III, MD**

*References*

1. Pegelow CH, Macklin EA, Moser FG, et al. Longitudinal changes in brain magnetic resonance imaging findings in children with sickle cell disease. *Blood.* 2002;99:3014-3018.
2. Machado RF, Barst RJ, Yovetich NA, et al. Hospitalization for pain in patients with sickle cell disease treated with sildenafil for elevated TRV and low exercise capacity. *Blood.* 2011;118:855-864.

---

**Platelet production and platelet destruction: assessing mechanisms of treatment effect in immune thrombocytopenia**
Barsam SJ, Psaila B, Forestier M, et al (Weill-Cornell Med College, NY; Kantonsspital Baden, Switzerland; et al)
*Blood* 117:5723-5732, 2011

---

This study investigated the immature platelet fraction (IPF) in assessing treatment effects in immune thrombocytopenia (ITP). IPF was measured on the Sysmex XE2100 autoanalyzer. The mean absolute-IPF (A-IPF) was lower for ITP patients than for healthy controls (3.2 vs $7.8 \times 10^9$/L, $P < .01$), whereas IPF percentage was greater (29.2% vs 3.2%, $P < .01$). All 5 patients with a platelet response to Eltrombopag, a thrombopoietic agent, but none responding to an anti-FcγRIII antibody, had corresponding A-IPF responses. Seven of 7 patients responding to RhoD immuneglobulin (anti-D) and 6 of 8 responding to intravenous immunoglobulin (IVIG) did not have corresponding increases in A-IPF, but 2 with IVIG and 1 with IVIG anti-D did. This supports inhibition of platelet destruction as the primary mechanism of intravenous anti-D and IVIG, although IVIG may also enhance thrombopoiesis. Plasma glycocalicin, released during platelet destruction, normalized as glycocalicin index, was higher in ITP patients than controls (31.36 vs 1.75, $P = .001$). There was an inverse correlation between glycocalicin index and A-IPF in ITP patients ($r^2 = -0.578$, $P = .015$), demonstrating the relationship between platelet production and destruction. Nonresponders to thrombopoietic agents had increased megakaryocytes but not increased A-IPF, suggesting that antibodies blocked platelet release. In conclusion, A-IPF measures real-time thrombopoiesis, providing insight into mechanisms of treatment effect.

▶ This report requires a bit of background. It was back in 1946 that Damashek and Miller[1] reported that numbers of megakaryocytes in patients with immune thrombocytopenia (ITP) were normal or increased, but only one-third or fewer of megakaryocytes showed evidence of platelet production. In addition, they found that the numbers of larger intermediate megakaryocytes, the promegakaryocytes, were decreased. They concluded that the thrombocytopenia in ITP might result from a severe reduction in platelet production by megakaryocytes. They obviously have been proven to be partially right. The debate about the mechanisms of thrombocytopenia in ITP took a turn in 1951 with an interesting experiment performed by Harrington et al.[2] In this seminal experiment, the investigators unequivocally demonstrated that ITP is characterized, at least in part, by reduced platelet survival related to a humoral factor later identified as antibodies against platelet glycoproteins.[2] In this experiment, Harrington et al[2] infused plasma from patients with ITP into himself. Besides reducing his own platelet count by such an experiment, he almost died. It has now been shown that platelet lifespan is markedly decreased in virtually all patients with ITP. Platelet turnover (a measure of platelet production) is frequently subnormal, however. It is now proposed that thrombocytopenia in patients with ITP results from both platelet destruction and antibody-mediated damage to megakaryocytes, limiting their ability to produce platelets.

In addition to treatment with agents that are designed to increase platelet lifespan, a conceptually different approach to the treatment of ITP has emerged in recent years with the introduction of second-generation thrombopoietin receptor (TPO-R) agonists, which aim at correcting the thrombocytopenia by stimulating platelet production through megakaryocyte proliferation and maturation. Two such agents, romiplostim and eltrombopag, recently have been licensed for use for management of ITP.

Barsam et al report their investigation of the patterns of both platelet production and platelet destruction in patients with ITP undergoing various pharmacologic treatments, including eltrombopag. These investigators found that TPO-R agonists help some patients but not others. It is suggested that in some patients, platelet formation and release by megakaryocytes is completely inhibited by platelet antibodies, and in some it is not or only partially inhibited. From a clinical perspective, strategies to overcome resistance to TPO-R agonists may involve adding conventional immunosuppressive agents to inhibit autoantibody production. This may be a practical tip for pediatric hematologists who care for patients responding poorly to second-generation thrombopoietic agents.

We have come a long way in the last 65 years understanding exactly how patients with ITP develop thrombocytopenia. To read more about all this, see the excellent commentary by Stasi.[3]

**J. A. Stockman III, MD**

*References*

1. Damashek W, Miller EB. The megakaryocytes in idiopathic thrombocytopenic purpura, a form of hypersplenism. *Blood*. 1946;1:27-51.
2. Harrington WJ, Minnich B, Hollingsworth JW, Moore CV. Demonstration of a thrombocytopenic factor in the blood of patients with thrombocytopenic purpura. *J Lab Clin Med*. 1951;38:1-10.
3. Stasi R. The stingy bone marrow and the wasteful peripheral blood: a tale of two ITPs. *Blood*. 2011;117:5553-5554.

### The role of vanin-1 and oxidative stress—related pathways in distinguishing acute and chronic pediatric ITP

Zhang B, Lo C, Shen L, et al (Stanford Univ, CA)
*Blood* 117:4569-4579, 2011

Pediatric immune thrombocytopenia (ITP) is usually self-limited. However, approximately 20% of children develop chronic ITP, which can be associated with significant morbidity because of long-term immunosuppression and splenectomy in refractory cases. To explore the molecular mechanism of chronic ITP compared with acute ITP, we studied 63 pediatric patients with ITP. Gene expression analysis of whole blood revealed distinct signatures for acute and chronic ITP. Oxidative stress—related pathways were among the most significant chronic ITP-associated pathways. Overexpression of *VNN1*, an oxidative stress sensor in epithelial cells, was most strongly associated with progression to chronic ITP. Studies of normal persons demonstrated *VNN1* expression in a variety of blood cells. Exposure of blood mononuclear cells to oxidative stress inducers elicited dramatic up-regulation of *VNN1* and down-regulation of *PPAR*γ, indicating a role for *VNN1* as a peripheral blood oxidative stress sensor. Assessment of redox state by tandem mass spectrometry demonstrated statistically significant lower glutathione ratios in patients with ITP versus healthy controls; lower glutathione ratios were also seen in untreated patients with ITP compared with recently treated patients. Our work demonstrates distinct patterns of gene expression in acute and chronic ITP and implicates oxidative stress pathways in the pathogenesis of chronic pediatric ITP.

▶ In children, immune thrombocytopenia (ITP) often appears after an infection or a vaccination, while in adults it is known to be associated with *Helicobacter pylori*, hepatitis C virus, human immunodeficiency virus, and other viral infections, although in both children and adults, the mechanism of the induction of ITP remains unknown. Exactly how the immune system is programmed to destroy platelets also remains unknown. Infection-related oxidative stress can induce peculiar immune responses, such as autoantibodies or immune complexes against platelets, thereby leading to early destruction of these cells by phagocytosis or by cytotoxic T cells in predisposed individuals.

Zhang et al tell us about the relationship between oxidative stress and ITP in children with a focus on gene expression and molecular-oxidative stress. These investigators have shown differences in the oxidative profile in patients with transient, self-limited ITP and chronic, long-term ITP in comparison with control individuals. Overexpression of the gene vanin-1 (*VNN1*)—an oxidative stress sensor—was associated with chronic ITP only. *VNN1* is characterized by its role in oxidative stress responses, and it mediates production of inflammatory cytokines by antagonizing what is known as peroxisome proliferative-activated receptor gamma. In fact, *VNN1* is the only gene variant that was detected in those patients who developed chronic ITP.

It appears that ongoing oxidative stress may be a significant factor in patients with chronic ITP. The importance of this report is that it may provide early prognostic estimation about whether an individual will have transient or long-term disease. If it is documented that part of the pathophysiologic mechanism of the ITP relates to oxidative stress, one might see new therapeutic approaches and medications put into our therapeutic armamentarium.

To read more about oxidative stress as related to ITP, see the excellent editorial comment by Imbach.[1]

**J. A. Stockman III, MD**

*Reference*

1. Imbach P. Oxidative stress may cause ITP. *Blood.* 2011;117:4405-4406.

---

**A randomized, double-blind study of romiplostim to determine its safety and efficacy in children with immune thrombocytopenia**

Bussel JB, Buchanan GR, Nugent DJ, et al (Weill Med College of Cornell Univ, NY; Univ of Texas Southwestern Med Ctr at Dallas; Children's Hosp of Orange County, CA; et al)
*Blood* 118.28-36, 2011

---

Romiplostim, a thrombopoietin-mimetic peptibody, increases and maintains platelet counts in adults with immune thrombocytopenia (ITP). In this first study of a thrombopoietic agent in children, patients with ITP of $\geq 6$ months' duration were stratified by age 1:2:2 (12 months-< 3 years; 3-< 12 years; 12-< 18 years). Children received subcutaneous injections of romiplostim (n — 17) or placebo (n = 5) weekly for 12 weeks, with dose adjustments to maintain platelet counts between $50 \times 10^9/L$ and $250 \times 10^9/L$. A platelet count $\geq 50 \times 10^9/L$ for 2 consecutive weeks was achieved by 15/17 (88%) patients in the romiplostim group and no patients in the placebo group ($P - .0008$). Platelet counts $> 50 \times 10^9/L$ were maintained for a median of 7 (range, 0-11) weeks in romiplostim patients and 0 (0-0) weeks in placebo patients ($P = .0019$). The median weekly dose of romiplostim at 12 weeks was 5 µg/kg. Fourteen responders received romiplostim for 4 additional weeks for assessment of pharmacokinetics. No patients discontinued the study. There were no treatment-related, serious adverse events. The most commonly reported adverse events in children, as in adults, were headache and epistaxis. In this short-term study, romiplostim increased platelet counts in 88% of children with ITP and was well-tolerated and apparently safe. The trial was registered with http://www.clinicaltrials.gov as NCT00515203.

▶ Immune thrombocytopenia (ITP) remains a common problem in children. It is an autoimmune disorder that is characterized by accelerated platelet destruction as well as suboptimal platelet production. In the United States, children are affected with ITP at a rate of 1.9 to 6.4 per 100 000 children-years.[1] Twelve months after diagnosis, only about 20% of youngsters affected with ITP will still be thrombocytopenic, most not requiring treatment. It is estimated that 5% to 10% of all pediatric ITP patients will have severe, chronic, or refractory disease. Therapeutic agents for childhood ITP—steroids, intravenous immunoglobulin, anti-D immunoglobulin, azathioprine and rituximab, and splenectomy—may be effective but have limitations with respect to long-term efficacy or safety.

Bussel et al tell us about the effectiveness of 2 new thrombopoietin receptor agonists that stimulate platelet production. These are romiplostim and eltrombopag. Both are approved for treatment of adults with chronic ITP. Bussel et al report on the first randomized study to evaluate romiplostim in the treatment of children with ITP. In this short-term study, romiplostim increased platelet counts in almost 90% of children with ITP. It was well tolerated and safe.

The report of Bussel et al was accompanied by an editorial by Despotovic and Ware.[2] We are reminded in this editorial that one of the risks of using recombinant products to stimulate the bone marrow is the development of antibodies against the product. This was seen with first-generation thrombopoietin receptor agonists. The second-generation agonist, romiplostim, has had a significantly lower incidence of antithrombopoietin receptor agonist antibody formation. One must keep an eye out for this problem, especially in young patients for whom long-term therapy would be considered likely. This aside, treatment with these new agents appears to be safe, well-tolerated, and efficacious for most severely affected children with refractory ITP.

**J. A. Stockman III, MD**

*References*

1. Terrell DR, Beebe LA, Vesely SK, Neas BR, Segal JB, George JN. The incidence of immune thrombocytopenia purpura in children and adults: a critical review of published reports. *Am J Hematol.* 2010;85:174-180.
2. Despotovic JM, Ware RE. Thrombopoiesis: new ITP paradigm? *Blood.* 2011;118:1-2.

---

**Romiplostim safety and efficacy for immune thrombocytopenia in clinical practice: 2-year results of 72 adults in a romiplostim compassionate-use program**

Khellaf M, Michel M, Quittet P, et al (Université Paris Est Créteil, France; CHU Lapéyronie, Montpellier, France; et al)
*Blood* 118:4338-4345, 2011

---

Romiplostim, a thrombopoietic agent with demonstrated efficacy against immune thrombocytopenia (ITP) in prospective controlled studies, was recently licensed for adults with chronic ITP. Only France has allowed romiplostim compassionate use since January 2008. ITP patients could receive romiplostim when they failed to respond to successive corticosteroids, intravenous immunoglobulins, rituximab, and splenectomy, or when splenectomy was not indicated. We included the first 80 patients enrolled in this program with at least 2 years of follow-up. Primary platelet response (platelet count $\geq 50 \times 10^9$/L and double baseline) was observed in 74% of all patients. Long-term responses (2 years) were observed in 47 (65%) patients, 37 (79%) had sustained platelet responses with a median platelet count of $106 \times 10^9$/L (interquartile range, 75-167 $\times 10^9$/L), and 10 (21%) were still taking romiplostim, despite a median platelet count of $38 \times 10^9$/L (interquartile range, 35-44 $\times 10^9$/L), but with clinical benefit (lower dose and/or fewer concomitant treatment(s) and/or diminished bleeding signs). A high bleeding score and use of concomitant ITP therapy were baseline factors predicting romiplostim failure. The most frequently reported adverse events were: arthralgias (26%), fatigue (13%), and nausea (7%). Our results confirmed that romiplostim use in clinical practice is effective and safe for severe chronic ITP. This trial was registered at www.clinicaltrials.gov as #NCT01013181.

▶ Patients with chronic immune thrombocytopenia (ITP) as young as 20 years of age were included in this report, and thus the information contained therein is applicable to teenagers with chronic ITP. Although chronic ITP is relatively infrequent in the young pediatric population, teens tend to act just like adults with respect to the development of chronic ITP. It is not a rare complication of ITP in this adolescent/young adult population.

Various strategies have been used to treat chronic ITP. Steroids are the first-line therapy but result in systemic and profound immunosuppression when used over the long haul. Intravenous immunoglobulin (IVIG) and Rhesus D antibodies can lead to a transient correction of platelet count because both compete with fragment crystallizable receptors on macrophages and thus block platelet destruction. Surgical splenectomy has historically been the second-line therapy for young and older adults with ITP, but it too is frequently ineffective. New drugs have been introduced, known as thrombopoietin mimetics. These trigger an increase in bone marrow platelet production. Therapeutic options available to patients with chronic and refractory ITP have recently expanded with the introduction of 2 thrombopoietic agents, romiplostim and eltrombopag.

Khellaf et al describe the results in 72 patients with chronic ITP treated with romiplostim. Half the patients treated had already been splenectomized. After 2 years of therapy with romiplostim, 65% of treated patients had achieved a clinical benefit with a rise in platelet count greater than $5 \times 10^9$/L. Only 2 patients were able to maintain a platelet response when romiplostim was discontinued. The romiplostim was generally well tolerated. Unfortunately, we have little long-term knowledge about the safety of this drug.

In the aggregate, in roughly one-third of patients with chronic ITP, the use of romiplostim results in no sustained improvement of platelet counts. These patients often tend to be those who have the worst bleeding problems. Despite these limitations, there is little doubt that romiplostim represents a major breakthrough in the management of chronic ITP. In addition to an increase in platelet count, decreased risk of bleeding, and reduction or discontinuation of concomitant ITP medications, patients responding to romiplostim also experience a dramatic improvement of health-related quality of life. This latter aspect of therapy cannot be underestimated.

This commentary concludes with another observation having to do with impropriety in the current medical literature. It is increasingly apparent that inappropriate "spin" of biomedical results is rife and could be countered in part by using a "propaganda index," so say some. Articles have been published that make a drug look better than the actual data support. This is achieved through choice of language or selective emphasis reporting certain parts of the research data. Investigators have examined 72 clinical trials all published in the same month (December 2006), which had a clear primary objective, but statistically insignificant findings. The investigators read the papers separately and noted phrases that clearly indicated "spin." For example, an article might say that the results "approached, but did not reach significance," or "would have been statistically significant if we had a bigger sample"—both of which mean the same thing, that the results were not statistically significant. To the casual reader, such spin may not be discernible. This spin was especially prominent in the conclusion sections of at least half of the articles reviewed. A proposed "propaganda index" would involve a statement of how much "spin" was actually present in a report. This is clearly a fascinating idea whose time has come.[1]

**J. A. Stockman III, MD**

*Reference*

1. Jones N. "Propaganda index" proposed for the medical literature. *Nature Medicine.* 2009;15:1100-1101.

---

### Incidence of factor VIII inhibitors throughout life in severe hemophilia A in the United Kingdom

Hay CRM, on behalf of United Kingdom Haemophilia Centre Doctors' Organisation (UKHCDO) (Manchester Royal Infirmary, UK; et al)
*Blood* 117:6367-6370, 2011

---

The age-adjusted incidence of new factor VIII inhibitors was analyzed in all United Kingdom patients with severe hemophilia A between 1990 and 2009. Three hundred fifteen new inhibitors were reported to the National Hemophilia Database in 2528 patients with severe hemophilia who were followed up for a median (interquartile range) of 12 (4-19) years. One hundred sixty (51%) of these arose in patients ≥5 years of age after a median (interquartile range) of 6 (4-11) years' follow-up. The incidence of new inhibitors was 64.29 per 1000 treatment-years in patients <5 years of age and 5.31 per 1000 treatment-years at age 10-49 years, rising significantly ($P = .01$) to 10.49 per 1000 treatment-years in patients more than 60 years of age. Factor VIII inhibitors arise in patients with hemophilia A throughout life with a bimodal risk, being greatest in early childhood and in old age. HIV was associated with significantly fewer new inhibitors. The inhibitor incidence rate ratio in HIV-seropositive patients was 0.32 times that observed in HIV-seronegative patients ($P < .001$). Further study is required to explore the natural history of later-onset factor VIII inhibitors and to investigate other potential risk factors for inhibitor development in previously treated patients.

▶ Anyone caring for a patient with hemophilia knows that the development of factor VIII inhibitor antibodies is the most important and serious complication of the treatment of severe hemophilia A. In most instances, factor VIII inhibitors arise after relatively few factor VIII exposure days, early in a patient's life, and the risk of inhibitor development is subsequently low after that period. Data from the United Kingdom suggest, however, that new inhibitors may present throughout the entire life span in patients with severe hemophilia, and this risk gradually increases in older patients. The development of early inhibitors is increased in certain situations, including a family history of inhibitors, nonwhite ethnicity, factor VIII mutation, and intense factor VIII replacement therapy

There is a registry for hemophilia A patients in Great Britain. Hay et al looked at the development of factor VIII inhibitor in some 2500 affected individuals who were followed for an average of 12 years. Three hundred fifteen patients of this group did develop inhibitors. The inhibitors evolved on an average in just 2 years. Half of the patients who developed inhibitors did so by 5 years of age. The incidence of inhibitors that were developing declined with increasing age before rising to a second peak of 10.5 new inhibitors per 1000 patient years at risk in patients 60 years of age or greater. Half of all reported inhibitors did occur in patients after the age of 5 years, a much higher proportion than commonly believed.

All this means is that if you have hemophilia A, you do not get out of childhood scot-free without a future risk of the development of factor VIII inhibitors. Older patients do require regular monitoring for the development of inhibitors, especially low-titer inhibitors, which need to be identified prior to surgery. As life expectancy increases in patients with hemophilia A, one can expect an increased prevalence of inhibitors in this population. It is good to forewarn our pediatric patients as they transition to adult care that even though they may not have inhibitors at that time, the risk of this problem continues well into later life.

**J. A. Stockman III, MD**

---

**Anti-Inhibitor Coagulant Complex Prophylaxis in Hemophilia with Inhibitors**
Leissinger C, Gringeri A, Antmen B, et al (Tulane Univ, New Orleans; Ospedale Maggiore Policlinico and Università degli Studi di Milano, Milan; Çukurova Univ, Adana; et al)
*N Engl J Med* 365:1684-1692, 2011

---

*Background.*—Patients with severe hemophilia A and factor VIII inhibitors are at increased risk for serious bleeding complications and progression to end-stage joint disease. Effective strategies to prevent bleeding in such patients have not yet been established.

*Methods.*—We enrolled patients with hemophilia A who were older than 2 years of age, had high-titer inhibitors, and used concentrates known as bypassing agents for bleeding in a prospective, randomized, crossover study comparing 6 months of anti-inhibitor coagulant complex (AICC), infused prophylactically at a target dose of 85 U per kilogram of body weight ( ± 15%) on 3 nonconsecutive days per week, with 6 months of on-demand therapy (AICC at a target dose of 85 U per kilogram [± 15%] used for bleeding episodes). The two treatment periods were separated by a 3-month washout period, during which patients received on-demand therapy for bleeding. The primary outcome was the number of bleeding episodes during each 6-month treatment period.

*Results.*—Thirty-four patients underwent randomization; 26 patients completed both treatment periods and could be evaluated per protocol for the efficacy analysis. As compared with on-demand therapy, prophylaxis was associated with a 62% reduction in all bleeding episodes ($P < 0.001$), a 61% reduction in hemarthroses ($P < 0.001$), and a 72% reduction in target-joint bleeding ($\geq 3$ hemarthroses in a single joint during a 6-month treatment period) ($P < 0.001$). Thirty-three randomly assigned patients received at least one infusion of the study drug and were evaluated for safety. One patient had an allergic reaction to the study drug.

*Conclusions.*—AICC prophylaxis at the dosage evaluated significantly and safely decreased the frequency of joint and other bleeding events in patients with severe hemophilia A and factor VIII inhibitors. (Funded by Baxter BioScience; Pro-FEIBA ClinicalTrials.gov number, NCT00221195.)

▶ There are few things less worrisome to the pediatric hematologist and to the patient with hemophilia A than the development of factor inhibitors. After exposure to factor VIII, antibodies (inhibitors) can develop that neutralize factor VIII clotting function. As many as 30% of patients with severe hemophilia A will develop some level of antibody against factor VIII. If the inhibitor level increases to greater than 5 Bethesda units, standard factor replacement will usually no longer allow a satisfactory response in a patient who is bleeding. In this circumstance, alternative forms of clotting concentrates, known as *bypassing agents*, are used to treat bleeding. Two bypassing agents are currently available. One is anti-inhibitor coagulant complex (AICC) The other is recombinant activated factor VII. About 80% of bleeding episodes in patients with high titer inhibitors are controlled with such bypassing agents. Control is frequently not perfect, however. In many cases, success rates are substantially less than the outcomes in patients who do not have factor VIII inhibitors who receive standard replacement therapy. For these reasons, patients with inhibitors are at significantly increased risk for bleeding that is difficult to control.

The report of Leissinger et al describes an attempt to use bypass therapy in a more innovative way than is traditionally used (the latter being episodic therapy). Prophylaxis, the routinely scheduled replacement of factor VIII, is standard therapy for patients who have severe hemophilia A without inhibitors because of its ability to prevent bleeding. However, for patients with inhibitors who have refractory bleeding with serious consequences and who could derive an even greater benefit from prevention of bleeding, traditional factor VIII prophylaxis is ineffective. Leissinger et al, however, designed a study to compare the efficacy and safety of AICC prophylaxis with ongoing demand therapy in patients with high titer inhibitor to see if it might be possible to prevent bleeding episodes in patients with high titer inhibitor before they actually start. In this report, patients with hemophilia A were enrolled in a study in which they received bypassing agents on a regular prophylactic basis on 3 nonconsecutive days of the week with 6 months of on-demand therapy, which was used for a control group of patients who had therapy given for bleeding episodes. The study also had a crossover phase between the treated and control group. AICC prophylaxis did significantly decrease the frequency of joint and other bleeding events in patients with severe hemophilia A who had high titered inhibitors. It also did this quite safely. All bleeding events, hemarthroses, and other events, were significantly reduced during AICC prophylaxis with the thrice-weekly dosing regimen.

These investigators also looked at the cost involved with the type of prophylaxis described. The cost of prophylaxis for patients who have hemophilia without inhibitors runs 2.4 to 3.1 times as high as the cost of on-demand therapy. Similarly, the cost of AICC prophylaxis in this study was 2.4 times as high as that of on-demand therapy ($493 633 vs $205 549 annually per patient based on an average cost of $1.56 per unit of AICC for patients in the United States and $1.13 per unit for patients in the European Union in this study). The cost of AICC ran $15 691 per bleeding episode during the on-demand period. After deducting the cost of bleeding episodes avoided and bleeding episodes treated during the prophylaxis period, the remaining cost for prophylaxis ran $288 081. The cost of bypassing therapy per bleeding episode avoided was $35 565 (or $585 per kilogram of body weight for a somewhat similar older patient population with a mean body weight of 60.8 kg). Of course, these costs do not reflect the potential benefits of avoiding hospitalization, potential subsequent surgeries, and days lost from work or school. They also do not include any dollar benefits from preventing long-term complications, such as worsening joint disease and disability.

This report is powerful and very well may change the way in which patients with factor VIII hemophilia who have high titered inhibitors are treated in the future. While everything comes down to money, if cost can be excluded from the equation, prophylaxis of high titered inhibitor patients seems to be the way to go, at least at this point. It will be interesting to see whether this report in fact does set a new trend in the management of these difficult-to-treat patients.

**J. A. Stockman III, MD**

---

**Genetic variation associated with plasma von Willebrand factor levels and the risk of incident venous thrombosis**
Smith NL, Rice KM, Bovill EG, et al (Univ of Washington, Seattle; Univ of Vermont, Burlington; et al)
*Blood* 117:6007-6011, 2011

---

In a recent genome-wide association study, variants in 8 genes were associated with VWF level, a risk factor for venous thrombosis (VT). In an independent, population-based, case-control study of incident VT, we tested hypotheses that variants in these genes would be associated with risk. Cases were 656 women who experienced an incident VT, and controls comprised 710 women without a history of VT. DNA was obtained from whole blood. Logistic regression was used to test associations between incident VT and single nucleotide polymorphisms (SNPs) in 7 genes not previously shown to be associated with VT. Associations with $P < .05$ were candidates for replication in an independent case-control study of VT in both sexes. Two of the 7 SNPs tested yielded $P < .05$: rs1039084 ($P = .005$) in *STXBP5*, a novel candidate gene for VT, and rs1063856 ($P = .04$) in *VWF*, a gene whose protein level is associated with VT risk. Association results for the remaining 5 variants in *SCARA5*, *STAB2*, *STX2*, *TC2N*, and *CLEC4M* were not significant. Both *STXBP5* and *VWF* findings were replicated successfully. Variation in genes associated with VWF levels in the genome-wide association study was found to be independently associated with incident VT.

▶ It has been known for some time that elevated plasma levels of factor VIII (FVIII) and von Willebrand factor (VWF) are risk factors for the development of venous thrombosis. Smith et al have demonstrated that genetic variants associated with the intermediate phenotype of plasma VWF: antigen (VWF:Ag) levels are associated with the risk of venous thromboses. Specifically, variants producing amino acid substitutions in *STXBP5* and *VWF*, among those most strongly associated with VWF:Ag levels, are also risk factors for venous thrombosis, at least in adult women and presumably in children. It appears that we are getting closer to knowing much more about what places some people at a greater risk of clotting than others.

This commentary closes with a few pearls for the hematologist aficionado. Are you aware of something known as the Weibel-Palade body? Back in 1964, Ewald Weibel and George Palade, using transmission electron microscopy, discovered "a hitherto unknown rod-shaped cytoplasmic component which consists of a bundle of fine tubules, enveloped by a tightly fitted membrane." This was regularly found in the endothelial cells of small arteries and various organs in man.[1] At the time of their discovery, the biological function of Weibel-Palade bodies was unknown. In the interval of almost 50 years, it has been determined that these bodies contain VWF and that the latter is secreted into blood in response to a variety of stimuli. In fact, VWF is the only protein readily detected in Weibel-Palade bodies, which are found in the endothelium of blood vessels. Various entities that disturb endothelial function can increase the release of VWF and may increase plasma levels of VWF and FVIII, both of which can be associated with an increased risk of arterial thrombosis, particularly in coronary heart disease, stroke, and venous thromboembolism. For a neat review of how all this works within our body, see the excellent review article by Valentijn et al.[2]

This commentary closes the Blood section with one more observation having to do with scientific publications. Have you ever heard of the term "coercive citation"? You are probably familiar with the term "impact factor" in reference to medical and other journal publishing. The frequency with which a journal is cited in the literature in part relates to how frequently that journal is either read or cited. This affects the journal's impact factor. The higher the impact factor, the more prominent a journal therefore is. The higher the impact factor, the more likely it is that that the journal will bring in advertisement revenue. When an article is submitted to a journal, it is common for the journal's editor to make suggestions to improve the article. It is also possible for the editor to suggest that the authors include additional references at the end of their article. Perhaps all too often the suggestion is to add a reference to a report previously published in that same journal. If this suggestion is made solely for the purpose of driving up the impact factor of that journal, this is known as "coercive citation." Wilhite et al have studied the issue of coercive citation by analyzing 6672 responses from a survey sent to researchers in economics, sociology, psychology, and many other scientific fields [3] Data were derived from 832 journals in the same disciplines. It was noted that coercion is uncomfortably common and appears to be practiced in an opportunistic way. Researchers in most of the business disciplines indicated that this is a likely phenomenon in comparison to other disciplines but it was present in all fields. In this study, editors were more likely to be coercive with assistant and associated professors than with higher ranking professors and to target articles with fewer authors The type of publisher also appears to be influential. Journals published by commercial, for-profit companies show significantly greater use of coercive tactics than journals from university presses. Academic societies also were more coercive than university presses. The more highly ranked impact a journal is, the more likely it was that the journal was coercive. Curiously, fewer than 7% of those surveyed indicated that they would refuse to add superfluous citations suggested by a journal editor. Thus a researcher can easily become both a victim and a coconspirator in the self-citation game.

**J. A. Stockman III, MD**

*References*

1. Weibel ER, Palade GE. New cytoplasmic components in arterial endothelia. *J Cell Biol.* 1964;23:101 112.
2. Valentijn KM, Sadler JE, Valentijn JA, Voorberg J, Eikenboom J. Functional architecture of Weibel-Palade bodies. *Blood.* 2011;117:5033-5043.
3. Wilhite AW, Fong EA. Coercive citation in academic publishing. *Science.* 2011; 335:542-543.

# 4 Child Development/ Behavior

---

**Trends in the Prevalence of Developmental Disabilities in US Children, 1997–2008**
Boyle CA, Boulet S, Schieve LA, et al (Natl Ctr on Birth Defects and Developmental Disabilities, Atlanta, GA; et al)
*Pediatrics* 127:1034-1042, 2011

---

*Objective.*—To fill gaps in crucial data needed for health and educational planning, we determined the prevalence of developmental disabilities in US children and in selected populations for a recent 12-year period.

*Participants and Methods.*—We used data on children aged 3 to 17 years from the 1997–2008 National Health Interview Surveys, which are ongoing nationally representative samples of US households. Parent-reported diagnoses of the following were included: attention deficit hyperactivity disorder; intellectual disability; cerebral palsy; autism; seizures; stuttering or stammering; moderate to profound hearing loss; blindness; learning disorders; and/or other developmental delays.

*Results.*—Boys had a higher prevalence overall and for a number of select disabilities compared with girls. Hispanic children had the lowest prevalence for a number of disabilities compared with non-Hispanic white and black children. Low income and public health insurance were associated with a higher prevalence of many disabilities. Prevalence of any developmental disability increased from 12.84% to 15.04% over 12 years. Autism, attention deficit hyperactivity disorder, and other developmental delays increased, whereas hearing loss showed a significant decline. These trends were found in all of the sociodemographic subgroups, except for autism in non-Hispanic black children.

*Conclusions.*—Developmental disabilities are common and were reported in ~ 1 in 6 children in the United States in 2006–2008. The number of children with select developmental disabilities (autism, attention deficit hyperactivity disorder, and other developmental delays) has increased, requiring more health and education services. Additional study of the influence of risk-factor shifts, changes in acceptance, and benefits of early services is needed.

▶ One of the last times there was an assessment of the prevalence of developmental disabilities among US children was in the 1998 National Health Interview

Survey, which indicated that 16.8% of children younger than 18 years of age had a lifelong condition arising in early childhood resulting in cognitive or physical impairment or a combination of both. Since that report, now more than 2 decades old, there have been more recent surveys suggesting that the numbers of children with developmental disabilities have been increasing with time.

Boyle et al have used information from the National Health Interview Survey (NHIS) to examine trends in a more in-depth way. The NHIS is an ongoing annual survey conducted by the Centers for Disease Control and Prevention, National Center for Health Statistics that uses a multistage probability sample to estimate the prevalence of a number of health conditions in the civilian noninstitutionalized population of the United States. Boyle used a current analysis of NHIS data for children age 3 to 17 years for the period 1997 to 2008. Children younger than 3 years were excluded because a number of developmental disabilities are not recognized or diagnosed before that age. The specific conditions assessed were attention deficit hyperactivity disorder (ADHD), cerebral palsy, autism, seizures, stammering/stuttering, mental retardation, moderate to profound hearing loss, blindness, learning disorders, and other developmental delays. The analysis noted that 15% of children age 3 years to 17 years, or nearly 10 million children in 2006 to 2008, had a developmental disability on the basis of information from the annual survey. This represented a 17% increase in prevalence over the 12-year period of the survey, with approximately 1.8 million more children with developmental disabilities in 2006 to 2008 when compared with a decade earlier. The largest percentage of change from 1997 to 1999 versus 2006 to 2008 was an almost 300% increase in the area of autism. Significant increases were also seen with ADHD and moderate to profound hearing loss.

Factors responsible for increases in autism and ADHD are numerous. Availability of services and how the service system classifies children with behavioral disorders have progressed as we have learned more about the advantages of early interventions. Improvements in clinical, parent, and societal recognition of and screening for these disorders have occurred. Another contributing factor may be the efficacy of medications and behavioral treatments for ADHD. The findings from this report have a direct bearing on the need for health education in social services, including the need for more specialized health services such as mental health services, medical specialists, therapists, and allied health professionals. The data from this report provide powder for the bullets of those who truly believe additional services need to be provided.

**J. A. Stockman III, MD**

---

## Memantine for dementia in adults older than 40 years with Down's syndrome (MEADOWS): a randomised, double-blind, placebo-controlled trial

Hanney M, on behalf of the MEADOWS trial researchers (King's College London, UK; et al)
*Lancet* 379:528-536, 2012

---

*Background.*—Prevalence of Alzheimer's disease in people with Down's syndrome is very high, and many such individuals who are older than

40 years have pathological changes characteristic of Alzheimer's disease. Evidence to support treatment with Alzheimer's drugs is inadequate, although memantine is beneficial in transgenic mice. We aimed to assess safety and efficacy of memantine on cognition and function in individuals with Down's syndrome.

*Methods.*—In our prospective randomised double-blind trial, we enrolled adults (> 40 years) with karyotypic or clinically diagnosed Down's syndrome, with and without dementia, at four learning disability centres in the UK and Norway. We randomly allocated participants (1:1) to receive memantine or placebo for 52 weeks by use of a computer-generated sequence and a minimisation algorithm to ensure balanced allocation for five prognostic factors (sex, dementia, age group, total Down's syndrome attention, memory, and executive function scales [DAMES] score, and centre). The primary outcome was change in cognition and function, measured with DAMES scores and the adaptive behaviour scale (ABS) parts I and II. We analysed differences in DAMES and ABS scores between groups with analyses of covariance or quantile regression in all patients who completed the 52 week assessment and had available follow-up data. This study is registered, number ISRCTN47562898.

*Findings.*—We randomly allocated 88 patients to receive memantine (72 [82%] had DAMES data and 75 [85%] had ABS data at 52 weeks) and 85 to receive placebo (74 [87%] and 73 [86%]). Both groups declined in cognition and function but rates did not differ between groups for any outcomes. After adjustment for baseline score, there were non-significant differences between groups of $-4\cdot1$ (95% CI $-13\cdot1$ to $4\cdot8$) in DAMES scores, $-8\cdot5$ ($-20\cdot1$ to $3\cdot1$) in ABS I scores, and $2\cdot0$ ($-7\cdot2$ to $11\cdot3$) in ABS II scores, all in favour of controls. 10 (11%) of 88 participants in the memantine group and six (7%) of 85 controls had serious adverse events ($p = 0\cdot33$). Five participants in the memantine group and four controls died from serious adverse events ($p = 0\cdot77$).

*Interpretation.*—There is a striking absence of evidence about pharmacological treatment of cognitive impairment and dementia in people older than 40 years with Down's syndrome. Despite promising indications, memantine is not an effective treatment. Therapies that are effective for Alzheimer's disease are not necessarily effective in this group of patients.

▶ Everyone in the practice of general pediatrics at some point will care for a child with Down syndrome, a very common disorder. Down syndrome affects 5.8 million individuals worldwide and is the most common cause of serious learning difficulties. We should all be aware that when a child with Down syndrome transitions into adulthood, the likelihood of developing dementia is very high. In fact, the dementia associated with Down syndrome is the single most common form of dementia in people younger than 50 years. Almost 40% of individuals with Down syndrome who are 60 years or older will have a diagnosis of dementia, although diagnosis is not straightforward because of an absence of validated approaches to evaluate people with intellectual disabilities. Despite antenatal screening, dementia in those with Down syndrome will continue to be an increasingly important clinical issue.

The MEADOWS (Memantine for dementia in adults older than 40 years with Down's syndrome) trial represents an important attempt to improve outcomes of adults with Down syndrome and Alzheimer disease. The trial looked at the benefits of memantine, a drug that improves cognitive function in older adults with moderate to severe Alzheimer disease in the general population. This drug was a rational choice for a trial of Alzheimer disease treatment in adults with Down syndrome for several reasons. It affects glutamate metabolism. Glutamate contributes to the pathogenesis of Alzheimer disease, in that high glutamate concentrations are thought to be neurotoxic and, in particular, to contribute to destruction of cholinergic neurons and therefore will worsen memory. Memantine is an agonist to the receptor responsible for signaling in the brain. Laboratory animals treated with this drug have shown improved learning and memory in models of Down syndrome. The entire length of chromosome 21 has now been sequenced, and we know that Down syndrome affects many aspects of brain development, brain function, and aging.

In the MEADOWS trial, 173 people with Down syndrome aged 40 years and older were randomized to treatment with memantine or placebo. Unfortunately, a year into the trial, there were no significant differences between the 2 groups in outcome measures assessing cognitive performance and function. These results are quite disappointing, but they help to exclude treatments of little benefit and prevent potential side effects and depletion of scarce resources. The findings are important because we might have assumed that patients with Down syndrome who show evidence of dementia might respond like any other patient with Alzheimer-like syndrome. Apparently they do not.

Despite the data from this report, there is optimism that the cognitive problems and neurodegeneration of Down syndrome previously regarded as intractable can be improved with pharmacological treatments, but there is a need for studies in animals to explore the potential effects of new treatment options more thoroughly before undertaking human clinical trials. The MEADOWS trial shows that randomized trials are possible in this population and should encourage future trials of potential drugs that are based on strong experimental evidence. We as pediatric care providers need to keep current with progress in this area. It is we who will inform parents of the long-term prognosis of the patients we care for with Down syndrome. With the risk of dementia being as high as it is as these patients age, it is important for us to know what lies ahead for these youngsters.

This commentary closes with an interesting observation about aging, always a relevant topic to child development and in particular to Down syndrome. PG Wodehouse and George Bernard Shaw were prolific authors who both continued writing well into old age. Researchers have examined the effect of age on linguistic markers and works by both authors using a measure of language called the MCU, mean clause per utterance.[1] This evaluation revealed no decline in language production with age for either writer. Both enjoyed good health, providing support for the age-old adage "use it or lose it" for written language production.

**J. A. Stockman III, MD**

*Reference*

1. Editorial comment. Effect of age on linguistic markers. *J Am Geriatr Soc.* 2011;59: 1567-1568.

---

**Pure Reasoning in 12-Month-Old Infants as Probabilistic Inference**
Téglás E, Vul E, Girotto V, et al (Central European Univ, Budapest, Hungary; Univ of California, San Diego, La Jolla; Univ IUAV of Venice, Italy; et al)
*Science* 332:1054-1059, 2011

---

Many organisms can predict future events from the statistics of past experience, but humans also excel at making predictions by pure reasoning: integrating multiple sources of information, guided by abstract knowledge, to form rational expectations about novel situations, never directly experienced. Here, we show that this reasoning is surprisingly rich, powerful, and coherent even in preverbal infants. When 12-month-old infants view complex displays of multiple moving objects, they form time-varying expectations about future events that are a systematic and rational function of several stimulus variables. Infants' looking times are consistent with a Bayesian ideal observer embodying abstract principles of object motion. The model explains infants' statistical expectations and classic qualitative findings about object cognition in younger babies, not originally viewed as probabilistic inferences (Fig 1).

▶ This is one of the most fascinating reports that I have read in the last several years. You will have to read it in detail, line by line, to follow the complexity of the study design, but the unequivocal results from the study indicate that preverbal infants' ability to reason about complex unseen events is surprisingly sophisticated: 12-month-olds can represent the crucial, spatial, temporal, and logical aspects of dynamic scenes with multiple objects in motion and integrate these cues with optimal context-sensitive weights to form rational expectations consistent with what much more mature adults will do in such circumstances. Having complete information with which to make predictions is a rarity and often is associated only in theoretical studies with paper and pencil. Téglás et al find that when 12-month-old infants view complex arrays of multiple moving objects, they do form rational probabilistic expectations about future events by integrating dynamic spatiotemporal cues present in a scene. To say this differently, we need to give the pretoddler a lot more respect than we may be accustomed to giving since they are in fact baby Einsteins.

While on the topic of early child development, one of the most overlooked developmental problems is something known as *development dyscalculia*. This is a mathematical disorder with an estimated prevalence of somewhere between 5% and 7%, roughly the same prevalence as developmental dyslexia. Recent neurobehavioral and genetic research suggest that dyscalculia is a coherent syndrome that reflects a single core deficit. The disability can be highly selective, affecting learners with normal or even high intelligence and normal working

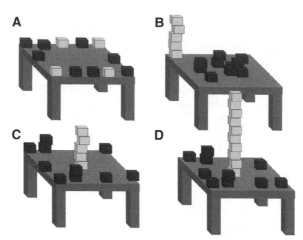

FIGURE 1.—Examples of common-sense predictions based on pure reasoning. If the table in this scene is bumped so that one block falls off the table onto the floor, is it more likely to be a red or a yellow block? Intuitions will vary according to the number of blocks of each type (A), their arrangement into more- or less-precarious stacks and their locations on the table (B), and interactions between all these factors (C and D). For interpretation of the references to color in this figure legend, the reader is referred to web version of this article. (From Téglás E, Vul E, Girotto V, et al. Pure Reasoning in 12-month-Old Infants as Probabilistic Inference. *Science*. 2011;332:1054-1059. Reprinted with permission from AAAS. Readers may view, browse, and/or download material for temporary copying purposes only, provided these uses are for noncommercial personal purposes. Except as provided by law, this material may not be further reproduced, distributed, transmitted, modified, adapted, performed, displayed, published, or sold in whole or in part, without prior written permission from the publisher.)

memory, although it frequently co-occurs with other developmental disorders, including reading disorders and attention deficit hyperactivity disorder. There are highly functioning adults who are severely dyscalculic, but still very good at geometry, using statistics packages, and doing degree-level computer programming. This low numeracy has been determined to be a substantial cost to nations. A positive one-half standard deviation in mathematics and science performance at the individual level implies, based on historical performance, an increase in annual growth rates of gross domestic product (GDP) per capita of 0.087%. Besides resulting in a reduced GDP growth, low numeracy is a substantial financial cost to governments and a personal cost to individuals. Affected individuals earn less, spend less, and are more likely to take time off for sick leave. They are also more likely to be in trouble with the law and need more help during their schooling years.[1]

To learn more about dyscalculia, see the excellent review of this topic by Butterworth et al.[2] Please note that between 2000 and 2010, the National Institutes of Health spent more than $100 million dollars on dyslexia research, but only $2.3 million dollars on dyscalculia.

This commentary closes with an observation having to do with child development. It appears that before they can even crawl, infants can distinguish between 2 languages they have never heard before just by looking at the face of a speaker. This ability is enhanced if they are raised in a bilingual household. Developmentalists at the University of British Columbia in Canada conducted a study on 8-month-old Spanish babies. Some were raised in homes in which only Spanish is spoken, some in homes whose residents spoke only Catalan, and some in bilingual homes. The investigators showed the babies a soundless video of 3 women who were bilingual speakers of French and English—languages the babies didn't know. Each was shown in turn speaking sentences in one of the languages. Eventually the babies got used to this and stopped watching. Then the language was changed. Babies raised in bilingual homes looked at the video again. The monolingual babies showed little reaction. These investigators speculate that the babies may be focusing on differences in lip shapes as the languages are spoken or can identify differing muscle movements in the face.[3] Also, it appears that 2-year-olds know more about grammar than they can actually say. Budding toddlers recognize the difference between nouns and verbs in simple sentences, even though the kids do not utter such sentences for at least another year, say investigators in Paris. Children begin to use 2 or more words at a time by age 2, but their statements are typically incomplete and show no signs of grammatical knowledge. Yet upon hearing a sentence in which a noun incorrectly replaces a verb or a verb incorrectly replaces a noun, toddlers display split second brain responses that signal awareness of the rule violation. In the study reported, youngsters were fitted with electrode caps allowing insight into brain responses after hearing mixed-up nouns and verbs. Electrical activity, mainly relegated to the left frontal brain, spiked when toddlers heard nouns in a verb position. Electrical responses farther back on the brain's left side, in the temporal lobe, jumped as toddlers heard verbs in a noun position. This experiment suggests that brain networks responsible for language processing get organized extremely early, showing striking similarities with the adult system long before children start producing adult language. Children could well have some basic syntactic knowledge by age 2, which continues to develop throughout early childhood as they identify the statistical regularities of their language.[4]

**J. A. Stockman III, MD**

*References*

1. Parsons S, Bynner J. *Does Numeracy Matter More? (National Research and Development Center for Adult Literacy and Numeracy)*. London, UK: Institute of Education; 2005.
2. Butterworth B, Varma S, Laurillard D. Dyscalculia: from brain to education. *Science*. 2011;332:1049-1053.
3. Editorial comment. Baby's watch which are say. *Science*. 2011;331:995.
4. Bower B. 2-year-olds don't talk in sentences but can still tell nouns from verbs. *Science News*. August 1, 2009:16.

## Stability of Cognitive Outcome From 2 to 5 Years of Age in Very Low Birth Weight Children

Munck P, the PIPARI Study Group (Turku Univ Hosp, Finland; et al)
*Pediatrics* 129:503-508, 2012

*Objective.*—This study assessed the stability of cognitive outcomes of premature, very low birth weight (VLBW; ≤1500 g) children.

*Methods.*—A regional cohort of 120 VLBW children born between 2001 and 2004 was followed up by using the Bayley Scales of Infant Development, Second Edition, at 2 years of corrected age and the Wechsler Preschool and Primary Scale of Intelligence—Revised at the age of 5 years. The Mental Development Index (MDI) and the full-scale IQ (FSIQ) were measured, respectively. A total of 168 randomly selected healthy term control children born in the same hospital were assessed for MDI and FSIQ.

*Results.*—In the VLBW group, mean ± SD MDI was $101.2 \pm 16.3$ (range: 50–128), mean FSIQ was $99.3 \pm 17.7$ (range: 39–132), and the correlation between MDI and FSIQ was 0.563 ($P < .0001$). In the term group, mean MDI was $109.8 \pm 11.7$ (range: 54–128), mean FSIQ was $111.7 \pm 14.5$ (range: 73–150), and the correlation between MDI and FSIQ was 0.400 ($P < .0001$). Overall, 83% of those VLBW children who had significant delay ($-2$ SD or less) according to MDI had it also in FSIQ. Similarly, 87% of those children who were in the average range in MDI were within the average range in FSIQ as well.

*Conclusions.*—Good stability of cognitive development over time was found in VLBW children and in term children between the ages of 2 and 5 years. This conclusion stresses the value and clinical significance of early assessment at 2 years of corrected age. However, we also emphasize the importance of a long-term follow-up covering a detailed neuropsychological profile of these at-risk children.

▶ Much has been written about the cognitive outcomes of low birth weight infants. This article reports on a regional cohort of very low birth weight infants born between 2001 and 2004. The importance of the study is that it recognizes that infants evaluated at 2 years of age are found to have cognitive performance that is virtually on par with that seen at 5 years of age, emphasizing the importance of the 2-year landmark.

We are also learning a great deal about behavioral outcomes of infants who were born preterm and who have suffered perinatal and neonatal insults. A recent article presented a broad systematic review of the type and probability of a range of neurodevelopmental sequelae showing a very high overall prevalence of at least 1 deficit in any domain of assessment of behavior.[1] Such studies are rarely seen in the literature. This is surprising because cognitive deficits are a cause of behavioral issues. It is likely that behavioral problems have been largely overtly ignored by investigators who have focused solely on cognitive assessments. In fact, behavioral problems are often the first sign for parents and caregivers that a child is not developing along the desired trajectory. There is an urgent need to understand and identify the signs better to achieve a fuller appreciation of the complex interactions of the neurodevelopmental sequelae of perinatal and neonatal insults. The most commonly seen sequelae that are referenced in the literature include learning difficulties, disturbed cognition, developmental delay, cerebral palsy, hearing impairment, and visual impairment. Each one of these is a risk factor for the development of behavioral disturbances.

For more on the interaction between neurodevelopmental outcomes and behavioral disturbances see the report of Mwaniki et al.[2] Last, this commentary closes with some observations on handedness. It has been observed that children age 8 who are mixed handed have a 2-fold increase in the odds of having difficulty with language and school performance, compared with right-handed children. Eight years later, these now 16-year-olds continue to have more language and school problems, often display the inattention symptoms of attention deficit hyperactivity disorder, and have symptoms scores indicating probable psychiatric disturbances. The authors suggest early identification of mixed-handed children could enable better recognition of problems.[3]

**J. A. Stockman III, MD**

*References*

1. Thompson LC, Gillberg C. Behavioural problems from perinatal and neonatal insults. *Lancet.* 2012;379:392-393.
2. Mwaniki MK, Atieno M, Lawn JE, Newton CR. Long-term neurodevelopmental outcomes after intrauterine and neonatal insults: a systematic review. *Lancet.* 2012;379:445-452.
3. Rodriguez A, Kaakinen M, Moilanen I, et al. Mixed-handedness is linked to mental health problems in children and adolescents. *Pediatrics.* 2010;125: e340-e348.

---

## Maternal Serum Vitamin D Levels During Pregnancy and Offspring Neurocognitive Development

Whitehouse AJO, Holt BJ, Serralha M, et al (Univ of Western Australia, Subiaco, Australia)
*Pediatrics* 129:485-493, 2012

---

*Objective.*—To determine the association between maternal serum 25(OH)-vitamin D concentrations during a critical window of fetal neurodevelopment and behavioral, emotional, and language outcomes of offspring.

*Methods.*—Serum 25(OH)-vitamin D concentrations of 743 Caucasian women in Perth, Western Australia (32°S) were measured at 18 weeks pregnancy and grouped into quartiles. Offspring behavior was measured with the Child Behavior Checklist at 2, 5, 8, 10, 14, and 17 years of age (*n* range = 412−652). Receptive language was assessed with the Peabody Picture Vocabulary Test—Revised at ages 5 (*n* = 534) and 10 (*n* = 474) years. Raw scores were converted to standardized scores, incorporating cutoffs for clinically significant levels of difficulty.

*Results.*—$\chi^2$ analyses revealed no significant associations between maternal 25(OH)-vitamin D serum quartiles and offspring behavioral/emotional problems at any age. In contrast, there were significant linear trends between quartiles of maternal vitamin D levels and language impairment at 5 and 10 years of age. Multivariate regression analyses, incorporating a range of confounding variables, found that the risk of women with vitamin D insufficiency (≤46 nmol/L) during pregnancy having a child with clinically significant language difficulties was increased close to twofold compared with women with vitamin D levels >70 nmol/L.

*Conclusions.*—Maternal vitamin D insufficiency during pregnancy is significantly associated with offspring language impairment. Maternal vitamin D supplementation during pregnancy may reduce the risk of developmental language difficulties among their children.

▶ Much has been written recently about the role of vitamin D. Data about vitamin D in the literature are no longer limited to the effects of this vitamin on bone and mineral metabolism. For example, there has also been a strong suspicion that maternal vitamin D insufficiency during pregnancy can have effects on fetal brain development. Studies in animals have linked low maternal 25-hydroxy-vitamin D levels during pregnancy with atypical behavior. If these data translate into the human situation, the impact could theoretically be quite high because it has been estimated that vitamin D insufficiency can be observed in up to 60% of white women. The rate among women with dark skin is estimated to be even higher.

These authors report on a large-scale longitudinal study of the association between maternal 25-dihydroxy-vitamin D concentrations measured during the second trimester and behavioral and language development of offspring to age 17 years. Enrollees in this study were from the Western Australian Pregnancy Cohort Study, a sample of pregnant women and their offspring from Perth, Western Australia. The current study investigated only white mothers and their offspring. Offspring behavior was measured with the Child Behavior Check List at 2, 5, 8, 10, 14, and 17 years of age. The study results represent the largest investigation to date of the association between maternal 1,25-dihydroxy-vitamin D status during pregnancy and offspring neurocognitive development. The study showed that there was no statistically significant association between maternal 25-dihydroxy-vitamin D concentrations during pregnancy and offspring behavioral and emotional difficulties. However, strong associations were observed with language impairment at 5 and 10 years of age. The risk of women with 25-dihydroxy-vitamin D insufficiency during pregnancy having a child with clinically significant language difficulties was increased close to 2-fold when compared with women who were vitamin D sufficient, even after taking into account all other significant variables.

This report is consistent with others suggesting that the developing fetus is completely reliant on maternal vitamin D stores, and thus the concentration of maternal circulating levels at 18 weeks' pregnancy would be expected to provide an accurate measure of fetal exposure during the second trimester. The study also supports the understanding that vitamin D does perform a number of biological functions that are fundamental to neurodevelopment, including a signaling role in the metabolism of neurotrophic factors and neurotoxins and a protective role against brain inflammation. Vitamin D may exercise this role through an interaction with a number of endocrine functions. The findings from this article also suggest a developing trend over the past 10 years of a reduction in vitamin D levels among women of reproductive age, at least in Western Australia. This has significant implications for offspring neurodevelopment and public health more generally. Randomized controlled trials of vitamin D supplementation are required to verify these observational data that suggest an adequate maternal vitamin D status during pregnancy is necessary for optimal language development in offspring.

This commentary closes with an observation about Tiny Tim and vitamin D. Recently, Russell Chesney commented on the condition that affected Tiny Tim in Charles Dickens's *A Christmas Carol*.[1] Chesney posits that an examination of the environment of London from 1820 to 1843, when the novella was written, provides important clues to Tiny Tim's condition. The blackened skies from coal burning, the crowding of people in tenements, the limited diet of the underclass, and the filth of London resulted in a haven for infectious diseases and rickets. Sixty percent of children at that time had rickets and nearly 50% had signs of tuberculosis. Chesney suggests that the key young character in Charles Dickens's novella had a combination of both diseases. It appears that Dickens was familiar with both rickets and tuberculosis and wrote about cod liver oil as a possible preventative treatment for both. Improved vitamin D status can result in enhanced macrophage synthesis of 25-dihydroxy-vitamin D. This component of the innate immune system has strong killing properties for the organism that causes tuberculosis. The combination of both rickets and tuberculosis therefore represented a crippling condition that could have been reversed by improved vitamin D status. That is Chesney's theory, and not a bad one at that!

**J. A. Stockman III, MD**

*Reference*

1. Chesney RW. Environmental factors in Tiny Tim's near fatal illness. *Arch Pediatr Adolesc Med.* 2012;166:271-275.

---

**Iron-Fortified vs Low-Iron Infant Formula: Developmental Outcome at 10 Years**
Lozoff B, Castillo M, Clark KM, et al (Univ of Michigan, Ann Arbor; Oakland Univ, Rochester, MI)
*Arch Pediatr Adolesc Med* 166:208-215, 2012

---

*Objective.*—To assess long-term developmental outcome in children who received iron-fortified or low-iron formula.

*Design.*—Follow-up at 10 years of a randomized controlled trial (1991-1994) of 2 levels of formula iron. Examiners were masked to group assignment.

*Setting.*—Urban areas around Santiago, Chile.

*Participants.*—The original study enrolled healthy, fullterm infants in community clinics; 835 completed the trial. At 10 years, 473 were assessed (56.6%).

*Intervention.*—Iron-fortified (mean, 12.7 mg/L) or low-iron (mean, 2.3 mg/L) formula from 6 to 12 months.

*Main Outcome Measures.*—We measured IQ, spatial memory, arithmetic achievement, visual-motor integration, visual perception, and motor functioning. We used covaried regression to compare iron-fortified and low-iron groups and considered hemoglobin level before randomization and sensitivity analyses to identify 6-month hemoglobin levels at which groups diverged in outcome.

*Results.*—Compared with the low-iron group, the iron-fortified group scored lower on every 10-year outcome (significant for spatial memory and visual-motor integration; suggestive for IQ, arithmetic achievement, visual perception, and motor coordination; 1.4-4.6 points lower; effect sizes, 0.13-0.21). Children with high 6-month hemoglobin levels (>12.8 g/dL [to convert to grams per liter, multiply by 10]) showed poorer outcome on these measures if they received iron-fortified formula (10.7-19.3 points lower; large effect sizes, 0.85-1.36); those with low hemoglobin levels (<10.5 g/dL) showed better outcome (2.6-4.5 points higher; small but significant effects, 0.22-0.36). High hemoglobin levels represented 5.5% of the sample (n = 26) and low hemoglobin levels represented 18.4% (n = 87).

*Conclusion.*—Long-term development may be adversely affected in infants with high hemoglobin levels who receive 12.7 mg/L of iron-fortified formula. Optimal amounts of iron in infant formula warrant further study.

*Trial Registration.*—clinicaltrials.gov Identifier: NCT01166451.

▶ These authors have written frequently over the years about the long-term effects of iron deficiency on child development. In this article, the authors report the findings of a long-term follow-up of children aged 10 years who were participants in a randomized controlled trial conducted from 1991 through 1994 in Santiago, Chile. The trial tested whether iron-fortified formula versus low-iron formula used at 6 to 12 months of age would make any difference in developmental outcome markers. The iron-fortified formula contained 12.7 mg/L iron. The low-iron formula contained just 2.3 mg/L iron. Curiously, the mean scores on tests of spatial memory and visual motor integration at 10 years of age were lower in the iron-fortified formula recipients compared with the control, although the actual effect of the difference was quite small. The former had significantly higher hemoglobin levels at all ages tested.

The importance of this study lies in the evaluation of the long-term developmental outcomes of an early infancy iron intervention program. Few such studies exist in the literature. The relation between iron deficiency and iron-deficiency anemia and developmental outcomes in children has been controversial. The authors of this report have made significant contributions to establish such a link and have demonstrated in longitudinal observational studies that iron deficiency early in life can result in cognitive and motor impairments that may be irreversible. They have previously also documented longer-term associations in 5-year-olds and 10-year-olds, showing poor developmental outcomes in children who were iron deficient and anemic in the first year of life. Christian et al[1] showed significant improvements in aspects of intelligence, executive function, including working memory and inhibitory control, and fine motor function with the use of antenatal iron—folic acid supplementation relative to a control in a prospective study of children aged 7 to 9 years whose mothers participated in an antenatal micronutrient supplementation trial in rural Nepal. That study suggests that it is just as important to supply adequate amounts of iron prior to birth as after birth.

Is there an explanation for the poor developmental outcome in children with high hemoglobin levels who have received high amounts of iron supplementation in the first year of life? Is there a link between high hemoglobin levels and poor developmental outcomes? Iron is not the only thing that can raise hemoglobin levels. Chronic hypoxia can as well. No information is provided in this report about the altitude at which the study subjects lived. Also, paternal smoking has been associated with poor developmental outcomes in some studies and can also elevate infant hemoglobin levels due to chronic mild hypoxia. It is also possible that under certain circumstances the growing brain may be vulnerable to iron. Iron is a catalyst in the auto-oxidation of fatty acids. Again this can be harmful in certain circumstances, particularly in hypoxic states. It is clear that iron is an essential nutrient of which both too little and too much are problematic.

Unfortunately, this study cannot be compared with other studies because there are no comparable studies. This study does indicate poorer long-term developmental outcome and infants with high hemoglobin concentrations who received formula fortified with iron at levels currently used in the United States. Needless to say this report is puzzling. A similar study in the United States is badly needed. Is it possible that iron, on occasion, is too much of a good thing?

This commentary closes with a somewhat unrelated topic on child development: the unfortunate circumstances facing "Baby Einstein." Cofounder of the company that introduced the popular Baby Einstein videos has sued to obtain records of researchers whose work casts doubt on the value of the series. William Clark, who founded the Baby Einstein company with his wife in 1996, has sued the University of Washington over warnings suggesting that TV-immersed toddlers may be at risk for the later development of attention problems and that watching baby videos could be associated with delays in language development. As an aside, the Clarks sold their business to Disney in 2001, which has toned down its claims about the value of Baby Einstein. In September 2009, facing the threat of a class-action suit, the company announced they would give refunds to dissatisfied parents.

To read more about this, see a review of the topic in *Science*.[2]

**J. A. Stockman III, MD**

*References*

1. Christian P, Murray-Kolb LE, Khatry SK, et al. Prenatal micronutrient supplementation and intellectual and motor function in early school-aged children in the Nepal. *JAMA*. 2010;304:2716-2723.
2. Holden C. Baby Einstein goes to court. *Science*. 2010;327:507.

## Early Diagnoses of Autism Spectrum Disorders in Massachusetts Birth Cohorts, 2001–2005

Manning SE, Davin CA, Barfield WD, et al (Bureau of Family Health and Nutrition, Boston, MA; Ctrs for Disease Control and Prevention, Atlanta, GA; et al)
*Pediatrics* 127:1043-1051, 2011

*Objective.*—We examined trends in autism spectrum disorder diagnoses by age 36 months (early diagnoses) and identified characteristics associated with early diagnoses.

*Methods.*—Massachusetts birth certificate and early-intervention program data were linked to identify infants born between 2001 and 2005 who were enrolled in early intervention and receiving autism-related services before age 36 months (through December 31, 2008). Trends in early autism spectrum disorders were examined using Cochran-Armitage trend tests. $\chi^2$ Statistics were used to compare distributions of selected characteristics for children with and without autism spectrum disorders. Multivariate logistic regression analyses were conducted to identify independent predictors of early diagnoses.

*Results.*—A total of 3013 children (77.5 per 10 000 study population births) were enrolled in early intervention for autism spectrum disorder by age 36 months. Autism spectrum disorder incidence increased from 56 per 10 000 infants among the 2001 birth cohort to 93 per 10 000 infants in 2005. Infants of mothers younger than 24 years of age, whose primary language was not English or who were foreign-born had lower odds of an early autism spectrum disorder diagnosis. Maternal age older than 30 years was associated with increased odds of an early autism spectrum disorder diagnosis. Odds of early autism spectrum disorders were 4.5 (95% confidence interval: 4.1–5.0) times higher for boys than girls.

*Conclusions.*—Early autism spectrum disorder diagnoses are increasing in Massachusetts, reflecting the national trend observed among older children. Linkage of early-intervention program data with population-based vital statistics is valuable for monitoring autism spectrum disorder trends and planning developmental and educational service needs.

▶ Massachusetts is among the few states that have collected excellent data on the prevalence of certain developmental disorders, including autism spectrum disorders (ASDs). Clearly autism is an important and growing public health concern with substantial impacts upon those affected and their families. Early identification of ASDs and initiation of developmental services can improve developmental and educational outcomes. Until this report from Massachusetts appeared, state-level, population-based estimates of ASD occurrence among children from birth through 3 years of age have been somewhat lacking. In 1998, Massachusetts created the Early Intervention Specialty Services Program to address the unique needs of children with ASDs. Approaching $11 million annually, the cost of ASD specialty services in Massachusetts has been increasing.

Data from Massachusetts show that among 388 644 children born in Massachusetts between 2001 and 2005 who survived to age 3 years, 3013 (78 per 10 000 births) were enrolled in early intervention for ASDs by 36 months of age. ASD incidence increased from 56 per 10 000 for the 2001 birth cohort to 93 per 10 000 for the 2005 cohort. Among boys, early ASD diagnoses increased more than 70% from 88 per 10 000 children for the 2001 birth cohort to 151 per 10 000 for the 2005 cohort. ASD diagnosis among girls increased by only 39% over the same period (from 23 per 10 000 to 32 per 10 000 children). Non-Hispanic white children had the highest incidence (63 per 10 000), 29% higher than non-Hispanic black children and 62% higher than non-Hispanic, other, including non-Hispanic Asian/Pacific Islanders and 90% higher than Hispanic children of any race. These findings indicate that 1 of every 129 children born in Massachusetts can be expected to be enrolled in an early intervention ASD program by 3 years of age. Having a baby when one is older than 30 years is also associated with significantly increased odds of an early diagnosis of ASD in a child by 3 years of age.

The obvious question, of course, is whether autism is actually increasing in both incidence and prevalence or whether our capability of diagnosing the disorder has improved. At the same time, society is placing greater demands on the appropriate diagnosis of this disorder. It should be noted that it was recently reported that the prevalence of autism among children age 7 to 14 years in South Korea is now 2.6%. That is more than twice the estimated rate overall in the United States.[1] It is interesting to note that children of Asian descent born in the United States have a much lower incidence of autism than those born overseas, for example, in South Korea.

**J. A. Stockman III, MD**

*Reference*

1. Editorial comment. Autism prevalence in South Korea. *Science*. 2011;332:775.

---

**The Prevalence of Gastrointestinal Problems in Children Across the United States With Autism Spectrum Disorders From Families With Multiple Affected Members**

Wang LW, Tancredi DJ, Thomas DW (Univ of California at Davis Med Ctr, Sacramento; Univ of California, Davis, Sacramento; Keck School of Medicine at the Univ of Southern California, Los Angeles)
*J Dev Behav Pediatr* 32:351-360, 2011

---

*Objective.*—To perform a large registry-based study to determine the relative prevalence of gastrointestinal (GI) problems in children with an autism spectrum disorder (ASD) from families with multiple affected members compared with their unaffected sibling(s).

*Methods.*—In-home structured retrospective medical history interviews by parent recall were conducted by a pediatric neurologist. Our analysis sample included information about GI health of 589 subjects with idiopathic, familial ASD and 163 of their unaffected sibling controls registered with Autism Genetic Resource Exchange. Individuals with ASD were subgrouped into 3 autism severity groups (Full Autism, Almost Autism, and Spectrum) based on their Autism Diagnostic Interview—Revised and Autism Diagnostic Observation Scale scores.

*Results.*—Parents reported significantly more GI problems in children with ASD (249/589; 42%) compared with their unaffected siblings (20/163; 12%) (*p* < .001). The 2 most common GI problems in children with ASD were constipation (116/589; 20%) and chronic diarrhea (111/589; 19%). Conditional logistic regression analysis showed that having Full Autism (adjusted odds ratio [AOR] = 14.28, 95% confidence interval [CI]: 6.22—32.77) or Almost Autism (AOR = 5.16, 95% CI 2.02—13.21) was most highly associated with experiencing GI problems. Increased autism symptom severity was associated with higher odds of GI problems (AOR for trend = 2.63, 95% CI: 1.56—4.45).

*Conclusions.*—Parents report significantly more GI problems in children with familial ASD, especially those with Full Autism, than in their unaffected children. Increased autism symptom severity is associated with increased odds of having GI problems.

▶ The aim of the Wang et al study was to determine the relative lifetime prevalence of gastrointestinal problems in a large cohort of children affected with autism spectrum disorder (ASD). The study also examined whether the prevalence of gastrointestinal symptoms differed between subgroups of children with ASD based on the severity of autism symptoms. The authors theorize that an increased prevalence of gastrointestinal problems would be observed in ASDs compared with unaffected siblings. The published literature has been inconsistent regarding the prevalence of gastrointestinal symptoms in children with ASD. The reported prevalence of gastrointestinal symptomatology in children with ASD has ranged from a low of about 10% to a high of almost 85%.[1]

The study of Wang et al collected information about gastrointestinal health from almost 600 subjects with idiopathic, familial ASD and used comparative data with unaffected sibling controls. The study represents the largest done to date comparing the relative lifetime prevalence of gastrointestinal problems in this population.

The results of this study document an increased lifetime prevalence of gastrointestinal problems in children with ASD. Increased autism symptom severity is associated with increased odds of having significantly more gastrointestinal problems reported. For example, the study shows that youngsters with full autism have a greater than 14-fold increased probability of having gastrointestinal problems in comparison with their non—ASD-affected siblings. The prevalence of gastrointestinal problems in the full autism group was 47%. The most common symptoms were constipation and chronic diarrhea. Ten percent of autistic children have a variety of other gastrointestinal problems, including colic, lactose intolerance, and vomiting related to motion sickness. Five percent have gastroesophageal reflux.

While on the topic of childhood-related developmental issues, would you believe that as recently as just 50 years ago, left-handed children were still being forced to attempt to write with their right hands? The origins of the latter go all the way back to the Zulus of South Africa. Among the Zulu tribes, eating with the left hand was taboo. It was noted that if a child ate porridge with his or her left hand, parents were taught that both hands of such a child should be put into the hot porridge as an object lesson.[2] The Zulus believed that the left hand was used for "mean" purposes such as scraping away dirt, so it must not be used for other purposes. Like the Zulus, many North and East African peoples attempted to "cure" left handedness. Similar practices have been identified by anthropologists in many other indigenous cultures. Over many centuries, a complicated picture has emerged in which early human cultures evolved into current ones with ambivalence toward left handedness, suggesting that suppression of left-handedness would in fact serve specific cultural agendas. As late as 1946, the chief psychiatrist of the New York City Board of Education, Abram Blau, warned that, unless retrained, left-handed children risked severe developmental and learning disabilities and insisted that children should be encouraged in their early years to adopt dextrality to become better equipped to live in our right-sided world.

For what it is worth, England's Duke of York, the future King George VI (1895-1952), had been forced to write with his right hand. As everyone now knows from the famous film *The King's Speech*, the Duke, who was naturally left-handed, also stuttered. Unfortunately, the poor Duke felt that part of his stuttering problem was related to a forced retraining of his left-handedness.

This commentary closes with mention of a recent report that suggests there may be some relationship between being born blind and the development of autism. Specifically, being born into a world of darkness seems to provide an unappreciated avenue to autism. Within the first few months of life babies have been shown to display a basic form of what researchers call joint attention. An infant will maintain a steady gaze with a nearby adult and imitate that adult's simple actions. By age 2, joint attention becomes more complex. Two children, for example, can convey with just a look that they know which toy is better. Developmental specialists view joint attention as a skill essential to forming relationships with others and communicating effectively. Blindness from birth can lead to difficulties that block emotional contact with others, fostering autism, at least as noted in one report. Autism-related blindness stems from the inability to see anyone or anything, making it exceedingly difficult to achieve joint attention. Fortunately, among blind children—related symptoms seem to diminish by adolescence. At British schools for the blind, a team of investigators assessed 24 congenitally blind children, ages 3 years through 9 years. Autism symptoms, such as lack of social and communication skills appeared in all the children. Half met the diagnostic criteria for autism. Compared with 9 sighted children with autism, low-functioning blind children with the developmental disorder showed slightly more engagement with others. Eight years later, all 9 sighted children were still considered to be autistic, compared with only 1 blind child. Thus the outlook for the autism (or autismlike) disorder seen in blind children is good.[3]

**J. A. Stockman III, MD**

*References*

1. Ibrahim SH, Voigt RG, Katusic SK, et al. Incidence of gastrointestinal symptoms in children with autism: a population-based study. *Pediatrics.* 2009;124:680-686.
2. Kushner HI. Retraining the King's left hand. *Lancet.* 2011;377:1998-1999.
3. Bower D. A blind path to childhood autism. Infants born without sight may have more social difficulties. *Science News.* November 7, 2009.

---

**Outcomes of population based language promotion for slow to talk toddlers at ages 2 and 3 years: Let's learn language cluster randomised controlled trial**

Wake M, Tobin S, Girolametto L, et al (Murdoch Childrens Res Inst and Univ of Melbourne, Parkville, Victoria, Australia; Univ of Toronto, Ontario, Canada; et al)
*BMJ* 343:d4741, 2011

---

*Objective.*—To determine the benefits of a low intensity parent-toddler language promotion programme delivered to toddlers identified as slow to talk on screening in universal services.

*Design.*—Cluster randomised trial nested in a population based survey.

*Setting.*—Three local government areas in Melbourne, Australia.

*Participants.*—Parents attending 12 month well child checks over a six month period completed a baseline questionnaire. At 18 months, children at or below the 20th centile on an expressive vocabulary checklist entered the trial.

*Intervention.*—Maternal and child health centres (clusters) were randomly allocated to intervention (modified "You Make the Difference" programme over six weekly sessions) or control ("usual care") arms.

*Main Outcome Measures.*—The primary outcome was expressive language (Preschool Language Scale-4) at 2 and 3 years; secondary outcomes were receptive language at 2 and 3 years, vocabulary checklist raw score at 2 and 3 years, Expressive Vocabulary Test at 3 years, and Child Behavior Checklist/1.5-5 raw score at 2 and 3 years.

*Results.*—1217 parents completed the baseline survey; 1138 (93.5%) completed the 18 month checklist, when 301 (26.4%) children had vocabulary scores at or below the 20th centile and were randomised (158 intervention, 143 control). 115 (73%) intervention parents attended at least one session (mean 4.5 sessions), and most reported high satisfaction with the programme. Interim outcomes at age 2 years were similar in the two groups. Similarly, at age 3 years, adjusted mean differences (intervention−control) were −2.4 (95% confidence interval −6.2 to 1.4; $P = 0.21$) for expressive language; −0.3 (−4.2 to 3.7; $P = 0.90$) for receptive language; 4.1 (−2.3 to 10.6; $P = 0.21$) for vocabulary checklist; −0.5 (−4.4 to 3.4; $P = 0.80$)

for Expressive Vocabulary Test; $-0.1$ ($-1.6$ to $1.4$; $P = 0.86$) for externalising behaviour problems; and $-0.1$ ($-1.3$ to $1.2$; $P = 0.92$) for internalising behaviour problems.

*Conclusion.*—This community based programme targeting slow to talk toddlers was feasible and acceptable, but little evidence was found that it improved language or behaviour either immediately or at age 3 years.

*Trial registration.*—Current Controlled Trials ISRCTN20953675.

▶ The report of Wake et al is from Australia. These investigators designed a study that included a randomized controlled trial of a community-based program to promote language skills in young children who were known to be slow to talk at 18 months of age. Children who scored below the 20th percentile at 18 months of age on standardized parent-reported checklists of expressive language were randomly assigned to an intervention group or to a usual care control group. The intervention comprised 6 two-hour group-based training sessions for parents that included coaching using video tapes of the parent and child to encourage effective child centered interaction over a 6-week period. The study found no significant differences between the groups and parent-reported measures of expressive language and behavior or blinded assessment of expressive and receptive language by professionals using standardized tests at 2 years and 3 years of age.

Despite the apparent negative results from this report, the study does provide insight into the feasibility of a secondary prevention program for language disorders. This large-scale population-based study cost just over $900 per family, targeted parents who were worried about their children's language development, and included children who were learning English as well as an additional language. The authors of this report suggested that the reason for finding little improvement in the intervention group may relate to the fact that 43% of families attended fewer than half of the available sessions, and only 57% attended 4 or more sessions.

In terms of the implications of this report for practice, the study highlights the importance of undertaking well-designed clinical trials to inform the best use of resources. It is also clear from the data from Australia that early and reliable identification of language delay prior to 24 months of age is problematic in all but the most severe cases. This probably relates to the wide variation that is seen in normal development. A significant proportion of the control group in this study who had "delayed" speech at 18 months of age had caught up with their typically developing peers by 36 months of age and did so without any intervention. The issue for the average family is whether watchful waiting is as good as treatments of the type described if there are no findings other than delayed speech at 18 months of age.

To read more about speech and language delays in preschool children, see the excellent editorial by Boyle.[1] This commentary closes with a query: you are seeing a 10-year-old for a routine office visit. His mother has an unusual question for you. It appears this child had an IQ test performed at school and the youngster was four standard deviations above the norm for IQ. The mother's question is "will this high IQ lead to a longer life for this youngster?" How would you answer this question? The answer may be found in a report of Lager et al.[2] It appears that in Malmo, Sweden, children back in the 1930s had IQ tests routinely performed at age 10. Data are available on all 1530 school children who had such IQ testing in 1938. This allowed a comparison of IQ with longevity. The results showed that for both sexes, one's personal educational attainment was clearly associated with survival, even beyond the importance of early IQ. With respect to schooling, each additional year in school was associated with a reduced risk of dying when IQ and father's education was adjusted for (hazard ratio for each additional year in school, 0.91 for men and 0.88 for women). Higher early IQ was also linked with a reduced mortality in men, even when educational attainment and father's education were adjusted for. In contrast, there was no crude effect of early IQ measurement on mortality for women, and women with above average IQ had an increased mortality when educational attainment was adjusted for, but only after the age of 60 (hazard ratio 1.60).

So the answer to this mother's query is that yes her son statistically is likely to live a bit longer than his peers. Why smart girls die younger than their not-so-brainy peers, however, remains a mystery. It is pretty obvious that sugar and spice and everything nice may not permit one to live long enough to enjoy dessert.

**J. A. Stockman III, MD**

*References*

1. Boyle J. Speech and language delays in preschool children. *BMJ*. 2011;343:d5181.
2. Lager A, Bremberg S, Vagero D. The association of early IQ and education with mortality: 65 year longitudinal study in Malmo, Sweden. *BMJ*. 2009;339:1432.

---

**GIT1 is associated with ADHD in humans and ADHD-like behaviors in mice**

Won H, Mah W, Kim E, et al (Korea Advanced Inst of Science and Technology (KAIST), Daejeon; et al)
*Nat Med* 17:566-572, 2011

---

Attention deficit hyperactivity disorder (ADHD) is a psychiatric disorder that affects ~5% of school-aged children; however, the mechanisms underlying ADHD remain largely unclear. Here we report a previously unidentified association between G protein–coupled receptor kinase–interacting protein-1 (GIT1) and ADHD in humans. An intronic single-nucleotide polymorphism in *GIT1*, the minor allele of which causes reduced *GIT1* expression, shows a strong association with ADHD susceptibility in humans. *Git1*-deficient mice show ADHD-like phenotypes, with traits including hyperactivity, enhanced electroencephalogram theta rhythms and impaired learning and memory. Hyperactivity in *Git1*$^{-/-}$ mice is reversed by amphetamine and methylphenidate, psychostimulants commonly used to treat ADHD. In addition, amphetamine normalizes enhanced theta rhythms and impaired memory. GIT1 deficiency in mice leads to decreases in ras-related C3 botulinum toxin substrate-1 (RAC1) signaling and inhibitory presynaptic input; furthermore, it shifts the neuronal excitation-inhibition balance in postsynaptic neurons toward excitation. Our study identifies a previously unknown involvement of GIT1 in human ADHD and shows that GIT1 deficiency in mice causes psychostimulant-responsive ADHD-like phenotypes.

▶ It has been believed for some time that attention deficit hyperactivity disorder (ADHD) has, at least in part, a hereditary basis. A solid 5% of children world-wide have the problem as defined by impaired attention, hyperactivity, and impulsivity. Although many factors are involved in ADHD, genes are known to have a key role because this condition is highly heritable. Psychostimulants, such as amphetamine and methylphenidate, are commonly used to treat ADHD, but serious long-term side effects make their widespread use controversial. This is why the hope is held out that the finding of ADHD-associated genes could lead to a better understanding of this condition and subsequently to new treatments with fewer side effects.

Several genes that are related to dopamine or other aspects of monoaminergic signaling have been associated with ADHD. On this basis, abnormalities in neurotransmitters might hold the solution to treatment of the problem. Stimulant drugs may act by increasing the amounts of dopamine and other neurotransmitters in the brain. Won et al have now identified GIT1 as a previously undescribed ADHD susceptibility gene in humans. Mice deficient in this gene show clinical findings similar to ADHD. The gene produces GIT1, a multifunctional adaptor protein. The protein regulates a number of central nervous system functions. Besides identifying GIT1 as a potential ADHD candidate gene, Won et al found 1 single nucleotide polymorphism (SNP) in GIT1 that was highly associated with ADHD susceptibility in children. They now report an association between this intronic SNP and ADHD susceptibility both in humans and in mice.

Needless to say, there are caveats in studies that involve modeling of psychiatric disorders, especially highly polygenic disorders such as ADHD. In addition to an SNP, ADHD is affected by environmental factors that yet remain unknown. Despite cautionary notes, it is obvious that mice with mutations in GIT1 will be invaluable tools to probe the mechanisms of hyperactivity. It is certain that you will be hearing much more from these investigators and their mice.

This commentary closes with an observation having to do with learning. College students have known for decades that information they try to learn just before sleep seems to be reinforced by sleep itself. This belief is now reinforced by recent studies. It turns out that people who have nap-time dreams about a task they have just practiced get a memory boost on the task upon awakening. In one study, 99 college students age 18 years to 30 years spent 45 minutes navigating a virtual 3D maze on a computer. They were instructed to remember the location of a particular tree in the maze, then were given a 5-hour break. For the first 90 minutes of the break, the students were assigned either to take a nap or to engage in quiet activities such as watching videos. In a second try at the maze, nappers who reported dreaming about the maze task—4 out of 50—found the tree much faster than they had in initial trials. These individuals describe dreams such as seeing people at particular locations in a maze or hearing music that had played in the laboratory during testing. In this case, a 90-minute snooze mostly involves non–rapid eye movement (NREM) sleep. Previous studies have found links between brain activity during NREM sleep and better learning by rats and people. Neural activity sparked by recent learning has not been observed during REM sleep, which often includes especially vivid and bizarre dreams. The researchers now plan to examine whether people who have REM dreams about a maze task during a full night's slumber navigate that maze better the next day.[1]

**J. A. Stockman III, MD**

*Reference*

1. Bower B. Practice. Dream. Improve. Repeat. Nap-time reveries may be the brain training itself to do better. *Science News*. May 22, 2010:12.

---

**Shyness Versus Social Phobia in US Youth**
Burstein M, Ameli-Grillon L, Merikangas KR (Natl Inst of Mental Health, Bethesda, MD)
*Pediatrics* 128:917-925, 2011

---

*Objectives.*—Scholars and the popular press have suggested that the diagnostic entity of social phobia "medicalizes" normal human shyness. In this study we examined the plausibility of this hypothesis by (1) determining the frequency of shyness and its overlap with social phobia in a nationally representative adolescent sample, (2) investigating the degree to which shyness and social phobia differ with regard to sociodemographic characteristics, functional impairment, and psychiatric comorbidity, and (3) examining differences in rates of prescribed medication use among youth with shyness and/or social phobia.

*Methods.*—The National Comorbidity Survey-Adolescent Supplement is a nationally representative, face-to-face survey of 10 123 adolescents, aged 13 to 18 years, in the continental United States. Lifetime social phobia was assessed by using a modified version of the fully structured World Health Organization Composite International Diagnostic Interview. Adolescents and parents also provided information on youth shyness and prescribed medication use.

*Results.*—Only 12% of the youth who identified themselves as shy also met the criteria for lifetime social phobia. Relative to adolescents who were characterized as shy, adolescents affected with social phobia displayed significantly greater role impairment and were more likely to experience a multitude of psychiatric disorders, including disorders of anxiety, mood, behavior, and substance use. However, those adolescents were no more likely than their same-age counterparts to be taking prescribed medications.

*Conclusions.*—The results of this study provide evidence that social phobia is an impairing psychiatric disorder, beyond normal human shyness.

Such findings raise questions concerning the "medicalization" hypothesis of social phobia.

▶ Where is the line between shyness and social phobia? Is there a line? All too often, the field of psychiatry has come under criticism for defining as pathology what otherwise is a truly normal variation in human behavior. This particular criticism has been highly evident for the condition known now as social phobia, particularly as it applies to children and adolescents. Some have suggested that the pharmaceutical industry and related scientific experts have sought to publicize social phobia in pursuit of particular pharmaceutical sales.[1]

Burstein et al note that only a minority of studies have examined the characteristics and associated impairments of social phobia in general population samples of young individuals, and none has investigated the degree to which shyness and social phobia differ with regard to those features. Based on this lack, the authors of this report designed a study to examine the frequency of shyness and its overlap with social phobia in a nationally representative sample of adolescents. They also investigated the potential differences between shyness and social phobia with respect to sociodemographic correlates; indices of impairment, and psychiatric comorbidity. Last, they examined rates of prescribed medication use among adolescents with shyness and/or social phobia. The diagnostic criteria used to define social phobia were the psychiatric classifications in *Diagnostic and Statistical Manual of Mental Disorders*, Fourth Edition, (*DSM-IV*). Data were gleaned from the National Comorbidity Survey Replication, Adolescent Supplement, a nationally representative, face-to-face survey of 10 123 adolescents aged 13 to 18 years.

In this report, we see that 46.7% of adolescents thought they were shy. In contrast, only 8.6% of adolescents met the *DSM-IV* criteria for social phobia at some point in their lifetimes. Of those individuals who identified themselves as shy, just 12.4% met the criteria for lifetime social phobia. Among youth who were not considered shy by their own reports or their parents' reports, about 5% met the criteria for social phobia.

The findings of this study strongly replicate previous investigations involving college students; those investigations found fairly low rates of social phobia among individuals who are shy. In addition, the report showed a nontrivial portion of youth who met the criteria for social phobia but who were not considered shy by either themselves or their parents. This is the first study to examine the rate of shyness and its overlap with social phobia in a nationally representative sample of US adolescents. It is also the first to investigate the degree to which features of these entities differ in the general population of adolescents. Social phobia is an impairing psychiatric disorder that goes beyond human shyness, but it must be carefully defined. It does appear that among many adolescents with true social phobia, very few ever seek or obtain professional help.

This commentary closes with a bit of psychology related to stock market traders. Stock market traders apparently regulate their emotional responses better because they are used to keeping market volatility in perspective, while the rest of us tend to fear potential loss more than we anticipate potential gain. A study has shown that the increased physiologic arousal and behavioral effects relating to this "loss aversion" are greatly ameliorated when people are advised to think more like stock traders. Count me on one end of the bell-shaped curve balanced on the other end by a Wall Street fellow named Gordon Gekko.[2]

**J. A. Stockman III, MD**

*References*

1. Lane LC. *Shyness: How Normal Behavior Became a Sickness.* New Haven, CT: Yale University Press; 2007.
2. Proceedings of the National Academy of Sciences 2009; Published online March 16. Doi: 10.1073/pnas.0806761106.

# 5 Dentistry and Otolaryngology (ENT)

**Medicaid Payment Levels to Dentists and Access to Dental Care Among Children and Adolescents**
Decker SL (Natl Ctr for Health Statistics, Hyattsville, MD)
*JAMA* 306:187-193, 2011

*Context.*—Although Medicaid removes most financial barriers to receipt of dental care among children and adolescents, Medicaid recipients may not be able to access dental care if dentists decline to participate in Medicaid because of low payment levels or other reasons.

*Objective.*—To describe the association between state Medicaid dental fees in 2 years (2000 and 2008) and children's receipt of dental care.

*Design, Setting, and Participants.*—Data on Medicaid dental fees in 2000 and 2008 for 42 states plus the District of Columbia were merged with data from 33,657 children and adolescents (aged 2-17 years) in the National Health Interview Survey (NHIS) for the years 2000-2001 and 2008-2009. Logit models were used to estimate the probability that children and adolescents had seen a dentist in the past 6 months as a function of the Medicaid prophylaxis fee and control variables including age group, race, poverty status, and state and year effects. The effect of fees on children with Medicaid relative to a control group, privately insured counterparts, served to separate Medicaid's effect on access to care from any correlation between the Medicaid fee or changes in fees by state and other attributes of states.

*Main Outcome Measure.*—Whether a child or adolescent had seen a dentist in the past 6 months.

*Results.*—On average, Medicaid dental payment levels did not change significantly in inflation-adjusted terms between 2000 and 2008, although a difference existed for some states, including in 5 states plus the District of Columbia, where payments increased at least 50%. In 2008-2009, more children and adolescents covered by Medicaid (55%, 95% confidence interval [CI], 53%-57%) had seen a dentist in the past 6 months than did uninsured children (27%, 95% CI, 24%-30%), but fewer than children covered by private insurance (68%, 95% CI, 67%-70%). Changes in state Medicaid dental payment fees between 2000 and 2008 were positively associated with use of dental care among children and adolescents covered by Medicaid. For example, a $10 increase in the Medicaid prophylaxis payment level (from $20 to $30) was associated with a 3.92 percentage point (95% CI, 0.54-7.50) increase in the chance that a child or adolescent covered by Medicaid had seen a dentist.

*Conclusion.*—Higher Medicaid payment levels to dentists were associated with higher rates of receipt of dental care among children and adolescents.

▶ Most of us do not pay a lot of attention to how the Medicaid system is structured to provide dental services to children. More than one-third of children are covered by public health insurance, primarily Medicaid and the Children's Health Insurance Program (CHIP). Medicaid, of course, was created by Title XIX of the Social Security Act enacted in 1965 and provides federal matching funds to states for coverage of health and long-term care services for low-income individuals. Eligibility rules in services covered are determined by states within federal guidelines. CHIP was created by the Balanced Budget Act of 1997 and reauthorized by Congress in 2009. It provides federal matching funds to states for coverage of children and some parents with incomes too high to qualify for Medicaid but for whom private health insurance was either unavailable or unaffordable. These programs are funded by states within guidelines set by the federal government. States may design their CHIP programs as independent programs separate from Medicaid (separate child health programs), use CHIP funds to expand their Medicaid programs (CHIP Medicaid expansion programs), or combine these approaches (CHIP combination programs).

Medicaid and CHIP do provide coverage of dental care for children and adolescents. Dental coverage is required for participating states, although states have wide latitude in setting payment rates for providers including dentists. These rates vary greatly by state. Very little work has been done to date on the effect of state dental fees on participation of dentists in the Medicaid program. Low reimbursement rates have been frequently cited as reasons for lack of participation of dentists in Medicaid in certain states. The report of Decker looks into this issue more deeply as an important contribution to the literature.

Decker et al examined data on Medicaid dental fees for 42 states plus the District of Columbia. They examined the year 2000 as well as the year 2008 and found that Medicaid dental payment levels did not change significantly in terms of inflation adjustments over that 8-year period. In some states, however, there were remarkable upward adjustments of 50% or more. Fig 1 in the original article shows the Medicaid prophylaxis fees in 2000 and 2008 with the fees in 2000 expressed in US dollars in 2008 using the Consumer Price Index. Looking first at the fees for 2008 on the vertical axis, it can be seen that the Medicaid prophylaxis fee varied widely across states from a low of less than $20.00 in New Jersey, Florida, Minnesota, Missouri, and Michigan to a high of $45.00 in Alaska, Kentucky, District of Columbia, Connecticut, and Arizona. The 2008 Medicaid dental fees were lower than the inflation-adjusted fees in 2000 in 23 states. Payment fees to dentists in 2008 were higher than that in 2000 in 19 states plus the District of Columbia. Fig 2 in the original article shows the probability that a child or adolescent had seen a dentist in the past 6 months. This varied by insurance. In 2008 to 2009, children covered by Medicaid were less likely (55%) than children with private insurance (68%) to have seen a dentist in the prior 6 months, although they were more likely to have seen one than were children or adolescents who had no insurance at all (27%).

Overall, Medicaid spent $3.2 billion on dental care in 2007. As the share of children and adolescents covered by Medicaid has increased from 16% to 26% from 2000 to 2008, the share of low-income children with dental insurance should have increased. However, providing children with Medicaid coverage does not cause them to see a dentist as frequently as privately insured children, even though Medicaid coverage for dental care for children is likely to be more comprehensive than at least some private dental insurance programs. Among the reasons the children and adolescents covered by Medicaid do not receive care are low payments to dentists for service, burdensome program administration requirements that are not required by other insurance carriers, and lack of patient education that can lead to frequently missed appointments. Also, in the current economic climate, many states are looking for ways to control costs in the Medicaid and CHIP programs. Although Medicaid requirements of states state that provider payments must be sufficient to enlist enough providers so that care and services are available, this requirement has generally not been enforced by the federal government.

All of us should be aware of what is happening to our dental colleagues and their reimbursement from federal support systems that provide for the underinsured and noninsured child. It is clear that there is a huge amount of unevenness across the states in support of dental services.

This commentary closes with a comment about the fact that it is apparent cavemen also craved carbs, just like us and it was not good for their teeth. Plaque stuck to the teeth of Neanderthals who died more than 35 000 years ago. No one knows why Neanderthals disappeared about 25 000 to 30 000 years ago as modern humans spread across Europe. Some data have suggested that they ate almost exclusively big game, which led to a hypothesis that they couldn't get enough calories to compete with modern humans. It seems, however, that their teeth tell a different story. Investigators have used dental tools to scrape tiny patches of calculus or hardened plaque deposits off Neanderthal teeth from museum collections. Through a microscope, the investigators showed grains of starch from seeds of cereal-like grasses, grains of cooked starch, legumelike starches, and hard structures, known as phytoliths, from date palms. This information shows that like moderate humans, Neanderthals ate what was available. As a result, they had dental problems just like we do from eating too many carbs![1]

**J. A. Stockman III, MD**

*Reference*

1. Editorial comment. Cavemen craved carbs, too. *Science.* 2011;331:13.

### Prospective Longitudinal Study of Signs and Symptoms Associated With Primary Tooth Eruption

Ramos-Jorge J, Pordeus IA, Ramos-Jorge ML, et al (Universidade Federal de Minas Gerais, Brazil; Universidade Federal dos Vales do Jequitinhonha e Mucuri, Diamantina, Brazil)
*Pediatrics* 128:471-476, 2011

*Objective.*—To assess the association between primary tooth eruption and the manifestation of signs and symptoms of teething in infants.

*Methods.*—An 8-month, longitudinal study was conducted with 47 non-institutionalized infants (ie, receiving care at home) between 5 and 15 months of age in the city of Diamantina, Brazil. The nonrandomized convenience sample was based on the registry of infants in this age range provided by the Diamantina Secretary of Health. Eligible participants were infants with up to 7 erupted incisors and no history of chronic disease or disorders that could cause an increase in the signs and symptoms assessed in the study. Tympanic and axillary temperature readings and clinical oral examinations were performed daily. A daily interview with the mothers was conducted to investigate the occurrence of 13 signs and symptoms associated with teething presented by the infants in the previous 24 hours.

*Results.*—Teething was associated with a rise in tympanic temperature on the day of the eruption ($P = .004$) and with the occurrence of other signs and symptoms. Readings of maximal tympanic and axillary temperatures were 36.8°C and 36.6°C, respectively. The most frequent signs and symptoms associated with teething were irritability (median: 0.60; $P < .001$), increased salivation (median: 0.50; $P < .001$), runny nose (median: 0.50; $P < .001$), and loss of appetite (median: 0.50; $P < .001$).

*Conclusions.*—Irritability, increased salivation, runny nose, loss of appetite, diarrhea, rash, and sleep disturbance were associated with primary tooth eruption. Results of this study support the concept that the occurrence of severe signs and symptoms, such as fever, could not be attributed to teething.

▶ There are a lot of misconceptions associated with the eruption of teeth. Teething can of course cause irritability, increased salivation, and sleep disturbance. Some have thought that it can cause fever, diarrhea, and loss of appetite. Unfortunately, teething occurs at a time in life when there may be other, more common and serious conditions taking place. There is little scientific evidence to tell us what signs and symptoms occur in association with the eruption of the primary teeth.

The authors of this report designed a study to investigate the association between tooth eruption in infants and a wide range of signs and symptoms while minimizing the limitations found in prior studies. Eleven dentists, well trained in handling temperature taking and performing oral examinations, conducted clinical examinations on infants enrolled in a study to determine tooth-eruption-related symptoms. Tympanic and axillary temperature readings in clinical oral examinations were performed daily around the time of tooth erup-tion. Also a daily interview with the infant's mother was undertaken to deter-mine the occurrence of some 13 signs and symptoms associated with teething.

The results of this study are quite interesting. It appears to be the first prospec-tive study in which temperature readings and oral clinical examinations were per-formed on a daily basis by trained examiners. The study confirmed the findings of previous studies that tooth eruption is associated with a slight rise in body temperature. Significant differences were found in mean tympanic temperature between noneruption days and the day of eruption, 1 day before eruption, and 1 day after eruption. However, there was a significant difference in axillary temperature only between noneruption days and day 1 after eruption. Despite these statistically significant associations, maximal tympanic temperature (36.8°C) and axillary (36.6°C) temperature did not characterize fever, because the variation in temperature remained within the normal range. There was a mean temperature increase of 0.12°C between noneruption days and the day of eruption. The results of the study did show a greater frequency of systemic manifestations (sleep disturbance, increased salivation, rash, runny nose, diar-rhea, loss of appetite, and irritability) on the day of eruption and 1 day after erup-tion compared with noneruption days. It is suggested that some of these signs and symptoms might be explained by the increase in inflammatory cytokine levels in the gingival fluids surrounding the teeth.

If there is a lesson to be learned from this report, it is that the presence of fever ( > 38.5°C) and some other clinically important symptoms are unlikely to be caused by tooth eruption. If you see a fever in a child who is teething, bite the bullet and think of something other than teething as a cause of the problem. Fever in association with teething is an old wives' tale.

**J. A. Stockman III, MD**

---

**Efficacy of Neonatal Release of Ankyloglossia: A Randomized Trial**
Buryk M, Bloom D, Shope T (Naval Med Ctr Portsmouth, VA)
*Pediatrics* 128:280-288, 2011

---

*Background.*—Ankyloglossia has been associated with a variety of infant-feeding problems. Frenotomy commonly is performed for relief of ankyloglossia, but there has been a lack of convincing data to support this practice.

*Objectives.*—Our primary objective was to determine whether frenot-omy for infants with ankyloglossia improved maternal nipple pain and ability to breastfeed. A secondary objective was to determine whether fre-notomy improved the length of breastfeeding.

*Methods.*—Over a 12-month period, neonates who had difficulty breast-feeding and significant ankyloglossia were enrolled in this randomized, single-blinded, controlled trial and assigned to either a frenotomy (30 infants) or a sham procedure (28 infants). Breastfeeding was assessed by a preintervention and postintervention nipple-pain scale and the Infant Breastfeeding Assessment Tool. The same tools were used at the 2-week follow-up and regularly scheduled follow-ups over a 1-year period. The infants in the sham group were given a frenotomy before or at the 2-week follow-up if it was desired.

*Results.*—Both groups demonstrated statistically significantly decreased pain scores after the intervention. The frenotomy group improved significantly more than the sham group ($P < .001$). Breastfeeding scores significantly improved in the frenotomy group ($P = .029$) without a significant change in the control group. All but 1 parent in the sham group elected to have the procedure performed when their infant reached 2 weeks of age, which prevented additional comparisons between the 2 groups.

*Conclusions.*—We demonstrated immediate improvement in nipple pain and breastfeeding scores, despite a placebo effect on nipple pain. This should provide convincing evidence for those seeking a frenotomy for infants with signficant ankyloglossia.

▶ Ankyloglossia is the 10-dollar name for "tongue-tie." Ankyloglossia defines a lingual frenulum that is unusually thick, tight, or short. The reported incidence of this condition among newborns in the United States runs between 1.7% and 4.8%, with a male-to-female ratio of approximately 3:1.[1] Having ankyloglossia would not matter much if it were not for some of its consequences. For example, duration of breastfeeding is shorter in infants with tongue-tie compared with those without it. At older ages, ankyloglossia can interfere with clear speech articulation. The most common treatment of ankyloglossia is frenotomy in the newborn period. Unfortunately, lacking clear definitions for the presence of ankyloglossia, the literature has not been very rewarding about success rates or even the necessity of frenotomy.

Buryk et al have designed a study to answer the question of whether frenotomy is efficacious for neonatal ankyloglossia and also to determine whether frenotomy for infants with ankyloglossia actually improves maternal nipple pain and the ability to breastfeed. The study also assessed whether frenotomy improved the length of breastfeeding. The study was a single-blinded, randomized controlled clinical trial of frenotomy for neonatal ankyloglossia and was conducted at the Naval Medial Center Portsmouth Newborn Nursery. This nursery handles about 350 newborn deliveries per month. Careful documentation of ankyloglossia was based on 5 appearance items (tongue appearance, frenulum elasticity, length of frenulum when tongue lifted, attachment of lingual frenulum to tongue, and attachment of frenulum to alveolar ridge) and 7 functional items (tongue lateralization, lift, extension, spread, cupping, peristalsis, and snapback).

Fifty-eight of 3025 normal newborns were identified as having ankylostoma. Half were treated with frenotomy, and half were not. Although frenotomy produced no benefit with respect to nipple pain, breastfeeding scores were significantly improved in the frenotomy group. All but 1 parent in the sham group elected to have frenotomy performed when their infant reached 2 weeks of age, thus preventing any additional comparison between the 2 study groups past that point in time.

This study is important because it addressed the methodologic problems of previous studies that have looked at frenotomy as part of the management of ankylostoma in the newborn period. The mean age of frenotomy in this report was 6.7 days, allowing time to establish breastfeeding patterns and time for mothers to demonstrate persistent problems with feeding despite lactation interventions. It can be concluded that when frenotomy is performed for clinically significant ankyloglossia, there is a clear and immediate improvement in reported breastfeeding scores. As in previous studies, the authors of this report found the procedure to be rapid, simple, and without complications. Frenotomy was performed by ear, nose, and throat specialists who elevated the tongue, exposed the frenulum, crushed the frenulum with a straight clamp to provide anesthesia and to decrease bleeding, and then incised the frenulum with a straight scissor. The average duration of crying by the infant was less than 10 seconds!

**J. A. Stockman III, MD**

*Reference*

1. Lalakea ML, Messner AH. Ankyloglossia: does it matter? *Pediatr Clin North Am.* 2003;50:381-397.

## Tongue Piercing: The Effect of Material on Microbiological Findings

Kapferer I, Beier US, Persson RG (Innsbruck Med Univ, Austria; Univ of Bern, Switzerland)
*J Adolesc Health* 49:76-83, 2011

*Purpose.*—Biofilms on oral piercings may serve as a bacterial reservoir and lead to systemic bacteremia or local transmission of pathogenic micro biota. The use of piercing materials which are less susceptible to biofilm accumulation could contribute to prevention of problems. The present study investigated whether there are microbiological differences in bacterial samples collected from tongue piercings made of different materials.

*Methods.*—A total of 85 subjects with tongue piercings participated in this study. After a baseline dental examination, sterile piercings of four different materials were randomly allocated to the study subjects. After 2 weeks, microbiologic samples were collected and processed by checkerboard deoxyribonucleic acid-deoxyribonucleic acid hybridization methods.

*Results.*—About 28.8% of subjects reported 61 lingual recessions (1.91 ± .96 mm), whereas 5% reported tooth chipping on one tooth each. With the exception of *Aggregatibacter actinomycetemcomitans* (Y4), *Fusobacterium nucleatum* species, and *Parvimonas micra*, bacteria associated with periodontitis were not commonly found in the samples from studs or piercing channels. Of the 80 bacterial species, 67 were found at significantly higher levels ($p < .001$) in samples from stainless steel than from polytetrafluoroethylene or polypropylene piercings.

*Conclusion.*—The low bacterial counts from piercing channels suggest that having a tongue pierced would not contribute to an increased risk for oral infection. The present study demonstrated that studs made of steel might promote the development of a biofilm, whereas those made of polytetrafluoroethylene or polypropylene may be rather inert to bacterial colonization. The finding of *Staphylococci* on steel and titanium studs may suggest an elevated risk for complication if the piercing channel is infected (Fig 1).

▶ Whoever said that a picture is not worth a thousands words? Take a gander at the image depicting piercing of the tongue and the upper lip. It is easy to see how unhygienic the tissues are through which the piercing materials have passed.

Currently, oral piercing involving the lips, tongue, and cheeks is increasingly common. This report from Europe reminds us that the prevalence of tongue piercing in adolescents and young adults runs on the order of 6.5%. Certainly from a medical perspective, the use of tongue jewelry cannot be considered a harmless fashion trend as it can produce undesirable local and general effects. Early complications include bacterial infection, pain, swelling, prolonged bleeding, and difficulties in swallowing, speech, and mastication. These are just the short-term effects. Late complications include chipped and fractured teeth, gingival trauma, localized periodontitis, persistent difficulties in oral function, and swallowing of the device. Some have also been concerned about how such piercings might affect biofilm formation. Changes in the composition of biofilms as a result of oral piercings could theoretically serve as a bacterial reservoir and lead to bacteremia and septic complications. Complications such as infective

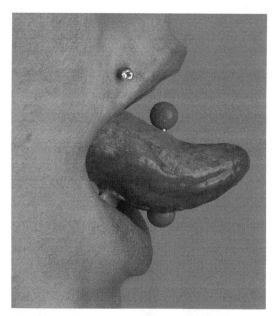

FIGURE 1.—Piercing of the tongue (and the upper lip). For interpretation of the references to colour in this figure legend, the reader is referred to the web version of this article. (Reprinted from Society for Adolescent Health and Medicine, Kapferer I, Beier US, Persson RG. Tongue Piercing: The Effect of Material on Microbiological Findings. *J Adolesc Health*. 2011;49:76-83. Copyright 2011, with permission from Elsevier.)

endocarditis, epidural abscess, chorioamnionitis, herpes simplex virus, hepatitis, hepatitis C virus infection, toxic shock syndrome, and cerebellar brain abscess can occur as complications of tongue piercing.

This report tells us about what the effects are on microbiological findings in the mouth related to various compositions of piercing materials. The most commonly used piercing materials include stainless steel, titanium, polytetrafluoroethylene, and polypropylene borealis. Stainless steel and titanium are well known to have good mechanical properties, high corrosion resistance, and excellent biocompatibility, whereas synthetic materials have very different characteristics, thus the importance of this report. Gold and silver commonly used for piercings in other parts of the body are rarely used in the mouth.

Kapferer et al studied microbiologic samples from the mouths of teens and young adults with various types of piercing materials in them. The study also demonstrated the occurrence of lingual recession at almost 30%, as well as tooth chipping occurring with a prevalence of 5%. The average age of the subjects studied was 22 years. No subject had evidence of periodontitis. Nonetheless, a number of pathogenic bacteria were observed associated with piercings, including *Actinomycetemcomitans*, *F nucleatum* species, *P micra*, and *T denticola*. In addition to these were many varieties of commonly found bacteria that could potentially become important pathogens if the biofilm of the mouth is disturbed by piercing.

The bottom line here is that this study has demonstrated some effects on the bacteriology of the mouth and tongue of teens and young adults who have tongue piercings. Interestingly, studs made of stainless steel appeared to promote the development of a biofilm over them, whereas studs made of synthetic materials appear to be rather inert to bacterial colonization. The finding of *Staphylococci* on stainless steel and titanium studs may suggest an elevated risk for complication if the piercing channel becomes infected.

**J. A. Stockman III, MD**

---

## Amoxicillin for Acute Rhinosinusitis: A Randomized Controlled Trial

Garbutt JM, Banister C, Spitznagel F, et al (Washington Univ School of Medicine, St Louis, MO)
*JAMA* 307:685-692, 2012

---

*Context.*—Evidence to support antibiotic treatment for acute rhinosinusitis is limited, yet antibiotics are commonly used.

*Objective.*—To determine the incremental effect of amoxicillin treatment over symptomatic treatments for adults with clinically diagnosed acute rhinosinusitis.

*Design, Setting, and Participants.*—A randomized, placebo-controlled trial of adults with uncomplicated, acute rhinosinusitis were recruited from 10 community practices in Missouri between November 1, 2006, and May 1, 2009.

*Interventions.*—Ten-day course of either amoxicillin (1500 mg/d) or placebo administered in 3 doses per day. All patients received a 5- to 7-day supply of symptomatic treatments for pain, fever, cough, and nasal congestion to use as needed.

*Main Outcome Measures.*—The primary outcome was improvement in disease-specific quality of life after 3 to 4 days of treatment assessed with the Sinonasal Outcome Test-16 (minimally important difference of 0.5 units on a 0-3 scale). Secondary outcomes included the patient's retrospective assessment of change in sinus symptoms and functional status, recurrence or relapse, and satisfaction with and adverse effects of treatment. Outcomes were assessed by telephone interview at days 3, 7, 10, and 28.

*Results.*—A total of 166 adults (36% male; 78% with white race) were randomized to amoxicillin (n = 85) or placebo (n = 81); 92% concurrently used 1 or more symptomatic treatments (94% for amoxicillin group vs 90% for control group; $P = .34$). The mean change in Sinonasal Outcome Test-16 scores was not significantly different between groups on day 3 (decrease of 0.59 in the amoxicillin group and 0.54 in the control group; mean difference between groups of 0.03 [95% CI, −0.12 to 0.19]) and on day 10 (mean difference between groups of 0.01 [95% CI, −0.13 to 0.15]), but differed at day 7 favoring amoxicillin (mean difference between groups of 0.19 [95% CI, 0.024 to 0.35]). There was no statistically significant difference in reported symptom improvement at day 3 (37% for amoxicillin group vs 34% for control group; $P = .67$) or at day 10 (78% vs 80%, respectively; $P = .71$), whereas at day 7 more participants treated with amoxicillin reported symptom improvement (74% vs 56%, respectively; $P = .02$). No between-group differences were found for any other secondary outcomes. No serious adverse events occurred.

*Conclusion.*—Among patients with acute rhinosinusitis, a 10-day course of amoxicillin compared with placebo did not reduce symptoms at day 3 of treatment.

*Trial Registration.*—clinicaltrials.gov Identifier: NCT00377403.

▶ This article discusses the benefits or lack of benefits of using amoxicillin for acute rhinosinusitis. This study included teenagers aged 18 years and older. Therefore, the results are valid, one can presume, for the overall teenage population. You will have to be the judge of whether the data can apply to a much younger pediatric age range. Chances are that because the organisms causing sinusitis are similar throughout much of the pediatric age spectrum, the information provided by this report would apply to most patients in a pediatric practice.

It is well known that the majority of cases of acute rhinosinusitis will have spontaneous improvement if careful clinical diagnostic criteria are applied. In adults, despite the controversy regarding their clinical benefit and concerns about antibiotic resistance, antibiotics for sinusitis account for about 20% of all prescriptions written for adults in the United States. The Centers for Disease Control and Prevention has guidelines for the evaluation and treatment of adults with acute rhinosinusitis that recommend using clinical criteria for diagnosis and reserving antibiotic treatment for patients with moderately severe or severe symptoms and treating patients with the most narrow-spectrum antibiotic activity against *Streptococcus pneumoniae* and *Haemophilus influenzae*.

The authors designed this study to determine the benefit of amoxicillin versus symptomatic treatment of acute rhinosinusitis. They enrolled 166 patients (aged 18-69 years) who were randomized to amoxicillin or placebo. A 10-day course of amoxicillin (1500 mg per day) or placebo was prescribed. The primary outcome was improvement in disease-specific quality of life after 3 or 4 days of treatment assessed by an objective outcomes scale. The diagnosis of acute rhinosinusitis required a history of maxillary pain or tenderness in the face or teeth, purulent nasal secretions, and rhinosinusitis symptoms for 7 days or more and 28 days or less that were not improving or worsening, or sinusitis symptoms lasting for less than 7 days that had significantly worsened after initial improvement. The data from this report showed that there were no statistically significant differences in reported symptomatic improvement at day 3 of treatment in the 2 groups (37% for amoxicillin-treated subjects vs 34% for controls). Days missed from work or unable to perform usual activities, rates of relapse and recurrence by 28 days, additional health care use, and satisfaction with treatment did not differ by study group. No adverse events occurred in either group.

The findings from this study support recommendations to avoid routine antibiotic treatment for patients with an uncomplicated acute rhinosinusitis in the age group studied. As noted, these results probably would apply to a significant proportion of the older pediatric age range as well. It should be noted that this is the first trial of antibiotic treatment for acute rhinosinusitis to assess improvement in disease specific quality of life as the primary outcome, the outcome that is most important to patients. It is true that the clinical criteria used to diagnose acute rhinosinusitis in this clinical trial are likely to be more rigorous than those routinely used in practice. Still, they failed to identify those for whom 10 days of treatment with amoxicillin provided any clinical benefit. It is unlikely that this finding was due to an inadequate dose of amoxicillin, because the prevalence of amoxicillin-resistant *Streptococcus pneumoniae* in the community where the study was performed was quite low, and there is no evidence that any other antibiotic is superior to amoxicillin when used for similar purposes.

This study adds to a considerable body of evidence from clinical trials conducted in the primary care setting that antibiotics provide little if any benefit for patients with clinically diagnosed acute rhinosinusitis, yet antibiotic treatment for upper respiratory tract infections is both expected by patients and all too frequently prescribed by physicians. The National Institute for Health and Clinical Excellence guidelines in the United Kingdom, and more recent guidelines here in the United States, suggest watchful waiting as an alternative approach to the management of patients for whom reassessment is possible; this approach delays and may preclude antibiotic treatment while providing symptomatic treatments and an explanation of the natural history of the disease. For specific guidelines related to pediatrics, go to the American Academy of Pediatrics website, which goes into this topic in great detail.

By the way, the primary clinical outcomes used in this study were measured using the modified Sinonasal Outcome Test-16, for which the abbreviation is SNOT-16, a delightfully creative and self-explanatory acronym! Last, this commentary closes with another observation having to do with the whales and what comes out of their noses. The 2010 Ig Noble Engineering Prize was awarded to investigators in London for perfecting a method to collect whale snot. This was done by using a remote control helicopter. Needless to say the helicopter had to be washed after each experiment.[1]

**J. A. Stockman III, MD**

*Reference*

1. Acevedo-Whitehouse K, Rocha-Gosselin A, Gendron D. A novel non-invasive tool for disease surveillance of free-ranging whales and its relevance to conservation programs. *Animal Conservation.* 2010;13:217-225.

## Tonsillectomy in Children with Periodic Fever with Aphthous Stomatitis, Pharyngitis, and Adenitis Syndrome

Garavello W, Pignataro L, Gaini L, et al (Univ of Milano-Bicocca, Monza, Italy; Univ of Milan; et al)
*J Pediatr* 159:138-142, 2011

*Objective.*—To seek evidence supporting a role for tonsillectomy or adenotonsillectomy in the management of affected children with periodic fever with aphthous stomatitis, pharnygitis, and adenitis (PFAPA) syndrome.

*Study Design.*—A comprehensive literature search was conducted to identify all published English-language observational and randomized studies evaluating the efficacy of tonsillectomy or adenotonsillectomy on PFAPA syndrome. A combination of keywords was used to identify relevant articles.

*Results.*—A total of 15 studies including 149 treated children were found, including 13 observational noncomparative studies and 2 randomized controlled trials. The pooled rate of complete resolution emerging from the combined analysis of all treated children was 83% (95% CI, 77%-89%). A meta-analysis of the two randomized controlled trials showed homogeneity of the results ($P = .37$, Breslow-Day test) and a common odds ratio for complete resolution of 13 (95% CI, 4-43; $P < .001$).

*Conclusions.*—Surgery appears to be a possible option for management of PFAPA syndrome. Available evidence is limited, however, and the precise role of surgery remains to be clarified. We suggest considering this option when symptoms markedly interfere with the child's quality of life and medical treatment has failed.

▶ Periodic fever with aphthous stomatitis, pharyngitis, and adenitis is a syndrome that has been around since 1987, achieving the acronym PFAPA some 2 years later.[1] The disorder typically occurs in young children (younger than age 5 years) and is characterized by short periods of illness lasting 3 to 4 days that recur regularly every 3 to 8 weeks for several years. The cycles occur on a strict and regular basis. In between, these youngsters feel perfectly well. PFAPA is frequently discussed together with other periodic fever syndromes, but its cause is unknown, and it is not understood whether this is primarily genetic in origin or due to some underlying initial infectious process. It produces disturbances in innate immunity that are quite complex. Flairs are accompanied by increased serum levels of activated T-lymphocyte chemokines and proinflammatory cytokines. Cases in family members with similar periodic episodes of fever are beginning to suggest a possible role of both genetics and the environment.

Given that the etiology of PFAPA remains an enigma, so too does the precise management. A possible treatment for PFAPA is a single dose of prednisone (1—2 mg/kg body mass) at the beginning of each fever episode. A single dose usually terminates the fever within several hours. However, in some children, steroids cause the fever episodes to occur more frequently (and more regularly). In such cases, care providers have switched to the use of colchicine, which is used in the treatment of familial Mediterranean fever. The role of tonsillectomy has remained uncertain. In one study, adenotonsillectomy was found to be totally effective in resolving symptoms.[2] A comprehensive review of the literature on PFAPA published in 2006, however, observed only weak evidence on the effectiveness of tonsillectomy in this syndrome and concluded that tonsillectomy should not be performed.[3]

Garavello et al have jumped into the tonsillectomy debate by doing an electronic database search of all objective studies published in the English language between January 1987 and May 2010 examining the effect of tonsillectomy or adenotonsillectomy in the management of PFAPA syndrome. The authors conducted 2 separate analyses to evaluate the magnitude of the effect of tonsillectomy. First they evaluated the benefits emerging from clinical series. The main objective was to determine the absolute rate of resolution combining all series on this topic. A binomial distribution model was used to calculate the 95% confidence interval of this rate. Second, the authors focused on controlled studies to assess the relative rate of resolution compared with medical management. To do so, they calculated a combined estimate of the odds ratio across studies determining the natural resolution of PFAPA.

The comprehensive literature review by Garavello et al documents that there remains insufficient evidence on the effectiveness of tonsillectomy for PFAPA syndrome. All studies reviewed had small sample sizes and, in most cases, the follow-up period was very short. Although there was a tendency for the benefits of surgery to be increasingly reported over the last decade or so, there was no evidence observed to definitively support the effectiveness of surgery. Also, there was no evidence to distinguish the effects of tonsillectomy versus adenotonsillectomy.[4]

Thus it is that most practitioners will continue to rely on the use of oral steroids to control flairs of PFAPA. In recent times, practitioners have also been using cimetidine. Cimetidine, a common H2 antagonist, has immune-modulating properties, inhibiting chemotaxis and T-cell activation and has been used with some success in doses of 150 mg once or twice a day and of 20 mg/kg/d to 40 mg/kg/d. According to 1 report, PFAPA syndrome will resolve in 28% to 44% of cases treated with cimetidine.[5] If nothing else, a tincture of time cures all, as PFAPA will ultimately resolve on its own albeit only after a number of years in some cases.

This commentary closes with mention about presidential illnesses, including one related to the upper airway. What president had more numerous illnesses/ conditions than any other in and about the time he was in office? The answer to this question is not Franklin Roosevelt (who had polio); it is George Washington (1732-1799). Historians count 10 bouts of serious illness as well as innumerable minor ailments that affected him. Obsessive about his health, GW meticulously detailed in his diaries his physical trials and triumphs and his favored remedies. An ardent fan of the humoral medicine of the day, he enthusiastically volunteered to be bled and blistered; but hedging his bets with numerous quack therapies on the market, he also bought a pair of Elisha Perkins's popular tractors with their persuasive claims for pain relief. It is noted that at 17 years of age he contracted the "Ague" (probably malaria) and two years later smallpox. An attack of pleurisy was followed by influenza and then dysentery. Downing large quantities of Dr James's powders—"the most excellent medicine in the world" —Washington found his complaints lingered "in spite of the efforts of all of the Sons of Aescu- lapius." By the time Washington took the oath of office in 1789, he sported glasses, was deaf to some degree, and wore false teeth. Within six weeks of his inaugural speech he was laid low again, with an abscess on his thigh that took 3 months to heal. Weathering further attacks of Agues and fevers, he survived his presidency to retire to his Mount Vernon estate in 1797 in the hope of a long and well-deserved rest. It was not to be. In December 1799, after riding all day in a storm, Washington took to his bed with a sore throat for which he gamely asked his overseer to bleed him in the absence of any professional aid. The next day his lifelong friend, Dr James Craik, and a fellow physician, Dr Gustavus Brown, bled the Founding Father twice more. Despite the objections of a third physician, Dr Elisha Dick, who proposed a tracheotomy to help the expiring pioneer to breathe, the doctors took a fourth donation of blood, amount- ing to a grand total of somewhere between 4 pints and 6 pints (just under three liters). Overwhelmed by his infection—possibly diphtheria or acute epiglottitis— and weak from blood loss, Washington died, making history by having the most numerous recorded presidential (including the pre- and postpresidential periods) illnesses/conditions.[6]

**J. A. Stockman III, MD**

*References*

1. Marshall GS, Edwards KM, Lawton AR. PFAPA syndrome. *Pediatr Infect Dis J.* 1989;8:658-659.
2. Licameli G, Jeffrey J, Luz J, Jones D, Kenna M. Effect of adenotonsillectomy in PFAPA syndrome. *Arch Otolaryngol Head Neck Surg.* 2008;134:136-140.
3. Leong SC, Karkos PD, Apostolidou MT. Is there a role for the otolaryngologist in PFAPA syndrome? A systematic review. *Int J Pediatr Otorhinolaryngol.* 2006;70: 1841-1845.
4. Thomas KT, Feder HM Jr, Lawton AR, Edwards KM. Periodic fever syndrome in children. *J Pediatr.* 1999;135:15-21.
5. Feder HM Jr. Cimetidine treatment for periodic fever associated with aphthous stomatitis, pharyngitis and cervical adenitis. *Pediatr Infect Dis J.* 1992;11: 318-321.
6. Moore W. The first George W. *BMJ.* 2009;338:362.

**Effectiveness of adenoidectomy in children with recurrent upper respiratory tract infections: open randomised controlled trial**
van den Aardweg MTA, Boonacker CWB, Rovers MM, et al (Univ Med Centre Utrecht, Netherlands)
*BMJ* 343:d5154, 2011

*Objective.*—To assess the effectiveness of adenoidectomy in children with recurrent upper respiratory tract infections.

*Design.*—Open randomised controlled trial.

*Setting.*—11 general hospitals and two academic centres.

*Participants.*—111 children aged 1-6 with recurrent upper respiratory tract infections selected for adenoidectomy.

*Intervention.*—A strategy of immediate adenoidectomy with or without myringotomy or a strategy of initial watchful waiting.

*Main Outcome Measure.*—Primary outcome measure: number of upper respiratory tract infections per person year calculated from data obtained during the total follow-up (maximum 24 months). Secondary outcome measures: days with upper respiratory tract infection per person year, middle ear complaints with fever in episodes and days, days with fever, prevalence of upper respiratory tract infections, and health related quality of life.

*Results.*—During the median follow-up of 24 months, there were 7.91 episodes of upper respiratory tract infections per person year in the adenoidectomy group and 7.84 in the watchful waiting group (difference in incidence rate 0.07, 95% confidence interval −0.70 to 0.85). No relevant differences were found for days of upper respiratory tract infections and middle ear complaints with fever in episodes and days, nor for health related quality of life. The prevalence of upper respiratory tract infections decreased over time in both groups. Children in the adenoidectomy group had significantly more days with fever than the children in the watchful waiting group. Two children had complications related to surgery.

*Conclusion.*—In children selected for adenoidectomy for recurrent upper respiratory tract infections, a strategy of immediate surgery confers no clinical benefits over a strategy of initial watchful waiting.

*Trial Registration.*—Dutch Trial Register NTR968: ISRCTN03720485.

▶ This report by van den Aardweg et al tells us about the effectiveness of adenoidectomy in children selected for surgery on the sole basis of upper respiratory infection. The randomized controlled trial of 111 children age 1 to 6 years compared immediate adenoidectomy, with or without myringotomy, with initial watchful waiting. The primary outcome was the total number of recurrent upper respiratory infections defined as 2 or more of the following symptoms during the first 2 years of follow-up: fever, diary scored, stuffiness or breathing through the mouth, nasal discharge, or cough. The investigators found no significant differences between the groups. Furthermore, no differences between the groups were found in the secondary outcomes of total number of days with upper respiratory tract infections a year, days with fever, or health-related quality of life. The report abstracted emanates from the Netherlands where adenoidectomy rates are more than 3 times higher than those in the United States.

The findings from this report are influencing public policy health care funding in the Netherlands. The report shows that adenoidectomy has no influence on the rate of sinusitis or otitis media or overall well being of a child. Tincture of time seems to be what cures without the need for surgery.

This commentary ends with some interesting information having to do with the sense of smell. It has been thought that women have sharper noses than men, but now researchers have found the first exception. Men are far better at detecting bourgeonal, a flowery compound used in perfumes. Scientists have engaged 500 participants, half of them male, to sniff increasingly concentrated solutions of bourgeonal as well as control odors. It turns out that men's threshold for bourgeonal was on average 13 parts per billion, whereas women needed twice this concentration to notice the distinctive lily-of-the-valley fragrance. This makes bourgeonal the first odorant ever for which human males are more sensitive than females. Curiously, in the laboratory, spermatozoa tend to make a beeline toward sources of bourgeonal as opposed to other control products, although scientists do not know if it is the very chemical that attracts sperm to the human egg. Because the olfactory receptors on sperm cells are also expressed in the human nose, and selective pressure for keener receptors would act on men, but not on women, it makes sense that men are more sensitive to the sperm attractant. The point of all this is that sperm and our noses share something in common, something that is uniquely more common to men and may help explain why sperm sniff their way to the egg.[1]

**J. A. Stockman III, MD**

*Reference*

1. Schenkman L. Nasal attraction. *Science.* 2010;328:673.

---

## Oral vs Intratympanic Corticosteroid Therapy for Idiopathic Sudden Sensorineural Hearing Loss: A Randomized Trial

Rauch SD, Halpin CF, Antonelli PJ, et al (Harvard Med School, Boston, MA; Univ of Florida, Gainesville; et al)
*JAMA* 305:2071-2079, 2011

---

*Context.*—Idiopathic sudden sensorineural hearing loss has been treated with oral corticosteroids for more than 30 years. Recently, many patients' symptoms have been managed with intratympanic steroid therapy. No satisfactory comparative effectiveness study to support this practice exists.

*Objective.*—To compare the effectiveness of oral vs intratympanic steroid to treat sudden sensorineural hearing loss.

*Design, Setting, and Patients.*—Prospective, randomized, noninferiority trial involving 250 patients with unilateral sensorineural hearing loss presenting within 14 days of onset of 50 dB or higher of pure tone average (PTA) hearing threshold. The study was conducted from December 2004 through October 2009 at 16 academic community-based otology practices. Participants were followed up for 6 months.

*Intervention.*—One hundred twenty-one patients received either 60 mg/d of oral prednisone for 14 days with a 5-day taper and 129 patients received 4 doses over 14 days of 40 mg/mL of methylprednisolone injected into the middle ear.

*Main Outcome Measures.*—Primary end point was change in hearing at 2 months after treatment. Noninferiority was defined as less than a 10-dB difference in hearing outcome between treatments.

*Results.*—In the oral prednisone group, PTA improved by 30.7 dB compared with a 28.7-dB improvement in the intratympanic treatment group. Mean pure tone average at 2 months was 56.0 for the oral steroid treatment group and 57.6 dB for the intratympanic treatment group. Recovery of hearing on oral treatment at 2 months by intention-to-treat analysis was 2.0 dB greater than intratympanic treatment (95.21% upper confidence interval, 6.6 dB). Per-protocol analysis confirmed the intention-to-treat result. Thus, the hypothesis of inferiority of intratympanic methylprednisolone to oral prednisone for primary treatment of sudden sensorineural hearing loss was rejected.

*Conclusion.*—Among patients with idiopathic sudden sensorineural hearing loss, hearing level 2 months after treatment showed that intratympanic treatment was not inferior to oral prednisone treatment.

*Trial Registration.*—clinicaltrials.gov Identifier: NCT00097448.

▶ Sudden deafness, also known as idiopathic sudden sensorineural hearing loss, can affect youngsters as well as adults. This series included patients in their teenage years, although the age of occurrence is mainly between 30 and 60 years of age. Given the fact that the effects of this problem can be devastating, sudden hearing loss should be treated as a medical emergency. About half of cases will spontaneously resolve on their own. The cause remains unknown. Possible causes include infections (ie, viruses, autoimmune disease, circulatory problems, and neurologic disease, including multiple sclerosis). There has been no defined treatment to date. Therapeutic options include oral steroids, intratympanic steroid injections, antiviral agents given by mouth, vasodilators, diuretics, hyperbaric oxygen therapy, and vitamins. The evaluation of what is the best treatment has been illusive, in part because of the rarity of the problem and the absence of validated tests for etiologic identification.

What Rauch et al have done is to describe the findings from the very first multi-institutional study of oral versus intratympanic corticosteroid therapy for hearing loss. Some 2400 patients were assessed for eligibility to enter the study. Ultimately, 250 agreed to participate and were randomly assigned to receive either 60 mg/dL oral steroids for 14 days with a 5-day taper or four 1-mL doses of 40 mg/dL of methylprednisolone injected into the middle ear over a 2-week period. The investigators were trying to determine whether intratympanic methylprednisolone is superior to oral steroids for the treatment of hearing loss of this type. The primary finding of this study was a 2.0-dB difference in the pure tone average between the 2 treatment groups at 2 months with a maximal difference of 6.6 dB seen in some patients. This value of 6.6 dB was below the required value of 10 dB to demonstrate clinical significance and reject the null hypothesis of inferiority (ie, intratympanic treatment is worse than oral prednisone). Overall, the 2 treatments were well tolerated, although 3.1% of patients had persistent tympanic membrane perforation from the injections and 4.7% had persistent otitis media in the middle ear injected versus 0.8% in the oral steroid group.

To read more about the steroids for sudden sensorineural hearing loss, see the editorial by Piccirillo.[1] Chances are no one will be switching to the routine use of intratympanic steroids versus the simple administration of oral prednisone.

This commentary closes with the observation of the results of a randomized trial that has compared the long-term effectiveness of using bulb syringes at home for self clearance of earwax as opposed to routine cleaning of the ears in a general family medicine practice.[2] In the two-year trial follow-up, more control patients returned with earwax buildup than patients who were irrigating their ears routinely at home. You will have to be the judge of why anyone would routinely want to do this on a regular basis. Ears are made for listening, not for inserting objects into them unless absolutely necessary.

**J. A. Stockman III, MD**

*References*

1. Piccirillo JF. Steroids for idiopathic sudden sensorineural hearing loss: some questions answered, others remain. *JAMA*. 2011;305:2114-2115.
2. Coppin R, Wicke D, Little P. Randomized trial of bulb syringes for earwax: impact on health service utilization. *Ann Fam Med*. 2011;9:110-114.

---

**Parental Smoking and the Risk of Middle ear Disease in Children: A Systematic Review and Meta-Analysis**
Jones LL, Hassanien A, Cook DG, et al (Univ of Nottingham, England; St George's Univ of London, England)
*Arch Pediatr Adolesc Med* 166:18-27, 2012

*Objective.*—A systematic review and meta-analysis of studies of the association between secondhand tobacco smoke (SHTS) and middle ear disease (MED) in children.

*Data Sources.*—MEDLINE, EMBASE, and CAB abstracts (through December 2010) and reference lists.

*Study Selection.*—Sixty-one epidemiological studies of children assessing the effect of SHTS on outcomes of MED. Articles were reviewed, and the data were extracted and synthesized by 2 researchers.

*Main Outcome Exposures.*—Children's SHTS exposure.

*Main Outcome Measures.*—Middle ear disease in children.

*Results.*—Living with a smoker was associated with an increased risk of MED in children by an odds ratio (OR) of 1.62 (95% CI, 1.33-1.97) for maternal postnatal smoking and by 1.37 (95% CI, 1.25-1.50) for any household member smoking. Prenatal maternal smoking (OR, 1.11; 95% CI,

0.93-1.31) and paternal smoking (OR, 1.24; 95% CI, 0.98-1.57) were associated with a nonsignificant increase in the risk of MED. The strongest effect was on the risk of surgery for MED, where maternal postnatal smoking increased the risk by an OR of 1.86 (95% CI, 1.31-2.63) and paternal smoking by 1.83 (95% CI, 1.61-2.07).

*Conclusions.*—Exposure to SHTS, particularly to smoking by the mother, significantly increases the risk of MED in childhood; this risk is particularly strong for MED requiring surgery. We have shown that per year 130 200 of child MED episodes in the United Kingdom and 292 950 of child frequent ear infections in the United States are directly attributable to SHTS exposure in the home.

▶ This report represents a systematic review and meta-analysis of the literature looking at studies that have attempted to assess the effect of secondhand smoke on the occurrence of middle ear disease in children. A systematic review performed more than 15 years ago did find a significant association between parents smoking and middle ear disease, but a lot has changed in the meantime.[1]

Jones et al were able to find more than 360 articles published since 1997 that have looked at a potential link between secondhand smoke and middle ear disease in children. Jones et al again documented an association between parent smoking and middle ear disease. In addition, they observed that smoking by any household member was statistically significantly associated with an increased risk of disease in children, which translates to an additional 130 000 episodes of middle ear disease per year in the United Kingdom and an additional almost 300 000 frequent ear infections (≥3 episodes in the previous 12 months) per year in children in the United States aged 3 to 11 years.

So what should be done about the problem? Surgical treatments of otitis media, such as grommet-pressure equalization tube insertion, have been shown to be questionable in their effectiveness and can be associated with complications and are costly. Primary prevention through reduction of risk factors, such as exposure to secondhand smoke, remains key to reducing the burden of middle ear disease in children. Middle ear disease as a consequence of secondhand smoke is still a problem despite the overall reduction in number of parents who smoke. The data from this report indicate that 7.5% of episodes of otitis media in the United Kingdom and 6.3% of such episodes in the United States are directly attributable to secondhand smoke exposure in the household. All these cases would be potentially avoidable.

This commentary closes with the observation that ear wax is actually good for something other than keeping bugs out of our ears. Hold the giant Q-tip. The waxy buildup in a whale's ears may contain interesting data about its exposure to contaminants. A wall of blubber and muscle protects a whale's ears from ocean water, sealing the wax inside. The wax plugs are laminated and made up of layers that can be matched roughly to a whale's age. This is sort of like tree rings. These layers can also be the repository of chemicals from seawater. Scientists have examined these earwax samples to determine any toxicological substances in waters that the whales may have been swimming in. Ear wax plugs must be taken from the dead whales, because marine mammals are protected by US law. Scientists have recently examined the earwax from a whale that died in 1969, the wax sample having been stored at the Smithsonian Institution in Washington DC.[2] The 6-centimeter long earplug contained the pesticide chlordane, banned in the United States in 1988, and also showed high levels of PCBs. As the various layers of the wax were examined, the levels of chlordane decreased with time while the levels of PCBs remained the same.

Thus it is, that earwax has more significance than you might have imagined.

**J. A. Stockman III, MD**

*References*

1. Strachan DP, Cook DG. Health effects of passive smoking. 4. Parental smoking, middle ear disease and adenotonsillectomy in children. *Thorax*. 1998;53:50-56.
2. Editorial comment. Tracking contaminants in whales—using there are earwax. *Science*. 2011;334:141.

---

## Occurrence of acute otitis media during colds in children younger than four years

Armengol CE, Hendley JO, Winther B (Univ of Virginia School of Medicine, Charlottesville)
*Pediatr Infect Dis J* 30:518-520, 2011

---

To determine how frequently acute otitis media (AOM) occurs, we enrolled children between 6 months and 3 years of age who returned several weeks before and 6 to 10 times during a cold for tympanometry and photography of the tympanic membrane. American Academy of Pediatrics (AAP) criteria were used to diagnose AOM. Children visited their physicians at their discretion. AOM occurred in 17 (55%) of 31 colds; in 12 (100%) colds with pre-existing middle ear effusion (MEE); and in 5 (26%) of 19 colds with no pre-existing MEE ($P < 0.0001$). Four patients received antibiotics from their physicians. Of 17 children with AOM, 12 did not seek care. AOM is common during colds, particularly with pre-existing MEE (Fig 1, Table 1).

▶ This is one neat little study. Its purpose was to determine whether and how frequently acute otitis media (AOM) actually occurs during the common cold in young children. These were children who had a baseline examination of the tympanic membrane prior to the onset of the cold and had a study pediatrician who both examined and photographed the tympanic membranes during the episode of a cold. This pediatrician had no role in the diagnosis or the management of acute otitis media. The diagnosis of acute otitis media was established by the study pediatrician who compiled the symptom data with tympanometry and the appearance of the tympanic membrane. The criteria used to make the diagnosis of AOM were the same as those published by the American Academy of Pediatrics several years back: (1) recent, abrupt onset of ear symptoms; (2) the presence of middle ear effusion; and (3) signs or symptoms of middle ear inflammation.

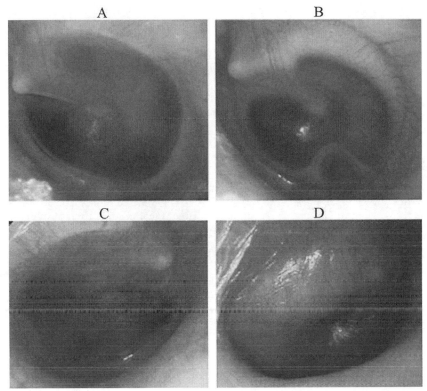

**FIGURE 1.**—Photographs of tympanic membranes. A, Normal TM (patient 17, baseline); B, Distinct erythema of the TM (no. 17, day 4 of illness, left ear); C, Middle ear effusion and erythema (no. 17, day 4 of illness, right ear); D, Bulging TM (no. 10, day 3 of illness). (Reprinted from Armengol CE, Hendley JO, Winther B. Occurrence of acute otitis media during colds in children younger than four years. *Pediatr Infect Dis J.* 2011;30:518-520.)

**TABLE 1.**—Frequency of AOM During 31 Colds in Children Less Than 4 Years of Age Based on the Presence of Middle Ear Effusion (MEE) at Baseline and Criteria for Middle Ear Inflammation

| Criteria for Middle Ear Inflammation | All Colds Cold Episodes (n = 31) | Occurrence of AOM MEE at Baseline Cold Episodes (n = 12) | No MEE at Baseline Cold Episodes (n = 19) |
|---|---|---|---|
| Symptoms and erythema | 11 (35)* | 8 (67)† | 3 (16) |
| Erythema | 14 (45) | 10 (83)‡ | 4 (21) |
| Symptoms | 14 (45) | 10 (83)‡ | 4 (21) |
| Symptoms or erythema | 17 (55) | 12 (100)§ | 5 (26) |
| Bulging TM appearance | 6 (19) | 5 (42) | 1 (5) |

AOM indicates acute otitis media.
*Number of colds with AOM (%).
†$P = 0.0070$ compared to no MEE at baseline.
‡$P = 0.0011$ compared to no MEE at baseline.
§$P < 0.0001$ compared to no MEE at baseline.

Thirty children were studied. They ranged in age from 11 months to 47 months. It was determined that AOM occurred in 55% of patients with a common cold. In 5 colds, AOM was present at a single visit; in the remaining 12, AOM was present at multiple visits. AOM occurred in 100% of colds if the youngster had preexisting middle ear effusion and in 26% of colds in which there was no preexisting middle ear effusion.

As is evident in other studies, the onset of AOM, when it occurs, does so early in the course of a cold. Given the high prevalence of AOM, one wonders what one should do about antibiotic management. The authors of this report suggest that the most prudent option for managing AOM would be emphasizing systemic and topical analgesia along with follow-up if the child does not improve quickly. Two recent trials, however, suggest that antibiotic therapy is associated with a faster recovery and a lower rate of clinical failure compared with placebo.[1,2] The trick here would be to identify cases severe enough to require immediate antibiotic treatment as opposed to more conservative approaches. That is a study still waiting to be done.

This commentary closes with another observation about ear wax. Investigators reporting in the *Annals of Family Medicine* tell us about a randomized trial comparing the long-term effectiveness of using a bulb syringe at home for self-clearance of ear wax in comparison with no such care. In the 2-year trial follow-up, more control patients returned with yearly wax buildup than patients who were irrigating the ears at home on a regular basis. Thus it is that the cleaning the potatoes out of your ears every once in a while is a stitch in time that saves nine.[3]

**J. A. Stockman III, MD**

*References*

1. Hoberman A, Paradise JL, Rockette HE, et al. Treatment of acute otitis media in children under 2 years of age. *N Engl J Med*. 2011;364:105-115.
2. Tähtinen PA, Laine MK, Huovinen P, Jalava J, Ruuskanen O, Ruohola A. A placebo-controlled trial of antimicrobial treatment for acute otitis media. *N Engl J Med*. 2011;364:116-126.
3. Editorial comment. Syringing wax from ears. *Ann Family Med*. 2011;9:110-114.

## Symptomatic Vocal Cord Paresis/Paralysis in Infants Operated on for Esophageal Atresia and/or Tracheo-Esophageal Fistula

Morini F, Iacobelli BD, Crocoli A, et al (Bambino Gesù Children's Res Hosp, Rome, Italy)
*J Pediatr* 158:973-976, 2011

*Objectives.*—To describe the prevalence and pathogenesis of symptomatic vocal cord paresis/paralysis (VCP) in patients treated for esophageal atresia (EA), tracheo-esophageal fistula (TEF) or both.

*Study Design.*—Retrospective study of all patients treated for EA/TEF in our center (1995 to 2009). Patients with and without symptomatic VCP were compared for gestational age, birth weight, associated anomalies, referrals, long-gap EA (>3 cm or 3 vertebral bodies), cervical esophagostomy, anastomotic leakage, length of ventilation, and major cardiac surgery. Prevalence or median (IQR) is reported.

*Results.*—Of 174 patients, 7 (4%) had symptomatic VCP. Prevalence of referrals (5/7 versus 21/167; $P = .0009$), long gap (5/7 versus 41/167; $P = .0146$), previous cervical esophagostomy (5/7 versus 7/167; $P < .0001$), and anastomotic leakage (3/7 versus 10/167; $P = .0097$) was higher, and ventilation longer (8.5 days [7.0 to 15.5] versus 6.0 days (5.0 to 7.0); $P = .0072$) in patients with VCP.

*Conclusions.*—In infants treated for EA/TEF, VCP should be ruled out in case of persistent respiratory morbidity or, when present, cautiously monitored. Surgical risk factors should be actively controlled. Further studies are needed to define the prevalence of acquired and congenital VCP in patients with EA/TEF.

▶ Vocal cord paresis/paralysis is a complication of certain surgical procedures. It is known to cause significant respiratory morbidity in infants and children, placing such children at increased risk of aspiration pneumonia because of impaired airway protection, swallowing difficulties, and gastroesophageal reflux. This is a result of injury to the vagus nerve or the recurrent laryngeal nerve. Esophageal surgery, in particular, can result in vocal cord paresis/paralysis. In adults who have undergone esophagectomy, the prevalence of vocal cord paresis/paralysis is as high as 80% depending on the surgical site (twice as high with a high cervical approach compared with an intrathoracic approach). In children, cardiovascular surgery, mainly for patent ductus ligation, is the most common cause of vocal cord paresis/paralysis with a prevalence ranging from 4% to 16%.[1]

What Morini et al have done is to perform a retrospective review of all patients consecutively treated for esophageal atresia and/or tracheoesophageal fistula to determine the presence or absence of asymptomatic vocal cord paresis/paralysis. Unfortunately, the results of this study documented that vocal cord paresis/paralysis is a highly overlooked complication resulting in significant morbidity when it is the result of surgery for esophageal atresia or tracheoesophageal fistula. Some 4% of children operated on for these disorders will have significant symptoms, many of which are underreported and place these youngsters at serious risk of associated morbidities.

While on the topic of things related to ear, nose, and throat issues, a baby's risk of being born with a cleft palate may depend on both the child's genes and whether the youngster's mother smoked, drank, or took vitamins during pregnancy. Researchers examining genetic risk combined with maternal smoking, drinking, and vitamin use found that environmental factors can interact with certain genes to either raise or lower the risk of the congenital malformation. Binge drinking and smoking early in pregnancy interact with some genes to raise the risk of clefts. Multivitamins interact with other genes to protect against clefts.[2]

This commentary closes with another brief remark about smell, in this case, the "smell of money." In Washington, DC, the smell of money might be as intoxicating as the smell of power. After studying money supplies in US cities and in countries worldwide, an investigator at the University of Massachusetts has reported finding cocaine traces in 95% of bank notes collected in Washington, DC. On average, 90% of US bank notes studied were contaminated compared with 85% of Canada's paper dollars and 80% of Brazil's reals. Of 234 bank notes from 17 US cities, those with the heaviest residues of cocaine (up to 1240 micrograms per bill — came from the largest cities with serious drug problems).[3] It would be interesting to use the "bill cocaine index" as a monitor of how well law enforcement is dealing with the drug problem throughout the United States and elsewhere.

**J. A. Stockman III, MD**

*References*

1. Smith ME, King JD, Elsherif A, Muntz HR, Park AH, Kouretas PC. Should all newborns who undergo patent ductus arteriosus ligation be examined for vocal cord mobility? *Laryngoscope.* 2009;119:1606-1609.
2. Editorial comment. Complex genes of cleft palates. *Science News.* March 12, 2011:19.
3. Raloff J. Drugged money. *Science News.* September 12, 2009:9.

---

**Endotracheal Tube and Laryngeal Mask Airway Cuff Pressures Can Exceed Critical Values During Ascent to Higher Altitude**

Miyashiro RM, Yamamoto LG (Univ of Hawaii John A. Burns School of Medicine, Honolulu; Kapi'olani Med Ctr for Women and Children, Honolulu, HI)

*Pediatr Emerg Care* 27:367-370, 2011

---

*Objectives.*—Tracheal mucosal perfusion is compromised at an endotracheal tube (ETT) cuff pressure of 30 cm $H_2O$, and blood flow is obstructed at a pressure of 50 cm $H_2O$.

*Methods.*—We measured the change in pressure of air-filled cuffs of 6.0 and 7.5 ETTs and a size 4 laryngeal mask airway (LMA) from sea level to 2400 m. The ETTs and LMA cuff measurements were done with the devices uncontained, and an additional 6.0 ETT was placed in a 10-mL syringe barrel to mimic placement in a trachea. This restricted cuff expansion simulating what would occur when it is placed within the trachea. The pressure of fluid-filled 6.0 ETT cuffs was also measured.

*Results.*—Intracuff pressure increases linearly with increasing altitude, in all air-filled ETT and LMAs. Water-filled cuffs demonstrated no significant change in pressure with changes in altitude. The rate of ETT cuff pressure increase was greater for the ETT restricted within the syringe barrel compared with the unrestricted ETT cuff. The rate of LMA cuff pressure increase was greater than the rate of increase for all the ETTs (restricted and unrestricted).

*Conclusions.*—This model indicates that ETT cuffs inflated before air transport are likely to exceed critical pressure levels rapidly during flight.

In addition, there will be loss of ETT cuff pressure, with loss of a good seal, during descent if a cuff is initially inflated at peak altitudes. Therefore, we suggest ETT cuff pressures should be monitored and adjusted continuously during ascent and descent.

▶ Have you ever wondered why when you are on a commercial airliner that your tummy may feel a bit uncomfortable or that your bag of pretzels (if the airlines distribute these anymore these days) is distended? The ambient air pressure onboard is less than the pressure that was originally inside your bowel and the pretzel bag at sea level. The same thing happens to any inflated object, including endotracheal tube and laryngeal mask airway cuffs during air transport of intubated patients.

Nonpressurized aircraft, such as helicopters, fly at an average altitude of 1700 m but on occasion up to 2500 m. During ascent, ambient pressure decreases and gas will expand. If an endotracheal cuff expands, one could expect complete obstruction of tracheal mucosal perfusion. Complications of overexpansion of a cuff include hoarseness, dysphasia, sore throat, inflammation, ulceration, granulation, and possibly stenosis and ischemia of tissue to the site of the endotracheal tube cuff. Ideal inflation cuff pressures vary within a fairly narrow range.

The report of Miyashiro and Yamamoto documents that endotracheal tube cuffs inflated before air transport may exceed critical pressure levels during air transport. Similarly, if ideal pressure is achieved during flight, loss of pressure will occur during descent if a cuff is initially inflated at peak altitudes. These data basically mean that on the way up and on the way down, careful attention needs to be paid to the proper inflation pressures in the cuffs associated with such airway tubes.

We close with some observations on an audiologic topic. There has been much interest over the years in the nature of Beethoven's deafness. Beethoven (1770–1827) first noted the onset of hearing loss in 1801. By 1812, people had to shout to make themselves understood. By 1825 it appeared that Beethoven's deafness was complete and that he could no longer even hear his Ninth Symphony. Medical discussions about Beethoven's health and deafness date back to the start of the 20th century. Although still debated, his symptoms of hearing problems suggest a sensorineural hearing loss with its origin in the organ of Corti. Recently, Saccenti et al[1] attempted to find out whether the evolution of Beethoven's deafness corresponded to his so-called 3 styles of musical composition. Beginning with the observation that Beethoven's hearing loss started off in the high tones, these investigators observed a distinct correlation between what Beethoven composed and his specific degree of hearing loss. For example, prior to the early loss of hearing, 8% of Beethoven's notes were in the high frequency range. During the period while hearing impaired, but not totally deaf, this percentage progressively decreased to just 1%. Once totally deaf, however, this all changed. It was obvious that Beethoven began to compose using his inner musical world. When he came to rely completely on his inner ear he was no longer compelled to produce music that he could actually hear when performed. When that happened, his third style of music emerged which included many more high notes once again.

Thus it is that Beethoven's music continues to inform us about hearing loss as well as the enjoyment of listening to 3 distinct styles of music. Were it not for his hearing loss, none of us would appreciate the richness and diversity of his compositions.

**J. A. Stockman III, MD**

*Reference*

1. Saccenti E, Smilde AK, Saris WHM. Beethoven's deafness and his 3 styles. *BMJ*. 2011;343:1298-1300.

# 6 Endocrinology

## Children and Adolescents With Gender Identity Disorder Referred to a Pediatric Medical Center

Spack NP, Edwards-Leeper L, Feldman HA, et al (Children's Hosp Boston, MA; et al)
*Pediatrics* 129.418-425, 2012

*Objectives.*—To describe the patients with gender identity disorder referred to a pediatric medical center. We identify changes in patients after creation of the multidisciplinary Gender Management Service by expanding the Disorders of Sex Development clinic to include transgender patients.

*Methods.*—Data gathered on 97 consecutive patients <21 years, with initial visits between January 1998 and February 2010, who fulfilled the following criteria: long-standing cross-gender behaviors, provided letters from current mental health professional, and parental support. Main descriptive measures included gender, age, Tanner stage, history of gender identity development, and psychiatric comorbidity.

*Results.*—Genotypic male:female ratio was 43:54 (0.8:1); there was a slight preponderance of female patients but not significant from 1:1. Age of presentation was $14.8 \pm 3.4$ years (mean $\pm$ SD) without sex difference ($P = .11$). Tanner stage at presentation was $4.1 \pm 1.4$ for genotypic female patients and $3.6 \pm 1.5$ for genotypic male patients ($P = .02$). Age at start of medical treatment was $15.6 \pm 2.8$ years. Forty-three patients (44.3%) presented with significant psychiatric history, including 20 reporting self-mutilation (20.6%) and suicide attempts (9.3%).

*Conclusions.*—After establishment of a multidisciplinary gender clinic, the gender identity disorder population increased fourfold. Complex clinical presentations required additional mental health support as the patient population grew. Mean age and Tanner Stage were too advanced for pubertal suppressive therapy to be an affordable option for most patients. Two-thirds of patients were started on cross-sex hormone therapy. Greater awareness of the benefit of early medical intervention is needed. Psychological and physical effects of pubertal suppression and/or cross-sex hormones in our patients require further investigation.

▶ The tendency for cross-gender behavior in children has been known for many years. Data from the Youth Self Report tell us that 5% to 13% of teenage boys and 20% to 26% of teenage girls report cross-gender behavior of some type.[1] Two percent to 5% of boys and 15% to 16% of girls report sometimes having a desire to be the opposite gender. In spite of this relatively high rate of cross-gender behavior, very few patients have presented for evaluation and treatment, even in countries such as the Netherlands where there is a well-established formal program for treatment of these youngsters.[2] The prevalence in that country is on the order of 0.01% (1:10 000—30 000). Many children seem to experiment with cross-gender behavior, but few follow through to request gender change as they mature.

Combining this relatively high prevalence of cross-gender behavior with widespread information in the public domain about the availability of new early treatment approaches using puberty blocking hormones has produced a rapid increase in the number of referrals, as noted in this article. There are guidelines for the evaluation and treatment of gender-variant children. Most guidelines make it clear that prepubertal children usually should not change gender before puberty because most of them will take another life path, often to homosexuality. Children should have time to explore both genders and gender roles before making a decision for a permanent change. This ambiguity is very hard on parents and sometimes leads to a referral to attempt to settle the matter quickly. The authors provide an extension of the decision time by medically turning off puberty, so the adolescent can have more time to mature and explore alternative possibilities, and even attend school in the new gender, without irreversibly changing his or her body. The authors suggest that the age of puberty, not the age of the child, should be the determining factor of when to begin medications to block puberty.

In this study, a gonadotropin-releasing hormone blocker was used to slow puberty. Because of the high cost and the frequent insurance denials for this particular drug, creating a significant hardship on families, a less-expensive treatment, medroxyprogesterone acetate, is being used by many other centers treating gender identity issues. Treatment with the latter less-expensive drug dates to the 1960s and 1970s when it was used to stop precocious puberty in children. It costs much less (approximately $10 for 90 10-mg tablets). Patients who take this drug must be monitored for weight gain, diabetes, hypertension, gallbladder problems, and, theoretically, adrenal suppression. The treatment does not seem to affect the normal progression of bone age.

All pediatricians should read this article. It explains that the gender ratio of children presenting to the gender identity clinic is 1:1. There was also a striking prevalence of psychiatric diagnoses and a history of self-harming behaviors in many of the patients. Transgender youths were found to be at higher risk of substance abuse, suicidal ideation, and suicidal attempts. Specifically, 44.3% had a prior history of psychiatric diagnoses, 37.1% were taking psychotropic medications, and 21.6% had a history of self-injurious behavior.

The rationale for using gonadotropin-releasing hormone inhibitors is to achieve a slow sexual development. For genotypic male individuals who identify as female, virilization of hair follicles, lowering of vocal pitch, and Adam's apple prominence are irreversible. For genotypic females who identify as males, preventing endogenous estrogen-driven epiphyseal plate closure is crucial to achieve male height. Preventing endogenous secondary sexual characteristics from fully developing not only relieves distress but also enables the individual with gender identity issues to live in the phenotype of the affirmed gender.

Finally, we see in this article the role that the pediatrician can play in this situation. The first discussion parents have about gender-variant behaviors is usually with their child's pediatrician. Many of the adolescent patients who present to the gender identity clinic report that it was their pediatrician who first asked if they were experiencing gender-related issues, which became the springboard to counseling and further medical evaluation. Even if patients are too young to receive medical treatment, they and their families can benefit from counseling to cope with the difficulties of being or raising a gender-variant child. Given the high prevalence of associated problems, patients with gender identity issues should be provided with care that helps prevent self-injurious behavior and suicidal ideation, among other psychiatric difficulties.

The authors were not necessarily proposing medical treatment of prepubertal children. They do advocate for early evaluation of these children by experienced professionals, however. Clues indicating gender identity issues in genotypic male children include preference for female clothing and underwear, always sitting to void, exclusive play with female toys when given a choice, and a desire for long hair. Clues indicating gender identity issues in genotypic female children include preference for wearing male underwear, breast binding, refusal to wear female swimsuits, and psychiatric decompensation at the onset of menstruation. Persistence or intensification of gender dysphoria into full Tanner stage 2 indicates that patients should be considered for medical treatment. Referrals can then be made to specialists who treat adolescents with gender identity issues. The role of the pediatrician is to understand all of this and to get these children to the right people for further care and evaluation and to do so in a timely manner.

**J. A. Stockman III, MD**

*References*

1. Landolt MA, Bartholomew K, Saffrey C, Oram D, Perlman D. Gender nonconformity, childhood rejection, and adult attachment: a study of gay men. *Arch Sex Behav.* 2004;33:117-128.
2. Smith TE, Leaper C. Self perceived gender typicality and the peer context during adolescence. *J Res Adolesc.* 2006;16:91-104.

---

**Antenatal Thyroid Screening and Childhood Cognitive Function**

Lazarus JH, Bestwick JP, Channon S, et al (Cardiff School of Medicine, UK; St David's Hosp, Cardiff, UK; Queen Mary Univ of London, UK; et al)
*N Engl J Med* 366:493-501, 2012

---

*Background.*—Children born to women with low thyroid hormone levels have been reported to have decreased cognitive function.

*Methods.*—We conducted a randomized trial in which pregnant women at a gestation of 15 weeks 6 days or less provided blood samples for measurement of thyrotropin and free thyroxine ($T_4$). Women were assigned to a screening group (in which measurements were obtained immediately) or a control group (in which serum was stored and measurements were obtained shortly after delivery). Thyrotropin levels above the 97.5th percentile, free $T_4$ levels below the 2.5th percentile, or both were considered a positive screening result. Women with positive findings in the screening group were assigned to 150 $\mu$g of levothyroxine per day. The primary outcome was IQ at 3 years of age in children of women with positive results, as measured by psychologists who were unaware of the group assignments.

*Results.*—Of 21,846 women who provided blood samples (at a median gestational age of 12 weeks 3 days), 390 women in the screening group and 404 in the control group tested positive. The median gestational age at the start of levothyroxine treatment was 13 weeks 3 days; treatment was adjusted as needed to achieve a target thyrotropin level of 0.1 to 1.0 mIU per liter. Among the children of women with positive results, the mean IQ scores were 99.2 and 100.0 in the screening and control groups, respectively (difference, 0.8; 95% confidence interval [CI], $-1.1$ to 2.6; $P = 0.40$ by intention-to-treat analysis); the proportions of children with an IQ of less than 85 were 12.1% in the screening group and 14.1% in the control group (difference, 2.1 percentage points; 95% CI, $-2.6$ to 6.7; $P = 0.39$). An on-treatment analysis showed similar results.

*Conclusions.*—Antenatal screening (at a median gestational age of 12 weeks 3 days) and maternal treatment for hypothyroidism did not result in improved cognitive function in children at 3 years of age. (Funded by the Wellcome Trust UK and Compagnia di San Paulo, Turin; Current Controlled Trials number, ISRCTN46178175.)

▶ Lazarus et al report the results of a randomized trial of thyroid function screening involving more than 20 000 pregnant women in Italy and throughout the United Kingdom. It is well known that maternal hypothyroidism in pregnancy is associated with a range of adverse outcomes including miscarriage, preterm delivery, and reduced cognitive function in offspring. Current guidelines recommend the testing of thyroid function only in women at increased risk rather than universal screening, but many obstetricians will do universal screening. The rub is that one does not know based solely on history, physical examination, or family history whether a pregnant woman is hypothyroid. An association between maternal hypothyroidism and reduced IQ testing performance in children has been known for many years. Most recently, children of women with an elevated thyrotropin level ( > 99.7 TH percentile) in the second trimester of pregnancy have been reported to have IQ scores at ages 7 years to 9 years that on average are 4 points lower than children of euthyroid women. About one-fifth of these children had IQ scores of less than 85.[1]

Lazarus et al obtained blood samples from all women enrolled in the study at a gestation age of 11 weeks to 14 weeks, but they immediately tested only the samples from those randomly assigned to screening and stored the remainder of samples until after delivery. Women in the screening group with a serum-free thyroxin (T4) level below the 2.5th percentile, a thyrotropin level above the 97.5th percentile, or both were treated with thyroxin at a starting dose of 150 $\mu$g daily, with dose adjustments based on subsequent thyroid function testing. The offspring of both groups then underwent IQ testing at 3 years of age. The authors found that antenatal screening and maternal treatment of hypothyroidism did not result in improved cognitive function in children at 3 years of age. In a commentary that accompanied this report, Brent et al suggested that the absence of a clinically significant effect of thyroxin treatment in the current study may be explained at least in part by the inclusion of women with milder hypothyroidism.[2] It is also suggested that thyroxin therapy started at an average age of 13 weeks may be too late to obtain maximum benefit from treatment, as during the first trimester the developing fetus is entirely dependent on maternal thyroxin and this is a critical period for the action of thyroid hormone on the developing brain. It is also possible that IQ testing at 3 years of age may not be sensitive enough to pick up differences between children born of hypothyroid mothers and those who are not.

As important as the results of this study are, the findings are not likely to influence those who advocate for universal testing. This is because of the late timing of treatment initiation and the relative crudeness of IQ testing at 3 years of age when done alone for assessing the effects of thyroid hormone on the developing brain. Many will continue to perform thyroid function screening based on the belief that earlier diagnosis and treatment will improve pregnancy outcomes. Needless to say, the findings from this report will be viewed as supporting the position of clinicians who have resisted the call for universal thyroid function screening in pregnancy based on guidelines published by the American Thyroid Association and the Endocrine Society. If you were an obstetrician, what would you do?

While on the topic of things endocrinologic, please be aware that a new growth hormone tests has finally nabbed its first doper. On February 22, 2010, Terry Newton became perhaps the world's best known rugby player—not for any accomplishment on the field. The UK Anti-Doping announced that Newton is the first athlete caught by a blood test designed to detect doping with human growth hormone (HCG) to boost muscle mass. The positive test, for which Newton accepted a 2-year ban from rugby, represents a warning to athletes who may have thought HCG use was undetectable. The current HCG blood test made a limited debut at the 2004 Athens Olympics, but because of a variety of difficulties, the assay is now only being widely used recently. It had been originally thought that the illicit use of the hormone was considered unstoppable, as the synthetic form of HCG is identical to the 22-kilodalton protein naturally made by the pituitary gland. It has been shown, however, that the pituitary makes other forms of growth hormone, notably a 20-kilodalton HCG and that analyzing the growth hormone isoform ratios in a blood sample could reveal if someone had spiked themselves with non-natural HCG. This isoform test was studied in athletes at the time of the 2004 and 2006 Olympic games. It should be noted that the test only spots abnormal isoform ratios within a day or so after HCG use, so it still is relatively easy for athletes to stop taking growth hormone a few days before an event. This makes the importance of randomized screening unrelated to sporting events necessary. That is how Newton was caught. There is no HCG urine test available as of this time.[3]

**J. A. Stockman III, MD**

*References*

1. Haddow JE, Palomaki GE, Allan WC, et al. Maternal thyroid deficiency during pregnancy and subsequent neuropsychological development of the child. *N Engl J Med.* 1999;341:549-555.
2. Brent GA. The debate over thyroid-function screening in pregnancy. *N Engl J Med.* 2012;366:562-563.
3. Travis J. Growth hormone test finally nabs first doper. *Science.* 2010;327:1185.

---

**Hypothyroidism Is a Rare Cause of Isolated Constipation**
Bennett WE Jr, Heuckeroth RO (Indiana Univ School of Medicine, Indianapolis; Washington Univ School of Medicine, St Louis, MO)
*J Pediatr Gastroenterol Nutr* 54:285-287, 2012

---

The prevalence of constipation in children is high and accounts for a large percentage of pediatric and pediatric gastroenterology visits. Thyroid testing is frequently ordered to evaluate constipation and other gastrointestinal complaints in children. We reviewed all of the patients with thyroid testing ordered by our pediatric gastroenterology division during a 5-year period. We found 873 patients on whom thyroid testing was performed, and 56 patients had evidence of hypothyroidism. Nine patients had constipation and clinically significant hypothyroidism in this group; however, only 1 child had constipation as their sole presenting symptom. The contribution of occult hypothyroidism to isolated constipation in children may have been previously overestimated.

▶ Constipation is a common problem in the pediatric population. Hypothyroidism, while not rare, is an uncommon problem. Every medical student is taught, however, that hypothyroidism can be associated with constipation. For this reason, thyroid studies are frequently obtained as part of the standard evaluation for children with constipation as well as for other problems presenting to the pediatric gastroenterologist. Interestingly, there have been no studies documenting the prevalence of hypothyroidism in pediatric patients referred for evaluation of constipation and thus we have little data to justify routine screening for hypothyroidism in constipated but otherwise healthy children, adolescents, and young adults.

Bennett et al have reviewed records for patients with free thyroxin (free T4) or thyroid-stimulating hormone (TSH) tests ordered by the Pediatric Gastroenterology Division at St Louis Children's Hospital between January 1, 2003, and January 1, 2008. A full chart review was performed for all patients with thyroid testing, which included review of clinical presentation (ie, indications for ordering thyroid test, as enumerated in the pediatric gastroenterology consultation note), medical history, medication history, other laboratory tests, radiologic evaluation, and consultation with other subspecialty services. It should be noted that the laboratory fee for performing a free T4 was $12.69 and was $23.64 for a TSH. Some institutions charge more than $200 for a TSH and almost $200 for a free T4, however. A free T4, TSH, or a combination of tests was ordered

1280 times during the 5-year period for a total of 873 unique patients. Overall, just 9 patients had a combination of constipation and clinically significant hypothyroidism, and only 1 child had constipation as a sole presenting symptom.

The authors of this report documented that laboratory testing for hypothyroidism in the patient population studied ran as high as $213 120. The total cost of screening of normal patients could have been as high as $147 159, depending on insurance reimbursements. The position statement from the North American Society for Pediatric Gastroenterology, Hepatology, and Nutrition states that thyroid hormone evaluation is recommended in children only in cases of severe, refractory constipation and in most cases before consultation with a pediatric gastroenterologist. Needless to say, the patients referred to a pediatric gastroenterologist in this report would more likely than not have fulfilled the criteria for thyroid screening. The data from the report, however, suggest that thyroid function tests are unlikely to be abnormal in the absence of other clinical indications or risk factors for hypothyroidism such as concomitant growth failure, certain medication use, or a genetic predisposition (such as in trisomy 21). The identification of the single case of hypothyroidism during this time period in a child who presented with constipation alone cost at least $18 653. One can argue that this is a reasonable price to pay to make the diagnosis. You will have to be the judge as to whether you want to screen every child with severe constipation with a free T4 and TSH study. The yield is going to be quite low if constipation is the only presenting symptom.

This commentary closes with an observation having to do with short stature. It is hard to say how the zebra got its stripes, but we now know how certain wiener-size dogs get their short legs. Height-challenged dog breeds—including dachshunds, corgis and basset hounds—can thank an extra copy of a normal gene for their diminutive stature. Researchers have focused on 8 breeds from more than a dozen known to have a trait called chondrodysplasia—having legs that are short relative to body size, curved and heavier-boned than normal. Researcher analyzed the genomes of 95 dogs from the 8 short-legged breeds and the genomes of 702 dogs from 64 breeds without the trait. It was possible to pinpoint an extra stretch of genae on chromosome 18 in every dog within the short-legged breeds. The extra DNA did not turn up in a closer analysis of the control dogs. The DNA sequence found is almost identical to another gene important for limb development called *FGF4*. Located at the opposite end of chromosome 18 in dogs, the original *FGF4* gene was duplicated at some point in the dog lineage, creating a new copy elsewhere called *fgf4* retrogene. Most pieces of genes that hop around a genome are not functional, but when it comes to short-legged breeds of dogs, apparently the retrogene is "hot," which causes, for example, the typical dachshund to be a hot dog and a small one at that.[1]

**J. A. Stockman III, MD**

*Reference*

1. Sanders L. Old gene learns new short-legged trick. Diminutive dogs owe short stature to duplicated stretch of DNA. *Science News*. August 15, 2009:8.

## Selenium and the Course of Mild Graves' Orbitopathy

Marcocci C, for the European Group on Graves' Orbitopathy (Univ of Pisa, Italy; et al)

*N Engl J Med* 364:1920-1931, 2011

*Background.*—Oxygen free radicals and cytokines play a pathogenic role in Graves' orbitopathy.

*Methods.*—We carried out a randomized, double-blind, placebo-controlled trial to determine the effect of selenium (an antioxidant agent) or pentoxifylline (an antiinflammatory agent) in 159 patients with mild Graves' orbitopathy. The patients were given selenium (100 $\mu$g twice daily), pentoxifylline (600 mg twice daily), or placebo (twice daily) orally for 6 months and were then followed for 6 months after treatment was withdrawn. Primary outcomes at 6 months were evaluated by means of an overall ophthalmic assessment, conducted by an ophthalmologist who was unaware of the treatment assignments, and a Graves' orbitopathy—specific quality-of-life questionnaire, completed by the patient. Secondary outcomes were evaluated with the use of a Clinical Activity Score and a diplopia score.

*Results.*—At the 6-month evaluation, treatment with selenium, but not with pentoxifylline, was associated with an improved quality of life ($P < 0.001$) and less eye involvement ($P = 0.01$) and slowed the progression of Graves' orbitopathy ($P = 0.01$), as compared with placebo. The Clinical Activity Score decreased in all groups, but the change was significantly greater in the selenium-treated patients. Exploratory evaluations at 12 months confirmed the results seen at 6 months. Two patients assigned to placebo and one assigned to pentoxifylline required immunosuppressive therapy for deterioration in their condition. No adverse events were evident with selenium, whereas pentoxifylline was associated with frequent gastrointestinal problems.

*Conclusions.*—Selenium administration significantly improved quality of life, reduced ocular involvement, and slowed progression of the disease in patients with mild Graves' orbitopathy. (Funded by the University of Pisa and the Italian Ministry for Education, University and Research; EUGOGO Netherlands Trial Register number, NTR524.)

▶ Most cases of Graves' disease occur in adults. Graves' disease can affect children and as in adults can have ocular involvement (Graves' orbitopathy). The typical bulging eyes of Graves' disease can have serious medical and psychological consequences. Moderately severe and active forms of Graves' orbitopathy usually can be managed with steroids, orbital irradiation (in adults) or both, whereas milder forms may improve spontaneously and generally require only local measures to control symptoms (ie, artificial tears, ointments, and prisms). The natural history of mild Graves' orbitopathy shows that spontaneous improvement occurs only in about 20% of patients. The eye remains static in about 65% of patients and progresses in about 15%. Thus, those with mild Graves'-associated orbitopathy should be considered for treatment. Two agents that may potentially inhibit pathogenic mechanisms believed to be relevant in Graves' orbitopathy are selenium and pentoxifylline.

Most of us are aware that selenium is a trace metal and is an essential nutrient for selenocysteine synthesis. The latter is important in the production of certain enzymes, particularly those that have antioxidant functioning. Several studies have suggested that increased generation of oxygen-free radicals may play a role in the development of the eye problem in patients with Graves' disease. Selenium also has an important effect on the immune system and may be beneficial in certain forms of autoimmune thyroid disease, including Graves' disease. Pentoxifylline is a phosphodiesterase inhibitor used for the treatment of intermittent claudication. It has anti-inflammatory and immune effects as well. These effects are relevant to the pathogenesis of Graves' orbitopathy.

The authors of this report are part of the European Group on Graves' Orbitopathy. The investigators have been engaged in a multicenter, randomized, double-blind, placebo-controlled clinical trial investigating whether selenium or pentoxifylline may be beneficial in patients with Graves' orbitopathy. These drugs were studied in a very controlled fashion and were administered orally for 6 months in a randomized, double-blind trial. Of the 2 drugs, only selenium was associated with an improved quality of life and less eye involvement. There was definite slowing of progression of Graves' orbitopathy with the use of selenium. The condition improved in 33 of 54 patients treated with selenium. Specifically, there was improvement in the soft tissue changes in and about the eye and a decrease in eyelid aperture.

Selenium was not a perfect treatment. Fifty-four patients given selenium had mild progression of the disease and required additional measures. Selenium, however, is cheap. It can be found in any health food store or on most pharmacy shelves. It is a pretty good antioxidant and may be useful for many different purposes.

While on the topic of the eye, were you aware that the human eye has a pivotal role in the evolution of human genomics? At least 90% of the genes in the human genome are expressed in the eyes. To read more about genomics and the eye, see the superb review article that appeared recently in the *New England Journal of Medicine*.[1]

**J. A. Stockman III, MD**

*Reference*

1. Sheffield VC, Stone EM. Genomics and the eye. *N Engl J Med*. 2011;364: 1932-1942.

### Iodine status of UK schoolgirls: a cross-sectional survey

Vanderpump MPJ, on behalf of the British Thyroid Association UK Iodine Survey Group (Royal Free Hampstead NHS Trust, London, UK; et al)
*Lancet* 377:2007-2012, 2011

*Background.*—Iodine deficiency is the most common cause of preventable mental impairment worldwide. It is defined by WHO as mild if the population median urinary iodine excretion is 50–99 µg/L, moderate if 20–49 µg/L, and severe if less than 20 µg/L. No contemporary data are available for the UK, which has no programme of food or salt iodination. We aimed to assess the current iodine status of the UK population.

*Methods.*—In this cross-sectional survey, we systematically assessed iodine status in schoolgirls aged 14–15 years attending secondary school in nine UK centres. Urinary iodine concentrations and tap water iodine concentrations were measured in June–July, 2009, and November–December, 2009. Ethnic origin, postcode, and a validated diet questionnaire assessing sources of iodine were recorded.

*Findings.*—810 participants provided 737 urine samples. Data for dietary habits and iodine status were available for 664 participants. Median urinary iodine excretion was 80·1 µg/L (IQR 56·9–109·0). Urinary iodine measurements indicative of mild iodine deficiency were present in 51% (n = 379) of participants, moderate deficiency in 16% (n = 120), and severe deficiency in 1% (n = 8). Prevalence of iodine deficiency was highest in Belfast (85%, n = 135). Tap water iodine concentrations were low or undetectable and were not positively associated with urinary iodine concentrations. Multivariable general linear model analysis confirmed independent associations between low urinary iodine excretion and sampling in summer ($p < 0.0001$), UK geographical location ($p < 0.0001$), low intake of milk ($p = 0.03$), and high intake of eggs ($p = 0.02$).

*Interpretation.*—Our findings suggest that the UK is iodine deficient. Since developing fetuses are the most susceptible to adverse effects of iodine deficiency and even mild perturbations of maternal and fetal thyroid function have an effect on neurodevelopment, these findings are of potential major public health importance. This study has drawn attention to an urgent need for a comprehensive investigation of UK iodine status and implementation of evidence-based recommendations for iodine supplementation.

▶ Vanderpump et al have shown that iodine nutrition, at least in the United Kingdom, is inadequate. These investigators have assayed urinary iodine in more than 700 girls attending secondary schools. Moderate-to-severe dietary iron deficiency causes goiter as well as hypothyroidism. As importantly, adequate concentrations of thyroid hormone are needed for normal neurodevelopment, both in utero and in early life. Iodine deficiency in pregnant or lactating women can lead to neurocognitive impairments in children. Currently, almost 2 billion individuals worldwide live in iodine-deficient areas.

So what went wrong in Great Britain? The United Kingdom, similar to other developed nations such as the United States, and, until recently, Australia and

New Zealand, has never mandated iodization of salt or other foods. In Great Britain, less than 5% of salt sold is iodized. Back in the 1930s, iodine was added to cattle feeds to improve milk production. Such iodization resulted in increased iodine content in cow's milk and therefore improved human nutrition with respect to iodine. Obviously the effect of feeding cows iodine has not produced a durable effect on iodine status, at least in teenage girls in Great Britain. Milk consumption or milk iodine content has decreased over the decades in Great Britain resulting in the reappearance of iodine deficiency.

In other parts of the world, we have seen this problem of iodine deficiency more directly addressed. In 2009, for example, Australia and New Zealand mandated iodization of salt in commercially baked bread to ensure adequate iodine nutrition in the general population. In the United States, dietary iodine sources are much more diverse, and the use of iodized salt, although not mandated, is much more widespread. Unfortunately, on US shores, dietary iodine intake has been estimated to have decreased by half between the early 1970s and the early 1990s, partly because of changes in the use of iodine by the dairy industry. While US iodine intake is currently substantially higher than that of the United Kingdom, there are now concerns that vulnerable populations in the United States might also be mildly iodine deficient.

Women who are pregnant are especially vulnerable to iodine deficiency as are lactating women. Women planning a pregnancy should be advised to take a daily vitamin supplement that contains iodine in the form of potassium iodide. This approach has been advocated by the American Thyroid Association in North America as well as by the Australian National Health and Medical Research Committee and the New Zealand Ministry of Health. Needless to say, whenever we are examining teens, it is best that we also keep a careful eye out for any clinical findings consistent with iodine deficiency, including the early development of goiter.

**J. A. Stockman III, MD**

---

**A 12-Month Phase 3 Study of Pasireotide in Cushing's Disease**
Colao A, for the Pasireotide B2305 Study Group (Univ of Naples Federico II, Italy; et al)
*N Engl J Med* 366:914-924, 2012

---

*Background.*—Cushing's disease is associated with high morbidity and mortality. Pasireotide, a potential therapy, has a unique, broad somatostatin-receptor–binding profile, with high binding affinity for somatostatin-receptor subtype 5.

*Methods.*—In this double-blind, phase 3 study, we randomly assigned 162 adults with Cushing's disease and a urinary free cortisol level of at least 1.5 times the upper limit of the normal range to receive subcutaneous pasireotide at a dose of 600 $\mu$g (82 patients) or 900 $\mu$g (80 patients) twice daily. Patients with urinary free cortisol not exceeding 2 times the upper limit of the normal range and not exceeding the baseline level at month 3 continued to receive their randomly assigned dose; all others received an additional 300 $\mu$g twice daily. The primary end point was a urinary free cortisol level at or below the upper limit of the normal range at month 6 without an increased dose. Open-label treatment continued through month 12.

*Results.*—Twelve of the 82 patients in the 600-μg group and 21 of the 80 patients in the 900-μg group met the primary end point. The median urinary free cortisol level decreased by approximately 50% by month 2 and remained stable in both groups. A normal urinary free cortisol level was achieved more frequently in patients with baseline levels not exceeding 5 times the upper limit of the normal range than in patients with higher baseline levels. Serum and salivary cortisol and plasma corticotropin levels decreased, and clinical signs and symptoms of Cushing's disease diminished. Pasireotide was associated with hyperglycemia-related adverse events in 118 of 162 patients; other adverse events were similar to those associated with other somatostatin analogues. Despite declines in cortisol levels, blood glucose and glycated hemoglobin levels increased soon after treatment initiation and then stabilized; treatment with a glucose-lowering medication was initiated in 74 of 162 patients.

*Conclusions.*—The significant decrease in cortisol levels in patients with Cushing's disease who received pasireotide supports its potential use as a targeted treatment for corticotropin-secreting pituitary adenomas. (Funded by Novartis Pharma; ClinicalTrials.gov number, NCT00434148.)

▶ Although this report largely deals with adults, children can develop Cushing disease, albeit rarely. The disease causes chronic hypercortisolism and is usually due to a corticotropin-secreting pituitary adenoma. The result is central obesity, osteoporosis, arterial hypertension, insulin resistance, glucose intolerance, diabetes mellitus, dyslipidemia, cardiovascular disease, growth failure in children, and increased mortality. In both children and adults, transsphenoidal surgery is the primary therapy in most patients. Unfortunately, not all patients respond. Up to 30% will have a relapse. The alternative then includes repeat pituitary surgery, radiation therapy, bilateral adrenalectomy, or medical therapy. In prior commentaries, I related a story of a family dog who developed Cushing syndrome and was treated medically with an agent that blocks cortisol production. Increasingly we have been seeing humans treated the same way medically. Adrenal adenomas express somatostatin receptors, predominantly somatostatin-receptor subtype 5. Activation of this subtype inhibits secretion of corticotropin, providing a potential therapeutic target for management of Cushing syndrome.

Pasireotide is a somatostatin analogue that targets 4 of the 5 somatostatin receptors. The investigators associated with the report abstracted enrolled patients 18 years of age and older with confirmed persistent or recurrent Cushing disease or newly diagnosed disease if they were not candidates for surgery. The enrollment was in a study in which patients were randomly assigned to receive subcutaneous medical treatment with pasireotide twice daily at 2 different doses. The primary endpoint was a reduction of urinary free cortisol to normal levels in the urine. Treatment continued for 12 months. This randomized, double-blind trial showed that just over 50% of patients had a substantial reduction in urinary cortisol levels by 6 months, including patients with very high baseline values. The majority of patients had moderate-to-severe Cushing syndrome at the start of this study. Normalization of adrenal function was more likely to be achieved in patients with lower baseline levels of urinary steroids. Many patients with severe disease also responded. Urinary cortisol levels decreased quickly with a mean reduction of steroid levels approximately 50% by 2 months. Patients who did not respond identified themselves quickly. The investigators suggest that additional medical therapy in combination with pasireotide would be helpful in refractory cases.

It should be noted that the patients who had reductions in urinary cortisol did lose body weight. They also experienced lower systolic and diastolic blood pressures and low-density lipid cholesterol levels, as well as improvements in scores for health-related quality of life indicators. The most common adverse event related to drug therapy was transient gastrointestinal discomfort. Approximately three-quarters of patients had some elevation in blood sugar. Six percent of patients discontinued the study treatment because of side effects. The elevation in blood sugar appears to be the result of decreased insulin and incretin secretion. In this study, hyperglycemia occurred despite declining cortisol levels. In all patients with this problem, blood glucose levels were able to be managed in a traditional way with insulin.

It can be concluded that there is now reasonably effective medical therapy available for patients, both young and old, with Cushing syndrome for whom surgical management, for one reason or another, is not the path to go, at least initially. This is good news. Last, this commentary closes with a question. Cushing syndrome is a known cause of diabetes. Who was the first individual to divide "diabetes" into diabetes mellitus and diabetes insipidus? It was apparent that the sweet test of diabetic urine escaped the attention of western physicians until 1679, when the English physician, Thomas Willis, used it to identify two forms of the disease: diabetes mellitus (the latter word from the Latin for honey) and diabetes insipidus (the latter word simply meaning without taste). For what it is worth, the Indian name for diabetes, *madhumea*, shows that Eastern medicine was aware of the sweet taste of the urine of diabetics long before Western physicians. Madhumea simply means "honey-urine disease."[1]

**J. A. Stockman III, MD**

*Reference*

1. Barnett R. Historical keyword: diabetes. *Lancet.* 2010;375:191.

---

**Recurrent *PRKAR1A* Mutation in Acrodysostosis with Hormone Resistance**
Linglart A, Menguy C, Couvineau A, et al (Hopital St Vincent de Paul, Paris, France; Universite Paris—DescartesFrance; et al)
*N Engl J Med* 364:2218-2226, 2011

---

The skeletal dysplasia characteristic of acrodysostosis resembles the Albright's hereditary osteodystrophy seen in patients with pseudohypoparathyroidism type 1a, but defects in the α-stimulatory subunit of the G-protein

(GNAS), the cause of pseudohypoparathyroidism type 1a, are not present in patients with acrodysostosis. We report a germ-line mutation in the gene encoding PRKAR1A, the cyclic AMP (cAMP)–dependent regulatory subunit of protein kinase A, in three unrelated patients with acrodysostosis and resistance to multiple hormones. The mutated subunit impairs the protein kinase A response to stimulation by cAMP; this explains our patients' hormone resistance and the similarities of their skeletal abnormalities with those observed in patients with pseudohypoparathyroidism type 1a.

▶ Acrodysostosis (Online Mendelian Inheritance in Man number 101800) is a rare form of skeletal dysplasia with severe brachydactyly, facial dysostosis, nasal hypoplasia, and short stature. Advanced skeletal maturation, decreased vertebral interpedicular distance, and obesity are also frequently observed. Autosomal dominant transmission has been reported in some families. Several forms of acrodysostosis are also present in patients with Albright hereditary osteodystrophy. Some patients will show resistance to either parathyroid hormone or thyrotropin. Given that these findings are not seen in all patients, it has been suspected that there are likely to be several forms of acrodysostosis.

This report of Linglart et al tells us about 3 unrelated patients with acrodysostosis and multihormone resistance and tests the hypothesis that a gene defect in the CaM-dependent protein kinase A signaling pathway downstream of GNAS might be involved. Protein kinase A is the enzyme that causes phosphorylation of specific proteins that mediate the physiologic effect of various hormones.

So why do we include an article such as this? It is important from time to time to provide information on complex reports to understand how far along science has come in identifying the underlying causes of various disorders and including uncommon ones. These authors have identified a novel genetic abnormality that results in resistance to stimulation of phosphorylation by protein kinase, thereby causing a serious bone disorder associated with resistance to several hormones. These findings open the door to a much better understanding of a variety of bone disorders that occur in children. We should pay attention to reports such as this when they appear even if it is unlikely that we are going to see a patient with the specific problem described.

While on the topic of things that affect bone and bone growth, in May 2011, a French appeals court threw out the charges of involuntary manslaughter and other crimes against 2 scientists involved in a growth hormone scandal that led to the deaths of 125 children from Creutzfeldt-Jakob disease (CJD), a fatal brain illness. This case has dragged on since the early 1990s, and 2 of the original defendants have since died. From 1959 to 1988, France treated almost 1700 growth-deficient children with hormone derived from pituitary glands taken from human cadavers, a practice that has been linked to the transmission of CJD, a prion disease. Prosecutors faulted the scientists involved for not doing enough to prevent CCJD by switching far too late to the much safer synthetic growth hormone in comparison to many other countries.

This commentary closes with a quiz having to do with growth. Can you name the world's smallest vertebrate? If you dropped a dime in the middle of an eastern

New Guinea rainforest you might squash a newly discovered frog species. *Paedophryne amanuensis* has taken the top spot as the world's smallest vertebrate. Adults attain an average size of just 7.7 mm in length, less than half the diameter of a US dime. That beats the former record holder, an Indonesian fish from the carp family whose females grow to about 7.9 mm. The new frog species eats rainforest leaf litter. Miniaturization is nothing new for frogs. The 29 smallest species all come in at under 13 mm. These tiny creatures have a distinct genetic advantage in that they can exploit the nooks and crannies in the vegetation of the floor of the rainforest.[1]

**J. A. Stockman III, MD**

*Reference*

1. Editorial comment. Meet the world's smallest vertebrate. *Science.* 2012;335:269.

# 7 Gastroenterology

**Fifty-three—year experience with pediatric umbilical hernia repairs**
Zendejas B, Kuchena A, Onkendi EO, et al (Mayo Clinic, Rochester, MN)
*J Pediatr Surg* 46:2151-2156, 2011

*Purpose.*—The aim of this study was to evaluate the long-term surgical and patient-reported outcomes of pediatric umbilical hernia (UH) repairs.

*Methods.*—A retrospective review of all children (<18 years old) who underwent UH repair at Mayo Clinic—Rochester in the last half century was done. Follow-up was obtained by mailed survey.

*Results.*—From 1956 to 2009, 489 children (boys, 251; girls, 238) underwent a primary UH repair. The mean age was 3.9 years (range, 0.01–17.8 years). Complicated UHs that required emergent repair (n = 34, or 7%) included recurrent incarceration (22), enteric fistula (7), strangulation (4), and evisceration (1). Mean UH size was 1.3 cm (range, 0.2-7.0 cm), varying by operative indication (1.0 cm emergent vs 1.5 cm elective repairs, *P* = .008) and decade of repair (2.2 cm, 1950s-60s vs 1.3 cm, 1990s-2000s; *P* = .001). Postoperative morbidity (2%) consisted of superficial wound infection (7), hematoma (3), and seroma (1). With a 66% survey response rate and mean follow-up of 13.0 years (range, 0-53.8 years), 8 (2%) patients experienced a recurrence. Most patients reported satisfaction (90%) with the cosmetic appearance of their umbilicus and are pain free (96%).

*Conclusion.*—Pediatric UH repairs have low morbidity and recurrence rates. Most patients are satisfied and pain free. Importantly, complicated UHs were more likely to be associated with smaller defects; therefore, parental counseling for signs of incarceration is recommended even in small defects.

▶ Every pediatric provider knows how common umbilical hernias are. In the white population, studies show at birth somewhere between 10% and 30% of infants will have an umbilical hernia. By contrast, rates as high as 85% have been reported for children of African descent and low birth weight infants.[1] Ninety percent of these defects will close by 4 years of age without consequence. Almost all hernias that are less than 0.5 cm will close by 2 years of age, whereas most that are greater than 1 cm do not close until the patient is near 4 years of age. Needless to say, since tincture of time takes care of the majority of umbilical hernias, usually repair for an umbilical hernia is advocated only if the defect persists beyond 4 to 5 years of age or if the defect is significantly larger than 1 to 2 cm, is enlarging, is symptomatic, or has been associated with a complication. In such cases, consideration for repair earlier than 4 years is entertained. Because there is always a risk in general anesthesia, if anesthesia is being given for another procedure, it might be desirable to close an umbilical hernia while under anesthesia for the unrelated surgery.

Investigators at Mayo Clinic have assessed the long-term outcomes of youngsters who have had an umbilical hernia repair. They identified all children younger than 18 years of age who underwent a primary umbilical hernia repair at Mayo Clinic from October 1956 through April 2007. Some 489 children underwent this procedure at Mayo. There were equal numbers of boys and girls. The average age at repair was just under 4 years. Twelve percent had a history of prematurity. Twenty-two percent had some comorbid problem. The most common indication for surgery was size or persistence, whereas 31% of infants had the surgery performed as part of a concomitant procedure. Just 7% of infants or youngsters had the repair done as part of an emergent problem. The average umbilical hernia size was 1.3 cm. Immediate postoperative morbidity consisted of superficial wound infection (1%), hematoma (1%), and seroma (1%), for an overall early postoperative morbidity rate of just 2%. During that period, 2% of patients experienced a recurrence. The median time to recurrence was 0.9 years. Hernia repair with nonabsorbable sutures (ie, silk) were nearly 6 times more likely to recur when compared with those repaired with absorbable sutures. Factors that did not appear to be associated with an increased risk of recurrence were repair technique; type of incision; hernia size; age at surgery; race/ethnicity; prematurity; sex; repair of a concomitant epigastric hernia; an umbilical hernia associated with an umbilical cyst, granuloma, or polyp; decade of surgery; and concomitant procedure. Most patients on follow-up said they were either satisfied (77%) or somewhat satisfied (13%) with the appearance of their umbilicus. Some 6% indicated that they were somewhat dissatisfied or very dissatisfied with the appearance of their umbilicus, with the remaining 14 patients (4%) neither being satisfied or dissatisfied. Girls were more likely to be dissatisfied compared with boys.

This is one of the most extensive follow-up studies of repair of umbilical hernia during infancy and childhood. The data from this report allow pediatricians to have an intelligent discussion with parents about the pros and cons of umbilical hernia repair as well as what the long-term outcome should be with such repairs, at least performed at a reputable institution. Overall, it is encouraging that umbilical pain or discomfort appears to be nearly nonexistent in patients who underwent an umbilical hernia repair as a child. It is important to adequately counsel both parents and patients (when age appropriate) in terms of setting realistic expectations regarding the final appearance of the umbilicus after an umbilical hernia repair because a small but real percentage, mostly girls, will not be happy with what they see in the mirror.

Given the low morbidity and recurrence rates (2%) and the fact that most patients are pain free and satisfied with the appearance of their umbilicus, it is reasonable to share such good news with parents of infants/toddlers/ young children who might be in need of such repair. Also, it should be noted that in contrast with the increasing use of mesh-based repairs in adult umbilical hernias, there seems to be no role whatsoever for their use in children undergoing primary umbilical hernia repair.

This commentary closes with a very ponderous query: why is it that some people accumulate navel fluff and others do not? This is a conundrum that few would dare to bother their doctors about, but it is still an interesting question. Abdominal hair appears to be responsible for navel lint, according to an article that appeared in *Medical Hypotheses*.[2] By definition, hair lint is largely a male phenomenon. Abdominal hair is thought to collect fibers from cotton shirts and direct them into the navel where they are compacted into a felt-like matter. If abdominal hair is shaved, lint no longer collects, so there is the therapy. Also, heavily washed tee-shirts and dress shirts produce less matter than new tee-shirts. A possible function of the lint may be to fulfill a cleaning function for the navel, or so it is hypothesized. Now there is a fact or two you might not want to remember about the belly button.

**J. A. Stockman III, MD**

*References*

1. Meier DE, OlaOlorun DA, Omodele RA, Nkor SK, Tarpley JL. Incidence of umbilical hernia in African children: redefinition of "normal" and reevaluation of indications for repair. *World J Surg.* 2001;25:645-648.
2. Steinhauser G. The nature of navel fluff. *Med Hypotheses.* 2009;72:623-625.

---

**Proton Pump Inhibitor Use in Infants: FDA Reviewer Experience**
Chen I-L, Gao W-Y, Johnson AP, et al (Ctr for Drug Evaluation and Res, Silver Spring, MD)
*J Pediatr Gastroenterol Nutr* 54:8-14, 2012

The Food and Drug Administration has completed its review of 4 clinical trials evaluating the use of proton pump inhibitors (PPIs) in infants (ages 1 month to <12 months) for the treatment of gastroesophageal reflux disease (GERD). An Advisory Committee meeting was held in November 2010 to discuss the potential reasons why PPI use in these trials failed to show a benefit in infants with GERD, and directions for future study. The present review summarizes the findings from the clinical trials. Potential mechanisms for the failed clinical trials are discussed. The safety of long-term use is also discussed. As a result of our analysis and review, the authors agree with the Advisory Committee members that PPIs should not be administered to treat the symptoms of GERD in the otherwise healthy infant without the evidence of acid-induced disease.

▶ The use of proton pump inhibitors in infants has been increasing in recent years. It's easy to see why. In infants compared with older children, gastric fluid enters the esophagus much more easily. In most infants, this does not cause problems other than simple gastroesophageal reflux (GER). If it does cause problems, we call it GERD (gastroesophageal reflux disease). In most instances, GERD will respond in time on its own. Sometimes simple measures are necessary to treat symptoms, though. The latter may include crying and arching of the back. Simple treatments, including thickened, frequent, and smaller feedings and frequent burping, usually work. If there is no response to such simple treatments, other etiologies should be looked for such as cow milk intolerance. Assuming none are found, treatment then often begins with an antacid and/or a protein pump inhibitor. It should be noted that as of 2012, no proton pump inhibitor has been approved by the US Food and Drug Administration for use in infants less than 12 months of age.

The review of Chen summarizes the efficacy results of trials that have taken place to date on proton pump inhibitors and shows information related to pharmacokinetics and safety in infants. Chen et al have examined the data on the 5 most commonly available proton pump inhibitors. The review clearly demonstrates that no deaths have occurred in infants treated with proton pump inhibitors. It is also clear that clinical trials to date have not revealed a serious safety signal.

It isn't clear why proton pump inhibitors are not effective in infants since they do suppress gastric acid. Nonetheless, clinical trials conducted to date have failed to demonstrate proton pump inhibitor efficacy in this population of young patients. Despite the lack of evidence to support their effectiveness in infant GERD, proton pump inhibitor use continues to increase over time. Among pediatric patients younger than 12 months, more than 400 000 prescriptions were dispensed to 145 000 patients nationally in 2009.[1] This represents an 11-fold increase in prescriptions from 2002. Curiously, the number of new prescriptions being written has not increased significantly but the numbers of prescriptions filled has, suggesting that proton pump inhibitors are being used on a chronic basis in many children. Chronic use of proton pump inhibitors does carry some possible risk. There have been rare reports of vitamin and electrolyte abnormalities, such as vitamin B12 deficiency and hypomagnesemia, in adults taking proton pump inhibitors chronically. Gastric acid is also important in the absorption of iron in the upper small bowel. Increasing concern exists about proton pump inhibitors as a cause of iron deficiency and iron deficiency anemia.

Chances are that those who provide care to children will continue to use proton pump inhibitors in infants with GER and GERD symptoms even though there is no clear-cut evidence that they work. That said, it is probably reasonable to use a short course of such agents for infants who have unexplained irritability or fussiness given the low-risk profile of short-term use. Sustained use, however, should not be undertaken without a thorough investigation of potential underlying causes of GERD symptoms.

This commentary closes with an interesting cause of a GI problem. See how you would handle the following situation. You are seeing a 17-year-old previously healthy boy, a member of a high school wrestling team, who presents with a 3-day history of progressive retrosternal chest pain, odynophagia and fever. He has been previously well. He is taking no medications. On physical examination, the patient is mildly uncomfortable, complaining of midsternal chest pain. The vital signs are normal. Routine laboratory studies show no abnormalities. An electrocardiogram and chest x-ray are both unremarkable. Suspecting that the patient may have esophagitis, you ask that an endoscopy be performed. This study reveals multiple ulcerations in the mid to lower esophagus. The person doing the procedure is smart enough to obtain one additional study at the time of the endoscopy. He does a viral culture. In view of the sporting activity of this youngster, what virus might be causing his esophagitis? If you answered herpes simplex virus, you would be right. Recently several cases of herpes simplex virus esophagitis in high school wrestlers were reported.[2] It has been well documented that herpes simplex virus skin infection can be endemic among high school and college wrestlers. Mode of transmission in such cases is skin-to-skin contact. The recently reported cases of herpes simplex virus esophagitis secondary to wrestling are the first in the literature, however. These cases demonstrate that herpetic esophagitis in the immunocompetent patient is self-limited and that supportive care without antiretroviral medication is usually sufficient for treatment. Remember this new entity: herpes simplex esophagitis gladiatorum.

**J. A. Stockman III, MD**

*References*

1. Vandenplas Y, Rudolph CD, Di Lorenzo C, et al. Pediatric gastroesophageal reflux clinical practice guidelines: joint recommendations of the North American Society for Pediatric Gastroenterology, Hepatology, and Nutrition (NASPGHAN) and the European Society for Pediatric Gastroenterology, Hepatology, and Nutrition (ESPGHAN). *J Pediatr Gastroenterol Nutr.* 2009;49:498-547.
2. Khlevner J, Beneri C, Morganstern JA. Wrestling and herpetic esophagitis. *Pediatr Infect Dis J.* 2011;30:911-912.

## Role of Gastroesophageal Reflux in Children With Unexplained Chronic Cough

Borrelli O, Marabotto C, Mancini V, et al (Great Ormond Street Hosp for Sick Children and Inst of Child Health, London, UK; "La Sapienza" Univ of Rome, Italy)

*J Pediatr Gastroenterol Nutr* 53:287-292, 2011

*Objective.*—The relation between respiratory symptoms and gastro-esophageal reflux (GER) is a matter of contention and debate, with limited data in children to substantiate or refute cause and effect. Moreover, there are few data on the relation between nonacid reflux and chronic cough in childhood. We aimed to describe the type and physical characteristics of reflux episodes in children with unexplained chronic cough.

*Patients and Methods.*—Forty-five children with chronic cough underwent 24-hour multichannel intraluminal impedance-pH monitoring (MII-pH monitoring). Symptom association probability (SAP) characterized the reflux-cough association. Twenty children with erosive reflux disease (ERD) served as controls.

*Results.*—Twenty-four children had cough-related reflux (CRR), with 19 having no gastrointestinal symptoms. Twenty-one had cough-unrelated reflux (CUR). CRR and ERD had increased acid (AR), weakly acidic (WAc), and weakly alkaline (WAlk) reflux. Esophageal acid exposure time and acid clearance time were higher in ERD than in CRR and CUR.

In the CRR group, of 158 cough episodes related to reflux episodes, 66% involved AR, 18% WAc, and 16% WAlk. Seventeen children had positive SAP, 7 for AR, 5 for both AR and WAc, 4 for both WAc and WAlk, and 1 for WAlk.

*Conclusions.*—In children with unexplained chronic cough, asymptomatic acid and nonacid GER is a potential etiologic factor. The increased acid exposure time and delayed acid clearance characteristic of ERD are absent in cough-related GER. MII-pH monitoring increases the likelihood of demonstrating a temporal association between the cough and all types of reflux.

▶ This report reminds us that gastroesophageal reflux (GER) can be a common cause of chronic cough in children. This is an important observation because many children who have this will have no other signs or symptoms specifically related to GER. The relation between respiratory symptoms and GER has been debated for a long time. In adults, it is widely accepted that reflux of gastric contents will potentially cause a chronic cough. To date there have been only limited data to support the association in children. In adults, when GER is a cause of chronic cough, in 75% of cases, there are no associated symptoms specifically related to GER itself. We see in this report that approximately 85% of patients in the pediatric age group who had cough related to GER had no complaints of typical reflux symptoms such as regurgitation, heartburn, and epigastric pain, documenting that in both children and adults, absence of typical GER symptoms in no way rules out GER as a cause of chronic cough.

There was one other interesting observation in this report. Although prolonged acid exposure can provide an explanation for why some patients develop esophagitis and others do not, the data from this study suggest that the proximal propagation of reflux material does not distinguish patients who develop respiratory symptoms such as cough from those with more typical esophageal symptoms. It seems likely, therefore, that mechanisms other than the type or proximal extension of the reflux episodes is the cause of cough. The actual volume of refluxate, the degree of esophageal distention, and the activation of different types of mechanical receptors may be involved in the generation of symptoms such as cough.

The lessons here are clear. As part of the evaluation of chronic cough, if nothing obvious jumps out at you, consider the possibility of otherwise asymptomatic GER.

This commentary closes with an observation on Charles Darwin's lifelong illness. It is now more than 200 years since the naturalist entered this world. Mr Darwin had a mysterious illness that endured throughout adulthood that was most manifested during his sail on the HMS Beagle in 1831. At the time his problem with vomiting was merely thought to be the result of sea sickness, but it was a major problem for Darwin to the extent that he was incapacitated for days at a time. Darwin's sea sickness was clearly more severe than normally experienced by anyone. This sickness continued after his voyage and was characterized by episodes of nausea, vomiting, intermittent abdominal pain, weakness, and lethargy and often was associated with headache and dizziness, visual disturbances, and palpitations. He complained of "inordinate flatulence" and at times diarrhea. These episodes were at times completely disabling. He went through many different treatments without lasting improvement from any. The nature of Darwin's illness has been the subject of much and varied speculation. Psychological diagnoses offered over the years have included hypochondria, neurasthenia, panic disorders, and agoraphobia. Psychoanalysts have put Darwin's illness down to repressed anger towards his father, nervousness about this relationship with his wife, and guilt over conflict with his earlier religious beliefs. Suggested physical diagnoses have included Ménière disease, arsenic poisoning from prescribed drugs, and Chagas disease resulting from an insect bite during his sojourn in South America. These diagnoses have all been disallowed for good reasons. The illness was not fatal. It was present probably for at least 50 years and became less severe in old age. Darwin died at age 73 with symptoms of cardiac ischemia and heart failure. The illness did not impair his fertility since as well as being the Father of Modern Biology, he fathered 10 children, all conceived during his long period of ill health.

A Darwin devotee in Melbourne, Australia, thinks he has solved the Darwin medical mystery.[1] It is now suggested that Darwin's symptoms most closely mimic those of cyclic vomiting syndrome. Although this is primarily a disease of children, it may persist into adulthood or may appear for the first time in adulthood. The disease is related to classic migraine and abdominal migraine, but is also linked to abnormalities of mitochondrial DNA with mutations in the MTTL1 gene. It was first described in the English literature in 1882. Affected individuals with cyclic vomiting syndrome experience abdominal, circulatory, and cerebral symptoms, including headaches, and anxiety. Symptoms overlap with those of classic and abdominal migraine, except for a lack of aura. The vomiting in most people is associated with severe abdominal pain. It should also be noted that many with cyclic vomiting syndrome also have eczema that may be related to various food allergies. A review of Darwin's family history indicates that his mother had vomiting spells as did her younger brother Tom.

Charles was not aware of mitochondria or of genes and genetic mutations, but he was very aware of random variations within species. This was the keystone for his theory of the "survival of the fittest," the driving mechanism of evolution. His personal inherited genetic variation made him substantially "less fit," but his survival prospects were greatly increased by his driving intelligence, loyal colleagues, devoted wife, family, and household servants, and personal wealth!

**J. A. Stockman III, MD**

*Reference*

1. Hayman JA. Darwin's illness revisited. *BMJ.* 2009;339:1413-1415.

---

### Identification of Specific Foods Responsible for Inflammation in Children With Eosinophilic Esophagitis Successfully Treated With Empiric Elimination Diet

Kagalwalla AF, Shah A, Li BUK, et al (Northwestern Univ, Chicago, IL; Children's Hosp of Wisconsin, Wauwatosa; et al)
*J Pediatr Gastroenterol Nutr* 53:145-149, 2011

---

*Objectives.*—Eosinophilic esophagitis (EoE) is an immune-mediated chronic inflammatory disorder triggered by food antigen(s). A 6-food elimination diet (SFED) excluding cow's milk, soy, wheat, egg, peanuts/tree nuts, and seafood has been shown to induce remission in a majority of children with EoE. The goal of the present study was to identify specific food antigens responsible for eosinophilic esophageal inflammation in children with EoE who had achieved histological remission with the SFED.

*Patients and Methods.*—In this analysis, we retrospectively analyzed children with EoE who completed subsequent single-food reintroductions that led to identification of foods causing disease recurrence. Repeat upper endoscopy with biopsies was performed after single-food introductions. Recurrence of esophageal eosinophilia following a food reintroduction identified that food antigen as a cause of EoE.

*Results.*—A total of 36/46 (25M/11F) children who were initially successfully treated with SFED completed this trial; the mean age was 7.6 ± 4.3 years. The most common foods identified were 25 to cow's milk (74%), 8 to wheat (26%), 4 to eggs (17%), 3 to soy (10%), and 1 to peanut (6%). Milk was 8 times more likely to cause EoE compared with wheat, the next most common food (95% confidence interval 2.41−26.62, $P = 0.0007$).

*Conclusions.*—Serial single-food reintroductions following induction of histological remission with the SFED can lead to the identification of specific causal food antigen(s) in EoE. Cow's milk was the most common food identified in subjects with EoE treated with SFED. A subset of children with EoE may develop tolerance to their food sensitivities while on the SFED.

▶ A quarter of a century ago, most pediatricians had never heard of eosinophilic esophagitis. It is now recognized as a disorder of both children and adults. Five years ago, a consensus report outlined recommendations for both diagnosis and treatment of individuals with this problem.[1] Most believe that eosinophilic esophagitis is a chronic immune-mediated inflammatory process, isolated to the esophagus, most likely triggered by exposure to food antigens. Exclusion of offending food antigens in many cases results in disease remission, and reexposure leads to recurrence. Given the varying antigens and responses to those antigens, currently no one-size-fits-all diet has been devised that can eliminate the disorder. Elemental diets that try to cover all bases tend to be costly and unpalatable. Some have suggested an alternative management with a "6-food elimination diet" (SFED). Kagalwalla et al tell us about the impact of this diet, which simultaneously eliminates milk, eggs, wheat, soy, fish/shellfish, and nuts without regard to the results of traditional allergy testing. Approximately 75% of children with eosinophilic esophagitis will experience a remission while avoiding these specific food types. The obvious advantage over an elemental diet is the retention of a substantial portion of the diet, which can be nutritionally complete when managed by a dietician.

We learn from this report about the frequency with which the individual antigens in the elimination diet are responsible for eosinophilic inflammation upon reintroduction of the antigen. Milk was the most common culpable antigen, but each of the antigens was an offender for some individuals, and some individuals adversely reacted to 2 or more of the foods. The latter is the basis for removing all 6 foods simultaneously at the onset. If the foods are removed individually, then none of the children who are intolerant of more than 1 antigen would show resolution because of the constant, although changing, presence of at least 1 offending food in their diet.

Unfortunately, there are no biomarkers to tell us who may have eosinophilic esophagitis without the need for biopsy. Noninvasive biomarkers such as cotaxin 3 or eosinophil-derived neurotoxin are currently under investigation. Eosinophilic esophagitis can result in lamina propria fibrosis, loss of compliance of the esophageal wall, or stricture. These can result in chronic dysphagia, the most common symptom in adolescents and adults. With early management, remodeling of the lamina propria is reversible and absolutely necessary to prevent complications.

It is likely that as a result of the report of Kagalwalla et al, we will see more implementation of the SFED diet early in the management of eosinophilic esophagitis in children. Patient education is crucial in this regard because therapy needs to be targeted to each child's needs.

This commentary closes with a query. Have you ever wondered whether a period of down economy might affect the value of the coinage that occasionally inadvertently trickles down the pediatric esophagus? Believe it or not, investigators have examined whether there is a relationship between societal wealth and the value of ingested foreign bodies. Firth et al looked at the relation of coins as foreign bodies in the esophagus and the Dow Jones Industrial average.[2] After ensuring that their institutional review board at Massachusetts General Hospital had a good sense of humor, the investigators compiled data on all numismatic and sundry detritus acquired (NASDAQ composite index) from childrens' gastrointestinal tract by the pediatric gastroenterology service at their hospital between August 2006 and July 2009. No patient, however rich or poor, was excluded. They calculated the total financial wealth swallowed and extracted as a fraction of the US dollar or 100 cents (FTSE 100 index), and the ratio of patients with coins versus all those with foreign objects removed (pecuniary extraction ratio, PE ratio). They then calculated the mean end-of-month closing value of the Dow Jones industrial average. The intent was to examine whether there was a change in the monthly mean NASDAQ, FTSE and PE ratio before and after the collapse of the Dow Jones Industrial Average of October 2008. The patients who had coinage removed were age 1 to 15 years. The bottom line was that there was no detectable difference in the total value of coins ingested, or ratio of coins to other objects swallowed, before or after the massive stockmarket crash.

It should be noted that for the coinage removed, there was a 27% penny aspiration rate significantly lower than the 36% penny pinching rate reported back in 1982 in other studies. Actually, if one corrects for inflation rates over time, this is exactly what one would expect, showing that our free market is indeed a free market in the United States. Assuming parents keep up with inflation over the decades then the coins left under pillows for exfoliated dentition also make sense. In any event, in times of extremely down economies, swallowing a coin is a safer way to save money…sort of like putting your money under your mattress instead of in the bank.

**J. A. Stockman III, MD**

*References*

1. Noel RJ, Putnam PE, Collins MH, et al. Clinical and immunopathologic effects of swallowed fluticasone for eosinophilic esophagitis. *Clin Gastroenterol Hepatol.* 2004;2:568-575.
2. Firth PG, Zheng H, Biller JA. Ingested foreign bodies and societal wealth: Three-year observational study of swallowed coins. *BMJ.* 2009;339:1400-1403.

## Ultrasonographic Quantitative Estimation of Hepatic Steatosis in Children With NAFLD

Shannon A, Alkhouri N, Carter-Kent C, et al (Cleveland Clinic, Cleveland, OH; et al)
*J Pediatr Gastroenterol Nutr* 53:190-195, 2011

*Background and Aims.*—The diagnostic accuracy of hepatic ultrasonography (US) for detection and grading of hepatic steatosis in children with suspected nonalcoholic fatty liver disease (NAFLD) remains poorly characterized. The aim of this study was to prospectively evaluate the clinical utility of ultrasonographic quantification of hepatic steatosis.

*Patients and Methods.*—Our cohort consisted of 208 consecutive pediatric patients with biopsy-proven NAFLD. Hepatic US was performed within 1 month of the liver biopsy procedure. Steatosis identified by US was scored using a 0 to 3 scale based on echogenicity and visualization of vasculature, parenchyma, and diaphragm, and compared to histological features based on Brunt's classification.

*Results.*—The median age at time of first visit was 10.8 years and 64% were boys. Sixty-nine percent had moderate to severe steatosis on histology. Ultrasonographic steatosis score (USS) had an excellent correlation with histological grade of steatosis (with a Spearman's coefficient of 0.80). The area under the receiver operating characteristic curve for ultrasonographic detection of moderate-to-severe steatosis was 0.87. The USS did not correlate significantly with inflammatory activity or fibrosis stage; however, there was significant correlation with the NAFLD activity score (NAS), albeit this was in large part the result of the strong correlation with the steatosis component of NAS. Serum alanine transaminase and aspartate transaminase were not associated with histological grade of steatosis and showed no correlation with USS.

*Conclusions.*—Our results, which represent the largest prospective pediatric study evaluating the role of hepatic US in children with biopsy-proven NAFLD, demonstrate the utility of this technique for noninvasive diagnosis and estimation of hepatic steatosis in children.

▶ Elsewhere, we have discussed the importance of nonalcoholic fatty liver disease (NAFLD). In children, the latter is mostly the consequence of obesity and can be associated with the metabolic syndrome and type 2 diabetes mellitus. Establishing a diagnosis of NAFLD is of utmost importance since it can lead to serious complications, including the development of cirrhosis. The diagnosis, however, can be a major challenge, because the liver disease itself is generally silent, and the gold standard for diagnosis is an invasive liver biopsy, a procedure that is not suitable for screening purposes. Other screening measures include monitoring of liver enzymes. Recently, the American Academy of Pediatrics recommended that serum aminotransferases (alanine transaminase [ALT] and aspartate transaminase [AST]) be performed in all overweight children starting at age 10 if the body mass index is ≥95th percentile or between the 85th and 94th percentile in those with risk factors. Unfortunately, liver enzymes perform poorly as a screening test for NAFLD diagnosis, with two-thirds of patients with NAFLD showing normal levels of serum ALT and AST.

The authors of the report abstracted have turned to examining ultrasonography as a possible screening tool to detect NAFLD. Using ultrasonography, they examined 208 pediatric patients who had biopsy-proven NAFLD. Radiologists scored the ultrasound scans. Steatosis score was calculated as follows: absent steatosis (score 0), defined as normal liver echotexture; mild steatosis (score 1) as slight and diffuse increase in fine parenchymal echoes with normal visualization of diaphragm and portal vein borders; moderate steatosis (score 2) as moderate and diffuse increase in fine echoes with slightly impaired visualization of portal vein borders and diaphragm; and severe steatosis (score 3) as fine echoes with poor or no visualization of portal vein borders, diaphragm, and posterior portion of the right lobe. The median age of children examined was just 10.8 years (range, 3.25–14.1 years). The principal findings of the study relate to the use of hepatic ultrasound scan for detection and quantification of hepatic steatosis in children with NAFLD. It is clear that ultrasound scan correlates closely with severity of steatosis on liver biopsy, suggesting that ultrasonographic examination is an excellent screening test for NAFLD in children and a useful noninvasive modality for quantifying hepatic steatosis. The authors also showed that serum liver enzymes have a poor predictive value regarding the presence or severity of fatty liver disease.

The current guidelines that recommend screening by ALT and AST are not helpful in indicating whether further workup should be done in obese children in whom fatty liver is suspected. It is clear, however, that ultrasound scan cannot differentiate between hepatic steatosis and the more advanced form of disease known as nonalcoholic steatohepatitis. The latter, nonetheless, does not occur in the absence of fatty infiltration of the liver; thus, ultrasound scan remains a good screening test for the early evolution to more severe forms of hepatitis that may lead to cirrhosis.

**J. A. Stockman III, MD**

---

**Factors Associated With Hepatic Steatosis in Obese Children and Adolescents**
Ruiz-Extremera Á, Carazo Á, Salmerón Á, et al (San Cecilio Univ Hosp, Granada, Spain; Instituto de Salud Carlos III, Majadahonda, Spain; Virgen de las Nieves University Hospital, Granada, Spain; et al)
*J Pediatr Gastroenterol Nutr* 53:196-201, 2011

---

*Objectives.*—Obesity is associated with high prevalence of hepatic steatosis. We speculate that determinant factors of susceptibility to hepatic steatosis in obesity could differ between children and adolescents.

*Patients and Methods.*—Blood biochemical parameters, systemic oxidative stress markers, proinflammatory cytokines, and adipokine levels were determined in 157 obese children and adolescents. The subjects were divided into 2 groups: children and adolescents, identified as such in accordance with Tanner stage and the measured level of dehydroepiandrosterone sulphate. Steatosis was evaluated by ultrasonography in 127 subjects.

*Results.*—Steatosis prevalence was 44.8%. In the "children" group, those with hepatic steatosis presented higher levels of erythrocyte oxidised glutathione (GSSG) and resistin, lower levels of high-density lipoprotein (HDL) cholesterol, and lower enzymatic activities of erythrocyte glutathione reductase (GRd) and glutathione oxidase (GPx). In the "adolescents" group, those with hepatic steatosis presented higher values for body mass index z score (BMIz), insulin, peptide C, homeostatic model assessment index (HOMA-IR), alanine aminotransferase (ALT), aspartate aminotransferase (AST), triglycerides, GSSG, and leptin. These subjects also presented lower values for soluble leptin receptor, GRd, and GPx. In the "children" group, the only independent factor of steatosis was a decrease in GRd activity (odds ratio [OR] 0.165, 95% CI 0.03–0.84, $P = 0.030$). Moreover, in the "adolescent" group, the independent factors were higher for GSSG (OR 6.8, 95% CI 1.6–28.7, $P = 0.010$) and HOMA-IR (OR 1.9, 95% CI 1.17–3.1, $P = 0.009$).

*Conclusions.*—Factors associated with hepatic steatosis differ between obese children and adolescents. Oxidative stress is seen to be the main process in children, whereas in adolescents oxidative stress and insulin resistance are significant factors for steatosis.

▶ Much is written these days about the metabolic syndrome. There is a distinct link between obesity, the metabolic syndrome, and nonalcoholic fatty liver disease (NAFLD), type 2 diabetes mellitus, and cardiovascular disease. NAFLD is a term that defines a spectrum of abnormalities. These abnormalities range from simple triglyceride accumulation into hepatocytes to hepatic steatosis with inflammation (nonalcoholic steatohepatitis). The latter can progress to scarring of the liver and frank cirrhosis. Some degree of NAFLD occurs in 50% of obese twins, primarily in boys but also in some girls. Most investigators believe that hepatic steatosis is the liver expression of the metabolic syndrome.

Ruiz-Extremera et al have studied the problem of hepatic steatosis and obesity to determine whether there is a different pathophysiologic mechanism linking the two in children as opposed to adolescents and young adults. Obesity was defined by these investigators as a body mass index greater than the 95th percentile. The investigators observed that aggravated oxidative stress on the liver was a relevant process in liver steatosis development in both children and adolescents. Free radical overproduction is believed to be a causative factor. The main sources of cellular oxidative stress are the endoplasmic reticulum and the mitochondrion. Mitochondrial dysfunction is closely associated with a hypercaloric diet.

Now that a good bit of the pathophysiology of the liver disease in obese children, including those with the metabolic syndrome, is understood, perhaps other therapeutic measures can be used in addition to caloric restriction. The latter is hard to achieve in many given social circumstances. Would it not be nice if there were a pill a day that would help spare the liver from converting itself into a fatty blob of cirrhotic tissue?

**J. A. Stockman III, MD**

---

## Weight Loss, Cardiovascular Risk Factors, and Quality of Life After Gastric Bypass and Duodenal Switch: A Randomized Trial

Søvik TT, Aasheim ET, Taha O, et al (Univ of Oslo, Norway; Sahlgrenska Univ Hosp, Gothenburg, Sweden)
*Ann Intern Med* 155:281-291, 2011

---

*Background.*—Gastric bypass and duodenal switch are currently performed bariatric surgical procedures. Uncontrolled studies suggest that duodenal switch induces greater weight loss than gastric bypass.

*Objective.*—To determine whether duodenal switch leads to greater weight loss and more favorable improvements in cardiovascular risk factors and quality of life than gastric bypass.

*Design.*—Randomized, parallel-group trial. (ClinicalTrials.gov registration number: NCT00327912).

*Setting.*—2 academic medical centers (1 in Norway and 1 in Sweden).

*Patients.*—60 participants with a body mass index (BMI) between 50 and 60 kg/m$^2$.

*Intervention.*—Gastric bypass ($n = 31$) or duodenal switch ($n = 29$).

*Measurements.*—The primary outcome was the change in BMI after 2 years. Secondary outcomes included anthropometric measures; concentrations of blood lipids, glucose, insulin, C-reactive protein, and vitamins; and health-related quality of life and adverse events.

*Results.*—Fifty-eight of 60 participants (97%) completed the study. The mean reductions in BMI were 17.3 kg/m$^2$ (95% CI, 15.7 to 19.0 kg/m$^2$) after gastric bypass and 24.8 kg/m$^2$ (CI, 23.0 to 26.5 kg/m$^2$) after duodenal switch (mean between-group difference, 7.44 kg/m$^2$ [CI, 5.24 to 9.64 kg/m$^2$]; $P < 0.001$). Total cholesterol concentration decreased by 0.24 mmol/L (CI, −0.03 to 0.50 mmol/L) (9.27 mg/dL [CI, −1.16 to 19.3 mg/dL]) after gastric bypass and 1.07 mmol/L (CI, 0.79 to 1.35 mmol/L) (41.3 mg/dL [CI, 30.5 to 52.1 mg/dL]) after duodenal switch (mean between group difference, 0.83 mmol/L [CI, 0.48 to 1.18 mmol/L]; 32.0 mg/dL [CI, 18.5 to 45.6 mg/dL]; $P \le 0.001$). Reductions in low-density lipoprotein cholesterol concentration, anthropometric measures, fat mass, and fat-free mass were also greater after duodenal switch ($P \le 0.010$ for each between-group comparison). Both groups had reductions in blood pressure and mean concentrations of glucose, insulin, and C-reactive protein, with no between-group differences. The duodenal switch group, but not the gastric bypass group, had reductions in concentrations of vitamin A and 25-hydroxyvitamin D. Most Short Form-36 Health Survey dimensional scores improved in both groups, with greater improvement in 1 of 8 domains (bodily pain) after gastric bypass. From surgery until 2 years, 10 participants (32%) had adverse events after gastric bypass and 18 (62%) after duodenal switch ($P = 0.021$). Adverse events related to malnutrition occurred only after duodenal switch.

*Limitation.*—Clinical experience was greater with gastric bypass than with duodenal switch at the study centers.

*Conclusion.*—Duodenal switch surgery was associated with greater weight loss, greater reductions of total and low-density lipoprotein cholesterol concentrations, and more adverse events. Improvements in other cardiovascular risk factors and quality of life were similar after both procedures (Fig 1).

▶ Although this report appears in the adult literature, the information gained clearly will be handed down to those who are involved with bariatric surgery in adolescents because the same procedures are often used. Bariatric procedures were devised to induce weight loss in patients who could not lose weight by diet and exercise alone. The first operation was the ill-fated jejunoileal bypass, a procedure that caused substantial nutrient malabsorption. Because jejunoileal bypass was the first successful treatment for morbid obesity, clinicians embraced it until its substantial complication profile became evident. Bacterial overgrowth in the bypassed intestinal limb led to damage to the liver and cirrhosis. Roux-en-Y gastric bypass and biliopancreatic diversion procedures were then devised to induce weight loss and avoid the long-term complications associated with jejunoileal bypass. It is clear that such operations should not be widely adopted until they have been studied in a controlled manner and over a number of years. Extensive reviews of bariatric surgery have provided irrefutable evidence showing that bariatric surgery does induce weight loss but also can cause harm.

Søvik et al report the 2-year results of a 2-center randomized trial comparing gastric bypass with duodenal switch in a cohort of very obese patients adding to the library of level-1 evidence in the bariatric literature. The figure demonstrates the anatomy of these procedures. The authors have shown that patients who had duodenal switch lost more weight than their gastric bypass counterparts

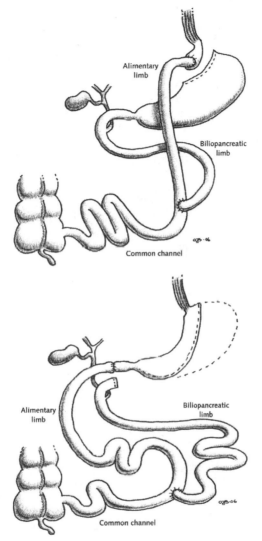

**FIGURE 1.**—Gastric bypass (*top*) and biliopancreatic diversion with duodenal switch (*bottom*). Bowel limb lengths for gastric bypass: alimentary limb, 150 cm; biliopancreatic limb, 50 cm; and common channel, variable length. Bowel limb lengths for duodenal switch: alimentary limb, 200 cm; biliopancreatic limb, variable length; and common channel, 100 cm. Figures by Ole-Jacob Berge, MD, and reproduced from reference 25 with permission. (Reprinted from Søvik TT, Aasheim ET, Taha O, et al. Weight Loss, Cardiovascular Risk Factors, and Quality of Life After Gastric Bypass and Duodenal Switch: A Randomized Trial. *Ann Intern Med.* 2011;155:281-291, with permission from the American College of Physicians.)

(reduction in body mass index, 24.8 kg/m$^2$ vs 17.3 kg/m$^2$). The investigators also found greater reductions in total and low-density lipoprotein cholesterol levels, waist circumference, and fat and fat-free mass.

The most striking observation in this report is the very high complication rate in both groups: 32% for gastric bypass and 62% for duodenal switch. Patients in both groups experienced vomiting, abdominal pain, and diarrhea. A worrisome observation was that among the 29 patients in the duodenal switch group, there were 3 cases of protein calorie malnutrition, 2 cases of night blindness necessitating treatment, and 1 case of severe iron deficiency requiring iron infusion. None of these events occurred in the gastric bypass cohort. Patients who underwent duodenal switch had lower levels of vitamin A and 25-hydroxy vitamin D. Patients in this study were young (the median age was about 35 years). Two-thirds of the duodenal switch group were women, many in their childbearing years. These women may later develop serious complications related to malabsorption. Night blindness is particularly worrisome for young women because it can lead to blindness in their children. Complications may take years to manifest.

In a commentary that accompanied this report, Livingston notes that short- and long-term complications of bariatric operations are inevitable.[1] Given the very high rate of lifelong complications and the minimal effect of these procedures on overall survival, improved longevity is probably not a reasonable cause for performing them. Bariatric operations, Livingston notes, probably should be done only to control an immediate medical problem that surgically induced weight loss is expected to resolve, such as diabetes and sleep apnea. In this context then, weight loss is not exactly the precise end goal but rather the elimination of comorbid conditions. It is also suggested that duodenal switch is not an appropriate operation, because the added weight loss compared with gastric bypass is offset by complications that far outweigh any potential benefits.

An editorial recently appeared in the *New England Journal of Medicine* that discussed bariatric surgery for adolescents with morbid obesity.[2] It is noted that by the late 1990s, only a few adolescents had undergone bariatric surgery, but its use since then has rapidly grown. It appears that somewhere between under 1000 and several thousand adolescents undergo bariatric procedures every year. There is no registry of these procedures. There are general guidelines that most accept that determine who is a suitable candidate for bariatric surgery. These are patients who are morbidly obese as defined by a body mass index of at least 40 in association with coexisting medical conditions (or at least 50 otherwise), have reached physical maturity (tanner stage 4 or 5), have evidence of emotional and cognitive maturity, and have been unable to achieve weight loss by all other methods. The presence of a supportive family is considered key. Guidelines currently state that prepubertal children, patients with Prader-Willi syndrome, and patients with untreated psychiatric disorders or eating disorders should not receive bariatric surgery. To read about these guidelines, see Barlow et al.[3] Roux-en-Y gastric bypass is the most commonly performed bariatric surgery for morbidly obese teens in the United States. A gastric sleeve operation is becoming more prevalent, but still accounts for a minority of surgical procedures. Alternatively, gastric banding can be done but is associated with less rapid and less profound weight loss but is considered more effective than lifestyle-based treatments. Alternatives such as an intragastric balloon, which is inflated and left in place for up to 6 months, or a gastric stimulator, in which electrodes are implanted and stimulated to lead to sense of satiety, have been recommended, but data in children and teens are minimal.

There are several prospective studies of bariatric surgery in progress in the United States. The Teen Longitudinal Assessment of Bariatric Surgery, which has nearly completed its enrollment, is obtaining extensive data on adolescents who have undergone any bariatric procedure. Hopefully, this and other prospective studies will answer the question of whether bariatric surgery in the young will prove more effective over time than less invasive approaches. Many practitioners believe that weight loss surgery is a better alternative than watching a morbidly obese youngster develop a myriad of complications.

**J. A. Stockman III, MD**

*References*

1. Livingston EH. Primum non nocere. *Ann Intern Med.* 2011;155:329-330.
2. Ingelfinger JR. Bariatric surgery in adolescents. *N Engl J Med.* 2011;365:1365-1367.
3. Barlow SE; Expert Committee. Expert committee recommendations regarding the prevention, assessment, and treatment of child and adolescent overweight and obesity: summary report. *Pediatrics.* 2007;120:S164-S192.

## Intussusception Risk and Health Benefits of Rotavirus Vaccination in Mexico and Brazil

Patel MM, López-Collada VR, Bulhões MM, et al (Ctrs for Disease Control and Prevention, Atlanta, GA; Natl Ctr for Child and Adolescent Health, Mexico City; Ministry of Health, Brasilia; et al)
*N Engl J Med* 364:2283-2292, 2011

*Background.*—Because postlicensure surveillance determined that a previous rotavirus vaccine, RotaShield, caused intussusception in 1 of every 10,000 recipients, we assessed the association of the new monovalent rotavirus vaccine (RV1) with intussusception after routine immunization of infants in Mexico and Brazil.

*Methods.*—We used case-series and case–control methods to assess the association between RV1 and intussusception. Infants with intussusception were identified through active surveillance at 69 hospitals (16 in Mexico and 53 in Brazil), and age-matched infants from the same neighborhood were enrolled as controls. Vaccination dates were verified by a review of vaccination cards or clinic records.

*Results.*—We enrolled 615 case patients (285 in Mexico and 330 in Brazil) and 2050 controls. An increased risk of intussusception 1 to 7 days after the first dose of RV1 was identified among infants in Mexico with the use of both the case-series method (incidence ratio, 5.3; 95% confidence interval [CI], 3.0 to 9.3) and the case–control method (odds ratio, 5.8; 95% CI, 2.6 to 13.0). No significant risk was found after the first dose among infants in Brazil, but an increased risk, albeit smaller than that seen after the first dose in Mexico — an increase by a factor of 1.9 to 2.6 — was seen 1 to 7 days after the second dose. A combined annual excess of 96 cases of intussusception in Mexico (approximately 1 per 51,000 infants) and in Brazil (approximately 1 per 68,000 infants) and of 5 deaths due to intussusception was attributable to RV1. However, RV1 prevented approximately 80,000 hospitalizations and 1300 deaths from diarrhea each year in these two countries.

*Conclusions.*—RV1 was associated with a short-term risk of intussusception in approximately 1 of every 51,000 to 68,000 vaccinated infants. The absolute number of deaths and hospitalizations averted because of vaccination far exceeded the number of intussusception cases that may have been associated with vaccination. (Funded in part by the GAVI Alliance and the U.S. Department of Health and Human Services.)

▶ Rotavirus infection remains the most important cause of severe diarrheal disease in young children. In less developed countries, it accounts for more than half a million childhood deaths annually. In developed countries, rotavirus is an infrequent cause of death, but a common cause of hospitalization and outpatient visits. The rotavirus vaccine, RotaShield, composed of 4 human × simian reassortants, has been recommended for universal pediatric use in the United States since 1998. All of us know that after the vaccine had been given to more than half a million children, it was found to cause a transient increased risk of intussusception (estimated to occur in 1 child in 10 000) in the first 10 days after the initial vaccination. RotaShield was rapidly withdrawn from the market before there was an opportunity for a detailed public discussion of the risks and benefits surrounding its use. Two second-generation rotavirus vaccine candidates were in development in 1999 and, after 7 additional years of study, were licensed in the United States and other countries. Both second-generation vaccines are effective and have undergone extensive safety trials. No association with intussusception has been detected in these trials.

With the reintroduction of the rotavirus vaccine, there has been a significant reduction in the rates of hospitalization and death from rotavirus in both developed and less-developed countries. As part of the post-licensure safety follow-up, the possible effect of the widespread use of these new vaccines on intussusception rates has been monitored in the United States and abroad. The report of Patel et al tells us about the results of safety assessments of the monovalent attenuated human rotavirus vaccine in Mexico and Brazil. This extensive post-licensure safety assessment shows that the monovalent vaccine is associated with a very small excess risk of intussusception (approximately 1 in 51 000 vaccinated children) and only in the first week after vaccination. The timing of this excess risk occurs at the peak of vaccine virus replication. A smaller excess risk has been observed after a second dose of the monovalent vaccine, but this excess risk occurs during the second and third week after vaccination, and its significance is unclear. A slightly decreased risk of intussusception was noted in Brazil compared with Mexico. In Brazil, the first dose of the monovalent vaccine is administered with the oral poliovirus vaccine, which somewhat suppresses rotavirus vaccine replication.

This report from Mexico and Brazil documents both the effectiveness and the safety of at least 1 of the 2 rotavirus vaccines currently on the market. As Patel et al point out, in Mexico alone, rotavirus vaccination would be expected to prevent 663 childhood deaths and 11 551 hospitalizations while causing 41 excess hospitalizations and 2 additional deaths due to intussusception. Similarly favorable ratios of benefit to risk would be expected to be found in virtually all less developed countries, where diarrheal illness remains a leading cause of death. The bottom line in the United States is that it seems both appropriate and advisable to continue to recommend rotavirus vaccine for children on the basis of increasingly well-documented and substantial benefits. To read more about rotavirus vaccination and intussusception, see the excellent editorial by Greenberg.[1]

**J. A. Stockman III, MD**

*Reference*

1. Greenberg HB. Rotavirus vaccination and intussusception—act two. *N Engl J Med.* 2011;364:2354-2355.

---

### Neonatal acute appendicitis: a proposed algorithm for timely diagnosis

Schwartz KL, Gilad E, Sigalet D, et al (Univ of Calgary, Alberta, Canada)
*J Pediatr Surg* 46:2060-2064, 2011

*Background.*—Neonatal appendicitis (NA) is a rare disease with a high mortality. The diagnosis has never been reported preoperatively and is notoriously difficult to make.

*Methods.*—Charts since 1995 were retrospectively reviewed for discharge or death diagnoses of appendicitis in neonates younger than 28 days. We report 3 cases of NA seen at our institution during this period.

*Results.*—All 3 infants were previously well, born at term, and presented with signs consistent with abdominal sepsis. The first 2 diagnoses were not made until autopsy. The third case survived after having an urgent computed tomographic scan, exploratory laparotomy, and appendectomy.

*Discussion.*—The literature summarizing common presenting features of NA is reviewed. We present an algorithm to guide the workup of these neonates to facilitate earlier diagnosis and potentially improve outcomes (Fig 3).

▶ Neonatal appendicitis is something that every pediatric care provider should be familiar with even though it is a rare condition. Missing the diagnosis is not good because neonatal appendicitis carries a high mortality rate. The mortality rate is as high as 28%.[1] Schwartz et al have retrospectively reviewed the medical records of the Alberta Children's Hospital, Calgary, Canada, for a 15-year period to determine the outcome of neonates with appendicitis. Three cases were found. All 3 cases showed rapid onset of symptoms and deterioration. None of the cases had bilious emesis or hematochezia. One infant was seen several times in an emergency department and discharged before presenting in septic shock requiring transfer to Alberta Children's Hospital. This patient died within 3 hours of transfer. A second case presented as neonatal peritonitis at 13 days of age. An initial ultrasound scan showed no abnormal appendix. This youngster died before surgery could be undertaken, and at autopsy it was shown that the tip

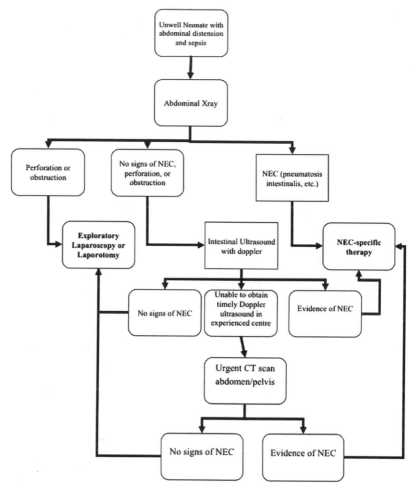

FIGURE 3.—Proposed algorithm for neonates with abdominal sepsis. (Reprinted from Journal of Pediatric Surgery, Schwartz KL, Gilad E, Sigalet D, et al. Neonatal acute appendicitis: a proposed algorithm for timely diagnosis. *J Pediatr Surg*. 2011;46:2060-2064. Copyright 2011, with permission from Elsevier.)

of the appendix had perforated. Given this infant's findings, the children's hospital instituted a policy that unexplained sepsis with a clinical suggestion of an abdominal source should be investigated immediately by laparotomy/ laparoscopy or computed tomographic (CT) scan. A third case presented with similar findings of sepsis and worsening distention that did not fit with the typical clinical presentation of necrotizing enterocolitis nor was there an improvement with intravenous antibiotics and supportive therapy. The patient was taken quickly to the operating room after a CT scan was performed, which revealed a grossly perforated appendix with no evidence of other bowel pathology. The patient did survive.

The authors of this report provided a protocol (Fig 3) that they now use that they anticipate will reduce the likelihood of morbidity and mortality related to the presence of neonatal hepatitis. The trick with this protocol is to move through it very quickly. It is clear that neonatal appendicitis may occur in healthy term neonates and that keeping the potential diagnosis on the radar screen early in the differential diagnosis is key to survivorship.

This commentary closes with a quiz. You are seeing a 6-month-old infant in follow-up for an umbilical discharge. The girl had been referred to pediatric surgeons a month ago with a persistent serosanguineous umbilical discharge and inflammation that had been present from 12 weeks of age. The provisional diagnosis at that time was a patent urachal duct. However, at surgery no abnormality was found. The problem has persisted. What simple test could you perform in your office that would help you make a diagnosis? Be aware that there are a number of dermatologic causes of umbilical discharge in an infant including eczema, bacterial omphalitis, and umbilical granuloma. Obviously this infant would have had these diagnoses excluded. What was not excluded was a residual vitelline duct containing ectopic gastric mucosa. This can contain gastrointestinal epithelium, which, like any other gastric epithelium, can discharge gastric acid. The diagnosis here could have readily been made by checking the pH of the umbilical discharge. The case described was a real one.[2] The care providers used a simple urine dipstick to determine the pH of the discharge which was very low. The next time you see an umbilical discharge in an infant, think about the remote possibility of ectopic gastric mucosa and reach for a dipstick!

**J. A. Stockman III, MD**

*References*

1. Karaman A, Cavuşoğlu YH, Karaman I, Cakmak O. Seven cases of neonatal appendicitis with a review of the English language literature of the last century. *Pediatr Surg Int.* 2003;19:707-709.
2. Browne F, Parashar K, Ogboli M, Moss C. Umbilical discharge: The acid test. *Arch Dis Child.* 2011;96:512.

## Risk of Intussusception Following Administration of a Pentavalent Rotavirus Vaccine in US Infants

Shui IM, Baggs J, Patel M, et al (Harvard Med School and Harvard Pilgrim Health Care Inst, Boston, MA; Ctrs for Disease Control and Prevention, Atlanta, GA; et al)
*JAMA* 307:598-604, 2012

*Context.*—Current rotavirus vaccines were not associated with intussusception in large prelicensure trials. However, recent postlicensure data from international settings suggest the possibility of a low-level elevated risk, primarily in the first week after the first vaccine dose.

*Objective.*—To examine the risk of intussusception following pentavalent rotavirus vaccine (RV5) in US infants.

*Design, Setting, and Patients.*—This cohort study included infants 4 to 34 weeks of age, enrolled in the Vaccine Safety Datalink (VSD) who received RV5 from May 2006-February 2010. We calculated standardized incidence ratios (SIRs), relative risks (RRs), and 95% confidence intervals for the association between intussusception and RV5 by comparing the rates of intussusception in infants who had received RV5 with the rates of intussusception in infants who received other recommended vaccines without concomitant RV5 during the concurrent period and with the expected number of intussusception visits based on background rates assessed prior to US licensure of the RV5 (2001-2005).

*Main Outcome Measure.*—Intussusception occurring in the 1- to 7-day and 1- to 30-day risk windows following RV5 vaccination.

*Results.*—During the study period, 786 725 total RV5 doses, which included 309 844 first doses, were administered. We did not observe a statistically significant increased risk of intussusception with RV5 for either comparison group following any dose in either the 1- to 7-day or 1- to 30-day risk window. For the 1- to 30-day window following all RV5 doses, we observed 21 cases of intussusception compared with 20.9 expected cases (SIR, 1.01; 95% CI, 0.62-1.54); following dose 1, we observed 7 cases compared with 5.7 expected cases (SIR, 1.23; 95% CI, 0.5-2.54). For the 1- to 7-day window following all RV5 doses, we observed 4 cases compared with 4.3 expected cases (SIR, 0.92; 95% CI, 0.25-2.36); for dose 1, we observed 1 case compared with 0.8 expected case (SIR, 1.21; 95% CI, 0.03-6.75). The upper 95% CI limit of the SIR (6.75) from the historical comparison translates to an upper limit for the attributable risk of 1 intussusception case per 65 287 RV5 dose-1 recipients.

*Conclusion.*—Among US infants aged 4 to 34 weeks who received RV5, the risk of intussusception was not increased compared with infants who did not receive the rotavirus vaccine.

▶ Anyone who has practiced pediatrics in recent years recalls the withdrawal of the rotavirus vaccine back in 1999 and then the reintroduction of 2 vaccines to prevent rotavirus infection in 2006. A postlicensure safety study performed in the United States after 2 years of surveillance did not find any evidence for an increased risk of intussusception in the 30 days following administration of the rotavirus vaccine, while at the same time 2 recent international postlicensure evaluations have observed an increased risk of intussusception in the first week after administration of the first dose of a rotavirus vaccine.[1,2] Shui et al now tell us what the current situation is in the United States. Shui et al looked at data related to three-quarters of a million doses of administered rotavirus vaccine to determine any adverse outcomes as the result of vaccine administration. The data from this report show that among US infants age 4 weeks to 34 weeks who received the rotavirus vaccine, the risk of intussusception was not increased compared with a control group of infants who did not receive the vaccine. At least on our shores, the rotavirus vaccine appears to be safe. The reasons for the inconsistent results between studies in the United States and overseas are unclear. Because intussusception is a rare event, one cannot rule out the chance of finding a risk in Australia and Mexico, where an increased risk was observed, as well as the possibility of not detecting a low-level risk in the United States or in Brazil, where findings similar to those in the United States have been reported. Another possible explanation might be environmental or genetic factors that influence the risk of intussusception in other countries.

It should be noted that the US Food and Drug Administration has approved a change in prescribing information by the manufacturers of the 2 currently available rotavirus vaccines. Prescribing information now notes that a previous episode of intussusception should be considered a contraindication to vaccination.[3] There are no data, however, on the actual risk of recurrent disease in such infants if they receive the vaccine. The warning seems to be a precautionary measure because around 5% to 10% of infants with intussusception in the past (before the vaccine was available) had a second episode of intussusceptions, making it impossible to tell for sure whether a second episode of intussusception might be related to vaccine administration

**J. A. Stockman III, MD**

*References*

1. Belongia EA, Irving SA, Shui IM, et al; Vaccine Safety Datalink Investigation Group. Real-time surveillance to assess risk of intussusception and other adverse events after pentavalent, bovine-derived rotavirus vaccine. *Pediatr Infect Dis J.* 2010;29:1-5.
2. Buttery JP, Danchin MH, Lee KJ, et al; PAEDS/APSU Study Group. Intussusception following rotavirus vaccine administration: post-marketing surveillance in the National Immunization Program in Australia. *Vaccine.* 2011;29:3061-3066.
3. Centers for Disease Control and Prevention (CDC). Addition of history of intussusception as a contraindication for rotavirus vaccination. *MMWR Morb Mortal Wkly Rep.* 2011;60:1427.

## Surgeon-performed ultrasound as a diagnostic tool in appendicitis

Burford JM, Dassinger MS, Smith SD (Arkansas Children's Hosp, Little Rock)
*J Pediatr Surg* 46:1115-1120, 2011

*Purpose.*—Diagnosing appendicitis may require adjunct studies such as computed tomography or ultrasound (US). Combining a clinical examination with surgeon-performed US (SPUS) may increase diagnostic accuracy and decrease radiation exposure and costs.

*Methods.*—A prospective study was conducted including children with a potential diagnosis of appendicitis. A surgery resident performed a clinical examination and US to make a diagnosis. Final diagnosis of appendicitis was confirmed by operative findings and pathology. Results were compared with radiology department US (RDUS) and a large randomized trial. Analysis was performed using Fisher exact test.

*Results.*—Fifty-four patients were evaluated and underwent SPUS. Twenty-nine patients (54%) had appendicitis. Overall accuracy was 89%, with accuracy increasing from 85% to 93% between the 2 halves of the study. Radiology department US was performed on 21 patients before surgical evaluation, yielding an accuracy of 81%. Surgeon-performed US on those 21 patients yielded an accuracy of 90%. No statistical differences were found between any groups ($P > .05$).

*Conclusion.*—Accuracy of SPUS was similar to RDUS and that of a large prospective randomized trial performed by radiologists. Furthermore, when the same clinician performs the clinical examination and US, a high level of accuracy can be achieved. With this degree of accuracy, SPUS may be used as a primary diagnostic tool and computed tomography reserved for challenging cases, limiting costs, and radiation exposure.

▶ We are hearing more and more about end-user performance of ultrasound as opposed to ultrasound performed by technicians in radiology departments or by radiologists themselves. This report by Burford et al tells us about how good surgical residents are in using ultrasound examinations to make a diagnosis of appendicitis. The study is an important one since we have been seeing much more in the way of liberal use of computed tomography (CT) as an imaging modality for the accurate diagnosis of both adult and pediatric patients suspected of having appendicitis. The use, however, of CT for appendicitis diagnosis has been questioned because of concerns over inefficiency, high cost, and the long-term effects of ionizing radiation. As a result, many have implemented clinical pathways using ultrasound as the primary imaging modality. However, such studies are operator-dependent and are typically performed in the radiology department where access may be limited after normal business hours.

The authors of this report recognize the increasingly widespread surgeon-performed ultrasound in trauma, endocrine, breast, and vascular surgery. Surgeons have been performing their own ultrasounds for the diagnosis of pyloric stenosis. This increasing familiarity with ultrasound techniques coupled with the lack of access to after-hours ultrasound led Burford et al to study the role of surgeon-performed ultrasound in the diagnosis of appendicitis.

In this report, third-year surgical residents were taught introductory abdominal ultrasonography over a 3-day period. In the institution where this study was undertaken, the third-year surgical residents performed ultrasounds of the abdomen in patients suspected of having appendicitis. Of course, the ultrasound was combined with a careful history and physical examination. When combined with history and physical examination, 27 of 29 patients were correctly diagnosed with appendicitis.

The diagnosis of appendicitis in children is more difficult than in adults. Imprecise histories and physical examinations are one cause of this. More children than adults tend to get adjunctive imaging. CT scans are likely to be used less frequently in the future because of data documenting the risk of radiation-induced malignancy. Ultrasound can be of help, but it does have lower sensitivity and specificities than CT. The authors of this report state, however, that surgeons do have a unique opportunity to be trained in this modality. It seems natural that surgeons would perform an ultrasound when initially evaluating a patient with possible appendicitis. The procedure takes less than 10 minutes. The accuracy when performed by trained surgical residents was virtually spot-on compared with ultrasonography performed by radiology technicians.

While on the topic of ultrasound versus radiologic procedures, a recent study has shown that using ultrasound instead of diagnostic contrast enemas in children suspected of having intussusception would result in a decrease of 79.3 and 59.7 cases of radiation-induced malignancy per 100 000 male and female children evaluated, respectively.[1]

Also, while on the topic of appendicitis, studies have been recently performed that have attempted to correlate findings on CT scan with white blood cell counts and CRP. It turns out that only changes in the appendix wall or abscess formation are significantly related to raised white blood cell count and CRP.[2] CT severity scores are more strongly correlated with CRP values than white blood cell counts, suggesting that CRP could be a useful predictor for perforated appendicitis. White blood cell counts are more useful in detecting early acute appendicitis.

**J. A. Stockman III, MD**

*References*

1. Bucher BT, Hall BL, Warner BW, Keller MS. Intussusception in children. cost effectiveness of ultrasound vs diagnostic contrast enema. *J Pediatr Surg.* 2011;46: 1099-1105.
2. Editorial comment. Appendicitis and CT scan findings. *Br J Radiol.* 2011;84: 1115-1120.

---

**Diagnostic Performance of Multidetector Computed Tomography for Suspected Acute Appendicitis**

Pickhardt PJ, Lawrence EM, Pooler BD, et al (Univ of Wisconsin School of Medicine and Public Health, Madison)
*Ann Intern Med* 154:789-796, 2011

---

*Background.*—Use of preoperative computed tomography for suspected acute appendicitis has dramatically increased since the introduction of multidetector CT (MDCT) scanners.

*Objective.*—To evaluate the diagnostic performance of MDCT for suspected acute appendicitis in adults.

*Design.*—Analysis of MDCT findings and clinical outcomes of consecutive adults referred for MDCT for suspected appendicitis from January 2000 to December 2009.

*Setting.*—Single academic medical center in the United States.

*Patients.*—2871 adults.

*Measurements.*—Interpretation of nonfocused abdominopelvic MDCT scans by radiologists who were aware of the study indication. Posttest assessment of diagnostic performance of MDCT for acute appendicitis, according to the reference standard of final combined clinical, surgical, and pathology findings.

*Results.*—675 of 2871 patients (23.5%) had confirmed acute appendicitis. The sensitivity, specificity, and negative and positive predictive values of MDCT were 98.5% (95% CI, 97.3% to 99.2%) (665 of 675 patients), 98.0% (CI, 97.4% to 98.6%) (2153 of 2196 patients), 99.5% (CI, 99.2% to 99.8%) (2153 of 2163 patients), and 93.9% (CI, 91.9% to 95.5%) (665 of 708 patients), respectively. Positive and negative likelihood ratios were 51.3 (CI, 38.1 to 69.0) and 0.015 (CI, 0.008 to 0.028), respectively. The overall rate of negative findings at appendectomy was 7.5% (CI, 5.8% to 9.7%) (54 of 716 patients), but would have decreased to 4.1% (28 of 690 patients) had surgery been avoided in 26 cases with true-negative findings on MDCT. The overall perforation rate was 17.8% (120 of 675 patients) but progressively decreased from 28.9% in 2000 to 11.5% in 2009. Multidetector computed tomography provided or suggested an alternative diagnosis in 893 of 2122 patients (42.1%) without appendicitis or appendectomy.

*Limitation.*—Possible referral bias, because some patients whose appendicitis was difficult to diagnose on clinical grounds may not have been referred for MDCT for evaluation of suspected appendicitis.

*Conclusion.*—Multidetector computed tomography is a useful test for routine evaluation of suspected appendicitis in adults.

▶ Since the clinical introduction of multidetector computed tomography (MDCT) in 1999, the use of CT in the diagnosis of suspected acute appendicitis has dramatically increased in both children and adults. In adult studies, it has been shown that preoperative CT is now being used in as many as 90% of suspected cases of appendicitis. Unfortunately, relatively few studies have evaluated the diagnostic performance of CT in the multidetector era for acute appendicitis. High sensitivity is critical to efficiently identify all patients who need an appendectomy, but it is also desirable to avoid unnecessary surgical procedures. Pickhardt et al have designed a study to assess the diagnostic performance of MDCT in a large adult cohort with suspected appendicitis. One can infer the likelihood of somewhat similar data were this study to have been done in children as well. Unfortunately, there is no such truly comparable study.

In this report, radiologists identified 708 patients as having acute appendicitis. Surgeons confirmed this diagnosis in 665 patients. The same radiologist ruled out the diagnosis of acute appendicitis in 2163 cases. Of the latter group, acute appendicitis was later diagnosed in 10. Increased use of MDCT over time coincided with fewer perforations (28.9% in 2000 vs 11.6% in 2009). This suggests that the scans aided earlier diagnosis and treatment and may have therefore reduced complication rates.

The data from this report do show that nonfocused abdominal MDCT is a highly sensitive and specific test for acute appendicitis in adult men and women in whom appendicitis is suspected clinically. In this setting, MDCT can effectively and efficiently identify the approximately one-quarter of patients with actual appendicitis who need urgent surgery, and it can often identify a probable alternative cause of symptoms in those who do not have appendicitis.

With MDCT, the rate of negative findings of appendectomy has fallen below 10% in adults.

It is somewhat difficult to translate the information from this report to the care of children. Chances are that MDCT would provide similar levels of sensitivity and specificity. The rub is the potential harms of CT level radiation in children. A one-time imaging in symptomatic adults with suspected appendicitis probably carries with it a favorable risk-benefit ratio in terms of the development of a secondary malignancy. The same may not be true of children who still have a lifetime to go in terms of accumulating radiation exposure. Fortunately, the radiation dosage—associated current standard MDCT has progressively fallen, and also emerging dose reduction strategies will probably soon result in lower doses of radiation. One would like to see more data comparing MDCT with ultrasonography. Most data to date show inferiority with ultrasonography. MRI is increasingly used for suspected appendicitis in pregnant women. Again, comparative data between MDCT and MRI is limited and even more limited with respect to data based on studies of children alone.

This commentary closes with a clinical pearl. Are you familiar with what is known as Amyand hernia? Recently, a man presented with a 5-day history of swelling and discomfort in the right inguinal region, which was followed by 24 hours of generalized abdominal pain, nausea, and vomiting. CT imaging of the abdomen revealed an inflamed appendix within a right-sided direct inguinal hernia. The appendix contained an appendicolith. The patient underwent a successful appendectomy and hernia repair and did well. An inguinal hernia containing a vermiform appendix is known as an Amyand hernia. Claudius Amyand, surgeon to King George II of England, is credited by some with performing the first documented successful appendectomy, in which he removed a perforated appendix from a right inguinal hernia sac in 1735. To learn more about Amyand hernia, see the interesting case report with an exquisite CT image in the *New England Journal of Medicine*.[1]

**J. A. Stockman III, MD**

*Reference*

1. Malayeri AA, Siegelman SS. Images in clinical medicine. Amyand's hernia. *N Engl J Med*. 2011;364:2147.

---

**Amoxicillin plus clavulanic acid versus appendicectomy for treatment of acute uncomplicated appendicitis: an open-label, non-inferiority, randomised controlled trial**

Vons C, Barry C, Maitre S, et al (Hôpital Antoine Béclère (Assistance Publique-Hôpitaux de Paris and Université Paris XI), Clamart, France; Université Paris-Sud and Université Paris Descartes, France; et de Radiologie, Clamart, France; et al)
*Lancet* 377:1573-1579, 2011

---

*Background.*—Researchers have suggested that antibiotics could cure acute appendicitis. We assessed the efficacy of amoxicillin plus clavulanic acid by comparison with emergency appendicectomy for treatment of patients with uncomplicated acute appendicitis.

*Methods.*—In this open-label, non-inferiority, randomised trial, adult patients (aged 18—68 years) with uncomplicated acute appendicitis, as assessed by CT scan, were enrolled at six university hospitals in France. A computer-generated randomisation sequence was used to allocate patients randomly in a 1:1 ratio to receive amoxicillin plus clavulanic acid (3 g per day) for 8—15 days or emergency appendicectomy. The primary endpoint was occurrence of postintervention peritonitis within 30 days of treatment initiation. Non-inferiority was shown if the upper limit of the two-sided 95% CI for the difference in rates was lower than 10 percentage points. Both intention-to-treat and per-protocol analyses were done. This trial is registered with ClinicalTrials.gov, number NCT00135603.

*Findings.*—Of 243 patients randomised, 123 were allocated to the antibiotic group and 120 to the appendicectomy group. Four were excluded from analysis because of early dropout before receiving the intervention, leaving 239 (antibiotic group, 120; appendicectomy group, 119) patients for intention-to-treat analysis. 30-day postintervention peritonitis was significantly more frequent in the antibiotic group (8%, n = 9) than in the appendicectomy group (2%, n = 2; treatment difference 5·8; 95% CI 0·3—12·1). In the appendicectomy group, despite CT-scan assessment, 21 (18%) of 119 patients were unexpectedly identified at surgery to have complicated appendicitis with peritonitis. In the antibiotic group, 14 (12% [7·1—18·6]) of 120 underwent an appendicectomy during the first 30 days and 30 (29% [21·4—38·9]) of 102 underwent appendicectomy between 1 month and 1 year, 26 of whom had acute appendicitis (recurrence rate 26%; 18·0—34·7).

*Interpretation.*—Amoxicillin plus clavulanic acid was not non-inferior to emergency appendicectomy for treatment of acute appendicitis. Identification of predictive markers on CT scans might enable improved targeting of antibiotic treatment.

▶ Who would have ever thought that one would see in the medical literature a study showing that antibiotic therapy could be effectively used to manage an episode of appendicitis without resorting to surgery? This report was undertaken in adults. The youngest patients were aged 18 years. Nonetheless, you can bet that the implications of this report will filter down to the pediatric age group. Many will be suggesting that a comparably designed study in children should be undertaken. Whether this is wise depends on how believable the results of this study are and whether they could be reproduced in children.

What the investigators have done is to undertake an open-label, noninferiority, randomized controlled trial involving 243 patients presenting to emergency rooms in France. Each patient entered the study with typical physical findings of appendicitis, confirmed with a CT scan. Patients with complicated appendicitis were excluded. The latter definition included those patients found to have appendicitis who had extra luminal gas, periappendiceal fluid, or disseminated intraperitoneal fluid. An appendix greater than 15 mm also was a criterion for exclusion because the latter finding is suggestive of an increased risk of malignancy. The endpoint of the study was whether at 30 days intervention was required in the antibiotic treatment group or not. Sixty-eight percent of patients in the category of uncomplicated appendicitis assigned to the antibiotic group did not need an appendectomy.

It is well worth the reader taking the time to read a commentary that accompanied this report. The author of the commentary reminds us that *Escherichia coli* remains the most common organism isolated from patients with appendicitis and that resistance of *E coli* to aminopenicillins, not only in Europe but elsewhere, runs high. For this reason, most would argue that amoxicillin-clavulanic acid should not be recommended in the nonoperative treatment of appendicitis.[1] Again, the story in children may turn out to be very different. Data thus far have been sufficiently meager to make recommendations one way or the other in this young age group.

This commentary closes with an interesting observation on an unrelated gastrointestinal problem: prolapsed bowel. Were you aware that a spoonful of sugar might be what the doctor orders for the latter? Recently a 62-year-old man presented to an emergency department in the Netherlands with a prolapsed ileostomy. He had undergone the ileostomy some 25 months earlier for treatment of mesenteric ischemia requiring an extended right hemicolectomy. The prolapse had occurred 12 hours before presentation and had no associated known cause. Manual reduction of the prolapse was unsuccessful. This patient had significant comorbidities, and general anesthesia with surgical reduction was considered risky. As had been described previously for the management of anal prolapse, plain granulated sugar was applied to the mucosa of the prolapsed ileum to promote the osmotic shift fluid out of the edematous tissue. Within 2 minutes, the edema had diminished sufficiently to allow spontaneous reduction of the prolapsed ileum. Twenty-four hours later, examination showed the patient was fine, and he was able to be discharged with no recurrence of the prolapse.

Yep, a spoonful of sugar works every time.[2]

**J. A. Stockman III, MD**

*References*

1. Mason RJ. Appendicitis: is surgery the best option? *Lancet.* 2011;377:1545-1546.
2. Brandt AR, Schouten O. Images in clinical medicine. Sugar to reduce a prolapsed ileostomy. *N Engl J Med.* 2011;364:1855.

---

**Diagnostic Medical Radiation in Pediatric Patients With Inflammatory Bowel Disease**
Huang JS, Tobin A, Harvey L, et al (Univ of California, San Diego; Rady Children's Hosp, San Diego, CA)
*J Pediatr Gastroenterol Nutr* 53:502-506, 2011

---

*Objectives.*—Certain diagnostic radiology procedures may expose patients with inflammatory bowel disease (IBD) to radiation and increase the risk for cancer. In the present study, we quantify the acute and cumulative effective dose of diagnostic radiation received by a cohort of pediatric patients with IBD.

*Patients and Methods.*—Patients with IBD were identified from the medical records of a pediatric tertiary care center. The number and type of radiology procedures for each patient were determined from medical record review. Cumulative effective radiation dose was calculated using radiation effective dose estimates.

*Results.*—One hundred five patients with IBD underwent radiation-associated abdominopelvic diagnostic radiology procedures with an average cumulative radiation exposure dose of 15 (18) [mean (SD)] mSv. Forty-two percent of the patients were exposed to acute radiation doses ≥10 mSv, and 6 patients (6%) were exposed to levels of cumulative radiation exposure ≥50 mSv, which has been associated with an increased risk of cancer development. Patients with Crohn disease, an increased number of hospital admissions, and a history of surgery were more likely to have been exposed to higher levels of cumulative radiation than their clinical counterparts.

*Conclusions.*—A majority of patients with IBD are exposed to radiation from typical diagnostic radiology procedures. Radiation-sparing procedures should be strongly considered in certain pediatric patients with IBD to reduce their risk for cancer given an already present increased lifetime malignancy potential.

▶ This report documents how much radiation exposure patients with a particular disorder (inflammatory bowel disease) might experience over their lifetime. A recent evaluation of diagnostic ionizing radiation exposure among a population-based sample of children with inflammatory bowel disease demonstrated that somewhere between 20% and 30% were exposed to moderate diagnostic radiation doses during a 2-year period (defined as 1 abdominal or pelvic CT and/or 3 fluoroscopic procedures [equivalent estimated radiation exposure ≥ 6 mSv]).[1] Unfortunately, there are no data published to date regarding the cumulative lifetime exposure to radiation among children and adolescents with inflammatory bowel disease resulting from routine diagnostic studies performed at initial evaluation and as part of chronic disease management. The report by Huang et al was designed to quantify the acute and cumulative effective dose of diagnostic radiation received by these patients.

In this report, a total of 114 patients diagnosed with Crohn disease, indeterminate colitis, or ulcerative colitis were identified. The records of these patients were reviewed and showed a total of 632 diagnostic radiologic procedures having been performed on the study subjects. In general, the patients underwent an average of 6 diagnostic radiology procedures, with an average of 4 procedures localized to the abdominopelvic region. Among these subjects, 42% were exposed to acute levels of radiation at or above 10 mSv. Acute doses of 10 to 50 mSv radiation are associated with an increase of cancer development.[2] Six percent of patients were exposed to levels of cumulative radiation exposure ≥50 mSv, clearly associated with an increased risk of cancer development. The investigators also demonstrated an increased risk for radiation exposure among black patients compared with nonblack patients. This may have reflected increased disease severity.

The findings of this report demonstrate that most pediatric patients with inflammatory bowel disease receive diagnostic radiology imaging procedures and have received acute radiation levels associated with potential increased risk for cancer. The authors suggest that patients presenting with chronic management that requires repeated imaging may benefit from additional aggressive dose-reduction strategies, including alternative imaging studies or further reductions in dose to minimize cumulative radiation dosing. These recommendations seem very wise indeed, given that many of these patients will likely be experiencing a lifelong disorder.

One closing comment, about MRI studies. Anyone who has had an MRI knows that all metallic objects must be removed from the body. Even things that contain small quantities of metal such as the pigment in tattoos can be a problem. A problem exists for two reasons. Metallic objects are attracted to the magnet and any object on or in the body that is metallic may be displaced if it is capable of reacting with the machine's magnet. Also, tiny metallic objects may vibrate enough in response to the magnet to generate fair amounts of heat. The latest object to hit the "do not enter with" an MRI unit is the transdermal patch. Some transdermal patches contain metal and may cause burns to the skin if patients wear them during an MRI procedure, according to the Food and Drug Administration. The nonadhesive backing of some drug patches contain aluminum or other metals that may become heated during an MRI. Many labels for such products already warn of this risk; however, the FDA was recently alerted that Teva Pharmaceutical fentanyl transdermal system lacked this warning. Further investigation by the agency revealed that a warning is also missing from the labels of a variety of other medical patches. The FDA has received at least two confirmed reports of patients developing a burn similar to a severe sunburn after wearing a nicotine patch during an MRI. In most instances, the metal in the patch was not visible. Some clear patches that appear to be plastic may in fact contain metal ions that heat during an MRI. Fortunately most MRI facilities do ask patients if they are wearing a transdermal patch and will ask them to remove it. Physicians referring a patient for an MRI are now asked to determine whether the patient uses a drug patch and, if so, provide advice on removal of the patch prior to the procedure. Such advice should also include proper disposal of the used patch and the procedure for reapplying a new patch following completion of the MRI.[3]

**J. A. Stockman III, MD**

*References*

1. Palmer L, Herfarth H, Porter CQ, Fordham LA, Sandler RS, Kappelman MD. Diagnostic ionizing radiation exposure in a population-based sample of children with inflammatory bowel diseases. *Am J Gastroenterol.* 2009;104:2816-2823.
2. Brenner DJ, Doll R, Goodhead DT, et al. Cancer risks attributable to low doses of ionizing radiation: assessing what we really know. *Proc Natl Acad Sci U S A.* 2003;100:13761-13766.
3. Kuehn BM. FDA warning: remove drug patches before MRI to prevent burns to the skin. *JAMA.* 2009;301:1328.

## Association of Crohn's Disease, Thiopurines, and Primary Epstein-Barr Virus Infection with Hemophagocytic Lymphohistiocytosis

Biank VF, Sheth MK, Talano J, et al (The Children's Hosp of Wisconsin, Milwaukee; et al)
*J Pediatr* 159:808-812, 2011

*Objective.*—To assess the incidence of hemophagocytic lymphohistiocytosis (HLH) in a well-defined population of children with inflammatory bowel disease (IBD) and evaluate the common clinical and laboratory characteristics of individuals with IBD who developed HLH.

*Study Design.*—We conducted a retrospective study of all children who developed HLH over an 8-year period. The incidence of HLH in patients with IBD was calculated using US census data and a statewide project examining the epidemiology of pediatric IBD.

*Results.*—Among children in Wisconsin, 20 cases of HLH occurred during the study period; 5 cases occurred in children with IBD. Common characteristics include: Crohn's disease (CD), thiopurine administration, fever lasting more than 5 days, lymphadenopathy, splenomegaly, anemia, lymphopenia, and elevated serum triglycerides and ferritin. Of the patients, 4 had primary Epstein-Barr virus infections. The incidence of HLH among all children in Wisconsin was 1.5 per 100 000 per year. The risk was more than 100-fold greater for children with CD ($P < .00001$).

*Conclusions.*—Pediatric patients with CD are at increased risk for developing HLH; primary Epstein-Barr virus infection and thiopurine administration may be risk factors (Table 1).

▶ At a recent morning report, a pediatric resident in the Department of Pediatrics at Duke University Medical Center presented a case of a teenager with hemophagocytic lymphohistiocytosis (HLH) who died as a result of this complex but interesting disorder. The trigger was an Epstein-Barr virus (EBV) infection. This is mentioned in this commentary simply to indicate that although HLH is a fairly rare disorder, it does occur and it is a disorder with which all of us should be familiar.

HLH is commonly a fatal disorder and one in which macrophages are inappropriately activated, resulting in phagocytosis of all bone marrow—derived cells. There are primary and secondary forms of HLH. Primary HLH is a rare autosomal-recessive disorder of the immune system that has been reported with a yearly incidence of 1.2 per 1 million population. Secondary HLH is more common and can present in a person of any age and has been documented in association with a variety of infections and systemic conditions. Both primary and secondary HLH result in the same activation of histiocytes with evidence of hemophagocytic activity in the bone marrow. Patients with HLH usually die as a result of pancytopenia. Criteria for the diagnosis of HLH have been developed by the Histiocyte Society and are now widely accepted (Table 1).

Biank et al report on an association between HLH and inflammatory bowel disease in children. The investigators conducting a retrospective chart analysis of all individuals with inflammatory bowel disease who developed HLH at

**TABLE 1.**—Diagnostic Guidelines for HLH: 2004

The diagnosis of HLH can be established if either 1 or 2 below is fulfilled:
 1. A molecular diagnosis consistent with HLH is present.
 2. Diagnostic criteria for HLH are fulfilled (5 of the 8 criteria below):
   A. Initial diagnostic criteria (to be evaluated in all patients with HLH):
       Fever
       Splenomegaly
       Cytopenias (affecting $\geq$ 2 of 3 lineages in the peripheral blood):
         Hemaglobin < 90 g/L
         Platelets < 100 × 10$^9$/L
         Neutrophils < 1.0 × 10$^9$/L
         Hypertriglyceridemia and/or hypofibrinogenemia:
         Fasting triglycerides $\geq$ 3 mmol/L (ie., $\geq$265 mg/d L)
         Fibrinogen $\leq$ 1.5 g/L
       Hemophagocytosis in bone marrow or spleen or lymph node
       No evidence of malignancy
   B. New diagnostic criteria
       Low or absent NK-cell activity (according to local laboratory references)
       Ferritin $\geq$ 500 $\mu$g/L
       Soluble CD-25 (ie., soluble interleukin-2 receptor) $\geq$ 2400U/mL

Adapted from Henter JI, Horne A, Arico M, Egeler RM, Filipovich AH, Imashuku S, et al. HLH-2004: diagnostic and therapeutic guidelines for hemophagocytic lymphohistiocytosis. *Pediatr Blood Cancer.* 2007;48:124-31.

Children's Hospital of Wisconsin over a period of 8.5 years and found a remarkably higher risk of HLH in patients with Crohn disease than in the general population. All the patients observed were receiving thiopurine therapies for their inflammatory bowel disease. All but 1 patient developing HLH had primary EBV infection. The math showed that the risk of a child with Crohn disease developing HLH was 100 times greater than the development of HLH in the general population. Only 1 of the patients in the Wisconsin study survived, a finding consistent with overall data published on reports of inflammatory bowel disease and HLH documenting that most patients succumb.

It is important to diagnose HLH quickly. There is no definitive therapy except bone marrow transplantation, which has been reported to markedly increase survivorship. If there is a viral etiology that triggers HLH, most commonly the virus will be EBV, although cytomegalovirus may be involved as well. The authors of this report strongly recommend that pediatric patients with inflammatory bowel disease, particularly those with Crohn disease, who are receiving thiopurine therapy and who present with 5 or more days of fever and adenopathy should be quickly screened for HLH. Demonstration of lymphopenia, serum ferritin levels above 500 ug/L, or evidence of EBV infection should prompt an additional evaluation for HLH and discontinuation of all immunosuppressive therapies and early referral to a hematologist-oncologist for bone marrow biopsy and consideration of more aggressive therapies. Based on the literature, these recommendations seem to be very appropriate.

This commentary closes with an interesting clinical observation having to do with the appendix. Have you ever heard of an autoappendectomy? This refers to the removal of one's own appendix by a trained person. Such an incidence occurred in 1961. The ship *OB*, with the Sixth Soviet Antarctic Expedition onboard, sailed from Leningrad on November 5, 1960. After 36 days, the occupants deboarded for an expedition onto the ice shelf on Princess Astrid Coast. Their task was to build a new Antarctic polar base inland at Schirmacher Oasis and to spend the winter there. One of the expedition's members was the 27-year-old Leningrad surgeon Leonid Ivanovich Rogozov. He had interrupted a promising scholarly career and left on the expedition shortly before he was due to defend his dissertation on new methods of operating on cancer of the esophagus. In the Antarctic he was first and foremost the team's doctor and only doctor, although he also served as a meteorologist and the driver of their terrain vehicle. By late April 1961, Rogozov fell ill. His symptoms were weakness, malaise, nausea, and later pain in the right lower quadrant of his abdomen. He diagnosed his own appendicitis. Over the next 24 hours things gradually began to go downhill as the "patient" became sicker. His situation was a cruel trick of fate. He knew that if he was to survive, he had to undergo an operation, but he was in the frontier conditions of a newly founded Antarctic colony on the brink of the polar night. Transportation was impossible. Flying was out of the question because of snowstorms and there was one further problem: he was the only physician on the base. Knowing the handwriting was on the wall, Rogozov bit the bullet, assembled a surgical team, sterilized to the extent possible his bedroom, instructed his assistants who were not medically oriented at all on how to help him. Using a local anesthetic and sitting in a semi-reclining position with his right hip slightly elevated, he disinfected and dressed the operating area and began to operate working without gloves in order to enhance his sense of touch since his ability to see well given the circumstances was limited. Using a local anesthetic and taking an hour and 45 minutes, Rogozov successfully removed his own almost ruptured appendix. After two weeks, he returned to his normal duties. A year later he left the Antarctic and returned to his clinical duties, having successfully defended his dissertation. He never returned to the Antarctic and died in St. Petersburg, as Leningrad had then become known, on September 21, 2000.

Rogozov's self operation was probably the first successful appendectomy undertaken in the wilderness, out of hospital settings, with no possibility of outside help and without any other medical professionals around. It remains an example of determination and the human will for life. In later years, Rogozov himself rejected all glorification of his deed. When thoughts like these were put to him, he usually answered with a smile and the words: "a job like any other, a life like any other."[1]

**J. A. Stockman III, MD**

*Reference*

1. Rogozov V, Bermel N. Autoappendectomy in the Antarctic. *BMJ*. 2009;339: 1420-1422.

### Cost-effectiveness Analysis of Adjunct VSL#3 Therapy Versus Standard Medical Therapy in Pediatric Ulcerative Colitis

Park KT, Perez F, Tsai R, et al (Packard Children's Hosp, Palo Alto, CA; Stanford Univ, Palo Alto, CA; et al)
*J Pediatr Gastroenterol Nutr* 53:489-496, 2011

*Background.*—Inflammatory bowel diseases (IBDs) are costly chronic gastrointestinal diseases, with pediatric IBD representing increased costs per patient compared to adult disease. Health care expenditures for ulcerative colitis (UC) are >$2 billion annually. It is not clear whether the addition of VSL#3 to standard medical therapy in UC induction and maintenance of remission is a cost-effective strategy.

*Patients and Methods.*—We performed a systematic review of the literature and created a Markov model simulating a cohort of 10-year-old patients with severe UC, studying them until 100 years of age or death. We compared 2 strategies: standard medical therapy versus medical therapy + VSL#3. For both strategies, we assumed that patients progressed through escalating therapies—mesalamine, azathioprine, and infliximab—before receiving a colectomy + ileal pouch anal anastamosis (IPAA) if the 3 medical therapy options were exhausted. The primary outcome measure was the incremental cost-effectiveness ratio (ICER), defined as the difference of costs between strategies for each quality-adjusted life-year (QALY) gained. One-way sensitivity analyses were performed on variables to determine the key variables affecting cost-effectiveness.

*Results.*—Standard medical care accrued a lifetime cost of $203,317 per patient, compared to $212,582 per patient for medical therapy + VSL#3. Lifetime QALYs gained was comparable for standard medical therapy and medical therapy + VSL#3 at 24.93 versus 25.05, respectively. Using the definition of ICER <50,000/QALY as a cost-effective intervention, medical therapy + VSL#3 produced an ICER of $79,910 per QALY gained, making this strategy cost-ineffective. Sensitivity analyses showed that 4 key parameters could affect the cost-effectiveness of the 2 strategies: cost of colectomy + IPAA, maintenance cost after surgery, probability of developing pouchitis after surgery, and the quality of life after a colectomy + IPAA. High surgical and postsurgical costs, a high probability of developing pouchitis, and a low quality of life after a colectomy + IPAA could make adjunct VSL#3 use a cost-effective strategy.

*Conclusions.*—Given present data, adjunct VSL#3 use for pediatric UC induction and maintenance of remission is not cost-effective, although several key parameters could make this strategy cost-effective. The quality of life after an IPAA is the single most important variable predicting whether this procedure benefits patients over escalating standard medical therapy.

▶ Probiotics are becoming very popular these days. They are being used for the management of a variety of gastrointestinal disorders. In particular, Miele et al[1] have suggested that a specific blend of high-dose probiotics, VSL#3, may be beneficial in the treatment of acute pediatric ulcerative colitis flairs and maintenance of remission. VSL#3 is composed of 8 strains of specific bacteria (1 strain of *Streptococcus thermophilus*, 3 strains of *Bifidobacterium*, and 4 strains of *Lactobacillus*). It contains 450 billion live probiotic bacteria per sachet.[1] This pediatric report by Park et al is consistent with adult studies that have shown efficacy of VSL#3 in the management of certain types of inflammation of the bowel, although its use as part of ulcerative colitis management is a more novel concept.[2]

Park et al have designed a study to determine whether use of VSL#3 is cost effective as part of the management of children with ulcerative colitis. This study is important because probiotics such as VSL#3 are rarely covered by insurance providers and out-of-pocket expenses for patients and families run in the neighborhood of about $200 per month. It is estimated that health care expenditures for ulcerative colitis run more than $2 billion annually, so it is important to understand whether the addition of VSL#3, which adds to this cost, is in fact an effective strategy.

Park et al performed a systematic review of the literature in which data from the literature were analyzed in 2 ways. The data looked at standard medical therapy plus VSL#3 versus standard medical therapy. The investigators found that among children with severe ulcerative colitis, the addition of VSL#3 to standard medical regimens is associated with a small gain in quality-adjusted life-years yet costs more than $50 000 per quality-adjusted life-year. To look at it in a somewhat different way, standard medical care over the lifetime of care of a patient with ulcerative colitis would run $203 317 per patient compared with $212 582 per patient for medical therapy that includes VSL#3.

From society's point of view, Park et al suggest that using adjunctive VSL#3 therapy does not in fact provide sufficient additional benefits over the lifetime of children with ulcerative colitis to justify the added cost. You can bet that health care plans will point to this particular report to continue not reimbursing for VSL#3 expenses. It will be difficult for individual families to decide whether it is worth paying several hundred dollars a month out of pocket for this particular adjunct to therapy. This is even made more complex since cost-effectiveness analysis is not without its own controversies, given that the thresholds for cost per quality of life-years are arbitrary when it comes to deciding what is worth it and what is not worth it to society.

For more on the topic about cost-effectiveness and the use of probiotics for children with inflammatory bowel disease, read the commentary by Samnaliev and Lightdale.[3]

**J. A. Stockman III, MD**

*References*

1. Miele E, Pascarella F, Giannetti E, Quaglietta L, Baldassano RN, Staiano A. Effect of a probiotic preparation (VSL#3) on induction and maintenance of remission in children with ulcerative colitis. *Am J Gastroenterol.* 2009;104:437-443.
2. Gionchetti P, Rizzello F, Venturi A, et al. Oral bacteriotherapy as maintenance treatment in patients with chronic pouchitis: a double-blind, placebo-controlled trial. *Gastroenterology.* 2000;119:305-309.
3. Samnaliev M, Lightdale JR. On the cost-effectiveness of the use of probiotics in inflammatory bowel disease. *J Pediatr Gastroenterol Nutr.* 2011;53:473.

**Infantile Colitis as a Novel Presentation of Familial Mediterranean Fever Responding to Colchicine Therapy**
Egritas O, Dalgic B (Gazi Univ School of Medicine, Ankara, Turkey)
*J Pediatr Gastroenterol Nutr* 53:102-105, 2011

*Background.*—Familial Mediterranean fever (FMF) is an autosomal recessive chronic inflammatory disease manifesting as recurrent fever and polyserositis attacks. FMF is common in Turks, Arabs, Armenians, and Jews. Carrier frequency in high-risk populations is among the highest for autosomal recessive diseases. Typically FMF attacks begin with instantaneous and rapidly escalating fever that continues for 12 to 72 hours and subside spontaneously. The gene causing FMF is located on the short arm of chromosome 16. Over 40 mutations have been identified thus far. FMF is diagnosed based on the clinical presentation, but patients with atypical features, younger patients, and patients with overlapping or associated disease such as vasculitis or inflammatory bowel disease (IBD) can present diagnostic challenges. Because IBD has been associated with FMF, infants with chronic ulcerative colonic disease should be investigated with FMF in mind. The clinical, laboratory, and follow-up characteristics of three patients who had findings suggestive of colitis were reported.

*Case Reports.*—Case 1: Girl, 3 months, had intermittent bloody mucoid diarrhea since age 2 weeks. Her uncle had FMF disease. Although her systemic examination and perianal inspection were normal, she had low hemoglobin and elevated platelets. Rich populations of leukocytes and erythrocytes were in her stool samples. Infectious agents were ruled out. Eliminating cow's milk from her diet helped partially but she still suffered intermittent episodes of abdominal pain and bloody mucoid stools. The patient was readmitted at age 2 years with pericardial effusion, elevated serum creatinine phosphokinase, and CK-MB. No specific cause for the pericarditis was found, but a DNA analysis for FMF was undertaken. One month later the patient was readmitted with intense bloody diarrhea, malaise, and fever; her percentiles for body weight and height had diminished significantly. She had a faint appearance but no bacterial, viral, or parasitic infections to account for the diarrhea. Several abnormal laboratory results were noted: mean corpuscular volume, white blood cells, platelets, albumin, total protein, erythrocyte sedimentation rate, and C-reactive protein levels. Although other tests were normal, colonoscopy showed hyperemia, fragility, and patchy ulcerations covered with white exudate in the colonic mucosa. Histopathologic analysis revealed a chronic active inflammatory process with polymorph leukocytes and eosinophils with no granuloma formation. DNA analysis revealed FMF mutation, and the patient was given colchicine, which produced normalization of findings within 1 week. The patient was diagnosed with Henoch-Schonlein purpura at age 3 years, with widespread ulceration in the bowels.

Steroid administration for 4 weeks produced a resolution of symptoms.

Case 2: Boy, 4, had intermittent bloody mucoid diarrhea since early infancy and experienced unexplained fever episodes over the preceding year. He weighed just 12.5 kg and height was 92 cm. His appearance was weak and faint. Leukocytes and erythrocytes were found on stool microscopy and several laboratory results were abnormal. Renal, liver, and gastrointestinal diseases were ruled out. Colonoscopy revealed edema, hyperemia, and patchy ulcerations covered with white exudate in colonic mucosa. Histopathology showed cryptitis and crypt abscess with leukocyte and mixed-type inflammation but no granuloma formation. IBD was diagnosed and steroid therapy begun. Azathioprine and mesalazine were added when steroids were reduced. An FMF analysis revealed a mutation, prompting colchicine therapy. The patient remained in remission for 4 years on colchicine and mesalazine treatment, but colchicine was discontinued to avoid azospermia during preadolescence. After 2 months the patient returned with severe colitis, erysipelas-like erythema of the lower extremities, and higher than normal acute-phase reactant levels. The colitis was considered FMF related and colchicine was restarted, returning symptoms and laboratory values to normal. The patient was eventually taken off mesalazine without relapse.

Case 3: Boy, 3, had fever and bloody mucoid diarrhea periods that lasted 3 to 4 days over the previous 6 months. He appeared anxious and faint, and laboratory results demonstrated several abnormalities. Colonoscopy found hyperemic edematous mucosa with nodularity, suggestive of follicular lymphoid hyperplasia. Cryptitis and mixed-type inflammation without granuloma were revealed on histopathologic evaluation. Within 4 days the boy's symptoms and laboratory test results resolved completely. This was considered an attack of FMF when combined with mutation analysis. Colchicine treatment was begun, with no further complaints over the following 2 years.

*Conclusions.*—Comorbidity of FMF and IBD is a common concern for both pediatric and adult gastroenterologists. The three patients reported had clinical colitis that responded to colchicine therapy, supporting the diagnosis of FMF. Symptoms usually begin before age 2 years. Isolated gastrointestinal involvement of FMF should be considered in high-risk ethnic groups, especially during infancy.

▶ Most of us are familiar with familial Mediterranean fever (FMF). This is an autosomal recessive chronic inflammatory disease with relapsing fever and polyserositis attacks. The gene causing FMF is located on the short arm of chromosome 16. Currently, the diagnosis of FMF is based almost solely on clinical grounds, with genetic testing reserved for patients with atypical presentations. The latter tend to occur in younger individuals and in patients with overlapping or associated disease, such as vasculitis and inflammatory bowel disease.

Many who provide care to pediatric patients may not realize it, but FMF can present as a form of infantile colitis. Egritas et al report on 3 infants with colitis documenting that colitis may be the only presenting finding for FMF. In each of these affected individuals, the terminal ileum was normal, but active inflammatory processes were seen in other segments of the colon. Cryptitis was noted in all. Fortunately, those providing care to these youngsters recognized the potential possibility that the colitis might be caused by FMF rather than by other forms of inflammatory bowel disease. All 3 cases responded to colchicine treatment without the need for other antiinflammatory or immunosuppressive drug therapy. In these patients, recurrence or relapse was not observed under colchicine therapy during extensive periods of follow-up.

It is important to make a correct diagnosis of FMF since the disorder may result in amyloidosis if not treated. Renal amyloidosis resulting in renal failure is the most notable type of FMF-associated amyloidosis.

If you have a patient with recurrent colitis, recall that it can arise in many conditions. Infectious states, allergic states, inflammatory bowel diseases (such as Crohn disease and ulcerative colitis), Behçet disease, immune deficiencies, microscopic colitis, and collagenous colitis are among the various causes of colitis. Do not forget, however, that FMF can also present as recurrent colitis.

**J. A. Stockman III, MD**

---

**Nonpharmacologic Treatments for Childhood Constipation: Systematic Review**
Tabbers MM, Boluyt N, Berger MY, et al (Emma's Children's Hosp/Academic Med Centre, Amsterdam, Netherlands; Univ Hosp Groningen, Netherlands)
*Pediatrics* 128:753-761, 2011

---

*Objective.*—To summarize the evidence and assess the reported quality of studies concerning nonpharmacologic treatments for childhood constipation, including fiber, fluid, physical movement, prebiotics, probiotics, behavioral therapy, multidisciplinary treatment, and forms of alternative medicine.

*Methods.*—We systematically searched 3 major electronic databases and reference lists of existing reviews. We included systematic reviews and randomized controlled trials (RCTs) that reported on nonpharmacologic treatments. Two reviewers rated the methodologic quality independently.

*Results.*—We included 9 studies with 640 children. Considerable heterogeneity across studies precluded meta-analysis. We found no RCTs for physical movement, multidisciplinary treatment, or alternative medicine. Some evidence shows that fiber may be more effective than placebo in improving both the frequency and consistency of stools and in reducing abdominal pain. Compared with normal fluid intake, we found no evidence that water intake increases or that hyperosmolar fluid treatment is more effective in increasing stool frequency or decreasing difficulty in passing stools. We found no evidence to recommend the use of prebiotics or probiotics. Behavioral therapy with laxatives is not more effective than laxatives alone.

*Conclusions.*—There is some evidence that fiber supplements are more effective than placebo. No evidence for any effect was found for fluid supplements, prebiotics, probiotics, or behavioral intervention. There is a lack of well-designed RCTs of high quality concerning non-pharmacologic treatments for children with functional constipation.

▶ If there is any diagnosis that proves that medicine is as much an art or craft as it is a profession, it is the diagnosis of common chronic constipation, a disorder that affects at least 1 in 30 in the US population. For as little as we know about many of the causes of constipation, even less is known about how best to manage it. Data show that only about half of children with functional chronic constipation recover after a year of laxative therapy, and despite intensive medical and behavioral therapy, 30% of patients who develop constipation before the age of 5 years continue to have severe complaints of constipation, infrequent painful defecation, and fecal incontinence beyond puberty.[1,2]

Early steps in the management of chronic constipation usually involve education, dietary advice, and behavioral modifications followed, if unsuccessful, by laxative therapy. Often there is little effect with such management, leading parents to explore alternative therapies, including acupuncture, homeopathy, mind-body therapy, osteopathic maneuvers, and spiritual therapies including yoga. What is lacking in the literature is an in-depth systematic review of the effectiveness of all nonpharmacologic treatments, such as fiber, fluid, physical movement, prebiotics and probiotics, behavioral therapy, multidisciplinary treatment, and forms of alternative medicine. This is where the report of Tabbers et al comes in. These investigators looked in a systematic manner to summarize the quantity and quality of current evidence on the effects of fiber, fluid, physical movement, prebiotics, probiotics, behavioral therapy, multidisciplinary therapy and alternative medical approaches including acupuncture, homeopathy, mind-body therapy, musculoskeletal manipulations such as osteopathic and chiropractic manipulations, and spiritual therapies including yoga.

So what did these investigators find as a result of their systematic review? The review unquestionably showed a lack of high-powered studies looking at the outcomes of nonpharmacologic treatment for chronic constipation. Their specific conclusions were as follows:

- Fiber therapy—some evidence does exist that fiber supplements are more effective than placebo.
- Fluid therapy and behavioral interventions—no evidence from trials exists that suggests any effect for fluid supplements or behavioral therapy.
- Prebiotics and probiotics—no evidence of effectiveness.
- Physical movement, multidisciplinary treatment, or any alternative medicine therapy—no evidence was found for effectiveness of any of these.

- Placebo—there is a paucity of placebo-controlled studies with a large patient sampling for pediatric patients with constipation. What appears in the literature shows a 60% success rate with placebos that could represent the natural evolution of the disease, fluctuations in symptoms, and regression to the mean.

It is fair to say that much of the negative information suggested by the conclusions of this report is the result of inadequately and underpowered studies in the literature. One would think that with a problem as common as constipation, a large national collaborative could readily be established to quickly assess therapies, discarding useless ones, and modifying ones that are suggested to be effective to achieve even better effectiveness. Such studies usually start with a high-quality registry. Let's get on with such a registry. Perhaps it should be called NPR (no, not National Public Radio; rather, the National Poo Registry).

This commentary closes with a quiz. How would you deal with the following situation? A 3-year-old girl is brought into your office by her father with a chief complaint of black, sticky stools. The patient had been dropped off at day care that morning without any complaints. While at day care, she experienced abdominal pain. The parents were contacted after she had a bowel movement that was black and tarry. On examination, the youngster is well appearing. She is not pale. Her vital signs are normal. The overall physical examination yields no findings. On rectal examination no masses are palpated. Only a small amount of dark-colored stool is seen on the examining glove. A hemoccult test is positive. Fortunately before you can order any additional studies, the patient's father indicates that the patient had ingested a traditional bowl of pork blood soup the evening before. The youngster's family is from Vietnam. You decide to simply watch the youngster carefully for several hours during which time she continues to do well. When her stool is retested several days later after the family had been warned not to give the child pork blood soup any longer, it was negative for blood. This case was recently reported in the literature as the first and only case of melena from ingestion of pork blood.[3] It should be noted, however, the blood is an ingredient in a wide variety of traditional dishes from different cultures. Duck blood soup is also commonly made in Vietnam. In Korea, soup is often made from ox blood. In Mexico, goat blood is frequently an ingredient in soups. Remember, all blood in the stool does not necessarily come from the patient's own vascular system.

**J. A. Stockman III, MD**

*References*

1. Pijpers MA, Bongers ME, Benninga MA, Berger MY. Functional constipation in children: a systematic review on prognosis and predictive factors. *J Pediatr Gastroenterol Nutr.* 2010;50:256-268.
2. Bongers ME, van Wijk MP, Reitsma JB, Benninga MA. Long-term prognosis for childhood constipation: clinical outcomes in adulthood. *Pediatrics.* 2010;126: e156-e162.
3. Alder MN, Timm NL. A "rare" case of melena in a 3-year-old. *Pediatr Emerg Care.* 2011;27:1084.

# 8 Genitourinary Tract

## Nocturnal Enuresis in Children: Prevalence, Correlates, and Relationship with Obstructive Sleep Apnea

Su MS, Li AM, So HK, et al (Wenzhou Med College Affiliated Second Hosp—Yuying Children's Hosp, Zhejiang, People's Republic of China; Prince of Wales Hosp, Shatin, Hong Kong; et al)
J Pediatr 159:238-242, 2011

*Objectives.*—To examine the prevalence and correlates of nocturnal enuresis (NE) in primary school children, and to compare the prevalence of NE in children with and those without obstructive sleep apnea (OSA).

*Study Design.*—Parents of children aged 6-11 years completed a questionnaire eliciting information on sleep-related symptoms, demography, and family and past medical history. Children screened due to high risk for OSA, along with a randomly chosen low-risk group, underwent overnight polysomnography (PSG).

*Results.*—A total of 6147 children (3032 girls) were studied. The overall prevalence of NE ($\geq 1$ wet night/month) was 4.6% (6.7% of boys and 2.5% of girls). Boys had a significantly greater prevalence across all age groups. In 597 children (215 girls) who underwent PSG, the prevalence of NE was not greater in children with OSA, but was increased with increasing severity of OSA in girls only. Boys with NE had longer deep sleep duration. Sex and sleep-related symptoms were associated with NE.

*Conclusions.*—This community-based study demonstrated a sex-associated prevalence of NE in relation to increasing OSA severity.

▶ Various mechanisms have been theorized as a potential cause for nocturnal enuresis. One is that there is delayed maturation of the nervous system controlling bladder function. Another is that youngsters with nocturnal enuresis have delayed development of bladder function. It has been suspected that decreased nighttime secretion of antidiuretic hormone might be 1 cause. There has also been some suspicion that youngsters with obstructive sleep apnea (OSA) have a higher prevalence of nocturnal enuresis. Children with OSA do have periods of increased negative intrathoracic pressure as a result of increased inspiratory effort during sleep. It has been suggested that the continual swing in intrathoracic pressure causes cardiac distention, which can lead to release of atrial natriuretic peptide, triggering enuresis.[1] Other studies have not supported a positive relationship between OSA and nocturnal enuresis.

The report abstracted is from the People's Republic of China. It aimed to identify the prevalence, sleep study characteristics, and risk factors associated with nocturnal enuresis in children while comparing the prevalence of nocturnal enuresis in children with and those without OSA. The youngsters studied ranged in age from 6 to 11 years. Both boys and girls were evaluated. All had histories of nocturnal enuresis and all were evaluated with overnight polysomnography. This study showed no difference in the rate of enuresis between children with OSA and those without. The study did note a differential sex response in nocturnal enuresis prevalence with increasing OSA severity in girls. The most important finding, however, was that children with nocturnal enuresis were shown to sleep more in deep sleep and were more likely to have other sleep-related symptoms.

This is an important study because the results were based on a large number of subjects with the use of validated and reliable questionnaires and methodologies used to study these subjects. It certainly allowed an accurate comparison of nocturnal enuresis prevalence in subjects with and without OSA. It is important for all of us to know that this report found no association between OSA and enuresis.

This commentary closes with an observation having to do with urination. The 2011 Ig Nobel Prize in Medicine was given to Mirjam et al for demonstrating that people make better decisions about some kinds of things—but worse decisions about other kinds of things—when they have a strong urge to urinate.[2] There was no mention at the time of the award whether the passing of one's water was affected by whether one was standing or sitting. One would think that the latter position, when used by Rodin's the "Thinker," would be more productive.

**J. A. Stockman III, MD**

*References*

1. Rittig S, Knudsen UB, Nørgaard JP, Gregersen H, Pedersen EB, Djurhuus JC. Diurnal variation of plasma atrial natriuretic peptide in normals and patients with enuresis nocturna. *Scand J Clin Lab Invest.* 1991;51:209-217.
2. Tuk M, Warlop J. Inhibitory spillover: Increased urination urgency facilitates impulse control in unrelated domains. *Psychol Sci.* May 2011:627-633.

---

## Persistent Asymptomatic Isolated Microscopic Hematuria in Israeli Adolescents and Young Adults and Risk for End-Stage Renal Disease

Vivante A, Afek A, Frenkel-Nir Y, et al (Israeli Defense Forces Med Corps, Tel Hashomer, Israel; Sheba Med Ctr, Tel Hashomer, Israel; et al)

*JAMA* 306:729-736, 2011

---

*Context.*—Few data are available on long-term outcomes among adolescents and young adults with persistent asymptomatic isolated microscopic hematuria.

*Objective.*—To evaluate the risk of end-stage renal disease (ESRD) in adolescents and young adults with persistent asymptomatic isolated microscopic hematuria.

*Design, Setting, and Participants.*—Nationwide, population-based, retrospective cohort study using medical data from 1 203 626 persons aged 16 through 25 years (60% male) examined for fitness for military service between 1975 and 1997 were linked to the Israeli treated ESRD registry. Incident cases of treated ESRD from January 1, 1980, to May 31, 2010, were included. Cox proportional hazards models were used to estimate the hazard ratio (HR) of treated ESRD among those diagnosed as having persistent asymptomatic isolated microscopic hematuria.

*Main Outcome Measures.*—Treated ESRD onset, defined as the date of initiation of dialysis treatment or the date of renal transplantation, whichever came first.

*Results.*—Persistent asymptomatic isolated microscopic hematuria was diagnosed in 3690 of 1 203 626 eligible individuals (0.3%). During 21.88 (SD, 6.74) years of follow-up, treated ESRD developed in 26 individuals (0.70%) with and 539 (0.045%) without persistent asymptomatic isolated microscopic hematuria, yielding incidence rates of 34.0 and 2.05 per 100 000 person-years, respectively, and a crude HR of 19.5 (95% confidence interval [CI], 13.1-28.9). A multivariate model adjusted for age, sex, paternal country of origin, year of enrollment, body mass index, and blood pressure at baseline did not substantially alter the risk associated with persistent asymptomatic isolated microscopic hematuria (HR, 18.5 [95% CI, 12.4-27.6]). A substantially increased risk for treated ESRD attributed to primary glomerular disease was found for individuals with persistent asymptomatic isolated microscopic hematuria compared with those without the condition (incidence rates, 19.6 vs 0.55 per 100 000 person-years, respectively; HR, 32.4 [95% CI, 18.9-55.7]). The fraction of treated ESRD attributed to microscopic hematuria was 4.3% (95% CI, 2.9%-6.4%).

*Conclusion.*—Presence of persistent asymptomatic isolated microscopic hematuria in persons aged 16 through 25 years was associated with significantly increased risk of treated ESRD for a period of 22 years, although the incidence and absolute risk remain quite low.

▶ Chances are that you will never see a study of this magnitude appearing in the literature again. The study provides information from a population-based analysis of more than 1.2 million people 16 to 25 years of age who had routine urine studies to detect the presence of microscopic hematuria. The weakness of the report has to do with the fact that the study involved those conscripted into military service in Israel and thus applies uniquely to a population of adolescent and young adult individuals of Jewish ancestry. Nonetheless, the information provided by this report is extremely powerful.

All military conscripts in Israel undergo an obligatory medical examination that includes a very thorough history, physical examination, and laboratory testing. The latter includes a routine urinalysis. In this report, those with isolated microscopic hematuria, defined as 5 or more red blood cells per high power field observed on 3 separate occasions, were followed up for more than 2 decades. It was possible to determine who among those with positive urine developed end-stage renal disease (ESRD), because in Israel there is a nationwide registry for ESRD. Individuals with microscopic hematuria were included in this study if at the time of detection of the problem they had normal serum creatinine values, were otherwise asymptomatic, and had no further abnormalities detected on renal imaging studies consisting of intravenous pyelographic contrast imaging (performed from 1975 into the late 1980s) and renal urinary tract and bladder ultrasound scan (performed from the late 1980s onward). When adjusted for confounding factors, the risk of development of end-stage renal disease was 18.5 times greater if microscopic hematuria was detected during adolescence or young adulthood compared with a control group without hematuria.

The issue with a study such as this is what to do with the information. We are helped in this regard by an excellent editorial by Brown[1] that accompanied the report. Brown indicates that if an individual is found to have persistent microscopic hematuria, the finding of acanthocytic red blood cells or red blood cell casts would suggest a glomerular source. If the latter are not present, a urologic examination is advised. Prior to the study by Vivante et al, patients with isolated microscopic hematuria and a negative evaluation were usually considered to have benign hematuria and required no follow-up. Now it seems reasonable to evaluate such patients every year or 2 for a possible increased incidence of proteinuria, hypertension, or renal insufficiency. If proteinuria or microalbuminuria evolves, there are convincing data now to show that these are modifiable risk factors in the evolution of ESRD for which therapies are available to improve adverse outcomes of chronic ESRD progression and cardiovascular disease. This is particularly true if treatment is begun early. For example, angiotensin-converting enzyme inhibitors or angiotensin II receptor blockers may reduce the relative risk of ESRD development, doubling of serum creatinine levels, or death by up to 40% in patients with nondiabetic nephropathy in association with proteinuria.

Brown et al[1] conclude that the time may have arrived for routine urine dipstick screening in adolescents and young adults. Again, the caveat is that this recommendation is based on a study that includes a fairly uniform population of young adults in Israel.

This commentary closes with a question for the reader. You are seeing a 5-year-old boy who has been referred to you by a family physician for evaluation of white, milky urine. The boy's mother reported 10-12 episodes of white-colored urine occurring during the previous 18 months. She described finding drops of whitish urine dried on his underwear that appeared white and crusty, like "dried Maalox." The boy was otherwise healthy, with no significant past medical history or family history. A physical examination was entirely normal. Initial laboratory examination of blood and urine, including electrolytes, blood urea nitrogen, creatinine, parathyroid hormone, vitamin D studies, alkaline phosphatase, and urine protein, were unremarkable, aside from an elevated urinary calcium-to-creatinine ratio of 0.36 mg/mg. His urine stained with Sudan was negative for fat, ruling out chyluria. The urine was initially cloudy. After the urine was allowed to sit for 30 minutes, a precipitate settled at the bottom of the sample that cleared after acidification with hydrochloric acid. Renal ultrasonography was unremarkable. Your diagnosis? If your diagnosis was hypercalciuria, you would have been correct. A 24-hour urine collection revealed hypercalciuria, as well as elevated supersaturations of calcium phosphate and calcium oxalate. This child was recently described in the literature.[2] The youngster represented the first case report of cloudy white urine due to mineral precipitation. White urine is most often secondary to chyluria, which results from an aberrant communication between the urinary tract and the lymphatic system, commonly due to filariasis. The child was treated with a low-sodium diet and no other restrictions, as well as a water intake of 1-1.5 L per day.

**J. A. Stockman III, MD**

*References*

1. Brown RS. Has the time come to include urine dipstick testing in screening asymptomatic young adults? *JAMA.* 2011;306:764-765.
2. Horner KB, Sas DJ. White urine in an otherwise asymptomatic child. *J Pediatr.* 2011;159:351.

## Prevalence of chronic kidney disease in China: a cross-sectional survey

Zhang L, Wang F, Wang L, et al (Peking Univ Inst of Nephrology, Beijing, China; Sichuan Provincial People's Hosp, Chengdu, China; et al)
*Lancet* 379:815-822, 2012

*Background.*—The prevalence of chronic kidney disease is high in developing countries. However, no national survey of chronic kidney disease has been done incorporating both estimated glomerular filtration rate (eGFR) and albuminuria in a developing country with the economic diversity of China. We aimed to measure the prevalence of chronic kidney disease in China with such a survey.

*Methods.*—We did a cross-sectional survey of a nationally representative sample of Chinese adults. Chronic kidney disease was defined as eGFR less than 60 mL/min per $1 \cdot 73$ m$^2$ or the presence of albuminuria. Participants completed a lifestyle and medical history questionnaire and had their blood pressure measured, and blood and urine samples taken. Serum creatinine was measured and used to estimate glomerular filtration rate. Urinary albumin and creatinine were tested to assess albuminuria. The crude and adjusted prevalence of indicators of kidney damage were calculated and factors associated with the presence of chronic kidney disease analysed by logistic regression.

*Findings.*—50 550 people were invited to participate, of whom 47 204 agreed. The adjusted prevalence of eGFR less than 60 mL/min per $1 \cdot 73$ m$^2$ was $1 \cdot 7\%$ (95% CI $1 \cdot 5 - 1 \cdot 9$) and of albuminuria was $9 \cdot 4\%$ ($8 \cdot 9 - 10 \cdot 0$). The overall prevalence of chronic kidney disease was $10 \cdot 8\%$ ($10 \cdot 2 - 11 \cdot 3$); therefore the number of patients with chronic kidney disease in China is estimated to be about $119 \cdot 5$ million ($112 \cdot 9 - 125 \cdot 0$ million). In rural areas, economic development was independently associated with the presence of albuminuria. The prevalence of chronic kidney disease was high in north ($16 \cdot 9\%$ [$15 \cdot 1 - 18 \cdot 7$]) and southwest ($18 \cdot 3\%$ [$16 \cdot 4 - 20 \cdot 4$]) regions compared with other regions. Other factors independently associated with kidney damage were age, sex, hypertension, diabetes, history of cardiovascular disease, hyperuricaemia, area of residence, and economic status.

*Interpretation.*—Chronic kidney disease has become an important public health problem in China. Special attention should be paid to residents in economically improving rural areas and specific geographical regions in China.

▶ The past decade has seen the remarkable development of China, which is now challenging the economic superiority of western European countries and the United States. The country that gave us the compass, gunpowder, and printing has already overtaken the United States and Europe in steel and energy consumption, mobile phone use, and car sales. China is projected to surpass the gross domestic product of the United States by 2018 and consumer spending by 2023.

Despite all these gains, China is now suffering from many of the afflictions associated with prosperity—namely, increasingly unhealthy diets and obesity as well as a rise in the incidence of hypertension and diabetes. Zhang et al present the first results of a comprehensive study exploring the prevalence of chronic kidney disease in China using a complex survey methodology that enables investigators to make nationally representative inferences about the prevalence of chronic renal disease in that nation. The results are noteworthy. The number of Chinese citizens with chronic kidney disease (prevalence 10.8%) dwarfs the number in the United States (119.5 million versus 20.3 million). Previous to this report, the United States was thought to have the highest prevalence of chronic kidney disease. If the findings from this report are correct, the results foreshadow a substantial emerging public health problem in China, because the health care resources in that country required to care for patients with advanced chronic kidney disease will likely increase exponentially in the near future. If China is an example of how health declines in a country with a rapidly emerging economy, then a few other countries that are currently doing better than they ever have will likely encounter the same problem. Hypertension, coronary artery disease, nephrosclerosis, and diabetes rapidly emerge when a society quickly becomes addicted to a bad diet and becomes obese. This is the lesson then to be learned from this report.

China's 3-year, $125-billion-dollar reform plan for health care, launched in 2009, is designed to achieve comprehensive universal health coverage in that country by 2020. The Chinese government's undertaking of systemic reform and its affirmation of its role in financing health care together with priorities for prevention, primary care, and redistribution of financial and human resources to poor regions are positive developments. Accomplishing nearly universal insurance coverage in such a short time is commendable. Nonetheless, transformation of financial and insurance coverage into cost-effective services is difficult when delivery of health care is hindered by waste, inefficiencies, poor quality of services, and scarcity and maldistribution of a qualified workforce. It is clear that China must reform its incentive structures for providers, improve its hospitals, and institute a stronger regulatory system. So far, it seems that China is up to the task, albeit an incredibly difficult one.

This commentary closes with a musical renal overture, in this instance, having to do with Mozart. For years, medical historians have wondered whether Mozart might have died of post *Streptococcal* glomerulonephritis. Wolfgang Amadeus Mozart died in Vienna on December 5, 1791, at age 35 years. From various descriptions, it seems that his illness may have been infectious, part of an epidemic, and characterized by a rapid onset of severe edema, pain of unknown localization, fever, and rash. From 1607 onward, all deaths in Vienna were registered in handwritten documents. The registry lists "Hitziges Frieselfieber" (fever and rash) as the cause of Mozart's death. However, of the 5011 deaths recorded in Vienna in 3 surrounding months, as well as in the corresponding periods of the preceding and following winter, only 4 were assigned to fever and rash as the official cause of death. In contrast, deaths from edema were remarkably common in the winter of 1791 in men aged 40 years or younger. A large proportion of these edema-related deaths occurred in a military hospital. We know that an inflammatory fever struck many Viennese people in the Autumn of 1791—possibly an epidemic of *Streptococcal* pharyngitis that may have originated in the military hospital. The infection may have led to complications in some people, resulting in an unusual peak of edema-related deaths that winter. Thus it is indeed possible that Mozart fell ill with *Streptococcal* pharyngitis, which was complicated by post *Streptococcal* glomerulonephritis, leading to acute nephritic syndrome and death.

What little many of us know about Mozart we learned from the film *Amadeus*. One of the remarkable things I learned from that film when I first saw it was that when Mozart was my age, he had been dead 12 years.[1]

**J. A. Stockman III, MD**

*Reference*

1. Zegars RHC, Weigl A, Steploe A. The death of Wolfgang Amadeus Mozart: An epidemiologic perspective. *Ann Intern Med.* 2009;151:274-278.

---

**Mycophenolate versus Azathioprine as Maintenance Therapy for Lupus Nephritis**
Dooley MA, for the ALMS Group (Univ of North Carolina, Chapel Hill; et al)
*N Engl J Med* 365:1886-1895, 2011

---

*Background.*—Maintenance therapy, often with azathioprine or mycophenolate mofetil, is required to consolidate remission and prevent relapse after the initial control of lupus nephritis.

*Methods.*—We carried out a 36-month, randomized, double-blind, double-dummy, phase 3 study comparing oral mycophenolate mofetil (2 g per day) and oral azathioprine (2 mg per kilogram of body weight per day), plus placebo in each group, in patients who met response criteria during a 6-month induction trial. The study group underwent repeat randomization in a 1:1 ratio. Up to 10 mg of prednisone per day or its equivalent was permitted. The primary efficacy end point was the time to treatment failure, which was defined as death, end-stage renal disease, doubling of the serum creatinine level, renal flare, or rescue therapy for lupus nephritis. Secondary assessments included the time to the individual components of treatment failure and adverse events.

*Results.*—A total of 227 patients were randomly assigned to maintenance treatment (116 to mycophenolate mofetil and 111 to azathioprine). Mycophenolate mofetil was superior to azathioprine with respect to the primary end point, time to treatment failure (hazard ratio, 0.44; 95% confidence interval, 0.25 to 0.77; $P = 0.003$), and with respect to time to renal flare and time to rescue therapy (hazard ratio, $< 1.00$; $P < 0.05$). Observed rates of treatment failure were 16.4% (19 of 116 patients) in the mycophenolate mofetil group and 32.4% (36 of 111) in the azathioprine group. Adverse events, most commonly minor infections and gastrointestinal disorders, occurred in more than 95% of the patients in both groups ($P = 0.68$). Serious adverse events occurred in 33.3% of patients in the azathioprine group and in 23.5% of those in the mycophenolate mofetil group ($P = 0.11$), and the rate of withdrawal due to adverse events was higher with azathioprine than with mycophenolate mofetil (39.6% vs. 25.2%, $P = 0.02$).

*Conclusions.*—Mycophenolate mofetil was superior to azathioprine in maintaining a renal response to treatment and in preventing relapse in patients with lupus nephritis who had a response to induction therapy. (Funded by Vifor Pharma [formerly Aspreva]; ALMS ClinicalTrials.gov number, NCT00377637.)

▶ Dooley et al report the results of the maintenance phase of the Aspreva Lupus Management Study (ALMS). This study compares the efficacy and safety of azathioprine and mycophenolate mofetil as maintenance therapy for patients with lupus nephritis who had responded to induction therapy either with mycophenolate mofetil or intravenous cyclophosphamide. After 3 years, mycophenolate mofetil appeared to be superior to azathioprine with respect to time to treatment failure, time to renal flare, and time to rescue therapy, regardless of how the initial episode of lupus nephritis was induced. Of note, among patients given mycophenolate mofetil for maintenance, those who had previously received induction therapy with intravenous cyclophosphamide had fewer treatment failures during the maintenance phase than did those who received mycophenolate mofetil for induction (11% vs 21%). This finding does suggest that intravenous cyclophosphamide continues to be an important option for induction of therapy for patients with lupus nephritis.

One important aspect of the report of Dooley et al is that it included pediatric-age patients as young as 12 years of age. It has only been within the last 10 to 15 years that clinical researchers have been able to extensively collaborate on the management of lupus and have carried out well-conducted controlled trials aimed at improving the efficacy and safety of immunosuppressive therapies. Indeed, advances have been achieved such as the use of more patient-friendly short-course induction regimens in which low-dose intravenous cyclophosphamide is followed by long-term azathioprine maintenance therapy and also the introduction of mycophenolate mofetil, an immunosuppressive drug used successfully for transplantation patients. The latter drug has been shown to be at least equivalent to cyclophosphamide in inducing an initial renal response, thereby rapidly earning itself a place in the armamentarium for the treatment of lupus nephritis at all ages, although long-term data on patients who have undergone induction therapy with mycophenolate mofetil are still awaited. The data of Dooley et al are truly important. Kidney involvement, mainly glomerulonephritis, occurs in at least one-third of patients with systemic lupus erythematosus. Kidney involvement significantly affects long-term survival. Somewhere between 10% and 20% of patients with lupus nephritis will ultimately require renal replacement therapy. Hopefully, the findings from this report indicate that mycophenolate mofetil is superior to azathioprine in maintaining the renal response to treatment and in preventing relapse in patients with active lupus nephritis.

**J. A. Stockman III, MD**

---

### *MYO1E* Mutations and Childhood Familial Focal Segmental Glomerulosclerosis

Mele C, for the PodoNet Consortium (Clinical Res Ctr for Rare Diseases, Bergamo, Italy; et al)

*N Engl J Med* 365:295-306, 2011

*Background.*—Focal segmental glomerulosclerosis is a kidney disease that is manifested as the nephrotic syndrome. It is often resistant to glucocorticoid therapy and progresses to end-stage renal disease in 50 to 70% of patients. Genetic studies have shown that familial focal segmental glomeruloslerosis is a disease of the podocytes, which are major components of the glomerular filtration barrier. However, the molecular cause in over half the cases of primary focal segmental glomerulosclerosis is unknown, and effective treatments have been elusive.

*Methods.*— We performed whole-genome linkage analysis followed by high-throughput sequencing of the positive-linkage area in a family with autosomal recessive focal segmental glomerulosclerosis (index family) and sequenced a newly discovered gene in 52 unrelated patients with focal segmental glomerulosclerosis. Immunohistochemical studies were performed on human kidney-biopsy specimens and cultured podocytes. Expression studies in vitro were performed to characterize the functional consequences of the mutations identified.

*Results.*—We identified two mutations (A159P and Y695X) in *MYO1E*, which encodes a non-muscle class I myosin, myosin 1E (Myo1E). The mutations in *MYO1E* segregated with focal segmental glomerulosclerosis in two independent pedigrees (the index family and Family 2). Patients were homozygous for the mutations and did not have a response to glucocorticoid therapy. Electron microscopy showed thickening and dis-organization of the glomerular basement membrane. Normal expression of Myo1E was documented in control human kidney-biopsy specimens in vivo and in glomerular podocytes in vitro. Transfection studies revealed abnormal subcellular localization and function of the A159P-Myo1E mutant. The

Y695X mutation causes loss of calmodulin binding and of the tail domains of Myo1E.

*Conclusions.*—*MYO1E* mutations are associated with childhood-onset, glucocorticoid-resistant focal segmental glomerulosclerosis. Our data provide evidence of a role of Myo1E in podocyte function and the consequent integrity of the glomerular filtration barrier.

▶ Focal segmental glomerulosclerosis (FSG), one of the most common glomerulopathies, typically presents with massive proteinuria, often associated with unremitting nephrotic syndrome and inexorable progression to end-stage renal disease. All too often, therapy is unsuccessful, with many patients not responding to treatment with glucocorticoids. The disease also frequently recurs after kidney transplantation. Although a small fraction of cases of FSG are familial, unraveling the molecular basis of these cases has informed the biology of renal podocyte function. The podocyte is the cell in the kidney that is critical to the development of FSG. The podocyte controls glomerular filtration by means of its slit-pore diaphragm and other properties. Podocytes surround and adhere to glomerular capillary loops. Over the last decade, mutations in nearly 20 different genes that affect multiple podocyte functions have been linked with FSG.

Mele et al describe 2 families with FSG that demonstrate distinct mutations in a gene known as *MYO1E*. This gene encodes myosin 1E, present in podocytes. Interestingly, all of the affected patients with this mutation are resistant to treatment with steroids, consistent with the course in most patients with FSG, yet most of these patients respond to cyclosporine. Cyclosporine has been known to cause remission in many patients with segmental glomerulosclerosis, but the mechanism underlying such remission has remained illusive. It has been suggested that cyclosporine may act by stabilizing the cytoskeleton of the podocyte. Another agent has recently been observed that is useful in the management of this disorder. This is rituximab, an anti-CD20 monoclonal antibody, which also stabilizes the podocyte actin cytoskeleton.

While this report provides us with knowledge of an infrequent familial cause of FSG, it does inform us about exactly how some patients develop this serious kidney disease and provides insights that may lead to new forms of therapy for a wider group of affected individuals.

**J. A. Stockman III, MD**

---

*INF2* **Mutations in Charcot–Marie–Tooth Disease with Glomerulopathy**
Boyer O, Nevo F, Plaisier E, et al (Hôpital Necker–Enfants Malades, Paris, France; et al)
*N Engl J Med* 365:2377-2388, 2011

---

*Background.*—Charcot–Marie–Tooth neuropathy has been reported to be associated with renal diseases, mostly focal segmental glomerulosclerosis (FSGS). However, the common mechanisms underlying the neuropathy and

FSGS remain unknown. Mutations in *INF2* were recently identified in patients with autosomal dominant FSGS. *INF2* encodes a formin protein that interacts with the Rho-GTPase CDC42 and myelin and lymphocyte protein (MAL) that are implicated in essential steps of myelination and myelin maintenance. We therefore hypothesized that *INF2* may be responsible for cases of Charcot—Marie—Tooth neuropathy associated with FSGS.

*Methods.*—We performed direct genotyping of *INF2* in 16 index patients with Charcot—Marie—Tooth neuropathy and FSGS who did not have a mutation in *PMP22* or *MPZ*, encoding peripheral myelin protein 22 and myelin protein zero, respectively. Histologic and functional studies were also conducted.

*Results.*—We identified nine new heterozygous mutations in 12 of the 16 index patients (75%), all located in exons 2 and 3, encoding the diaphanous-inhibitory domain of INF2. Patients presented with an intermediate form of Charcot—Marie—Tooth neuropathy as well as a glomerulopathy with FSGS on kidney biopsy. Immunohistochemical analysis revealed strong INF2 expression in Schwann-cell cytoplasm and podocytes. Moreover, we demonstrated that INF2 colocalizes and interacts with MAL in Schwann cells. The INF2 mutants perturbed the INF2—MAL—CDC42 pathway, resulting in cytoskeleton disorganization, enhanced INF2 binding to CDC42 and mislocalization of INF2, MAL, and CDC42.

*Conclusions.*—*INF2* mutations appear to cause many cases of FSGS-associated Charcot—Marie—Tooth neuropathy, showing that *INF2* is involved in a disease affecting both the kidney glomerulus and the peripheral nervous system. These findings provide new insights into the pathophysiological mechanisms linking formin proteins to podocyte and Schwann-cell function. (Funded by the Agence Nationale de la Recherche and others.)

▶ Charcot-Marie-Tooth disease refers to a heterogeneous group of inherited peripheral motor and sensory neuropathies. Individuals affected with this disorder typically present with progressive distal muscle weakness and atrophy along with reduced tendon reflexes and foot and hand deformities. There are 3 forms of the disease, characterized by means of electrophysiological and neuropathologic studies—a glial myelinopathy (type 1) showing slow motor nerve conduction velocities and demyelinating neuropathy, an axonal form (type 2) associated with normal or subnormal nerve conduction velocities and axonal degeneration, and an intermediate form with demyelinating and axonal features in which patients from the same family may have either subnormal or reduced nerve conduction velocities. There are more than 40 different gene loci that have been associated with Charcot-Marie-Tooth disease. The most common genetic form is autosomal dominant type 1 with mutations in the peripheral myelin protein 22 gene and the myelin protein 0 gene.

As time has passed, we have seen more and more written about the presence of neuropathies, particularly focal segmental glomerular sclerosis (FSGS) in patients with Charcot-Marie-Tooth disease. Not understood is what the link might be between the neurologic manifestations and the renal manifestations. It is known that FSGS is an histologic pattern of renal damage associated with a spectrum of primary and secondary glomerular diseases, including isolated proteinuria and glucocorticoid-resistant nephrotic syndrome. Mutations in the INF2 gene account for somewhere between 12% and 17% of autosomal dominant cases of FSGS. The authors of this report hypothesize that INF2 mutations may be causal for the association between FSGS and Charcot-Marie-Tooth neuropathy. They have documented that INF2 mutations are a major cause of Charcot-Marie-Tooth disease associated with FSGS, accounting for approximately 75% of all cases. These findings shed new light on the genetic basis of the dual neurologic and renal manifestations of Charcot-Marie-Tooth disease.

The clinical link between the kidney and the nervous system was first described more than 45 years ago.[1] We now see that although INF2 mutations are known to be the major cause of autosomal dominant FSGS, accounting for up to 17% of all cases, the prevalence of this exact set of mutations in association with FSGS and Charcot-Marie-Tooth is much higher than this. This report provides insight into the role of cellular machinery and podocytes (foot processes in the kidney) and Schwann cells in the central nervous system, even though these 2 highly specialized cell types have distinct functions.

**J. A. Stockman III, MD**

*Reference*

1. Lemieux G, Neemeh JA. Charcot-Marie-Tooth disease and nephritis. *Can Med Assoc J*. 1967;97:1193-1198.

---

**Sterile Cerebrospinal Fluid Pleocytosis in Young Febrile Infants With Urinary Tract Infections**

Schnadower D, for the Pediatric Emergency Medicine Collaborative Research Committee of the American Academy of Pediatrics (Columbia Univ College of Physicians and Surgeons, NY; et al)
*Arch Pediatr Adolesc Med* 165:635-641, 2011

---

*Objectives.*—To determine the prevalence of and to identify risk factors for sterile cerebrospinal fluid (CSF) pleocytosis in a large sample of febrile young infants with urinary tract infections (UTIs) and to describe the clinical courses of those patients.

*Design.*—Secondary analysis of a multicenter retrospective review.

*Setting.*—Emergency departments of 20 North American hospitals.

*Patients.*—Infants aged 29 to 60 days with temperatures of 38.0°C or higher and culture-proven UTIs who underwent a nontraumatic lumbar puncture from January 1, 1995, through May 31, 2006.

*Main Exposure.*—Febrile UTI.

*Outcome Measures.*—Presence of sterile CSF pleocytosis defined as CSF white blood cell count of 10/µL or higher in the absence of bacterial meningitis and clinical course and treatment (ie, presence of adverse events, time to defervescence, duration of parenteral antibiotic treatment, and length of hospitalization).

*Results.*—A total of 214 of 1190 infants had sterile CSF pleocytosis (18.0%; 95% confidence interval, 15.9%-20.3%). Only the peripheral white blood cell count was independently associated with sterile CSF pleocytosis, and patients with a peripheral white blood cell count of 15/μL or higher had twice the odds of having sterile CSF pleocytosis (odds ratio, 1.97; 95% confidence interval, 1.32-2.94; $P = .001$). In the subset of patients at very low risk for adverse events (ie, not clinically ill in the emergency department and without a high-risk medical history), patients with and without sterile CSF pleocytosis had similar clinical courses; however, patients with CSF pleocytosis had longer parenteral antibiotics courses (median length, 4 days [interquartile range, 3-6 days] vs 3 days [interquartile range, 3-5 days]) ($P = .04$).

*Conclusion.*—Sterile CSF pleocytosis occurs in 18% of young infants with UTIs. Patients with CSF pleocytosis at very low risk for adverse events may not require longer treatment with antibiotics.

▶ There have been reports from time to time about the finding of white blood cells in the cerebrospinal fluid (CSF) of young infants with urinary tract infections (UTIs) who are experiencing fever. The literature in this regard has been somewhat murky. The prevalence of sterile CSF pleocytosis and its causes in febrile infants with UTIs remains controversial. What to do about such findings is even more controversial.

Schnadower et al designed a study to determine a more precise estimate of the prevalence of sterile CSF pleocytosis in a large sample of febrile infants with UTIs aged 29 to 60 days. In doing so, the investigators also sought to identify potential risk factors for sterile CSF pleocytosis and also attempted to describe the clinical course and treatment of these infants. Data from 20 North American emergency departments that are part of the Pediatric Emergency Medicine Collaborative Research Committee were collected. A UTI was defined as growth of a single pathogen with colony counts meeting at least 1 of the following 3 criteria: 100 colony-forming units (CFU)/mL or more for urine cultures obtained by suprapubic aspiration, 50 000 CFU/mL or more from a catheterized specimen, or 10 000 CFU/mL from a catheterized specimen in association with a positive urinalysis result. A positive urinalysis was defined by any organism visualized on gram stain, trace or greater result for leukocyte esterase or nitrite on dipstick or laboratory-based urinalysis, or 5 or more white blood cells per high-powered field using standard light microscopy. CSF pleocytosis was defined as a CSF white blood cell count of 10 cells/μL or higher.

Using the parameters described, it was observed that CSF pleocytosis occurs in 18% of febrile infants with UTIs aged 29 to 60 days. These data are consistent with most prior studies on this topic, although the sample size in the study reported far exceeds that of prior studies. The authors of this report also attempted to see what factors might be associated with the finding of CSF pleocytosis in the presence of fever and a urinary tract infection in a young infant. Only the peripheral white blood cell count was independently associated with the risk of CSF pleocytosis, suggesting a possible inflammatory cause of sterile CSF pleocytosis. It should be noted that the presence of sterile CSF pleocytosis appears to have affected the clinical decision making of the care providers of the infants in this study. More than 20% of the infants with UTIs and sterile CSF pleocytosis who did not have a high-risk medical history and who were not clinically ill in the emergency department received at least 7 days of intravenous antibiotics. These patients defervesced as rapidly as those without CSF pleocytosis and were no more likely to have adverse outcomes when compared with those without sterile CSF pleocytosis, suggesting that prolonged antibiotic therapy was unnecessary.

Perhaps the data from this report will help all of us relax a bit more the next time we see a young infant with fever and a urinary tract infection who has some white blood cells in his or her CSF. If the infant is otherwise well looking, he or she should probably be treated as any other infant with a UTI, ignoring, to the extent possible, the implications of a CSF pleocytosis.

This commentary ends with a clinical case scenario and asks for your diagnosis. You are seeing a 14-year-old girl with diffuse abdominal pain. She complains of dysuria. She is afebrile. Lacking a clear diagnosis, you obtain a plain film of the abdomen. This shows air throughout the urinary tract. There is a large bubble of air in the bladder. The ureters are bilaterally filled with air as are the collecting systems of the kidneys. Your diagnosis? Your diagnosis should be that of acute emphysematous cystitis. A patient has been described with these exact findings and the urine culture grew *Escherichia coli*. The patient had an excellent response to antibiotic treatment. In most patients with acute emphysematous cystitis, the underlying diagnosis is diabetes mellitus where a predisposition exists to complicated urinary tract infections such as emphysematous cystitis, which is thought to be caused by fermentation of glucose by bacterial and fungal pathogens.[1]

**J. A. Stockman III, MD**

*Reference*

1. Lu CC, Cheng TC. Air in the urinary tract. *N Engl J Med*. 2009;361:388.

---

### Characteristics of First Urinary Tract Infection With Fever in Children: A Prospective Clinical and Imaging Study

Ismaili K, Wissing KM, Lolin K, et al (Université Libre de Bruxelles (ULB), Brussels, Belgium; Universitairé Ziekenhuis Brussels-Vrije Universitéit Brussel (VUB), Belgium; et al)
*Pediatr Infect Dis J* 30:371-374, 2011

---

*Background.*—Our objective is to provide the clinical characteristics, uropathogen frequencies, and antimicrobial resistance rates of first urinary tract infection (UTI) diagnosed in febrile Belgian children. The ability of noninvasive ultrasound to detect renal abnormalities and vesicoureteral reflux (VUR) in these patients was also assessed.

*Methods.*—We prospectively followed (median, 20 months) 209 children treated for first febrile UTI. Renal ultrasound (US) and voiding cystourethrography examinations were performed in all patients.

*Results.*—Among these children, 63% were females and 37% were males, and 75% of them had their first UTI before the age of 2 years. The most common causative agent was *Escherichia coli* (91% of cases) with high rate resistance to ampicillin (58%) and trimethoprim/sulfamethoxazole (38%). Of these children, 25% had evidence of VUR (15 boys and 38 girls). VUR was of low grade in 85% of cases. The overall performance of renal US as a diagnostic test to detect significant uropathies excluding low-grade VUR was excellent; the sensitivity attained 97% and the specificity 94%.

*Conclusion.*—Girls represent 63% of cases with first UTI. For 91% of UTIs, *Escherichia coli* is held responsible with a high rate of resistance to ampicillin and trimethoprim/sulfamethoxazole. US is an excellent screening tool that allows avoidance of unjustified voiding cystourethrography studies.

▶ After all these years, we are still learning more about the presentation and management of urinary tract infections (UTIs). This report reminds us that approximately 8% of girls and 2% of boys will experience at least 1 UTI by 7 years of age. The report from Belgium tells us about the design of a prospective study intended to describe the characteristics and clinical evolution of first UTI as diagnosed by systematic screening in an emergency department of febrile children in whom UTI was considered a possible diagnosis on clinical grounds. The study also aimed to characterize the frequency of specific uropathogens and their antimicrobial resistance rates to evaluate the options for empiric antibiotic therapy. Over a 2-year period, more than 200 children (median age of 10 months) with a clinically proven first episode of UTI were included in the study. UTI was initially suspected based on the definition of the presence of a combination of 2 of the following criteria: C-reactive protein $\geq 4.0$ mg/dL, leukocytosis $\geq 15\,000$ mm$^3$, signs of systemic infection with a deteriorating health condition, vomiting and poor feeding in infants, and back pain and chills in older children. A positive urinalysis finding was defined as a trace or greater result for leukocytes esterase or nitrite on dipstick or the presence of $\geq 35$ µL leukocytes in uncentrifuged urine. A positive urine culture was diagnosed if the child had $\geq 100\,000$ colony-forming units per milliliter in urine culture. In urine samples obtained by suprapubic aspiration, any growth of enteric gram-negative pathogens was considered significant.

As one might suspect, most UTIs in this report were caused by gram-negative organisms (*Escherichia coli*, being the most common organism isolated accounting for up to 80% of infections). Resistance rates to this organism to ampicillin were as high as 58%. These types of resistance rates are commonly seen throughout Europe as a whole. In this series, 85% of patients with a new UTI showed evidence of vesicoureteral reflux (VUR) on voiding cystourethrography examination; 85% of the latter were of a low grade VUR. Relapses were seen in only 11% of patients within a median period of 7 months after presentation.

At least in this series, with the majority of children with UTI having a low risk of recurrence or of high-grade VUR, one can question the extent to which these children should be submitted to unnecessary investigations. Studies have suggested that in febrile children < 2 years of age with UTI, ultrasound scan might not be required because of the widespread use of prenatal ultrasound scan in areas where this is undertaken. The authors of this report document the widespread belief, perhaps true, that antenatal ultrasound examinations are not reliable for the purpose of ruling out significant renal problems. The authors suggest that if some type of renal imaging is desired, ultrasound scan is the way to go. They have shown that all children with high-grade VUR will have renal abnormalities that are visible on ultrasound scan. One final observation from this study is that of the 11% of children who have a recurrence of infection in their series, half of these patients will have normal urinary tract findings on extensive imaging.

**J. A. Stockman III, MD**

---

## Impact of a More Restrictive Approach to Urinary Tract Imaging After Febrile Urinary Tract Infection

Schroeder AR, Abidari JM, Kirpekar R, et al (Santa Clara Valley Med Ctr, San Jose, CA)
*Arch Pediatr Adolesc Med* 165:1027-1032, 2011

---

*Objectives.*—To determine the impact of using an algorithm requiring selective rather than routine urinary tract imaging following a first febrile urinary tract infection (UTI) on imaging use, detection of vesicoureteral reflux (VUR), prophylactic antibiotic use, and UTI recurrence within 6 months.

*Design.*—Retrospective review comparing outcomes during periods before algorithm use (September 1, 2006, to August 31, 2007) and after algorithm use (September 1, 2008, to August 31, 2009). The new algorithm, which adapted recommendations from the United Kingdom's National Institute for Health and Clinical Excellence 2007 guidelines, was implemented in 2008. The algorithm calls for renal ultrasonography in most cases and restricts voiding cystourethrography for use in patients with certain risk factors.

*Setting.*—County health system.

*Participants.*—Children younger than 2 years with a first febrile UTI.

*Intervention.*—Selective algorithm for urinary tract imaging.

*Main Outcome Measures.*—Urinary tract imaging use, detection of VUR, prophylactic antibiotic use, and UTI recurrence within 6 months.

*Results.*—After introduction of the new algorithm, voiding cystourethrography and prophylactic antibiotic use decreased markedly. Rates of UTI recurrence within 6 months and detection of grades 4 and 5 VUR did not change, but detection of grades 1 to 3 VUR decreased substantially. Patients in the prealgorithm group with grades 1 to 3 VUR who would have been missed with selective screening underwent no interventions other than successive urinary tract imaging and prophylactic antibiotic use.

*Conclusions.*—By restricting urinary tract imaging after an initial febrile UTI, rates of voiding cystourethrography and prophylactic antibiotic use decreased substantially without increasing the risk of UTI recurrence within 6 months and without an apparent decrease in detection of high-grade VUR. Clinicians can be more judicious in their use of urinary tract imaging.

▶ It was in 1999 that the American Academy of Pediatrics issued a practice parameter dealing with the evaluation of youngsters with urinary tract infections (UTIs). There was a recommendation for renal ultrasonography and voiding cystourethrography (VCUG) in all children with a first-time febrile UTI. The guideline further recommended daily antibiotic prophylaxis after initial UTI treatment until imaging studies were completed and the results were returned as normal. These recommendations have come under quite a bit of scrutiny in recent years, raising the issue of whether routine imaging, especially VCUG and antibiotic prophylaxis were truly necessary. In 2007, the United Kingdom's National Institute for Health and Clinical Excellence (NICE) established new guidelines for the management of UTI in children. These guidelines recommend more selective use of ultrasonography and VCUG based on age and other risk factors. The figure shows the essence of the United Kingdom's guidelines.

The report of Schroeder et al summarizes a study that assesses the impact of the new guidelines emanating from across the pond related to imaging use (specifically, renal ultrasound scan and VCUG), prophylactic antibiotic use, and UTI recurrence within 6 months. The study looked at only children younger than 2 years because this age is consistent with the upper age limit cutoff for the American Academy of Pediatrics UTI Practice Parameter. The study reported was not from the United Kingdom, rather from the Santa Clara Valley Medical Center in San Jose, California. Specifically, the investigators followed an algorithm that calls for renal ultrasound scan in most cases and the more selective use of VCUG based on the following risk factors according to the NICE guidelines: bacteremia with the UTI, inadequate response of the UTI to antibiotic treatment within 48 hours, non-*Escherichia coli* pathogen, poor urine flow, elevated serum creatinine level, palpable abdominal or pelvic mass, or abnormal renal ultrasound scan findings. Prophylactic antibiotic use was discouraged. The main outcome measures were urinary tract imaging use, detection of reflux, prophylactic antibiotic use, and UTI recurrence within 6 months.

This report represents the first study that has assessed the effect of a more selective approach to imaging after a first febrile UTI in children. It demonstrates that VCUG use in particular can be reduced substantially without affecting the risk of UTI reoccurrence within 6 months and without compromising the detection of high-grade reflux. With the British algorithm in place, rates of UTI recurrence within 6 months and detection of grades 4 and 5 reflux did not change, but detection rates of 1–3 reflux decreased substantially. This study also looked at the outcome of discouraging the routine use of antibiotic prophylaxis in low-risk patients. There was no outcome difference when antibiotic prophylaxis, used in a routine manner, was eliminated.

Because low-grade reflux in infants and young children with UTI is common, any algorithm, such as the one used at the Santa Clara Medical Center, or the British guidelines that significantly restrict the use of VCUG, will by design diagnose fewer instances of low-grade reflux. Missing these cases seems in no way to harm the long-term outcome of these youngsters. Eliminating unnecessary VCUG studies has many benefits since the procedure is invasive, painful, and expensive and does carry radiation risk. It has been calculated that the lifetime risk of a fatal cancer as a result of a single study is 1 in 10 000 patients. Eliminating performing a VCUG also avoids the later temptation of repeating the study just to see whether low-grade reflux has improved. The average cost of a VCUG study, at least as performed in California, runs $2000, a cost that can be averted in many instances.

Shortly after the Schroeder et al article appeared, the American Academy of Pediatrics (AAP) issued new guidelines for the management of urinary tract infection. These guidelines continue to support the 1999 AAP guideline recommending renal/bladder ultrasound examination after a first febrile UTI to rule out anatomical abnormalities. The recommendation most dramatically different from the 1999 guideline is that VCUG should not be routinely performed after a first febrile UTI. The main reason for this change is the accumulation of evidence, such as that of Schroeder et al, casting doubt on the benefit of making a diagnosis of low-grade reflux. The report suggests that the risk, cost, and discomfort of VCUG are not justified, because there is no evidence the patients benefit from having reflux diagnosed. To read more about the new AAP urinary tract infection guideline, see the commentary by Newman.[1]

**J. A. Stockman III, MD**

*Reference*

1. Newman TB. The new American Academy of Pediatrics urinary tract infection guideline. *Pediatrics.* 2011;128:572-575.

---

**National Ambulatory Antibiotic Prescribing Patterns for Pediatric Urinary Tract Infection, 1998–2007**
Copp HL, Shapiro DJ, Hersh AL (Univ of California, San Francisco; Univ of Utah, Salt Lake City)
*Pediatrics* 127:1027-1033, 2011

---

*Objective.*—The goal of this study was to investigate patterns of ambulatory antibiotic use and to identify factors associated with broad-spectrum antibiotic prescribing for pediatric urinary tract infections (UTIs).

*Methods.*—We examined antibiotics prescribed for UTIs for children aged younger than 18 years from 1998 to 2007 using the National Ambulatory Medical Care Survey and National Hospital Ambulatory Medical Care Survey. Amoxicillin-clavulanate, quinolones, macrolides, and second-and third-generation cephalosporins were classified as broad-spectrum antibiotics. We evaluated trends in broad-spectrum antibiotic prescribing patterns and performed multivariable logistic regression to identify factors associated with broad-spectrum antibiotic use.

*Results.*—Antibiotics were prescribed for 70% of pediatric UTI visits. Trimethoprim-sulfamethoxazole was the most commonly prescribed antibiotic (49% of visits). Broad-spectrum antibiotics were prescribed one third of the time. There was no increase in overall use of broadspectrum antibiotics ($P = .67$); however, third-generation cephalosporin use doubled from 12% to 25% ($P = .02$). Children younger than 2 years old (odds ratio: 6.4 [95% confidence interval: 2.2—18.7, compared with children 13—17 years old]), females (odds ratio: 3.6 [95% confidence interval: 1.6—8.5]), and temperature ≥100.4°F (odds ratio: 2.9 [95% confidence interval: 1.0—8.6]) were independent predictors of broadspectrum antibiotic prescribing. Race, physician specialty, region, and insurance status were not associated with antibiotic selection.

*Conclusions.*—Ambulatory care physicians commonly prescribe broad-spectrum antibiotics for the treatment of pediatric UTIs, especially for febrile infants in whom complicated infections are more likely. The doubling in use of third-generation cephalosporins suggests that opportunities exist to promote more judicious antibiotic prescribing because most pediatric UTIs are susceptible to narrower alternatives.

► A great deal continues to be written about antibiotic use and otitis media, but less so do we see much written about what pediatricians are doing with respect to antibiotic use and urinary tract infections. When one realizes that between 3% and 4% of children in the United States are diagnosed annually with urinary tract infections (UTIs), you can see the importance of any information regarding the antibiotics that are being used to treat this problem and whether the antibiotics selected are appropriate. The report of Copp et al is the first that examines ambulatory antibiotic prescribing patterns in the United States for children with UTIs. Studies performed in adults have documented a marked increase in the use of broad-spectrum antibiotics for the management of this type of infection, raising serious concerns about the development of antibiotic resistance.

Copp et al analyzed data from the Ambulatory Medical Care Survey and the National Hospital Ambulatory Medical Care Survey for the periods 1998 through 2007 to determine whether at the time of outpatient visit, pediatric care providers were prescribing antibiotics for UTIs. The survey documented an estimated 16 million visits for UTIs in children younger than 18 years. Most of these visits were by female patients with an acute problem. Less than 1% of the total visits for pediatric UTIs required hospital admission. Antibiotics were prescribed for 70% of these pediatric UTIs. Parenteral therapy was used in slightly more than 10% of such visits. Third-generation cyclosporins contributed to the majority of parenterally administered antibiotics (77%) and, among these, ceftriaxone was selected 95% of the time. Trimethoprim-sulfamethoxazole was prescribed in 49% of UTI antibiotic visits and was the single most commonly prescribed antibiotic throughout the entire study period. First-generation cephalosporins and urinary antiinfective agents comprised less than 5% and 8% of antibiotics prescribed for UTIs, respectively. In 32% of UTI antibiotic visits, a broad-spectrum antibiotic was prescribed, and there was no change in the percentage of broad-spectrum antibiotics prescribed over time. Amoxicillin-clavulanate use ranged from 4% and 9% of UTI visits with no significant change in trend over time. The alarming circumstance described, however, was the doubling of use of third-generation cephalosporins from 12% in 1998 to 2000 to 25% in 2005 to 2007.

The use of third-generation cephalosporins began to be popular in the late 1990s when it was suggested that oral cefixime was safe and effective for outpatient treatment of pyelonephritis. However, more recent evaluations for this problem in children suggest that there is no difference in the effectiveness of oral therapy with third-generation cephalosporins compared with amoxicillin-clavulanate. In fact, third-generation cephalosporins may no longer afford the assured antimicrobial coverage for patients with complicated UTIs that they once did. Third-generation cephalosporins, in particular ceftriaxone, have become popular because of the latter drug's availability as a parenteral formulation with once-daily dosing. A 1-time dose of a parenteral antibiotic in combination with the same drug given orally is a commonly used strategy now for the outpatient management of pyelonephritis.

The data from this report are extremely important. When a single disease, such as a urinary tract infection, accounts for more than 1.5 million visits annually in the United States, we have to know the best ways of managing the problem with the least adverse consequences. The authors of this report note that the findings from this report support the need for interventions that promote judicious antibiotic selection for the treatment of pediatric UTIs.

This commentary closes with an interesting observation about the urine output of house staff while on call. Recently reported was an evaluation of 18 residents responsible for covering day shifts on inpatient services. These residents were determined to be oliguric (defined as mean urine output <0.5 mL/kg/h over 6 hours or more of measurement) on 22% of 87 shifts.[1] These residents were more likely to be oliguric than the patients they took care of. The urine output in one resident was consistent with "renal injury." Fortunately, the mortality among such house staff was astonishingly low, at 0%. Evian rules!

**J. A. Stockman III, MD**

*Reference*

1. Solomon AW, Kirwan CJ, Alexander NDE, et al. Urine output on an intensive care unit: case-control study. *BMJ*. 2010;341:c6761.

---

## Association Between Smoking and Risk of Bladder Cancer Among Men and Women

Freedman ND, Silverman DT, Hollenbeck AR, et al (Natl Cancer Inst, Rockville, MD; AARP, Washington, DC)
*JAMA* 306:737-745, 2011

---

*Context.*—Previous studies indicate that the population attributable risk (PAR) of bladder cancer for tobacco smoking is 50% to 65% in men and 20% to 30% in women and that current cigarette smoking triples bladder cancer risk relative to never smoking. During the last 30 years, incidence rates have remained stable in the United States in men (123.8 per

100 000 person-years to 142.2 per 100 000 person-years) and women (32.5 per 100 000 person-years to 33.2 per 100 000 person-years); however, changing smoking prevalence and cigarette composition warrant revisiting risk estimates for smoking and bladder cancer.

*Objective.*—To evaluate the association between tobacco smoking and bladder cancer.

*Design, Setting, and Participants.*—Men (n = 281 394) and women (n = 186 134) of the National Institutes of Health-AARP (NIH-AARP) Diet and Health Study cohort completed a lifestyle questionnaire and were followed up between October 25, 1995, and December 31, 2006. Previous prospective cohort studies of smoking and incident bladder cancer were identified by systematic review and relative risks were estimated from fixed-effects models with heterogeneity assessed by the $I^2$ statistic.

*Main Outcome Measures.*—Hazard ratios (HRs), PARs, and number needed to harm (NNH).

*Results.*—During 4 518 941 person-years of follow-up, incident bladder cancer occurred in 3896 men (144.0 per 100 000 person-years) and 627 women (34.5 per 100 000 person-years). Former smokers (119.8 per 100 000 person-years; HR, 2.22; 95% confidence interval [CI], 2.03-2.44; NNH, 1250) and current smokers (177.3 per 100 000 person-years; HR, 4.06; 95% CI, 3.66-4.50; NNH, 727) had higher risks of bladder cancer than never smokers (39.8 per 100 000 person-years). In contrast, the summary risk estimate for current smoking in 7 previous studies (initiated between 1963 and 1987) was 2.94 (95% CI, 2.45-3.54; $I^2 = 0.0$%). The PAR for ever smoking in our study was 0.50 (95% CI, 0.45-0.54) in men and 0.52 (95% CI, 0.45-0.59) in women.

*Conclusion.*—Compared with a pooled estimate of US data from cohorts initiated between 1963 and 1987, relative risks for smoking in the more recent NIH-AARP Diet and Health Study cohort were higher, with PARs for women comparable with those for men.

▶ Teens who smoke should be aware of this report showing an association between smoking and a later risk in life of the development of bladder cancer. Bladder cancer is not a rare diagnosis in adults. More than 350 000 individuals worldwide are diagnosed with bladder cancer each year. Tobacco smoking is the best established risk factor for bladder cancer in both men and women. Although rates of bladder cancer have remained stable during the last 30 years, the prevalence of cigarette smoking in the United States has substantially decreased during the same period. During this same interval, the composition of cigarettes has changed, leading to a reduction in tar and nicotine concentrations in cigarette smoke but also to an apparent increase in the concentration of specific carcinogens, including β-naphthylamine, a known bladder carcinogen, and tobacco-specific nitrosamines. Similar to the findings with bladder cancer incidence, concurrent with the decreasing prevalence of smoking in the United States and the smoking of cigarettes with lower tar content, epidemiologic studies have observed high relative risk associated with cigarette smoking for lung cancer, again suggesting that an increase in concentration of specific carcinogens may be the problem.

Freedman et al mined data from a large prospective National Institutes of Health (NIH)-American Association of Retired Persons (AARP) Diet and Health Study to estimate the strength of the association between tobacco smoking and bladder cancer. This study involves a questionnaire that is mailed to 3.5 million AARP members age 50 to 71 years residing in 8 states. The survey obtained careful smoking histories. The investigators also identified the prevalence of cancers by linking the NIH-AARP Diet and Health Study cohort with the Cancer Registry Databases of 10 states. The survey information was originally initiated in 1995 and 1996, so a follow-up period of 10 years was possible.

In the NIH-AARP prospective cohort study, cigarette smoking was unequivocally and strongly associated with bladder cancer risk in both men and women, explaining at least half of the occurrence of bladder cancer in both sexes. The relative risk of the development of bladder cancer was in excess of 4-fold among smokers. Compared with other similar studies, it appeared that changes in the constituents of cigarette smoke, including apparent increased concentrations of $\beta$-naphthylamine, a known bladder carcinogen, and tobacco-specific nitrosamines, strengthened the cigarette smoking-bladder cancer association.

In this report, the median age at smoking initiation was 17 years in both men and women. The study did not provide sufficient information to say whether if one stopped smoking after a period of time, the risk of the development of bladder cancer would be lessened. In any event, teens should be aware that there is a risk of development of bladder cancer if they start smoking at any time during their life and that this risk appears to be increasing with time in the United States. What was once thought to be a good thing, reducing tar in cigarettes, has not solved the problem. Tobacco is a dirty weed and teens need to know that.

This commentary closes with an observation having to do with the genitourinary tract. One of the most common surgical procedures performed these days is inguinal hernia repair. In adults and in some children, hernioplasty is undertaken using a synthetic mesh. The availability and cost of such mesh are generally prohibitive to both surgeons and patients in poorly developed countries. Recently, Stephenson and Kingsnorth described a very cost-effective method as an alternative.[1] Instead of using medical grade synthetic mesh, they decided to cut mosquito netting into appropriate sized pieces, comparing the surgical outcomes with a comparable number of patients in whom surgical grade synthetic mesh was used. This study was reported from Ghana. No differences in outcomes were observed. The cost of mosquito netting mesh for a single patient was negligible and estimated at about $2. This price is significantly lower than that in the developed world for a similar-sized piece of mesh produced commercially ($40-$50). By the way, the same surgeons, instead of using commercial nylon suture, resorted to using sterilized nylon fishing line bought locally.

**J. A. Stockman III, MD**

*Reference*

1. Stephenson B, Kingsnorth A. Inguinal hernioplasty using mosquito net mesh in low income countries. *BMJ.* 2011;343:1334-1335.

## The Seasonality of Testicular Torsion

Grushevsky A, Allegra JR, Eskin B, et al (Morristown Memorial Hosp Emergency Dept, NJ)
*Pediatr Emerg Care* 27:1146-1147, 2011

*Objective.*—Previous studies of the seasonality of testicular torsion have yielded conflicting results. Our goal was to examine this issue in a large emergency department (ED) database. We also hypothesized that seasonal patterns would be similar in younger and older patients.

*Methods.*—This was a retrospective cohort of ED visits. This study was performed on 20 New Jersey and New York EDs. The subjects are consecutive patients seen by ED physicians from January 1, 1996, to December 31, 2009. The authors identified visits with testicular torsion using *International Classification of Disease, Ninth Revision* codes. We then determined the number of testicular torsion visits by month, correcting for the total number of days over the study period in each month. We compared the corrected number of visits for the winter (December—February) compared with the summer (June—August) using the Student *t* test, with α set at 0.05. We also calculated these visits for the older and younger half of the patients. Finally, we determined the correlation between mean monthly testicular torsion visits and ambient temperatures.

*Results.*—Of the 8,545,979 visits in the database, 768 (0.009%) had an ED diagnosis of testicular torsion. The median age was 15.5 years (interquartile range, 11.7—20.8 years). We found that testicular torsion visits were 39% (95% confidence interval, 24%—57%) more likely in the winter compared with the summer, and this was similar when the older and younger half of the patients were analyzed separately. The correlation coefficient between mean monthly testicular torsion visits and ambient temperature was $r^2 = 0.54$ ($P = 0.006$).

*Conclusions.*—Testicular torsion visits are more frequent in the winter than in the summer months (Figs 1 and 2).

▶ Anything we can learn about testicular torsion is of value to the clinical practice of pediatrics. This disorder is the third most common cause of malpractice suits in adolescent boys 12 to 17 years of age.[1] Regarding major liabilities for paid claims related to testicular torsion, the most common incorrect diagnosis was epididymitis (72%). Urologists were named most frequently (48%). Atypical presentations of testicular torsion were common (31%). Part of the problem is that torsion of the testicle is a relatively rare condition occurring with an annual incidence of 4.5 in 100 000 males 1 to 25 years of age. Consequently, the incidence of testicular torsion presenting to emergency departments is low in contrast to other complaints in and about the genitalia of adolescents. Thus, there are signs and symptoms that mimic testicular torsion. The literature confirms that it is not possible to consistently and accurately differentiate testicular torsion from epididymo-orchitis and other scrotal pathologic abnormalities by physical examination and history alone. It is an old wives tale that the presence of a cremasteric reflex essentially rules out a testicular torsion, for example.

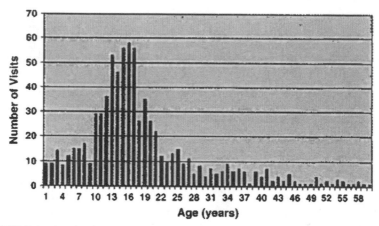

FIGURE 1.—Age distribution of patients with testicular torsion. (Reprinted from Grushevsky A, Allegra JR, Eskin B, et al. The seasonality of testicular torsion. *Pediatr Emerg Care*. 2011;27:1146-1147, with permission from Lippincott Williams & Wilkins.)

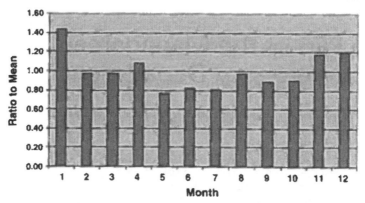

FIGURE 2.—Ratio of mean monthly testicular torsion visit to month (normalized for length of month). (Reprinted from Grushevsky A, Allegra JR, Eskin B, et al. The seasonality of testicular torsion. *Pediatr Emerg Care*. 2011;27:1146-1147, with permission from Lippincott Williams & Wilkins.)

There are also misconceptions about whether a testicle is salvageable if a testicular torsion has been present for more than 6 hours. One cannot be laissez faire about an aggressive approach, even if signs and symptoms of testicular torsion have been present for many hours. Even imaging using color Doppler ultrasound scan is an inconsistently reliable tool for confirming the diagnosis of testicular torsion. The failure of both history and physical examination and color Doppler ultrasound scan to definitively make a diagnosis in a significant percentage of patients was demonstrated in a 2007 multicenter study by Kalfa et al.[2] Thus, it is that one must use every bit of information one has available to make a correct diagnosis of testicular torsion.

The report of Grushevsky et al tells us about the seasonality of the occurrence of testicular torsion and possibly gives information about clues to its etiology.

These investigators looked at the records of patients diagnosed with testicular torsion during the period of January 1996 through December 2009. The patients presented to emergency rooms in New Jersey. Of 8 545 879 emergency room visits looked at, 768 had a diagnosis of testicular torsion. The median age of patients diagnosed was 15.5 years. Some 40% of cases of testicular torsion occurred in the months December through February compared with summer months (June—August). Fig 1 shows the age spectrum of patients with testicular torsion, and Fig 2 shows evidence of seasonality. Similar seasonal effects have been found in other countries in the northern hemisphere.

The data from this report are intriguing and suggest some possible mechanisms that might be etiologic for testicular torsion. It has been postulated that spasm of the cremasteric muscle by reflex activity may result in testicular torsion. Obviously, any guy knows that colder months accentuate this reflex, possibly increasing the likelihood that testicular torsion will develop. The lesson is that if you are evaluating a patient who might have a testicular torsion, if it is winter, the odds will be higher that this problem is the cause of the scrotal findings

This commentary closes with some observations having to do with fertility. While bioethicists continue to agonize over whether women should be compensated for donating oocytes to research, the US market for eggs for assisted reproduction is flourishing. In a recent report it is noted that some donors are offered tens of thousands of dollars and having a high SAT score may be more important than appearance or ethnicity in determining the value of a student's oocytes. Investigators have obtained copies of student newspapers from 366 colleges and universities around the country. They found 111 ads that solicited eggs in 65 different student newspapers, in what is believed to be the first national cross-sample of such ads. It was observed that top fees were offered at the institutions with the highest average SAT scores of incoming students and it was calculated that every increase of 100 SAT points increased the bounty by some $1930. That amount roughly doubled if the advertisements were placed on behalf of a specific couple. One ad, which ran in *The Harvard Crimson, The Daily Princetonian*, and *Yale Daily News*, offered $35 000 to an attractive, athletic donor with an SAT score over 1400.

I have academic appointments at both Duke and the University of North Carolina (UNC). The study that looked at the student newspapers showed 2 ads at Duke for donor eggs. The amounts being offered were $10 000 and $15 000 respectively. At nearby UNC, oocytes were sought for only $2500. One should note that the difference in tuition at Duke versus UNC is approximately 4-fold higher. I offer no comment about any potential difference in the SAT scores of entering students at either university.[3]

**J. A. Stockman III, MD**

*References*

1. Selbst SM, Friedman MJ, Singh SB. Epidemiology and etiology of malpractice lawsuits involving children in US emergency departments and urgent care centers. *Pediatr Emerg Care.* 2005;21:165-169.
2. Kalfa N, Veyrac C, Lopez M, et al. Multicenter assessment of ultrasound of the spermatic cord in children with acute scrotum. *J Urol.* 2007;177:297-301.
3. Holden C. The price of eggs. *Science.* 2010;328:149.

# 9 Heart and Blood Vessels

## Childhood Adiposity, Adult Adiposity, and Cardiovascular Risk Factors

Juonala M, Magnussen CG, Berenson GS, et al (Univ of Turku and Turku Univ Hosp, Finland; Tulane Univ, New Orleans, LA; et al)
*N Engl J Med* 365:1876-1885, 2011

*Background.*—Obesity in childhood is associated with increased cardiovascular risk. It is uncertain whether this risk is attenuated in persons who are overweight or obese as children but not obese as adults.

*Methods.*  We analyzed data from four prospective cohort studies that measured childhood and adult body-mass index (BMI, the weight in kilograms divided by the square of the height in meters). The mean length of follow-up was 23 years. To define high adiposity status, international age-specific and sex-specific BMI cutoff points for overweight and obesity were used for children, and a BMI cutoff point of 30 was used for adults.

*Results.*—Data were available for 6328 subjects. Subjects with consistently high adiposity status from childhood to adulthood, as compared with persons who had a normal BMI as children and were nonobese as adults, had an increased risk of type 2 diabetes (relative risk, 5.4; 95% confidence interval [CI], 3.4 to 8.5), hypertension (relative risk, 2.7; 95% CI, 2.2 to 3.3), elevated low-density lipoprotein cholesterol levels (relative risk, 1.8; 95% CI, 1.4 to 2.3), reduced high-density lipoprotein cholesterol levels (relative risk, 2.1; 95% CI, 1.8 to 2.5), elevated triglyceride levels (relative risk, 3.0; 95% CI, 2.4 to 3.8), and carotid-artery atherosclerosis (increased intima–media thickness of the carotid artery) (relative risk, 1.7; 95% CI, 1.4 to 2.2) ($P \leq 0.002$ for all comparisons). Persons who were overweight or obese during childhood but were nonobese as adults had risks of the outcomes that were similar to those of persons who had a normal BMI consistently from childhood to adulthood ($P > 0.20$ for all comparisons).

*Conclusions.*—Overweight or obese children who were obese as adults had increased risks of type 2 diabetes, hypertension, dyslipidemia, and carotid-artery atherosclerosis. The risks of these outcomes among overweight or obese children who became nonobese by adulthood were similar to those among persons who were never obese. (Funded by the Academy of Finland and others.)

▶ The report by Juonala et al provides information from long-term studies of individuals over many decades. The report adds considerably to our understandings about the relationship of cardiovascular disease and obesity, suggesting that cardiovascular risk in adulthood is reduced if obesity is treated or prevented in childhood. In this study of 6328 subjects, those with persistently high adiposity from childhood into adulthood had a significantly increased risk of diabetes, hypertension, lipid abnormalities, and carotid-artery atherosclerosis. Fortunately, the study also showed that the risks of these outcomes among overweight or obese children who became nonobese adults did not differ significantly from the risk among those who were never obese. This finding that childhood obesity does not permanently increase cardiovascular risk appears valid.

This report has to be understood in light of prior studies. For example, Bibbins-Domingo et al,[1] using information on the prevalence of obese adolescents in the 2000 National Health and Nutrition Examination Surveys (NHANES), were able to estimate the likely prevalence of obesity among 35-year-olds in 2020. Using this estimate in a computer simulation model of coronary heart disease, these investigators were able to predict the likely annual excess incidence and prevalence of coronary heart disease that resulted from obesity from 2020 through 2035. It was predicted that by 2035, the prevalence of coronary heart disease in adults would increase by 5% to 16% and that more than 100 000 excess cases of coronary heart disease would be directly linked to childhood obesity.

To gain a better understanding of the findings from the Juonala et al report, see the excellent editorial by Rocchini.[2] Childhood obesity is still a great predictor of adult obesity, and once in place, obesity is difficult to treat. Nonetheless, some children in adolescence with a high body mass index do become nonobese adults, and this change is associated with a reduction in cardiovascular risk.

This commentary closes on the topic of atherosclerosis. Bet you were not aware that evidence now exists that heart disease plagued ancient Egyptians as well as modern members of our society. Full body CT scans of 22 mummies dating from 2000 to 3500 years ago turned up 16 with hearts or arteries preserved well enough to study. Of those, 9 had clear evidence of blockage from atherosclerosis. These findings appeared to be most prevalent in those mummies who were thought to have lived past 45 years of age. The most ancient mummy to have suffered from heart disease, Lady Rai, died in her 30s, around 1530 BC. She was nursemaid to Queen Amrose Nefertari. These findings are interesting because it is believed that none of the mummies were likely to have been overweight in life so their atherosclerosis was probably a combination of bad diet and little exercise.[3]

**J. A. Stockman III, MD**

*References*

1. Bibbins-Domingo K, Coxson P, Pletcher MJ, Lightwood J, Goldman L. Adolescent overweight and future adult coronary heart disease. *N Engl J Med.* 2007;357:2371-2379.
2. Rocchini AP. Childhood obesity and coronary heart disease. *N Engl J Med.* 2011;365:1927-1929.

3. Beil L. Heart disease plagued ancient Egyptians: CTs of mummies reveal evidence of clogged arteries. *Science News.* December 19, 2009:14.

**Television Viewing and Risk of Type 2 Diabetes, Cardiovascular Disease, and All-Cause Mortality: A Meta-Analysis**

Grøntved A, Hu FB (Univ of Southern Denmark, Odense; Harvard Med School and Brigham and Women's Hosp, Boston, MA)

*JAMA* 305:2448-2455, 2011

*Context.*—Prolonged television (TV) viewing is the most prevalent and pervasive sedentary behavior in industrialized countries and has been associated with morbidity and mortality. However, a systematic and quantitative assessment of published studies is not available.

*Objective.*—To perform a meta-analysis of all prospective cohort studies to determine the association between TV viewing and risk of type 2 diabetes, fatal or nonfatal cardiovascular disease, and all-cause mortality.

*Data Sources and Study Selection.*—Relevant studies were identified by searches of the MEDLINE database from 1970 to March 2011 and the EMBASE database from 1974 to March 2011 without restrictions and by reviewing reference lists from retrieved articles. Cohort studies that reported relative risk estimates with 95% confidence intervals (CIs) for the associations of interest were included.

*Data Extraction.*—Data were extracted independently by each author and summary estimates of association were obtained using a random-effects model.

*Data Synthesis.*—Of the 8 studies included, 4 reported results on type 2 diabetes (175 938 individuals; 6428 incident cases during 1.1 million person-years of follow-up), 4 reported on fatal or nonfatal cardiovascular disease (34 253 individuals; 1052 incident cases), and 3 reported on all-cause mortality (26 509 individuals; 1879 deaths during 202 353 person-years of follow up). The pooled relative risks per 2 hours of TV viewing per day were 1.20 (95% CI, 1.14-1.27) for type 2 diabetes, 1.15 (95% CI, 1.06-1.23) for fatal or nonfatal cardiovascular disease, and 1.13 (95% CI, 1.07-1.18) for all-cause mortality. While the associations between time spent viewing TV and risk of type 2 diabetes and cardiovascular disease were linear, the risk of all-cause mortality appeared to increase with TV viewing duration of greater than 3 hours per day. The estimated absolute risk differences per every 2 hours of TV viewing per day were 176 cases of type 2 diabetes per 100 000 individuals per year, 38 cases of fatal cardiovascular disease per 100 000 individuals per year, and 104 deaths for all-cause mortality per 100 000 individuals per year.

*Conclusion.*—Prolonged TV viewing was associated with increased risk of type 2 diabetes, cardiovascular disease, and all-cause mortality.

▶ Although this report deals largely with adults and their viewing habits in relationship to the risks of developing type 2 diabetes, other cardiovascular disorders and all-cause mortality, you can bet that the information is also critically important for pediatricians. If adults in the family are watching a lot of television, you can be guaranteed their offspring will be as well.

The data from this report remind us that the problem of excessive TV viewing is not unique to the United States. On average, 40% of daily free time is occupied by TV viewing in several European countries and 50% in Australia.[1,2] This corresponds to a TV viewing time of anywhere from 3.5 to 4 hours. The data from the United States suggest that the average daily hours of TV viewings is 5 hours.[3] The rub with such extensive TV viewing is not merely the fact that one is not expending a lot of energy. TV viewing is associated with other poor habits, such as munching on fried foods, processed meats, drinking sweetened beverages, and lower intakes of fruit, vegetables, and whole grains. This is true of both adults and children. Sedentary habits and poor quality of eating are known to be associated with type 2 diabetes, excess cardiovascular disease risk factors, and all-cause mortality.

Grøntved et al performed a meta-analysis of all prospective cohort studies to examine the association between TV viewing and the risk of type 2 diabetes, cardiovascular disease, and all-cause mortality. The results of this study yielded 8 solid cohort investigations that observed the habits of several million individuals. These studies documented a straight line association between time viewing television and the prevalence of type 2 diabetes. All-cause mortality began to increase when TV viewing became greater than 3 hours per day. The authors observed relative risks of 1.20 for type 2 diabetes, 1.15 for cardiovascular disease, and 1.13 for all-cause mortality for every 2-hour increase in TV viewing per day. Given the incidence rates in the United States, it is estimated that the absolute risk difference (cases per 100 000 individuals per year) per 2 hours of TV viewing per day was 176 for type 2 diabetes, 38 for fatal cardiovascular disease, and 104 deaths for all-cause mortality.

Although the authors of this report cannot exclude the possibility of residual confounding and bias due to misclassification in these cohort studies, they did their very best to control for various known factors that might have affected the data outcome. Their conclusions, therefore, appear to be solid. It is biologically plausible that prolonged TV viewing is associated with type 2 diabetes, cardiovascular disease, and all-cause mortality. Several randomized controlled trials have shown beneficial effects of reducing TV viewing time. One randomized school-based study of 9-year-old children found that reducing TV viewing time and video game playing slowed increases in body mass index (BMI) and decreased the number of meals eaten in front of the TV but was not associated with a change in self-reported physical activity.[4] Another study of 70 children with BMIs above the 75th percentile showed that reducing TV viewing and computer time by 50% over 2 years resulted in a significant reduction of BMI and energy intake but did not increase subjectively measured physical activity.[5]

Although some of us are not allowed to ask about gun ownership in a house, there is nothing that precludes us from asking how many TVs there are in the home or how many hours a day a child in our practice watches these TVs. The data from this report are extraordinarily powerful in discussing the overall topic with parents. It is noted that there is one other risk factor for cardiovascular disease that has been recently reported: loneliness. Very lonely women are more prone to heart disease, but lonely men appear to not be, according to a study in *Psychosomatic Medicine*. This single risk factor persisted in women after controlling for a multitude of other known factors such as smoking, hypertension, marital status, diabetes, high cholesterol, physical activity, education, and age. The authors conclude that loneliness is worthy of further clinical attention.[6]

This commentary closes with an observation having to do with cardiovascular fitness. A number of times a month I cross a busy intersection in front of Duke University Hospital. One readily notices that the timing of the lights is such that pedestrians have only a minimal time to cross the intersection and then if only moving at a good clip. I have seen disabled individuals struggle with that timing, which raises the question, do lights at pedestrian crossings give the disabled and older individuals enough time to cross safely? Actually this question has been addressed in the literature. After measuring the walking speed of patients attending a geriatric assessment center, investigators calculated that with current timings at most intersections, many 80-year-olds are unable to make it across a road more than 22 meters wide. Although matching crossing times to the walking speeds of older people may seem unrealistic, in the European Union, nearly 40% of pedestrians killed are age 65 and older, a percentage far in excess of the proportionate age population.[7]

**J. A. Stockman III, MD**

*References*

1. Office for Official Publications of the European Communities. Time use at different stages of life: Results from 13 European countries. July 2003. http://epp.eurostat.ec.europa.eu/cache/ITY_OFFPUB/KS-CC-03-001/EN/KS-CC-03-001-EN.pdf. Accessed May 16, 2011.
2. Australian Bureau of Health Statistics. *How Australians use their time*. Canberra: Commonwealth of Australia; 2008.
3. Nielson CO. TV usage trends: Q3 and Q4 2010. http://www.nielsen.com/content/dam/corporate/us/en/reports-dowloads/2011-Reports/State%20of%20the%20Media%20TV%20Q3%20Q4%202010.pdf. Accessed May 16, 2011.
4. Robinson TN. Reducing children's television viewing to prevent obesity: a randomized controlled trial. *JAMA*. 1999;282:1561-1567.
5. Epstein LH, Roemmich JN, Robinson JL, et al. A randomized trial of the effects of reducing television viewing and computer use on body mass index in young children. *Arch Pediatr Adolesc Med*. 2008;162:239-245.
6. Thurston RC, Kubzansky LD. Women, loneliness, and incident coronary heart disease. *Psychosom Med*. 2009;71:836-842. http://dx.doi.org/10.1097/psy.0b013e3181b40efc.
7. Romero-Ortuno R, Cogan L, Cunningham CU, Kenny RA. Do older pedestrians have enough time to cross roads in Dublin? A critique of the Traffic Management Guidelines based on clinical research findings. *Age Ageing*. 2010;39:80-86.

### Fasting Might Not Be Necessary Before Lipid Screening: A Nationally Representative Cross-sectional Study

Steiner MJ, Skinner AC, Perrin EM (Univ of North Carolina, Chapel Hill)
*Pediatrics* 128:463-470, 2011

*Background.*—There are barriers to fasting lipid screening for at-risk children. Results of studies in adults have suggested that lipid testing might be reliably performed without fasting.

*Objective.*—To examine population-level differences in pediatric lipid values based on length of fast before testing.

*Methods.*—We used the National Health and Nutrition Examination Survey (1999–2008) to examine total cholesterol (TC), HDL (high-density lipoprotein), LDL (low-density lipoprotein), and triglyceride cholesterol components on the basis of the period of fasting. Young children fasted for varying times before being tested, and children older than 12 years were asked to fast; however, adherence was variable. We used ordinary least-squares regression to test for differences in lipid values that were based on fasting times, controlling for weight status, age, race, ethnicity, and gender.

*Results.*—TC, HDL, LDL, or triglyceride values were available for 12 744 children. Forty-eight percent of the TC and HDL samples and 80% of the LDL and triglyceride samples were collected from children who had fasted $\geq 8$ hours. Fasting had a small positive effect for TC, HDL, and LDL, resulting in a mean value for the sample that was 2 to 5 mg/dL higher with a 12-hour fast compared with a no-fast sample. Fasting time had a negative effect on triglycerides ($\beta = -0.859; P = .02$), which resulted in values in the fasting group that were 7 mg/dL lower.

*Discussion.*—Comparison of cholesterol screening results for a nonfasting group of children compared with results for a similar fasting group resulted in small differences that are likely not clinically important. Physicians might be able to decrease the burden of childhood cholesterol screening by not requiring prescreening fasting for these components (Figs 1 and 2).

▶ This report should be of as much interest to the health of the reader as it is to the care of children. Currently, the American Academy of Pediatrics and the American Heart Association have recommended that if one is to screen children for lipid disorders, it should be done in a fasting state. Needless to say, screening of children for lipid disorders presents rather unique challenges. It is pretty rare to be able to get a child to fast before a routine physician office visit. Most fasting lipid panels therefore either are planned for very early morning visits or are checked at subsequent office visits or additional visits to outpatient phlebotomy centers in the early morning. These arrangements may require parents to miss work and children to miss school to arrive for an early morning test. These children also wind up having to eat before heading off for school. Fasting of 8 to 12 hours has been recommended before lipid screening because of theoretical dynamic changes that might occur in test results for some lipid components with a postprandial test. The worry has been about triglycerides in particular. In many laboratories, the

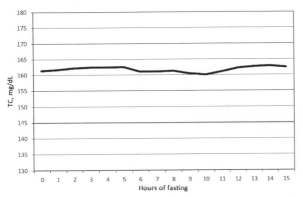

FIGURE 1.—Predicted values of TC based on hours of fasting before testing. (Reproduced with permission from Pediatrics, Steiner MJ, Skinner AC, Perrin EM. Fasting might not be necessary before lipid screening: a nationally representative cross-sectional study. *Pediatrics.* 2011;128:463-470. Copyright © 2011 by the American Academy of Pediatrics.)

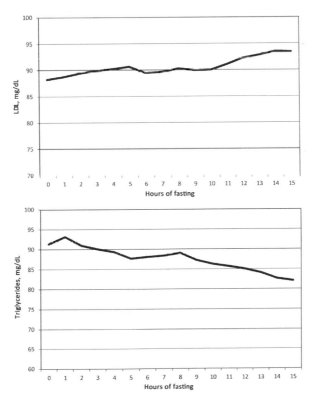

FIGURE 2.—Predicted values of LDL cholesterol and triglycerides based on hours of fasting before testing. (Reproduced with permission from Pediatrics, Steiner MJ, Skinner AC, Perrin EM. Fasting might not be necessary before lipid screening: a nationally representative cross-sectional study. *Pediatrics.* 2011;128:463-470. Copyright © 2011 by the American Academy of Pediatrics.)

low-density lipoprotein (LDL) level is merely estimated from a formula based on determination of total cholesterol minus high-density cholesterol minus triglyceride levels divided by 5. Thus LDL levels would be affected if the triglyceride level is artifactually high after eating.

Recent research in adults has raised questions regarding the importance of fasting before lipid measurements. Researchers have suggested that for the majority of people who take in an average-sized meal, the overall lipid profile will have minimal change after eating. Interestingly, some research in adult patients has also suggested that abnormal postprandial triglyceride levels might actually be more highly associated with cardiovascular disease than abnormal fasting levels.

The authors of this report sought to determine the effect of fasting on complete lipid panels in children because of the added burden of fasting before screening and the emerging research data that call into question the value of fasting before lipid assessment of cardiovascular risk in adults. They used data from the National Health and Nutrition Survey to undertake their study. They included children aged 3 to 17 years who had at least 1 of the 4 common lipid measurements available in the Survey. Fig 1 shows little or no variation in total cholesterol levels based on hours of fasting before testing. Fig 2 shows predictive values of LDL cholesterol and triglycerides based on hours of fasting before testing. In the aggregate, fasting had a very small positive effect for total cholesterol, high-density lipoprotein, and LDL, resulting in a mean value for the sample that was slightly higher with a 12-hour fast compared with a no-fast sample. Fasting time had a negative effect on triglycerides, which resulted in values in the fasting group that were approximately 7 mg/dL lower. None of these differences are likely to be of any clinical importance.

The conclusion of this report is in some ways quite reassuring in that, at least in this instance, children are little adults. Both adults and children can, in most cases, have their lipid profile assessed with some degree of accuracy either in the fasting or nonfasting state. Not having to fast will decrease the burden of childhood cholesterol screening.

This commentary ends with a tidbit about myocardial infarctions. For some time it has been thought that there was a significantly higher rate of myocardial infarctions during the winter months. A German analysis of data collected over 10 years has shown a bit of a peak as a result of the "cold effect" on incidence of myocardial infarction making a heart attack more likely during winter months, but at the same time a relationship was documented between high temperatures and myocardial infarct occurrence seen during the summer. The effect was most pronounced in years with the highest variations in average temperatures.[1] To paraphrase the words of the songstress Carole King, "winter, spring, summer, fall, all you've got to do is call and I'll be there"—with an MI, that is.

**J. A. Stockman III, MD**

*Reference*

1. Guigliano RP, Braunwald E. The year in non-ST-segment elevation acute coronary syndrome. *Circulation.* 2009;120:735-742.

### Effect of Supplementation With High-Selenium Yeast on Plasma Lipids: A Randomized Trial

Rayman MP, Stranges S, Griffin BA, et al (Univ of Surrey, Guildford, UK; Univ of Warwick Med School, Coventry, UK; Carlos III Inst of Health, Madrid, Spain; et al)

*Ann Intern Med* 154:656-665, 2011

*Background.*—High selenium status has been linked to elevated blood cholesterol levels in cross-sectional studies.

*Objective.*—To investigate the effect of selenium supplementation on plasma lipids.

*Design.*—Randomized, placebo-controlled, parallel-group study stratified by age and sex. Participants, research nurses, and persons assessing outcomes were blinded to treatment assignment. (International Standard Randomised Controlled Trial Number Register registration number: ISRCTN25193534).

*Setting.*—4 general practices in the United Kingdom.

*Participants.*—501 volunteers aged 60 to 74 years.

*Intervention.*—Participants received selenium, 100 mcg/d ($n = 127$), 200 mcg/d ($n = 127$), or 300 mcg/d ($n = 126$), as high-selenium yeast or a yeast-based placebo ($n = 121$) for 6 months.

*Measurements.*—Total and high-density lipoprotein (HDL) cholesterol concentrations were measured in nonfasting plasma samples stored from participants in the UK PRECISE (United Kingdom PREvention of Cancer by Intervention with SElenium) Pilot Study at baseline ($n = 454$) and at 6 months ($n = 394$). Non-HDL cholesterol levels were calculated.

*Results.*—Mean plasma selenium concentration was 88.8 ng/g (SD, 19.2) at baseline and increased statistically significantly in the treatment groups. The adjusted difference in change in total cholesterol levels for selenium compared with placebo was −0.22 mmol/L (−8.5 mg/dL) (95% CI, −0.42 to −0.03 mmol/L [−16.2 to −1.2 mg/dL]; $P = 0.02$) for 100 mcg of selenium per day, −0.25 mmol/L (−9.7 mg/dL) (CI, −0.44 to −0.07 mmol/L [−17.0 to −2.7 mg/dL]; $P = 0.008$) for 200 mcg of selenium per day, and −0.07 mmol/L (−2.7 mg/dL) (CI, −0.26 to 0.12 mmol/L [−10.1 to 4.6 mg/dL]; $P = 0.46$) for 300 mcg of selenium per day. Similar reductions were observed for non-HDL cholesterol levels. There was no apparent difference in change in HDL cholesterol levels with 100 and 200 mcg of selenium per day, but the difference was an adjusted 0.06 mmol/L (2.3 mg/dL) (CI, 0.00 to 0.11 mmol/L [0.0 to 4.3 mg/dL]; $P = 0.045$) with 300 mcg of selenium per day. The total-HDL cholesterol ratio decreased progressively with increasing selenium dose (overall $P = 0.01$).

*Limitation.*—The duration of supplementation was limited, as was the age range of the participants.

*Conclusion.*—Selenium supplementation seemed to have modestly beneficial effects on plasma lipid levels in this sample of persons with relatively low selenium status. The clinical significance of the findings is unclear and should not be used to justify the use of selenium supplementation as additional or alternative therapy for dyslipidemia. This is particularly true for persons with higher selenium status, given the limitations of the trial and the potential additional risk in other metabolic dimensions.

▶ The relationship between low serum selenium levels and high plasma lipid levels has been bantered about for quite some time. Since 1982 when Salonen et al showed a significant 2- to 3-fold increase in cardiovascular morbidity and mortality for people with low serum selenium concentrations, there has been interest in the link between selenium status and cardiovascular disease.[1] Many in society have been taking selenium supplements since that time, and some parents are giving supplements to their offspring. In theory, potential cardiovascular benefits are supported by the ability of selenoproteins, such as glutathione peroxidase and selenoprotein S, to combat the oxidative modification of lipids, inhibit platelet aggregation, and reduce inflammation.

Despite what seems like a solid biological rationale for a beneficial effect of selenium on cardiovascular health, evidence that selenium status in any way alters one's lipid profile or confers some benefit on risk of coronary artery disease has been equivocal, at least in the literature. Rayman et al decided to investigate the effect of selenium supplementation on plasma lipid levels, performing a randomized, placebo-controlled, parallel-grouped study stratified by age and sex. This study was performed in the United Kingdom and included adult study subjects, although the information garnered for this report would seem to apply equally to a younger age group as well. Study participants received selenium, 100 mcg/day, 200 mcg/day, or 300 mcg/day as high-selenium yeast or a yeast-based placebo for a period of 6 months. With selenium supplementation, depending on the levels of selenium given, there were improvements in total cholesterol levels ranging from 2.7 mg/dL to 8.5 mg/dL. There were no apparent differences in HDL cholesterol levels on 100 mcg and 200 mcg of selenium per day and slight improvement on 300 mcg of selenium per day. This study shows that selenium supplementation in the form of yeast does have a modest beneficial effect on plasma lipid levels in a group of subjects who began with relatively low selenium status. The clinical findings of this report are unclear, however, and the data should not be used to justify the widespread use of selenium supplementation as an additional or alternative therapy for dyslipidemia. This statement is true simply because there are perfectly adequate alternative ways of managing lipid levels in the vast majority of patients and because there is some potential risk with the use of very high-dose selenium.

This report was included in the pediatric literature to keep our reading audience aware of what is going on in the world of lipid disorder management. Selenium supplementation does not appear to be the way to go in adults and is certainly not the way to go in children.

This commentary closes with a query. Does laughter influence arterial stiffness? Recently a randomized, single-blind, crossover study assessed 18 healthy individuals on three separate occasions: watching a 30-minute segment of a film to induce laughter, watching a 30-minute segment of a film to induce stress; and observing during a 30-minute period when no film was screened. Researchers found that laughter decreased pulse wave velocity—an index of arterial stiffness—whereas stress actually increased pulse wave velocity.[2] Laughter, by the way, also reduced cortisol levels and increased total oxidative status. If there is a lesson in all this, it is to go out and have the time of our lives if one wants to stay healthy.

**J. A. Stockman III, MD**

*References*

1. Salonen JT, Alfthan G, Huttunen JK, Pikkarainen J, Puska P. Association between cardiovascular death and myocardial infarction and serum selenium in a matched-pair longitudinal study. *Lancet.* 1982;2:175-179.
2. Vlachopoulos C, Xaplanteris P, Alexopoulos N, et al. Divergent effects of laughter and mental stress on arterial stiffness and central hemodynamics. *Psychosom Med.* 2009;71:446-453.

## Minimum amount of physical activity for reduced mortality and extended life expectancy: a prospective cohort study

Wen CP, Wai JPM, Tsai MK, et al (Natl Health Res Insts, Zhunan, Taiwan; Natl Taiwan Sport Univ, Taoyuan; et al)

*Lancet* 378:1244-1253, 2011

*Background.*—The health benefits of leisure-time physical activity are well known, but whether less exercise than the recommended 150 min a week can have life expectancy benefits is unclear. We assessed the health benefits of a range of volumes of physical activity in a Taiwanese population.

*Methods.*—In this prospective cohort study, 416 175 individuals (199 265 men and 216 910 women) participated in a standard medical screening programme in Taiwan between 1996 and 2008, with an average follow-up of 8·05 years (SD 4·21). On the basis of the amount of weekly exercise indicated in a self-administered questionnaire, participants were placed into one of five categories of exercise volumes: inactive, or low, medium, high, or very high activity. We calculated hazard ratios (HR) for mortality risks for every group compared with the inactive group, and calculated life expectancy for every group.

*Findings.*—Compared with individuals in the inactive group, those in the low-volume activity group, who exercised for an average of 92 min per week (95% CI 71—112) or 15 min a day (SD 1·8), had a 14% reduced risk of all-cause mortality (0·86, 0·81—0·91), and had a 3 year longer life expectancy. Every additional 15 min of daily exercise beyond the minimum amount of 15 min a day further reduced all-cause mortality by 4% (95% CI 2·5—7·0) and all-cancer mortality by 1% (0·3—4·5). These benefits were applicable to all age groups and both sexes, and to those with cardiovascular disease risks. Individuals who were inactive had a 17% (HR 1·17, 95% CI 1·10—1·24) increased risk of mortality compared with individuals in the low-volume group.

*Interpretation.*—15 min a day or 90 min a week of moderate-intensity exercise might be of benefit, even for individuals at risk of cardiovascular disease.

▶ While diehard exercisers may poo-poo the thought that someone should look for the minimum amount of exercise that makes a true cardiovascular difference, some of us would call the search for the latter a search for efficiency. Most of the literature on exercise suggests that 150 minutes or more a week of leisure time physical activity has substantial health benefits. Guidelines from the 2008 Physical Activity Guidelines for Americans and the World Health Organization's 2010 Global Recommendations on Physical Activity for Health have drawn attention to the health benefits of a moderate amount of weekly exercise.[1,2] Because barriers exist to this 30-minutes-a-day, 5-days-a-week recommendation, the actual amount of physical activity minimally needed to produce health benefits has remained largely unstudied.

Wen et al sought to look at whether there is a lesser amount of exercise that would be easier to achieve that does reduce mortality. The suggestion is that patients might be more readily motivated to exercise if health care providers could recommend a more manageable amount of exercise with a simple health message. In a prospective cohort study that involved almost half a million individuals, these investigators showed that those participating in a low volume level of activity (as opposed to none) who exercised for an average of 92 minutes per week, or just 15 minutes a day, had a 14% reduced risk of all-cause mortality and a 3-year longer life expectancy. More exercise did help. For every additional 15 minutes of daily exercise, one saw a further reduction of all-cause mortality by 4%. It should be noted that all cancer mortality was also reduced by 1% for each 15-minute increment upward in exercise.

The bottom line with this report is that there is hope for all of us, even the most sedentary of couch potatoes who might just get up and move around a bit for a quarter of an hour a day. We should be grateful to Wen et al for showing us how we can wen our way to better health with just a dribble of physical activity. Less may not be more, but less can still be healthful and maybe enough to make a difference.

This commentary closes with an observation. Readers know that I abhor exercise as much as I do asparagus and cats. We are indeed born with a fixed number of heartbeats that should not be wasted on exercise. For similar believers who may be subject to criticism for not exercising, a product that has been on the market for a bit of time may do the trick. It is called Rom, the ad for which periodically appears in Scientific American. The 4800 Rom machine is made in an 82 000 square foot factory in North Hollywood, California, and is said to be able to produce a complete body workout in just 4 minutes, a workout equivalent to the more traditional 30- to 60-minute workout. The rub is the equipment costs $14 615, but you can try it out for 30 days on rental for just $2500 (rental applies to purchase price). The ads for the equipment say that Tom Cruise and Tony Robbins have both purchased one and see what it has done for them. Tom is capable of leaping onto couches in a single bound. You may view this equipment at www.fastworkout.com.

Before doing so, you should first look up the rationalization for how $14 615 is actually a cheap price to pay. This rationalization may be found at www. pleasedothemath.com.

**J. A. Stockman III, MD**

*References*

1. Physical Activity Guidelines Advisory Committee. Physical Activity Guidelines Advisory Committee Report and 2008 Physical Activity Guidelines for Americans. http://www.health.gov/paguidelines/committeereport.aspx. http://www.health.gov/paguidelines/pdf/paguide.pdf. Accessed November 27, 2011.
2. World Health Organization. Global Recommendations on Physical Activity for Health. http://www.who.int/dietphysical/activity/factsheet_recommendations/en/index.html. Accessed November 27, 2011.

---

## Management of Pediatric Chest Pain Using a Standardized Assessment and Management Plan

Friedman KG, Kane DA, Rathod RH, et al (Children's Hosp Boston, MA)
*Pediatrics* 128:239-245, 2011

---

*Objectives.*—Chest pain is a common reason for referral to pediatric cardiologists and often leads to an extensive cardiac evaluation. The objective of this study is to describe current management practices in the assessment of pediatric chest pain and to determine whether a standardized care approach could reduce unnecessary testing.

*Patients and Methods.*—We reviewed all patients, aged 7 to 21 years, presenting to our outpatient pediatric cardiology division in 2009 for evaluation of chest pain. Demographics, clinical characteristics, patient outcomes, and resource use were analyzed.

*Results.*—Testing included electrocardiography (ECG) in all 406 patients, echocardiography in 175 (43%), exercise stress testing in 114 (28%), event monitoring in 40 (10%), and Holter monitoring in 30 (7%). A total of 44 (11%) patients had a clinically significant medical or family history, an abnormal cardiac examination, and/or an abnormal ECG. Exertional chest pain was present in 150 (37%) patients. In the entire cohort, a cardiac etiology for chest pain was found in only 5 of 406 (1.2%) patients. Two patients had pericarditis, and 3 had arrhythmias. We developed an algorithm using pertinent history, physical examination, and ECG findings to suggest when additional testing is indicated. Applying the algorithm to this cohort could lead to an ~20% reduction in echocardiogram and outpatient rhythm monitor use and elimination of exercise stress testing while still capturing all cardiac diagnoses.

*Conclusions.*—Evaluation of pediatric chest pain is often extensive and rarely yields a cardiac etiology. Practice variation and unnecessary resource use remain concerns. Targeted testing can reduce resource use and lead to more cost-effective care.

▶ There is not a single person in clinical practice who has not been confronted with the dilemma about how far to go in evaluating a youngster complaining of chest pain. The latter is one of the most common presenting complaints to pediatricians, pediatric cardiologists, and pediatric emergency departments. Most such cases will turn out to have either no etiology or a noncardiac etiology. Despite the low prevalence of serious cardiac pathology in children, the undertaking of extensive and costly referral and cardiac evaluation is all too common. There are relatively few studies that have evaluated practice variation in the diagnosis of pediatric chest pain. At Children's Hospital Boston, a standardized approach to pediatric chest pain currently is being implemented as part of a broader quality improvement initiative that has been named Standardized Clinical Assessment and Management Plans (SCAMP). The goal of the SCAMP initiative, including the chest pain SCAMP, is to decrease practice variation, improve patient care, and reduce unnecessary resource use.

Friedman et al describe a study that is designed to tell us about current practice trends in the evaluation of chest pain by pediatric cardiologists, evaluating whether a mechanism to standardize care actually leads to a reduction in unnecessary resource use while still capturing all important cardiac etiologies of chest pain. The investigators reviewed the records of all patients, age 7 years to 21 years, presenting to the outpatient division of pediatric cardiology at Children's Hospital Boston in 2009 for initial evaluation of chest pain. Past medical history, family history, and presenting symptoms, including chest-pain characteristics and associated symptoms, were collected. All patients had an electrocardiogram (ECG) performed at all clinic visits. Other studies were performed based on history and clinical findings using an algorithm that uses history, physical examination, and ECG as the starting point (Fig 1 in the original article). During the 1-year period, 417 patients were evaluated using this algorithm. A cardiac etiology for chest pain was found in just 5 of 406 patients (1%). Two of 5 patients had pericarditis. Both of these patients presented with friction rub on examination, positional chest pain, ST-segment, and T-wave changes consistent with pericardial disease and echocardiograms showing small pericardial effusions. Two patients had supraventricular tachycardia, and 1 patient had short runs of nonsustained ventricular tachycardia, which were identified using outpatient rhythm monitors. All 3 of these patients with arrhythmias presented with palpitations as a significant complaint in addition to chest pain. The remaining 401 cases (99%) were thought to be noncardiac chest pain, most commonly nonspecific musculoskeletal pain or costochondritis, or were respiratory/asthma related. Several patients had cardiac diagnoses discovered during their chest pain evaluation that were completely unrelated to the presenting complaint of chest pain. Incidental diagnoses included Wolff-Parkinson-White syndrome, mild subaortic stenosis, small atrial septal defect, small muscular ventricular septal defect, mitral valve prolapse and dilated aortic root (one each of the aforementioned), and a small coronary artery to pulmonary artery fistula ($n = 3$).

For the patients evaluated, the total estimated charges for the chest pain evaluations ran $1 166 465. Clinic visits alone accounted for one-third of all charges and cardiac testing for about 70% of the total patient care charges. The echocardiograms obtained accounted for about half of the laboratory testing. No cardiac testing other than ECGs was performed in 172 patients (43%), all of whom were felt to have noncardiac chest pain. Despite having no adjunctive testing, the subgroup still accounted for nearly $150 000 in charges.

Overall, the cardiologists at Children's Hospital Boston suggest that implementation of a pediatric chest pain SCAMP could lead to an approximate 21% reduction in charges. Reducing the number of unnecessary echocardiograms, exercise stress tests, and outpatient rhythm monitors are the main source of projected savings. The authors indicate that the serious causes of cardiac chest pain, including anomalous coronary origins, cardiomyopathy, pulmonary hypertension, myocarditis, and pericarditis, are readily diagnosed by suggestive history, cardiac examination, ECG, and selective use of echocardiography. Thus, echocardiography is the diagnostic test of choice for patients with concerning past medical or family histories or abnormal ECG or physical examination findings in this study. The authors also propose eliminating exercise stress tests in the routine evaluation of pediatric chest pain. These studies add little to the evaluation of pediatric chest pain, unlike in adults. Studies have suggested that a normal exercise stress test in no way rules out an anomalous coronary artery. Additional findings from this report include the fact that Holter and Event monitors are unlikely to be helpful in the evaluation of chest pain in the absence of palpitations or syncope.

We should be grateful to the cardiologists at Children's Hospital Boston for sharing with us the information from this very important report. All too often, pediatricians are caught in the dilemma of trying to figure out how far to go in the evaluation of such children. A detailed history, including a family history, a careful physical examination, and an ECG can go a long way in deciding whether anything further needs to be done as part of the evaluation. Whether the first parts of the algorithm described (Fig 1 in the original article) require a cardiology consultation clearly depends on the confidence and skill set of the primary care provider.

This commentary closes with an observation and question having to do with exercise. Just what is the risk of cardiac arrest associated with running a marathon or half-marathon? The answer to the question comes from a report that recently appeared in the New England Journal of Medicine.[1] Investigators assessed the incidence and outcomes of cardiac arrest associated with marathon and half-marathon races in the United States from January 1, 2000 to May 31, 2010. Of 10.9 million runners, 59 experienced a cardiac arrest. The average age of cardiac arrest was 42 years. 51 of the 59 were men. Cardiovascular disease accounted for the majority of cardiac arrests. There were a few cases of severe dehydration and hyperthermia. The incidence rate was significantly higher during marathons in comparison to half-marathons. Unfortunately, of the 59 cases of cardiac arrest, 71% were fatal. Among the 31 cases with complete clinical data, initiation of bystander-administered cardiopulmonary resuscitation and an underlying diagnosis other than hypertrophic cardiomyopathy were strong predictors of survival. Thus it is that marathons and half-marathons are associated with a risk of cardiovascular arrest and sudden death but this risk appears to be low. For some reason, the incidence rate in the young adult male experiencing cardiac arrest while running has increased during the past 10 years. The specific incidence rates of cardiac arrest and sudden death during long-distance running, such as in a marathon, is one event per 184 001 and 259 000, respectively. These estimates translate to 0.2 cardiac arrests and 0.14 sudden deaths per 100 000 runner-hours at risk, using average running times of 4 and 2 hours for marathon and half-marathon, respectively. Even more interesting is that the overall death rates among marathon and half-marathon runners are relatively low, as compared with other athletic populations, including collegiate athletes (1 death per 43 770 per year), triathlon participants (1 death per 52 630 participants), and previously healthy middle-aged joggers (1 death per 7620 participants). These data suggest that the risk associated with long-distance-running events is equivalent to or lower than the risk associated with other vigorous physical activity. Thus it is that the first person to run from Athens to Marathon, who started all this stuff, had a very good chance of arriving at this destination alive.

**J. A. Stockman III, MD**

*Reference*

1. Kim JH, Malhotra R, Chiampas G, et al. Cardiac arrest during long-distance running races. *N Eng J Med.* 2012;366:130-140.

---

**Is Pocket Mobile Echocardiography the Next-Generation Stethoscope? A Cross-Sectional Comparison of Rapidly Acquired Images With Standard Transthoracic Echocardiography**

Liebo MJ, Israel RL, Lillie EO, et al (Scripps Clinic, La Jolla, CA; Scripps Translational Science Inst, La Jolla, CA; West Wireless Health Inst, La Jolla, CA)
*Ann Intern Med* 155:33-38, 2011

---

*Background.*—A pocket mobile echocardiography (PME) device is commercially available for clinical use, but public data documenting its accuracy compared with standard transthoracic echocardiography (TTE) are not available.

*Objective.*—To compare the accuracy of rapidly acquired PME images with those acquired by standard TTE.

*Design.*—Cross-sectional study. At the time of referral for TTE, ultrasonographers acquired PME images first in 5 minutes or less. Ultrasonographers were not blinded to the clinical indication for imaging or to the PME image results when obtaining standard TTE images. Two experienced echocardiographers and 2 cardiology fellows who were blinded to the indication for the study and TTE results but not to the device source interpreted the PME images.

*Setting.*—Scripps Clinic Torrey Pines and Scripps Green Hospital, La Jolla, California.

*Patients.*—Convenience sample of 97 patients consecutively referred for echocardiography.

*Measurements.*—Visualizability and accuracy (the sum of proportions of true-positive and true-negative readings and observer variability) for ejection fraction, wall-motion abnormalities, left ventricular end-diastolic dimension, inferior vena cava size, aortic and mitral valve pathology, and pericardial effusion.

*Results.*—Physician-readers could visualize some but not all echocardiographic measurements obtained with the PME device in every patient (highest proportions were for ejection fraction and left ventricular end-diastolic dimension [95% each]; the lowest proportion was for inferior vena cava size [75%]). Accuracy also varied by measurement (aortic valve was 96% [highest] and inferior vena cava size was 78% [lowest]) and decreased when nonvisualizability was accounted for (aortic valve was 91% and inferior vena cava size was 58%). Observer agreement was fair to moderate for some measurements among less-experienced readers.

*Limitation.*—The study was conducted at a single setting, there was no formal estimate of accuracy given the small convenience sample of patients, and few abnormal echocardiographic measurements occurred.

*Conclusion.*—The rapid acquisition of images by skilled ultrasonographers who use PME yields accurate assessments of ejection fraction and some but not all cardiac structures in many patients. Further testing of the device in larger patient cohorts with diverse cardiac abnormalities and with untrained clinicians obtaining and interpreting images is required before wide dissemination of its use can be recommended.

▶ Most of us have seen the ads for hand-held ultrasound equipment. The most popular of these is made by General Electric. The unit is small enough to slip into a "white coat" pocket. There has been a lot of debate in recent years about end-user performance of ultrasound scan (as opposed to radiology technician/radiologist control of such instrumentation). We are seeing more and more emergency room physicians trained to perform their own routine ultrasound scans for many diagnostic procedures. In a sense, portable ultrasonography then becomes merely an extension of one's physical examination, and a good one at that.

The report by Liebo et al suggests that pocket mobile echocardiography (PME) may in fact be the next generation of the stethoscope. A PME device is roughly the size of a mobile phone and easily fits into a pocket (weight 3.8 ounces; dimensions, 5.3 × 2.9 × 1.1 inches). The first of these was released to the medical community in February 2010, but without documentation of the instrument's accuracy compared with standard transthoracic echocardiography (TTE). Liebo et al compared the accuracy of PME as a quick assessment for clinical and subclinical cardiovascular disease with standard TTE by using blinded assessments from several cardiologists. They looked at things such as cardiac ejection fraction, wall-motion abnormalities, left ventricular end diastolic dimension, inferior vena cava size, aortic and mitral valve pathology, and pericardial effusion. Ninety-five percent of the time, ejection fractions and left ventricular end diastolic dimensions were able to be measured. The lowest accuracy was for inferior vena cava size (75%). Even amateurs were able to detect something in a very high percentage of patients with aortic and mitral valve abnormalities.

The bottom line from the study of Liebo et al is that the rapid acquisition of images using PME yields accurate assessments in most, though not all, cardiac structures. With these limitations in mind, one can bet that we will see more use of end-user mobile devices such as echocardiography. The proof, however, will be whether individuals can be as skillfully trained, particularly for ultrasonography.

**J. A. Stockman III, MD**

---

**Accuracy of Interpretation of Preparticipation Screening Electrocardiograms**
Hill AC, Miyake CY, Grady S, et al (Stanford Univ, CA; Pediatric Cardiology Associates, San Jose, CA)
*J Pediatr* 159:783-788, 2011

---

*Objective.*—To evaluate the accuracy of pediatric cardiologists' interpretations of electrocardiograms (ECGs).

*Study Design.*—A series of 18 ECGs that represented conditions causing pediatric sudden cardiac death or normal hearts were interpreted by 53 members of the Western Society of Pediatric Cardiology. Gold-standard diagnoses and recommendations were determined by 2 electrophysiologists (100% concordance).

*Results.*—The average number of correct ECG interpretations per respondent was 12.4 ± 2.2 (69%, range 34%-98%). Respondents achieved a sensitivity of 68% and a specificity of 70% for recognition of any abnormality. The false-positive and false-negative rates were 30% and 32%, respectively. Based on actual ECG diagnosis, sports participation was accurately permitted in 74% of cases and accurately restricted in 81% of cases. Respondents gave correct sports guidance most commonly in cases of long QT syndrome and myocarditis (98% and 90%, respectively) and least commonly in cases of hypertrophic cardiomyopathy, Wolff-Parkinson-White syndrome, and pulmonary hypertension (80%, 64%, and 38%, respectively). Respondents ordered more follow-up tests than did experts.

*Conclusions.*—Preparticipation screening ECGs are difficult to interpret. Mistakes in ECG interpretation could lead to high rates of inappropriate sports guidance. A consequence of diagnostic error is overuse of ancillary diagnostic tests (Fig 1).

▶ A great deal has been written this year about sudden death in athletes. Preparticipation screening is in place in most public school systems and at the collegiate level to assist in determining which athletes are potentially at risk for sudden death. Among the controversies that have existed, however, with respect to preparticipation screening, is whether there is a role for screening electrocardiograms (ECGs). Part of the debate was catalyzed when other countries, particularly in Europe, began to mandate ECGs as part of participation screening. The annual rate of sudden cardiac death in the Venuto region of Italy (northwest Italy, encompassing Padua, Venice) decreased significantly with the introduction of ECG

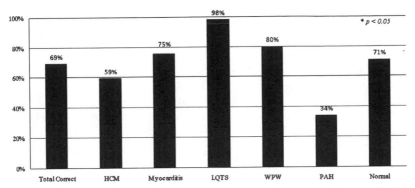

**FIGURE 1.**—Percentage of correct ECG interpretations: respondents' scores of accurate findings in ECG interpretation broken down by underlying disease. (Reprinted from Journal of Pediatrics, Hill AC, Miyake CY, Grady S, et al. Accuracy of interpretation of preparticipation screening electrocardiograms. *J Pediatr.* 2011;159:783-788. Copyright 2011, with permission from Elsevier.)

screening, which allowed for the detection of arrhythmogenic right ventricular cardiomyopathy.[1] The American Heart Association has not changed its position, which states that it is not prudent to recommend routine ECGs because of the large number of athletes in the United States, the low frequency of diseases leading to sudden cardiac death, the low rate of sudden cardiac death itself, and the frequent false-positives that can occur with ECGs that might lead to unnecessary anxiety among athletes and their families as well as to unjustified exclusion from sports or even from life insurance coverage. The American Heart Association currently recommends taking a thorough history and performing a physical examination for competing athletes every 2 years.

Hill et al have entered this debate, raising the question about whether or not preparticipation ECGs can in fact be accurately read and interpreted. The study was organized specifically to assess the accuracy of pediatric cardiologists' interpretations of ECGs in demonstrating diseases that commonly underlie sudden cardiac death. The investigators selected eighteen 12-lead ECGs from the ECG database at Lucille Packard Children's Hospital and asked members of the Western Society for Pediatric Cardiology to link to an e-mail site in which they were requested to read the ECGs. The ECGs contained information from patients with normal hearts as well as from those with long QT syndrome, hypertrophic cardiomyopathy, Wolff-Parkinson-White syndrome, pulmonary hypertension, and myocarditis. Fig 1 shows the percentage of correct ECG interpretations among the 212 individuals who were queried, of whom 53 responded.

It is clear that ECGs demonstrating diseases that underlie sudden cardiac death are difficult to interpret, even for seasoned pediatric cardiologists (94% were board certified). Their accuracy in this study was just 69%. The accuracy rate did not differ significantly among respondents despite variations in length of time practicing pediatric cardiology, number of ECGs read per month, or practice type. It does appear that one factor that influences the accuracy of ECG interpretation is the amount of clinical history offered to the reading cardiologist. Less experienced cardiologists interpret ECGs more accurately when given clinical history than do more experienced cardiologists, whose accuracy is not affected by the presence of clinical history. Also, respondents in these studies scored lowest when interpreting ECGs showing ventricular hypertrophy, pulmonary artery hypertension, hypertrophic cardiomyopathy, and Wolfe-Parkinson-White syndrome, probably because of the similarities in these pathologies and the normal changes seen in athletes' hearts. In addition, the cardiologists disagreed substantially in diagnosing ventricular hypertrophy on the basis of ECGs.

Some have suggested that expert pediatric electrophysiologists read all the pre-participation screening ECGs. This would be essentially impractical in the United States. With some 10.7 million athletes on our shores and approximately 200 electrophysiologists, the latter would have to read 223 ECGs per day in addition to their regular workload. That aside, proponents of including ECGs in preparticipation screening still point to the data from Italy. In Italy, mandatory preparticipation screening including ECGs for all athletes has correlated with an 89% decline in sudden cardiac death. However, the sudden death rate in Italy was 2.5-fold higher to begin with when this law was first implemented in 1982, compared with similar US populations. By 2004, the rate of sudden cardiac death in Italy was not significantly different from that in the United States, despite the performance of ECGs in Italy and the absence of such preparticipation screening in the United States. There is a significant difference also in the way preparticipation screening takes place in Italy. In Italy, the history, physical examination, and ECG (including interpretation) are performed by a sports cardiologist who has completed a 4-year training program, works in a sports medicine facility, and sees athletes for these examinations on a regular basis. This system is in contrast to the American system, in which a general pediatrician usually does the history and physical examination and then, if an ECG is desired, faxes the ECG to a pediatric cardiologist for interpretation.

It is clear that preparticipation ECGs do not have perfect sensitivity or specificity, and the interpretations are difficult, even for pediatric cardiologists. The follow-up after false-positive findings suggests that with 10.7 million participants younger than 40 years in amateur and competitive sports, the cost of unnecessary tests would be more than $1 billion annually. The difficulty in ECG interpretation also clearly identifies the need for reevaluation of pediatric cardiology training. According to the American College of Cardiology/American Heart Association recommendations, all physicians must interpret 500 supervised ECGs to attain initial competency. Beyond general training, cardiology fellows should interpret 3500 supervised ECGs to obtain competency, according to the Accreditation Council for Graduate Medical Education Residency Review Committee for cardiovascular diseases. Despite these recommendations, pediatric cardiology fellowship programs do not have a standardized curriculum for teaching ECG interpretation or formal testing of interpretation competency.

For more on preparticipation screening ECGs, see the commentary on this topic by Washington.[2] It is noted that the annual cost of such screening in the United States would run $7.5 million, a cost associated with an additional $750 million for secondary evaluations to follow up on ECGs initially suspected to be abnormal. As an aside, each month, *Pediatric Emergency Medicine* publishes a column edited by Dr Stephen Selbst that discusses medicolegal issues. In the October 2011 edition of the journal, the case of a 19-year-old who experienced sudden death while playing in a college basketball game was reviewed. This teen had had a pre-participation examination that detected for the first time a slight systolic murmur, and an ECG was ordered. The physician never followed up to be sure that an ECG had been performed (it was not), but he signed off on the teen's having no physical restrictions. A lawsuit ensued and a jury found in favor of the plaintiff, awarding the family $1.6 million. It should be noted that this patient's sudden cardiac event occurred 4 years after the initial physical examination.

This commentary closes with a few historical observations having to do with the discovery of the electrocardiogram (ECG). It was back in 1841, in Pisa, that Matteucci demonstrated that each heartbeat in an animal is accompanied by an electric current, which he could document by transforming the contraction of the heart muscle to electrical activity. The next step in the understanding of electrical conduction system in the heart was made in 1856 when Koelliker and Müller applied a galvanometer to the base and apex of an exposed ventricle and observed a muscle twitch just prior to ventricular systole, followed by a much smaller twitch after the systole. Later these two twitches were found to be caused by the electrical currents of the QRS and T waves, respectively. The electrical currents that are produced by the heart were then investigated with the capillary electrometer invented by Lippman, which made it possible to actually register the QRS and T phases. The first human actual ECG was recorded by Waller in 1887 with the use of this capillary electrometer.

It was Willen Einthoven, however, who developed the modern ECG after having attended a demonstration in 1889 by Waller of the technique that he had named electrocardiography. He developed an improved galvanometer and discovered that electrical currents could be registered on the skin from the heart, skeletal muscle and the brain as well as on the cornea from the retina, findings which are not only the basis of the ECG, but also electromyography and electroretinography. Unfortunately, the instruments that were available for this purpose at the end of the 19th century were not suitable for registering weak signals, but Einthoven designed something called a string galvanometer. The principle of the string galvanometer is that a thin thread is stretched in a magnetic field when an electric current passes. The sensitivity of this string galvanometer was found to be approximately 1000 times greater than that of the most sensitive mirror galvanometer, thus making it possible to analyze the currents that were produced by the heart muscles in different planes using three recording leads. It thus became possible to measure the direction and magnitude of the variations in the electrical potential within the heart. It was in 1905 that Einthoven began clinical studies in his laboratory using patients' ECG recordings and the following year he published the first description of normal and abnormal ECG recordings with the use of the string galvanometer. Within 5 years of his invention, the instrument was used in clinical cardiology.

Einthoven (1860-1927) was born in Java, which at the time belonged to the Dutch East Indies. His father was an Army doctor who died when Einthoven was 6 and the family then returned to Holland. He spent most of his professional career at the University of Leiden. In 1924 he was awarded the Nobel Prize for the discovery of the mechanisms underlying the ECG.[3]

**J. A. Stockman III, MD**

*References*

1. Chaitman BR. An electrocardiogram should not be included in routine preparticipation screening of young athletes. *Circulation.* 2007;116:2610-2614.
2. Washington RL. Pre-participation screening electrocardiograms-still not a good idea. *J Pediatr.* 2011;159:712-713.
3. Zetterstrom R. Nobel Prize to Willem Einthoven in 1924 for the discovery of the mechanisms underlying the electrocardiogram (ECG). *Acta Paediatrica.* 2009;98: 1380-1382.

---

**Long-Term Follow-Up of Children and Adolescents Diagnosed with Hypertrophic Cardiomyopathy: Risk Factors for Adverse Arrhythmic Events**

Moak JP, Leifer ES, Tripodi D, et al (Children's Natl Med Ctr, Washington, DC; Natl Heart, Lung, and Blood Inst, Bethesda, MD)

*Pediatr Cardiol* 32:1096-1105, 2011

---

Our aim was to identify prognostic factors for an arrhythmic event (AE) in children with hypertrophic cardiomyopathy (HCM) without a previous AE. One hundred thirty-one nonconsecutive patients (≤20 years) with HCM but no previous AE were evaluated at the NIH Clinical Center from 1980 to 2001. At a median follow-up of 6.4 years, 22 patients experienced an AE [sudden death (SD) ($n = 12$), resuscitated cardiac arrest ($n = 3$), clinical sustained ventricular tachycardia (VT) ($n = 2$), and implantable cardiac defibrillator discharge ($n = 5$)], resulting in a 2% annual AE rate. Baseline factors that were most predictive in univariate risk analysis included ventricular septal thickness (ST) ($P = 0.01$), VT induction by programmed ventricular stimulation (PVS) ($P = 0.01$), age ($P = 0.05$), and presyncope/syncope ($P = 0.05$). In multivariate analysis, ST, age, presyncope/syncope, and PVS were not independently predictive of risk for an AE. However, the 5-year event rates for AE was 15% (95% CI: 5–23%) if ST ≥ 20 mm, 19% (95% CI: 6–31%) when age ≥ 13 years and ST ≥ 20 mm were combined together, and 23% (95% CI: 3–39%) when PVS and ST ≥ 20 mm were combined together. Of the various risk factors that were considered in our pediatric HCM cohort, ST and inducible VT were the most significant univariate predictors of risk for an AE. More traditional risk factors identified in older patients (family history of SD, VT on Holter, and exercise-induced hypotension) were not predictive of an AE in patients age under 21 years.

▶ Once a youngster is diagnosed with hypertrophic cardiomyopathy (HCM), the patient, the parents, and the care providers all will be worried about what the future holds for the affected individual. HCM is common enough that everyone knows someone who has had some experience with affected individuals. Currently, the prevalence in the overall pediatric population runs 0.2%. Affected children have a significant risk of mortality, ranging up to 6% per year. For those at particularly high risk, an implantable cardiac defibrillator (ICD) is the management of choice but carries with it significant psychological burden and some potential morbidity. Somewhere between 20% and 30% of individuals with an ICD will have inappropriate shock from the device. Also, the device does not always work to convert an episode of ventricular fibrillation. Thus, it is important to understand which youngsters in the population of those with HCM are the ones that are likely to benefit from defibrillator therapy to minimize the associated morbidity.

Moak et al designed a study to determine whether risk factors for sudden cardiac events that had been established for adults would have predictive value in children and, if not, what clinical parameters would identify subgroups of children and adolescents that might benefit the most from ICD implantation. The investigators examined the records of 144 children (less than 20 years of age) diagnosed with HCM between 1980 and 2001, all of whom were evaluated at the cardiology branch of the National Heart, Lung and Blood Institute, National Institutes of Health (NIH). Each of these patients had undergone an electrophysiology study (EPS). HCM was diagnosed by echocardiographic demonstration of a hypertrophied nondilated left ventricle in the absence of another cause of left ventricular hypertrophy. These youngsters were followed up for many years with annual visits to the NIH.

The data from this study showed that the annual rate of arrhythmic event (AE) as defined by sudden death, resuscitated cardiac arrest, sustained ventricular tachycardia, or defibrillator discharge in children with HCM, but no prior episode of arrhythmic event, was 2% per year. Analysis of the data identified sudden death (SD) segment elevation $\geq 20$ mm and inducible ventricular tachycardia during electrophysiologic (EP) study as significantly associated with a higher arrhythmic event risk. A family history of sudden death, exercise-induced hypotension, nonsustained ventricular tachycardia on Holter monitoring, and myocardial ischemia were not significant risk factors. The combination of inducible ventricular tachycardia and SD segment $\geq 20$ mm or patient age $\geq 13$ years and ventricular septal thickness (ST) $\geq 20$ mm had the highest 5-year acute arrhythmic event rates. In contrast, patients with ST less than 20 mm had a 5-year event rate of 0%.

Also, as one might suspect, the 13 children in the NIH database who had a prior history of an arrhythmic event had a significantly higher subsequent arrhythmic event rate. Finally, the data from this report provide evidence for an increased risk of arrhythmic events in children when the septal thickness was $\geq 20$ mm. This risk was markedly compounded in the presence of inducible ventricular tachycardia and older age.

The bottom line is that the data from this report suggest that an ICD implantation is probably warranted when the ventricular septal thickness is $\geq 20$ mm, and there is positive evidence at the time of EP study of inducible ventricular tachycardia. The combined likelihood of an acute cardiac event in such circumstances ran 23%. Nevertheless, it must be said that when the septal thickness was greater than 20 mm and the EP study was negative, the 5-year cardiac event still ran 10%. The authors of this report concluded that newer technologies using smaller ICD leads and devices with improved algorithms for ventricular tachycardia detection might suggest that a septal thickness $\geq 20$ mm alone would be sufficient to justify ICD implantation.

To read more about the quality of life experienced by adolescents and young adults affected with congenital heart disease, see the interesting report of Teixeira et al.[1]

While on the topic of things having to do with the heart, virtually all care providers now are learning or have learned proper cardiopulmonary resuscitation (CPR) techniques. One way to get CPR correct, we are told by folks in Great Britain, is to listen to music during CPR training. In Great Britain, guidelines for adult basic life support recommend a compression ratio of 100 per minute, with a repeating sequence of 30 compressions followed by two rescue breaths. With this approach it is important to maintain chest compression rates and reduce interruptions to compressions as failure to do so is associated with a reduced chance of survival. Estimating a rate of 100 beats per minute can be difficult. A pilot study involving listening to the song *Stayin' Alive* by the Bee Gees while performing CPR has suggested this helps professionals maintain a compression rate around 100 beats per minute. Rawlins et al decided to update the literature by seeing if folks in training mentally "singing" the children's nursing tune *Nellie the Elephant* would also keep the CPR 100 compressions per minute because of the appropriate rhythm and tempo of this nursery tune.[2] They compared this tune with *That's The Way (I like it)*. The conclusion of the study was that there was a significant increase in the proportion of participants providing an appropriate compression rate while listening to themselves sing *Nellie the Elephant* compared with no music or *That's The Way (I like it)*. It should be noted that listening to *That's The Way (I like it)* caused no significant decrease in the proportion achieving the desired compression rates compared with no music.

*Nellie the Elephant* is not all that particularly popular as a nursery rhyme in the United States. You can look it up, however, on YouTube®. Potential tunes on our shores that would likely meet the standard of *Nellie the Elephant* would include *Another One Bites the Dust (Queen), Quit Playing Games With My Heart (Backstreet Boys)*, and *Achy Breaky Heart (Billy Rae Cyrus)*. Conceptually these tunes would seem to be better suited to resuscitating a patient who has had a heart attack given the fact that most such patients already describe a sensation of having an elephant on their chest.

**J. A. Stockman III, MD**

*References*

1. Teixeira FM, Coelho RM, Proença C, et al. Quality of life experienced by adolescents and young adults with congenital heart disease. *Pediatr Cardiol.* 2011;32:1132-1138.
2. Rawlins L, Woollard M, Williams J, Hallam P. Effective listening to Nellie the Elephant during CPR training on performance of chest compressions by lay people: randomized crossover trial. *BMJ.* 2009;339:1429-1431.

### Deadly Proposal: A Case of Catecholaminergic Polymorphic Ventricular Tachycardia

Heiner JD, Bullard-Berent JH, Inbar S (Brooke Army Med Ctr, San Antonio, TX; Mary Bridge Children's Hosp, Tacoma, WA; Univ of New Mexico, Albuquerque)
*Pediatr Emerg Care* 27:1065-1068, 2011

Catecholaminergic polymorphic ventricular tachycardia (CPVT) is a rare adrenergically mediated arrhythmogenic disorder classically induced by exercise or emotional stress and found in structurally normal hearts. It is an important cause of cardiac syncope and sudden death in childhood. Catecholaminergic polymorphic ventricular tachycardia is a genetic cardiac channelopathy with known mutations involving genes affecting intracellular calcium regulation. We present a case of a 14-year-old boy who had cardiopulmonary arrest after an emotionally induced episode of CPVT while attempting to invite a girl to the school dance. Review of his presenting cardiac rhythm, induction of concerning ventricular arrhythmias during an exercise stress test, and genetic testing confirmed the diagnosis of CPVT. He recovered fully and was treated with β-blocker therapy and placement of an implantable cardioverter-defibrillator. In this report, we discuss this rare but important entity, including its molecular foundation, clinical presentation, basics of diagnosis, therapeutic options, and implications of genetic testing for family members. We also compare CPVT to other notable cardiomyopathic and channelopathic causes of sudden death in youth including hypertrophic cardiomyopathy, arrhythmogenic right ventricular dysplasia, long QT syndrome, short QT syndrome, and Brugada syndrome.

▶ This report is included in case you might not be familiar with the disorder known as catecholaminergic polymorphic ventricular tachycardia (CPVT). CPVT is a rare arrhythmogenic disorder that was first described in 1995 with the report of 4 children with catecholamine induced ventricular tachycardia causing syncope. This malignant arrhythmogenic disorder occurs in structurally normal hearts with a normal baseline electrocardiogram. It is a characteristic ventricular tachyarrhythmias classically induced by exercise or emotional distress. The cause is a cardiac channelopathy with known molecular mechanisms and genetic mutations that are often inherited. Unfortunately, while most care providers are familiar with sudden death as a result of hypertrophic cardiomyopathy, long QT syndrome, Brugada syndrome, and others, CPVT seems to be low on the recognition scale, thus the importance of the report of this 14-year-old boy who suddenly collapsed as a result of CPVT.

The report of Heiner et al tells us about a healthy 14-year-old boy who suddenly collapsed and lost consciousness at school while inviting a girl to a school dance. He was found to be pulseless. Basic life support was begun by school personnel and fellow students with cardiopulmonary resuscitation using the school's automated external defibrillator. A shock was advised by the defibrillator and he was defibrillated once, but required continued cardiopulmonary resuscitation for an additional 15 minutes until arrival of paramedics. Defibrillation was repeated, and the patient was orotracheally intubated. A normal sinus rhythm and hemodynamic stability were obtained at the school and he was transported by ambulance to a local hospital. Review of the cardiac rhythms captured by the automated external defibrillator revealed polymorphic ventricular tachycardia in addition to ventricular fibrillation. Once at the hospital, the patient was induced into a level of deep sedation followed by 24 hours of therapeutic hypothermia. A day later he was able to be extubated and regained normal cognitive function. An echocardiogram showed no structural abnormalities. A stress test was used to induce tachycardia at which time the patient had several premature ventricular beats. These progressed to ventricular bigeminy. A diagnosis of CPVT was suspected, and an implantable cardioverter-defibrillator was placed in addition to maximally tolerated β-blocker therapy. Further testing found that he possessed a mutation affecting the cardiac ryanodine receptor, a mutation documenting an autosomal dominant form of CPVT. Other family members were found to be heterozygous for the disorder.

A diagnosis of CPVT primarily rests with progressive polymorphic ventricular arrhythmias during exercise or a catecholamine stress test. The arrhythmias characteristically occur between 100 and 120 beats per minute. CPVT differs from many other inherited forms of cardiac arrhythmias because it has a normal electrocardiogram (ECG) associated with it as well as normal imaging studies. While not as common as hypertrophic cardiomyopathy (the latter affects 1:500 people), it is not totally rare either.

The mainstay of treatment of those with CPVT is the use of a β-blocker. This has been recommended for the prophylactic treatment of identified genetic carriers of the mutation causing CPVT in those who have no personal history of syncope, cardiac arrhythmias, or concerning findings on exercise stress testing. Patients who do not respond to β-blockers or who otherwise seem at particularly high risk are candidates for placement of an implantable cardioverter-defibrillator. Someone who has had a sudden untoward event would be an immediate candidate for the latter because beta blockers are effective only about 60% of the time in the prevention of sudden untoward events.

The lethality of CPVT, its possible role in sudden unexplained deaths, and its impact on undiagnosed family members have been underscored by recent studies. The importance of this report is that it provides an increased awareness of CPVT that may motivate more prompt referral and follow-up despite a reassuring evaluation and normal ECG. A normal ECG does not rule out an inherited potential for death from a tachyarrhythmia. If the simple stress of asking for a date can trigger an episode leading to death, you can see how important it is to know about CPVT.

This commentary closes with a fictitious clinical scenario. You and your family are returning to the United States from a month-long vacation to Australia. You are flying on Quantus Airlines and are somewhere over the Pacific when the ever-distressing call comes over the plane intercom: "Is there a doctor on the plane?" You are somewhat hesitant to respond since you are in administrative medicine and have not practiced in a bit of time. The question is, are you required to do so by law? Obviously, every physician is morally obliged to render assistance wherever possible and to the degree one's skills can be applied. This question, however, is one of the laws itself and the issue of medical liability. The answer to the question is actually specific to the country where that law applies. According to British, Canadian, and US laws, medical professionals are not required to volunteer assistance during an in-flight medical event, unless they have a preexisting clinical relationship with the passenger in question. In contrast, however, the laws of Australia and many Asian, European, and Middle Eastern countries require a physician to provide assistance. On international flights, the country where the aircraft is registered has the legal jurisdiction except when the aircraft is on the ground in another country or in sovereign airspace. Since you are flying on Quantus Airlines, the official airline of Australia/New Zealand, you are required to provide assistance. Medical assistance during an in-flight medical event is protected under Good Samaritan laws and no physician has ever been held liable for his or her action while providing such medical care. The 1998 US Aviation Medical Assistance Act limits liability for volunteering physicians under the assumption they act in good faith, receive no monetary compensation, and provide reasonable care. This law pertains to events that occur within US airspace and aircraft registered within the US. Gifts, such as seat upgrades and liquors, are not considered compensation. Furthermore, many airlines indemnify volunteering physicians and the captain should provide written confirmation upon request.[1]

**J. A. Stockman III, MD**

*Reference*

1. Silverman D, Gendreau M. Medical issues associated with commercial flights. *Lancet.* 2009;373:2067-2077.

---

**Plasma Hydrogen Sulfide in Differential Diagnosis between Vasovagal Syncope and Postural Orthostatic Tachycardia Syndrome in Children**

Zhang F, Li X, Stella C, et al (Peking Univ First Hosp, Beijing, China; Univ of California—San Diego, La Jolla; et al)
*J Pediatr* 160:227-231, 2012

*Objective.*—To explore the predictive value of plasma hydrogen sulfide ($H_2S$) in differentiating between vasovagal syncope (VVS) and postural orthostatic tachycardia syndrome (POTS) in children.

*Study Design.*—Patients were divided between the POTS group (n — 60) and VVS group (n = 17) by using either the head-up test or head-up tilt test. Twenty-eight healthy children were selected for the control group. Plasma concentrations of $H_2S$ were determined for children in all groups (POTS, VVS, and control).

*Results.*—Plasma levels of $H_2S$ were significantly higher in children with VVS (95.3 ± 3.8 μmol/L) and POTS (100.9 ± 2.1 μmol/L) than in children in the control group (82.6 ± 6.5 μmol/L). Compared with the VVS group, the POTS group had plasma levels of $H_2S$ that were significantly increased. The receiver operating characteristic curve for the predictive value of $H_2S$ differentiation of VVS from POTS showed a $H_2S$ plasma level of 98 $\mu$mol/L as the cutoff value for high probability of distinction. Such a level produced both high sensitivity (90%) and specificity (80%) rates of correctly discriminating between patients with VVS and patients with POTS.

*Conclusion.*—$H_2S$ plasma level has both high sensitivity and specificity rates to predict the probability of correctly differentiating between patients with VVS and patients with POTS.

▶ Postural orthostatic tachycardia syndrome and vasovagal syncope are common causes of orthostatic intolerance in children. Postural orthostatic tachycardia operationally is defined by symptoms of orthostatic intolerance in association with excessive tachycardia. On the other hand, vasovagal syncope is defined by a characteristic transient loss of consciousness and postural tone caused by cerebral hypoperfusion. Some believe these are simply part of a spectrum of disorders, while others feel very differently that there are significant differences in the pathophysiology and clinical presentation of the 2 disorders. Often, postural orthostatic tachycardia syndrome manifests itself as a chronic day to day form of orthostatic intolerance, whereas vasovagal syncope is most often infrequent and episodic. This is not to say, however, that postural orthostatic tachycardia syndrome cannot produce sudden transient loss of consciousness, because it does on occasion. At the same time, patients with vasovagal syncope can have chronic symptoms of orthostatic intolerance. One is left with the difficulty, therefore, of distinguishing these 2 entities solely on the basis of their clinical symptomatology.

Zhang et al have studied hydrogen sulfide as an agent that could possibly distinguish between these causes of orthostatic intolerance. While hydrogen sulfide can be a toxic gas, in recent times it has also been looked at as a novel endogenous gasotransmitter. It is produced in human and other mammalian tissues from L-cystine by mainly 3 enzymes: cystathione, beta-synthetase, cystathione gamma-lyase, and 3-mercaptosulfurotransferase. Hydrogen sulfide produces regulatory effects on vascular smooth muscle cells and endothelial cells and is produced by these cells. It causes endothelium-dependent vasorelaxation and exerts regulatory effects on the pathogenesis of various diseases including hypertension, pulmonary hypertension, and shock. The potential link between hydrogen sulfide and orthostatic intolerance is based on the fact that abnormal vascular relaxation and cardiothoracic hypovolemia are thought to be mechanisms of postural orthostatic tachycardia syndrome. The reason Zhang et al studied this relationship was the theory that increased hydrogen sulfide levels might be different between postural orthostatic tachycardia syndrome and vasovagal syncope. They looked at plasma levels of hydrogen sulfide in children affected by these disorders and in controls.

The results obtained by these investigators were quite interesting. The results of their study indicated that children with postural orthostatic tachycardia syndrome and vasovagal syncope had higher hydrogen sulfide plasma levels than healthy children. Therefore, evidence continues to suggest that hydrogen sulfide functions as an endothelium-derived relaxing factor in the vascular bed of mesenteric arteries. It is suggested that hydrogen sulfide may be one of the vasorelaxants of splanchnic vessels during the process of standing up, resulting in decreased effective blood volume and symptoms of orthostatic intolerance. The data suggest that plasma levels of hydrogen sulfide have both high sensitivity and specificity to predict patients with postural orthostatic tachycardia syndrome and vasovagal syncope and could provide a useful method for identifying these 2 kinds of diseases. Hydrogen sulfide is not specific to these diseases, as there are other conditions, such as chronic obstructive lung disease, coronary heart disease, hypertension, pulmonary hypertension, and type 1 and type 2 diabetes, in which hydrogen sulfide production is altered. Nonetheless, each of these disorders presents differently than postural orthostatic tachycardia syndrome or vasovagal syncope.

We now have 3 gaseous transmitters to think about in medicine. Hydrogen sulfide joins nitric oxide and carbon monoxide as agents affecting a wide variety of physiologic processes including memory, nociception, insulin secretion, liver function, kidney function, and gastrointestinal function while playing a role in vascular tone regulation. All this may be more than you ever wanted to know about something that smells like rotten eggs, but you should be forewarned that there will be much more written about this noxious-smelling substance.

**J. A. Stockman III, MD**

---

**Postural Tachycardia in Children and Adolescents: What is Abnormal?**
Singer W, Sletten DM, Opfer-Gehrking TL, et al (Mayo Clinic, Rochester, MN)
*J Pediatr* 160:222-226, 2012

---

*Objectives.*—To evaluate whether the use of adult heart rate (HR) criteria is appropriate for diagnosing orthostatic intolerance (OI) and postural tachycardia syndrome (POTS) in children and adolescents, and to establish normative data and diagnostic criteria for pediatric OI and POTS.

*Study Design.*—A total of 106 normal controls aged 8-19 years (mean age, 14.5 ± 3.3 years) underwent standardized autonomic testing, including 5 minutes of 70-degree head-up tilt. The orthostatic HR increment and absolute orthostatic HR were assessed and retrospectively compared with values in 654 pediatric patients of similar age (mean age, 15.5 ± 2.3 years) who were referred to our Clinical Autonomic Laboratory with symptoms of OI.

*Results.*—The HR increment was mildly higher in patients referred for OI/POTS, but there was considerable overlap between the patient and control groups. Some 42% of the normal controls had an HR increment of ≥30 beats per minute. The 95th percentile for the orthostatic HR increment in the normal controls was 42.9 beats per minute. There was a greater and more consistent difference in absolute orthostatic HR between the 2 groups, although there was still considerable overlap.

*Conclusion.*—The diagnostic criteria for OI and POTS in adults are unsuitable for children and adolescents. Based on our normative data, we propose new criteria for the diagnosis of OI and POTS in children and adolescents.

▶ One of the characteristic features of orthostatic intolerance and postural tachycardia syndrome is an excessive orthostatic rise in heart rate. For a diagnosis of orthostatic intolerance, current criteria suggest the presence of an orthostatic heart rate increment of at least 30 beats per minute (BPM) within 5 minutes of active standing or passive head-up tilt, associated with symptoms of lightheadedness or faintness. For a diagnosis of postural orthostatic tachycardia syndrome, most cardiologists believe that the heart rate must increase to a level of at least 120 BPM in addition to the criteria for orthostatic intolerance. There is controversy surrounding such definitions, but that is the state of the art as it exists in pediatric cardiology beliefs right now. These criteria are largely based on adult studies. Pediatric cardiologists have suggested higher asymptomatic orthostatic increases in heart rate in normal adolescents, which only confuses the matter. Thus the report by Singer et al is useful in that the authors raise the question of whether it is appropriate to use adult criteria for a diagnosis of orthostatic intolerance and postural orthostatic tachycardia syndrome in pediatric and adolescent patients. They designed a study to look at orthostatic heart rates and increases in heart rates with head-up tilt in an otherwise-normal pediatric population. The data derived create normative data and criteria that can be used as a baseline for the diagnosis of pediatric and adolescent postural orthostatic tachycardia syndrome and orthostatic intolerance.

The authors of this report looked at more than 100 girls and boys with an average age of 15.5 years. They also looked at heart rate increments in patients referred for orthostatic intolerance and postural orthostatic tachycardia syndrome. At 5 minutes of passive head-up tilt, 33% of normal control adolescents had an increase in their average heart rate of 30 BPM or more in comparison with those with orthostatic intolerance or postural orthostatic tachycardia syndrome, the latter two having heart rate increases of 30 BPM or more in 55% of instances. Specifically, the 5-minute orthostatic heart rate was 107 ± 18 BPM in patients versus 95 ± 16 BPM in controls.

This study fills an important gap in our knowledge of what is normal and abnormal when evaluating heart rate and heart rate response with head-up tilt in children and adolescents when studied in an autonomic function laboratory. The study demonstrates that an orthostatic heart rate increase of 30 BPM, the main diagnostic criterion for orthostatic intolerance in adults, is still well within the normal range for children and adolescents. Use of this increment figure would result in very low specificity if applied to children and adolescents. The findings from this report suggest that an orthostatic heart rate increment exceeding 40 to 45 BPM would be considered excessive.

The authors of this report suggest the following diagnostic criteria for pediatric orthostatic intolerance/postural orthostatic tachycardia syndrome.

Pediatric orthostatic intolerance: (1) symptoms of orthostatic intolerance such as lightheadedness and palpitations, occurring frequently (> 50% of the time) when assuming the upright position, and (2) orthostatic heart rate increments ≥ 40 BPM within 5 minutes of head-up tilt.

Pediatric postural orthostatic tachycardia syndrome: (1) symptoms and heart rate increment fulfilling criteria for pediatric orthostatic intolerance and (2) absolute orthostatic heart rate ≥ 130 BPM (for age ≤ 13 years) or absolute orthostatic heart rate ≥ 120 BPM (for age ≥ 14 years) within 5 minutes of head-up tilt.

While these guidelines represent the beliefs of the authors, they do seem to make sense. The findings do not necessarily replace more sophisticated assessment such as tilt table testing. When autonomic dysfunction is suspected by the generalist caring for these children, referral to a specialist is probably wise. These disorders are very complicated entities.

**J. A. Stockman III, MD**

---

**A Prospective Evaluation of a Protocol for Magnetic Resonance Imaging of Patients With Implanted Cardiac Devices**

Nazarian S, Hansford R, Roguin A, et al (Johns Hopkins Univ, Baltimore, MD; Rambam Med Ctr, Haifa, Israel; Natl Insts of Biomedical Imaging and Bioengineering, Bethesda, MD)
*Ann Intern Med* 155:415-424, 2011

---

*Background.*—Magnetic resonance imaging (MRI) is avoided in most patients with implanted cardiac devices because of safety concerns.

*Objective.*—To define the safety of a protocol for MRI at the commonly used magnetic strength of 1.5 T in patients with implanted cardiac devices.

*Design.*—Prospective nonrandomized trial. (ClinicalTrials.gov registration number: NCT01130896).

*Setting.*—One center in the United States (94% of examinations) and one in Israel.

*Patients.*—438 patients with devices (54% with pacemakers and 46% with defibrillators) who underwent 555 MRI studies.

*Intervention.*—Pacing mode was changed to asynchronous for pacemaker-dependent patients and to demand for others. Tachyarrhythmia functions were disabled. Blood pressure, electrocardiography, oximetry, and symptoms were monitored by a nurse with experience in cardiac life support and device programming who had immediate backup from an electrophysiologist.

*Measurements.*—Activation or inhibition of pacing, symptoms, and device variables.

*Results.*—In 3 patients (0.7% [95% CI, 0% to 1.5%]), the device reverted to a transient back-up programming mode without long-term effects. Right ventricular (RV) sensing (median change, 0 mV [interquartile range {IQR}, −0.7 to 0 V]) and atrial and right and left ventricular lead impedances (median change, −2 Ω [IQR, −13 to 0 Ω], −4 Ω [IQR, −16 to 0 Ω], and −11 Ω [IQR, −40 to 0 Ω], respectively) were reduced immediately after MRI. At long-term follow-up (61% of patients), decreased RV sensing (median, 0 mV, [IQR, −1.1 to 0.3 mV]), decreased RV lead impedance (median, −3 Ω, [IQR, −29 to 15 Ω]), increased RV capture threshold (median, 0 V, IQR, [0 to 0.2 Ω]), and decreased battery voltage (median, $-0.01$ V, IQR, $-0.04$ to 0 V) were noted. The observed changes did not require device revision or reprogramming.

*Limitations.*—Not all available cardiac devices have been tested. Long-term in-person or telephone follow-up was unavailable in 43 patients (10%), and some data were missing. Those with missing long-term capture threshold data had higher baseline right atrial and right ventricular capture thresholds and were more likely to have undergone thoracic imaging. Defibrillation threshold testing and random assignment to a control group were not performed.

*Conclusion.*—With appropriate precautions, MRI can be done safely in patients with selected cardiac devices. Because changes in device variables and programming may occur, electrophysiologic monitoring during MRI is essential.

▶ Although this report contains data mostly on adults, many in the pediatric population also have implanted cardiac rhythm management devices (CRMDs). Most patients who have these implanted are over 60 years of age, but all of us are familiar with the horror stories in teenagers who develop sudden cardiac arrest as a result of a congenital or acquired cardiac rhythm abnormality. Hypertrophic cardiomyopathy that cannot be managed otherwise is sometimes treated with a CRMD. Those in the pediatric age group face the same problem adults face if they need an MRI study. For many years, the presence of a CRMD has been widely considered an absolute contraindication to MRI as a result of several hypothetical risks to the function of CRMDs in an MRI environment, as well as reports of harm, including death, caused by MRI in patients with CRMDs. These concerns about the safety of MRI are well founded. The electromagnetic fields generated by MRI machines, with or without active scanning, can interact with pacemakers and implantable cardioverter-defibrillators (ICDs) in multiple and sometimes unpredictable ways. One concern is the displacement of the device generator or its leads by the MRI-generated magnetic field. The leads, however, are composed of mostly nonmagnetic material, and the ferromagnetic force applied to the generator is insufficient to cause pain or movement. As a precaution, MRI should be delayed for at least 6 weeks after device implantation until its location is stable. Also, a magnetic field may trigger activation of the device switch. In most ICDs, the magnet response has no effect on pacing variables, but it temporarily suspends the detection and treatment of ventricular arrhythmias. Thus, simply bringing a patient with a CRMD into an MRI suite can alter the function of his or her device. It has also been theorized that the strong electromagnetic fields associated with MRI may cause the ferromagnetic component implanted leads to heat.

Many of the potential risks noted here, with the exception of lead heating, can be mitigated by careful reprogramming of the CRMD before MRI, including changing to an asynchronous pacing mode in pacemaker-dependent patients and suspending tachycardia detection and therapy in patients with ICDs. These were among the main precautions taken by the authors of the report. Nazarian et al found that 1.5-T MRI, done according to their study protocol, in this widely represented population of devices was remarkably safe. In 555 scans performed in 438 patients, there was no serious incidence of harm. Changes in the devices' performance variables were in general small and clinically insignificant. It should be noted that in the Nazarian et al study, only pacemakers manufactured after 1998 and ICDs manufactured after 2000 were included.

In an editorial that accompanied this report, it was noted that the data from the report suggest that the risks of MRI in the presence of CRMDs, although potentially serious, have probably been overestimated and can be managed effectively in many cases. In the authors' opinion, the presence of a CRMD should no longer be considered an absolute contraindication to MRI; rather, the risks and benefits of MRI in a patient with CRMD should be assessed on an individual basis as would be done with any important medical decision. All the criteria used by Nazarian et al should be followed. This means that only 1.5-T machines should be used; CRMD devices should have been in place for at least 6 weeks; no epicardial or nonfunctioning leads should be present; and patient selection, monitoring, and follow-up should be carefully and cautiously planned. Most important, the equipment and experienced personnel necessary to manage any eventuality must be immediately available.

Yes, some children with CRMD will need an MRI study, and if the procedure is carefully done, it should be possible to undertake the scan without undue harm to the patient. What was once an absolute contraindication to MRI no longer is.

This commentary closes with an observation that has relatively little to do with pediatrics, but does involve technology that pediatric cardiologists are familiar with: the implantable cardioverter-defibrillator. Indications for implantable cardioverter-defibrillators have expanded greatly, mostly in the care of adults, but also in the care of children with certain diseases that can cause sudden cardiac death. Have you ever wondered what happens to these devices during end-of-life care? Interestingly Goldstein et al studied this problem in hospices in the United States.[1] Patients admitted to hospice in the United States must have a life expectancy of only a few months or fewer and must agree to forgo life-prolonging treatment. What investigators did was to examine the processes of 900 randomly selected hospices to see what their policies are with respect to deactivating an implantable cardioverter-defibrillator upon admission to the hospice. Surprisingly, just 10% of hospices had a policy that addressed such deactivation and 58% of hospices reported that in the preceding year a patient with such a device had been shocked by the device during their terminal hospice care. It appears that fewer than half the patients admitted to hospice with an implantable device had their devices deactivated while receiving hospice care.

The United States is an amazing country, isn't it? In order to be "green," we all learn to turn lights off as we leave a room, but forget to turn off a life-sustaining device in somebody who is in the natural process of dying.

**J. A. Stockman III, MD**

*Reference*

1. Goldstein N, Carlson M, Livote E, Kutner JS. Brief communication. Management of implantable cardioverter-defibrillators in hospice: A nationwide study. *Ann Intern Med.* 2010;152:296-299.

### Bevacizumab in Patients With Hereditary Hemorrhagic Telangiectasia and Severe Hepatic Vascular Malformations and High Cardiac Output

Dupuis-Girod S, Ginon I, Saurin J-C, et al (Hôpital Louis Pradel, Bron, France; Centre Hospitalier Lyon Sud, Pierre-Bénite, France; Hospices Civils de Lyon, France; et al)

*JAMA* 307:948-955, 2012

*Context.*—The only treatment available to restore normal cardiac output in patients with hereditary hemorrhagic telangiectasia (HHT) and cardiac failure is liver transplant. Anti–vascular endothelial growth factor treatments such as bevacizumab may be an effective treatment.

*Objectives.*—To test the efficacy of bevacizumab in reducing high cardiac output in severe hepatic forms of HHT and to assess improvement in epistaxis duration and quality of life.

*Design, Setting, and Patients.*—Single-center, phase 2 trial with national recruitment from the French HHT Network. Patients were 18 to 70 years old and had confirmed HHT, severe liver involvement, and a high cardiac index related to HHT.

*Intervention.*—Bevacizumab, 5 mg per kg, every 14 days for a total of 6 injections. The total duration of the treatment was 2.5 months; patients were followed up for 6 months after the beginning of the treatment.

*Main Outcome Measure.*—Decrease in cardiac output at 3 months after the first injection, evaluated by echocardiography.

*Results.*—A total of 25 patients were included between March 2009 and November 2010. Of the 24 patients who had echocardiograms available for reread, there was a response in 20 of 24 patients with normalization of cardiac index (complete response [CR]) in 3 of 24, partial response (PR) in 17 of 24, and no response in 4 cases. Median cardiac index at beginning of the treatment was 5.05 L/min/m$^2$ (range, 4.1-6.2) and significantly decreased at 3 months after the beginning of the treatment with a median cardiac index of 4.2 L/min/m$^2$ (range, 2.9-5.2; $P < .001$). Median cardiac index at 6 months was significantly lower than before treatment (4.1 L/min/m$^2$; range, 3.0-5.1). Among 23 patients with available data at 6 months, we observed CR in 5 cases, PR in 15 cases, and no response in 3 cases. Mean duration of epistaxis, which was 221 minutes per month (range, 0-947) at inclusion, had significantly decreased at 3 months (134 minutes; range, 0-656) and 6 months (43 minutes; range, 0-310) ($P = .008$). Quality of life had significantly improved. The most severe adverse events were 2 cases of grade 3 systemic hypertension, which were successfully treated.

*Conclusion.*—In this preliminary study of patients with HHT associated with severe hepatic vascular malformations and high cardiac output, administration of bevacizumab was associated with a decrease in cardiac output and reduced duration and number of episodes of epistaxis.

*Trial Registration.*—clinicaltrials.gov Identifier: NCT00843440.

▶ This report describes a potential new therapy to treat patients with hereditary hemorrhagic telangiectasia. Because this disorder is a multivisceral disease that may be caused by disturbances in angiogenesis, the use of a vascular endothelial growth factor inhibitor such as bevacizumab could be an effective treatment.

Hereditary hemorrhagic telangiectasia is a dominantly inherited genetic vascular disorder characterized by recurrent epistaxis, cutaneous telangiectasia, and visceral arteriovenous malformations. The latter can affect many organs, including the lungs, gastrointestinal tract, liver, and brain. The criteria for diagnosis are spontaneous and recurrent epistaxis, telangiectasia, a family history, and visceral lesions. Hepatic involvement is observed in as many as 74% of patients, but no more than 6% of affected patients, mainly women, have symptomatic liver shunting. Liver malformations result in 3 complications: high output cardiac failure (in most cases) and, more rarely, portal hypertension and biliary necrosis. Hepatic shunting, like other extracardiac systemic shunts, is thought to be associated with increased cardiac preload and decreased peripheral vascular resistance, leading to an adaptive increase in cardiac output. High-output cardiac failure usually starts with a progressive increase in cardiac output, in turn leading to elevated left ventricular filling pressures, dyspnea, heart failure, and pulmonary hypertension. Two genes are associated with hereditary hemorrhagic telangiectasia: *ENG* and *ACRLV1*. Mutations in either of these genes account for most clinical cases. These genes encode endothelial cell protein transporter that is responsive to growth factors that stimulate vascular formations. Thus it has been hypothesized that hereditary hemorrhagic telangiectasia is related to an imbalance between forces that foster blood vessel formation and those that inhibit blood vessel formation. Vascular endothelial growth factor is a pro-angiogenesis factor.

The authors of this report have studied the efficacy of bevacizumab in severe hepatic forms of hereditary hemorrhagic telangiectasia associated with high cardiac output and report the results of this treatment with a 6-month follow-up. This agent is an inhibitor of vascular endothelial growth factor. The results showed that, 3 months after the beginning of treatment, this agent was effective in 80% of patients in decreasing cardiac output related to hepatic shunting, resulting in normalization of cardiac output in 12% of patients. There was also clinical improvement in dyspnea and normalization of pulmonary pressure in those with pulmonary hypertension before treatment. The suggestion is that the improvement is due to normalization of liver vascularization. Presumably, the drug acts on liver capillaries, reducing shunting and resulting in decreases in cardiac output. Also, nosebleeds are a major life-threatening complication of hereditary hemorrhagic telangiectasia. This report showed that the total duration of epistaxis significantly improved 6 months after the beginning of treatment in 87% of patients. No surgery was needed for nosebleeds during the study.

Toxic effects of drug therapy in this report were low and easily managed. The drug used is generally well tolerated, although it can cause systemic hypertension in as many as 16% of patients. The authors of this report remarked that they did not know whether this treatment could be definitive or merely a bridging therapy while patients are awaiting a liver transplant. Longer follow-up studies are necessary to determine the duration of hereditary hemorrhagic telangiectasia treatment effectiveness and whether maintenance therapy is required. Given that there are other disorders related to defects in angiogenesis, the progress made in this disease hopefully provides a new way of thinking about vascular problems of this type.

**J. A. Stockman III, MD**

### Congenital Heart Defects and Major Structural Noncardiac Anomalies, Atlanta, Georgia, 1968 to 2005

Miller A, Riehle-Colarusso T, Alverson CJ, et al (Ctrs for Disease Control and Prevention, Atlanta, GA)
*J Pediatr* 159:70-78, 2011

*Objective.*—To identify the proportion of major structural noncardiac anomalies identified with congenital heart defects (CHDs).

*Study Design.*—Records of infants with CHDs in the Metropolitan Atlanta Congenital Defects Program who were born during the period 1968 through 2005 were classified as having isolated, syndromic, multiple CHD (ie, having an unrecognized pattern of multiple congenital anomalies or a recognized pattern of multiple congenital anomalies of unknown etiology), or laterality defects. Frequencies of associated noncardiac anomalies were obtained.

*Results.*—We identified 7984 live-born and stillborn infants and fetuses with CHDs. Among them, 5695 (71.3%) had isolated, 1080 (13.5%) had multiple, 1048 (13.1%) had syndromic, and 161 (2.0%) had laterality defects. The percentage of multiple congenital anomalies was highest for case with atrial septal defects (18.5%), cardiac looping defects (17.2%), and conotruncal defects (16.0%), and cases with atrioventricular septal defects represented the highest percentages of those with syndromic CHDs (66.7%).

*Conclusions.*—Including those with syndromes and laterality defects, 28.7% of case infants with CHDs had associated major noncardiac malformations. Thus, infants with CHDs warrant careful examination for the presence of noncardiac anomalies (Table 2).

▶ It is interesting that to date there has been no uniform understanding of what the rate of noncardiac abnormalities is in youngsters with congenital heart defects. Previous reports have suggested that noncardiac structural anomalies among children with congenital heart disease range from a low of 14.5% to as much as 66% depending on the type of analysis that is performed. The highest percentage of additional anomalies has been observed in studies based on autopsy reports. Miller et al tell us the frequency of such noncardiac abnormalities using an active surveillance system in which clinicians classify cardiac and noncardiac defects in a standardized manner. They identified all live-born infants, stillborn infants, and elective terminations of pregnancy in which a diagnosis of congenital heart disease was made during the period 1968 through 2005 based on information from the Metropolitan Atlanta Congenital Defects Program (MACDP). In this study, live-born and stillborn infants' records were reviewed and classified by experts in pediatric cardiology. Clinical information was also

**TABLE 2.**—Distribution of Congenital Heart Defects According to the Presence and Type of Associated Noncardiac Anomalies, Metropolitan Atlanta Congenital Defects Program, 1968 to 2005

| Class of Defect | All CHDs* n (%) | Cardiac Looping Defects n (%) | Conotruncal Defects n (%) | TOF† n (%) | AVSDs‡ n (%) | LVOTOs§ n (%) | Coarctation of Aorta n (%) | HLHS¶ n (%) | RVOTOs‖ n (%) | Pulmonary Valve Stenosis n (%) | ASDs** n (%) | ASDs Secundum n (%) | VSDs†† n (%) | VSDs Muscular n (%) | VSDs Perimembranous n (%) | Cell Growth n (%) | Ebstein Anomaly n (%) |
|---|---|---|---|---|---|---|---|---|---|---|---|---|---|---|---|---|---|
| Isolated | 5695 (71.3) | 123 (72.8) | 851 (70.7) | 383 (67.1) | 109 (24.4) | 777 (75.4) | 377 (73.2) | 249 (77.3) | 557 (80.3) | 412 (82.1) | 606 (59.4) | 405 (60.5) | 2,752 (76.9) | 1306 (85.0) | 580 (69.5) | 129 (82.2) | 60 (90.9) |
| MCAs‡‡ | 1080 (13.5) | 29 (17.2) | 193 (16.0) | 102 (17.9) | 40 (8.9) | 157 (15.2) | 84 (16.3) | 49 (15.2) | 99 (14.3) | 65 (12.9) | 189 (18.5) | 114 (17.0) | 458 (12.8) | 146 (9.5) | 115 (13.8) | 20 (12.7) | 4 (6.1) |
| Syndromes§§ | 1048 (13.1) | 17 (10.1) | 159 (13.2) | 85 (14.9) | 298 (66.7) | 97 (9.4) | 54 (10.5) | 24 (7.5) | 37 (5.3) | 25 (5.0) | 224 (22.0) | 150 (22.4) | 369 (10.3) | 84 (5.5) | 140 (16.8) | 8 (5.1) | 2 (3.0) |
| Trisomy 21 | 536 (6.7) |  | 27 (2.2) | 19 (3.3) | 258 (57.7) | 14 (1.4) | 12 (2.3) | 1 (0.3) | 6 (0.9) | 5 (1.0) | 127 (12.5) | 102 (15.2) | 176 (4.9) | 38 (2.5) | 83 (9.9) | 1 (0.6) | 1 (1.5) |
| Trisomy 18 | 134 (1.7) | 6 (3.6) | 23 (1.9) | 12 (2.1) | 19 (4.3) | 18 (1.7) | 7 (1.4) | 8 (2.5) | 3 (0.4) | 5 (1.0) | 13 (1.3) | 5 (0.9) | 73 (2.0) | 5 (0.3) | 26 (3.1) |  |  |
| Trisomy 13 | 63 (0.8) | 2 (1.2) | 19 (1.6) | 9 (1.6) | 7 (1.6) | 7 (0.7) | 3 (0.6) | 2 (0.6) | 2 (0.3) | 3 (0.6) | 23 (2.3) | 13 (1.9) | 23 (0.6) | 3 (0.2) | 6 (0.7) | 1 (0.6) |  |
| 22q11 deletion | 54 (0.7) |  | 43 (3.6) | 19 (3.3) |  | 2 (0.2) |  | 1 (0.3) |  | 1 (0.2) | 6 (0.5) | 6 (0.9) | 7 (0.2) | 3 (0.2) | 4 (0.5) | 2 (1.3) |  |
| Laterality defects | 161 (2.0) |  |  |  |  |  |  |  |  |  |  |  |  |  |  |  |  |
| Total | 7984 (100) | 169 (100) | 1204 (100) | 571 (100) | 447 (100) | 1031 (100) | 515 (100) | 322 (100) | 694 (100) | 502 (100) | 1020 (100) | 669 (100) | 3579 (100) | 1536 (100) | 835 (100) | 157 (100) | 66 (100.0) |

*Congenital heart defects.
†Tetralogy of Fallot.
‡Atrioventricular septal defects.
§Left ventricular outflow tract obstructions.
¶Hypoplastic left heart syndrome.
‖Right ventricular outflow tract obstructions.
**Atrial septal defects.
††Ventricular septal defects.
‡‡Multiple congenital anomalies.
§§Chromosomal syndromes, single-gene disorders, and recognized conditions.

reviewed by a geneticist. Of 7984 live-born and stillborn infants and fetuses meeting the definition of having congenital heart disease, 71.3% had isolated cardiac disease and 13.5% had an undefined pattern of notable extra cardiac anomalies, 13.1% had specific syndromes, and 2% had other findings (Table 2). As one might suspect, the frequency of additional noncardiac anomalies varied with the different types of congenital heart disease with the highest proportion of noncardiac anomalies being observed among those with atrial septal defects, cardiac looping defects, and conotruncal defects. These findings are consistent with those of other reports. The results also show that the most frequent noncardiac anomalies include skeletal defects (35%), gastrointestinal abnormalities (25%), and renal defects (23%). Needless to say, a number of those with noncardiac abnormalities fell into syndromic/genetic categories, including Down syndrome.

The conclusion of this report is that any infant diagnosed with a congenital heart defect should have a very careful physical examination and other studies performed as warranted to detect the presence of noncardiac abnormalities.

This commentary ends with the fact that if you are evaluating a patient for a chronic cough for which there appears to be no explanation, you might think about a cardiac arrhythmia as a potential etiology. A prospective study of 120 patients without organic heart disease who were referred for the management of symptomatic premature ventricular complexes (PVC) found that 10 had a chronic cough. After fully investigating possible causes of the cough, just one patient's cough was put down solely to PVC, while another 5 had PVCs plus another cause. PVC-related cough stopped in 6 patients after antiarrhythmic treatment or spontaneous remission of the PVCs.[1]

**J. A. Stockman III, MD**

*Reference*

1. Stec SM, Grabczak EM, Bielicki P, et al. Diagnosis and management of premature ventricular complexes-associated chronic cough. *Chest.* 2009;135:1535-1541.

---

**The Contribution of Chromosomal Abnormalities to Congenital Heart Defects: A Population-Based Study**
Hartman RJ, Rasmussen SA, Botto LD, et al (Natl Ctr on Birth Defects and Developmental Disabilities, Atlanta, GA; Univ of Utah School of Medicine, Salt Lake City; et al)
*Pediatr Cardiol* 32:1147-1157, 2011

---

We aimed to assess the frequency of chromosomal abnormalities among infants with congenital heart defects (CHDs) in an analysis of population-based surveillance data. We reviewed data from the Metropolitan Atlanta Congenital Defects Program, a population-based birth-defects surveillance system, to assess the frequency of chromosomal abnormalities among live-born infants and fetal deaths with CHDs delivered from January 1, 1994, to December 31, 2005. Among 4430 infants with CHDs, 547 (12.3%) had a chromosomal abnormality. CHDs most likely to be associated with a chromosomal abnormality were interrupted aortic arch (type B and not otherwise specified; 69.2%), atrioventricular septal defect (67.2%), and double-outlet right ventricle (33.3%). The most common chromosomal abnormalities observed were trisomy 21 (52.8%), trisomy 18 (12.8%), 22q11.2 deletion (12.2%), and trisomy 13 (5.7%). In conclusion, in our study, approximately 1 in 8 infants with a CHD had a chromosomal abnormality. Clinicians should have a low threshold at which to obtain testing for chromosomal abnormalities in infants with CHDs, especially those with certain types of CHDs. Use of new technologies that have become recently available (e.g., chromosomal microarray) may increase the identified contribution of chromosomal abnormalities even further.

▶ We tend to do chromosomal studies based on findings of clusters of phenotypic abnormalities observed in patients. This report suggests that simply having a congenital heart defect alone may warrant looking for chromosomal abnormalities. The association between congenital heart defects and chromosomal abnormalities is well recognized, but estimates of the proportion of congenital heart disease cases associated with a chromosomal anomaly vary widely from a low of 9% to 18% in the literature, depending on study location, inclusion criteria for infants with congenital heart defects, and whether the analysis was clinic based or population based. Most estimates of the prevalence of chromosomal abnormalities have included aneuploidies, whereas other somewhat common chromosomal abnormalities, such as 22q11.2 deletions, have not been included.

Investigators in Atlanta have reviewed data from the Metropolitan Atlanta Congenital Defects Program to determine the prevalence of chromosomal abnormalities in infants born with congenital heart defects. Some 4400 infants with congenital heart defects were observed over a period from 1994 through 2005. The prevalence of congenital heart disease in the Atlanta region was 7.9 per 1000 live births, consistent with historical data elsewhere. Among infants with congenital heart defects, 12.3% had a chromosomal anomaly, and most of these infants (77.1%) had only 1 type of congenital heart disease. Congenital heart diseases most likely to be associated with a chromosomal anomaly were interrupted aortic arch (69.2%), atrioventricular septal defect (67.2%), double-outlet right ventricle (33.3%), partial anomalous pulmonary venous return (33.3%), and truncus arteriosus (32.3%). Congenital heart defects that were the least likely to have a chromosomal abnormality diagnosed were heterotaxy (2.2%), Epstein anomaly (2.6%), and pulmonary valve stenosis (3.3%). The most commonly observed chromosomal anomalies among infants with congenital heart defects were trisomy 21 (52.8%), trisomy 18 (12.8%), 22q11.2 deletion (12.2%), and trisomy 13 (5.7%). The proportion of infants with congenital heart defects who had a chromosomal abnormality did not differ by infant sex or gestational age. Infants with more than 1 congenital heart defect were more likely to have a chromosomal abnormality. Fetal deaths with congenital heart defects were 3 times as likely to have a chromosomal abnormality diagnosed as live born infants (33.9% vs 12.1%).

The bottom line here is that about 1 in 8 newborns with congenital heart disease will have a chromosomal anomaly detected by G-banding analysis or targeted fluorescence in situ hybridization technology. These findings support the hypothesis that genetic loci on many different chromosomes are involved in the causation of congenital heart disease. The findings from this report also suggest that clinicians should maintain a low threshold at which to obtain testing for chromosomal anomalies in infants with congenital heart disease, especially in infants with specific types of congenital heart disease or those with multiple congenital heart defects. Certainly more studies will appear in the future looking at microarrays in addition to traditional chromosomal studies, and these will yield even more information about the relationship between chromosomal abnormalities and congenital heart disease.

**J. A. Stockman III, MD**

---

### Patent Foramen Ovale in Children with Migraine Headaches

McCandless RT, Arrington CB, Nielsen DC, et al (Primary Children's Med Ctr and the Univ of Utah, Salt Lake City)
*J Pediatr* 159:243-247, 2011

*Objective.*—To determine the prevalence of patent foramen ovale (PFO) in children with migraine.

*Study Design.*—Children aged 6.0 to 18.0 years with migraine headache were evaluated for PFO and right-to-left shunting with color-flow Doppler scanning, saline solution contrast transthoracic echocardiography, and contrast transcranial Doppler scanning.

*Results.*—The population consisted of 109 children with migraine; 38 (35%) with aura and 71 (65%) without aura. The overall PFO prevalence was 35%, similar to the general population (35% vs 25%; $P = .13$). However, compared with the general population (25%), the PFO prevalence was significantly greater in subjects with aura (50%, $P = .0004$) but similar in those without aura (27%, $P = .73$). Atrial shunt size was not associated with the presence or absence of aura.

*Conclusion.*—Children with migraine with aura have a significantly higher prevalence of PFO compared with those without aura or the general population. These data suggest that PFO may contribute to the pathogenesis of migraine with aura in children and have implications for clinical decision making.

▶ Migraine is common in both adults and children. It has been estimated that migraine affects about 15% of the pediatric population. About 1 in 3 children with migraine will have an aura. It has also been noted that somewhere between 10% and 25% of the general population will have a foramen ovale that remains patent. A number of studies done in adults with migraine with aura have found a significantly higher prevalence of patent foramen ovale ranging from 41% to 62%. This has led to the hypothesis that a right-to-left shunt across the atrial septum may allow metabolic or microembolic triggers that would normally be cleared by the lungs to pass unfiltered into the cerebral circulation, perhaps leading to the evolution of a migraine episode. No comparable studies have been published in children, thus the value of this report of McCandless.

McCandless et al, from the Primary Children's Medical Center in Salt Lake City, hypothesized that children with migraine with aura would have a higher prevalence of patent foramen ovale compared with the general population. They designed a study to determine the prevalence of patent foramen ovale in pediatric patients with migraine and investigated the relationships between the amount of right-to-left atrial shunting and the type of migraines that patients experienced. They used Doppler transthoracic echocardiography and transcranial Doppler scanning to assess shunting across the atrial septum, utilizing agitated saline solution contrast. Recordings were obtained with normal breathing and with a Valsalva maneuver to increase right atrial pressure maximizing detection of right-to-left atrial shunting through a patent foramen ovale. The agitated saline solution contains small bubbles that are readily detectible by echocardiography.

The study of McCandless et al found a significantly higher prevalence of patent foramen ovale in children with migraine with aura compared with the general population and provides a basis for further research on the role of patent foramen ovale in pediatric migraines. Independent reports of migraine cessation in adults after patent foramen ovale closure for nonmigraine indications such as stroke or decompression illness have led to the hypothesis that a patent foramen ovale may permit vasoactive metabolic or microembolic triggers to enter the cerebrocirculation, directly bypassing the pulmonary circulation. There are several studies in the adult literature showing that closure of patent foramen ovale will reduce the occurrence of migraines along the order of 70% to 100%. Other studies, however, have not shown such dramatic responses. No such studies have been done in children, but the results of the study of McCandless et al do document that the prevalence of patent foramen ovale in migraine with aura is roughly double that found in migraine without aura.

There is a lot written in the adult literature these days about the use of patent foramen ovale closure as a therapy for migraines, particularly in those patients for whom medical management has failed. Despite the absence of rigorous evidence supporting patent foramen ovale closure as a safe and effective treatment for migraines, increasing numbers of children are being referred to pediatric cardiologists for patent foramen ovale evaluation and potential closure. It would be premature to say that the surgical treatment of medically refractive migraine is an acceptable alternative in children, at least as of this time, but the results of the report abstracted are similar to those of adults showing a much higher probability of the presence of a patent foramen ovale in patients with migraine and aura. Spontaneous patent foramen ovale closure must be rare after about 6 years of age.

It is important for general pediatricians to be aware of studies such as this because parents of children with migraine will research the literature and find data on the association between patent foramen ovale and migraine with and without aura.

This commentary closes with an interesting clinical observation. You are covering an emergency room and in comes a young adult with a history of recurrent syncope. During the latter episodes she is profoundly hypoxic. No arrhythmias are noted and computed tomography shows no pulmonary emboli. A transesophageal echocardiogram, however, shows a patent foramen ovale with intermittent right to left shunt. When standing this patient develops hypoxemia. When lying supine the hypoxia goes away. Your diagnosis? If you diagnose platypnea orthodeoxia, you would be correct. This is a syndrome of hypoxia which occurs in the upright position that is relieved when supine. It can be associated with a patent foramen ovale. In the patient described, a real patient, surgery corrected the problem.[1]

**J. A. Stockman III, MD**

*Reference*

1. Pearman CM, Andron M. Hypoxia induced by standing up. *BMJ.* 2010;341: c3975.

## Incidence of Aortic Complications in Patients With Bicuspid Aortic Valves

Michelena HI, Khanna AD, Mahoney D, et al (Mayo Clinic, Rochester, MN; et al)
*JAMA* 306:1104-1113, 2011

*Context.*—Bicuspid aortic valve (BAV), the most common congenital heart defect, has been thought to cause frequent and severe aortic complications; however, long-term, population-based data are lacking.

*Objective.*—To determine the incidence of aortic complications in patients with BAV in a community cohort and in the general population.

*Design, Setting, and Participants.*—In this retrospective cohort study, we conducted comprehensive assessment of aortic complications of patients with BAV living in a population-based setting in Olmsted County, Minnesota. We analyzed long-term follow-up of a cohort of all Olmsted County residents diagnosed with definite BAV by echocardiography from 1980 to 1999 and searched for aortic complications of patients whose bicuspid valves had gone undiagnosed. The last year of follow-up was 2008-2009.

*Main Outcome Measure.*—Thoracic aortic dissection, ascending aortic aneurysm, and aortic surgery.

*Results.*—The cohort included 416 consecutive patients with definite BAV diagnosed by echocardiography, mean (SD) follow-up of 16 (7) years (6530 patient-years). Aortic dissection occurred in 2 of 416 patients; incidence of 3.1 (95% CI, 0.5-9.5) cases per 10 000 patient-years, age-adjusted relative-risk 8.4 (95% CI, 2.1-33.5; $P = .003$) compared with the county's general population. Aortic dissection incidences for patients 50 years or older at baseline and bearers of aortic aneurysms at baseline were 17.4 (95% CI, 2.9-53.6) and 44.9 (95% CI, 7.5-138.5) cases per 10 000 patient-years, respectively. Comprehensive search for aortic dissections in undiagnosed bicuspid valves revealed 2 additional patients, allowing estimation of aortic dissection incidence in bicuspid valve patients irrespective of diagnosis status (1.5; *95% CI*, 0.4-3.8 cases per 10 000 patient-years), which was similar to the diagnosed cohort. Of 384 patients without baseline aneurysms, 49 developed aneurysms at follow-up, incidence of 84.9 (*95% CI*, 63.3-110.9) cases per 10 000 patient-years and an age-adjusted relative risk 86.2 (*95% CI*, 65.1-114; *P* < .001 compared with the general population). The 25-year rate of aortic surgery was 25% (*95% CI*, 17.2%-32.8%).

*Conclusions.*—In the population of patients with BAV, the incidence of aortic dissection over a mean of 16 years of follow-up was low but significantly higher than in the general population.

▶ This report dealing with complications in patients with bicuspid aortic valves includes pediatric-age patients and thus its importance for us who provide care to such individuals, particularly given that bicuspid aortic valve is the most common form of congenital heart defect affecting 1.3% of children and adults. A little known fact, at least in pediatrics, is that bicuspid aortic valve is responsible for more deaths than all other forms of congenital heart defects combined. The reason for this is that bicuspid aortic valves commonly cause pathology in the aorta resulting in aortic dissection. Michelena et al have studied the problem of aortic dissection in patients with bicuspid aortic valve as diagnosed by echocardiography.

Olmstead County, Minnesota, is a unique area of our country that has provided us with much information on population data related to disease states. Olmstead County contains a well-defined population with few clinicians or hospitals delivering health care in the community. For example, all echocardiograms are reviewed by 1 laboratory, and all cardiovascular surgeries are performed at 1 institution. This has allowed Michelena et al to follow a cohort of 416 consecutive patients from this county who had bicuspid aortic valve diagnosed by echocardiography. Patients were followed up for an average of 16 years. This included patients diagnosed with this congenital heart defect in childhood. It should be noted that Mayo Clinic is in Olmstead County and was the source of the data for this report. The data are the first published in the literature to show the incidence of aortic dissection related to bicuspid aortic valve. The risk of aortic dissection appears to be 8 times higher in those with bicuspid aortic valve compared with the general population. Because aortic dissection is generally rare to begin with, the overall prevalence in bicuspid aortic valve therefore is low in terms of absolute prevalence (1.3%). Despite a low occurrence of dissection, patients with bicuspid aortic valve incurred significant morbidity, with 25-year risks of aortic surgery of 25%, aneurysm formation of 26%, and valve replacement of 53%. This study confirms that aortic valve replacement remains the most common complication of patients with bicuspid aortic valve.

The bottom line from this report is that there is a clinical aortopathy associated with bicuspid aortic valve with associated excess risk of aneurysm formation and aortic dissection. Fortunately the incidence of actual dissection is low. This incidence of dissection is highest in patients older than 50 years and higher in those with baseline aortic aneurysms, highlighting the importance of close monitoring and current guideline implementation for periodic echocardiography in this patient population. Ultimately more than 25% of patients with the most common form of congenital heart disease will require some surgery during their lifetime to manage complications of the problem. What we as pediatricians consider to be a benign form of congenital heart disease is actually not so benign when one adds up all the numbers over a whole life span.

This commentary closes with mention of a new device related to blood vessels, specifically how to puncture one. Every year hundreds of thousands of people develop medical complications such as nerve injury when hypodermic needles penetrate deeper than they should. A novel needle devised by researchers at Harvard Medical School and their colleagues automatically stops itself from going too far. The force of the first push of the device's plunger goes only to a blunt, flexible wire inside the hollow needle. As long as this filament remains unbent, a special clutch keeps the rest of the needle from advancing. On entering resistance from tissue, the wire buckles and the clutch permits the entire needle to move forward. On reaching a target cavity, such as a blood vessel, the filament no longer faces resistance and so straightens out, preventing the needle from proceeding, but uncovering the tip to allow medicine out. This is described by Choi.[1] As of this writing, the device is not yet on the market.

**J. A. Stockman III, MD**

*Reference*

1. Choi CQ. Medical devices: point taken. *Scientific American.* June 2009:31.

---

### A right-to-left shunt in children with arterial ischaemic stroke

Perkovič-Benedik M, Zaletel M, Pečarič-Meglič N, et al (Univ Med Centre Ljubljana, Slovenia)
*Arch Dis Child* 96:461-467, 2011

---

*Objective.*—To compare the prevalence and grade of right-to-left shunt (RLS) in children with arterial ischaemic stroke (AIS) and in controls.

*Design.*—Prospective study.

*Setting.*—Tertiary paediatric referral centre.

*Patients.*—30 consecutive children with AIS.

*Intervention.*—Contrast transcranial Doppler (cTCD) with Valsalva manoeuvre was performed in children with AIS and in controls.

*Main Outcome Measures.*—Detection and quantification of RLS.

*Results.*—Logistic regression analysis showed that RLS was significantly associated with AIS and prothrombotic disorders or with AIS of undetermined aetiology (OR 6.10; 95% CI 1.41 to 26.3; $p = 0.015$). The prevalence of RLS was significantly higher in a group of children with AIS and prothrombotic disorders or with AIS of undetermined aetiology compared to controls ($p < 0.05$). Significantly more microembolic signals (MES) were detected in a group of children with AIS and prothrombotic disorders or with AIS of undetermined aetiology than in controls ($p < 0.005$).

*Conclusions.*—Both the prevalence of RLS and number of detected MES were significantly higher in a group of children with AIS and prothrombotic disorders or with AIS of undetermined aetiology compared to controls. These findings suggest that paradoxical embolism may be an underestimated cause of AIS in children, particularly those with AIS and prothrombotic disorders or with AIS of undetermined aetiology.

▶ Pediatricians do not often see youngsters with arterial ischemic strokes, but they do occur in infants, children, and adolescents. If a stroke occurs, one should be thinking about the possibility that the patient might have a patent foramen ovale (PFO). All too often, the etiology of an arterial ischemic stroke remains undetermined, but recently paradoxical embolism across the PFO has been suggested as a possible etiology of many of these children. This is particularly true of children who have a genetic or acquired tendency toward venous thromboembolism. All it takes, at the wrong point in time, is a Valsalva maneuver, and such patients may have a right-to-left shunt at the atrial level resulting in a thromboembolism.

Perkovič-Benedik et al have studied this problem. It appears that transcranial Doppler with bubble contrast and Valsalva appears to be a more sensitive technique than echocardiography for detecting PFO in both children and adults. The technique described allows the detection of paradoxical embolism from the systemic venous circulation to the right side of the heart and then on to the brain. There are well-documented case reports in series of PFO associated with such strokes, both in neonates and in older children, thus the value of a good diagnostic test to rule the problem in or out.

While on the topic of things cardiologic, a new iPhone app provides tons of fun for physician care providers. The app is the "iStethoscope" that monitors the heartbeat through sensors in the phone. This application has been downloaded in droves since a free version was introduced in September 2010.[1]

I close with the observation on how in ancient times, the heart was held in high esteem. A review of ancient Greek philosophical and medical texts notes that earlier primitive beliefs attributed great significance to the heart and accounted for cannibalistic behaviors such as possessing and eating a defeated enemy's heart. Mental functions such as thinking and feeling have been attributed to the heart since the times of Greek mythology. The brain's role was underestimated, probably because it was "silent" compared with the beating heart—even after Galen discovered the course of the cranial and spinal nerves.[2]

**J. A. Stockman III, MD**

*Reference*

1. iPhone app to replace the stethoscope. *The Telegraph*. http://www.telegraph.co.uk/technology/apple/7971950/iPhone-app-to-replace-the-stethoscope.html. Published August 31, 2010. Accessed November 10, 2011.
2. Editorial comment. How the heart was viewed in ancient times. *BMJ*. 2011;342: 390.

# 10 Infectious Diseases and Immunology

**Markers for bacterial infection in children with fever without source**
Manzano S, Bailey B, Gervaix A, et al (Université de Montréal, Quebec, Canada; Children's Hosp HUG, Geneva, Switzerland)
*Arch Dis Child* 96:440-446, 2011

*Objectives.*—To compare the diagnostic properties of procalcitonin (PCT), C reactive protein (CRP), total white blood cells count (WBC), absolute neutrophil count (ANC) and clinical evaluation to detect serious bacterial infection (SBI) in children with fever without source.

*Design.*—Prospective cohort study.

*Setting.*—Paediatric emergency department of a tertiary care hospital.

*Participants.*—Children aged 1–36 months with fever and no identified source of infection.

*Intervention.*—Complete blood count, blood culture, urine analysis and culture. PCT and CRP were also measured and SBI probability evaluated clinically with a visual analogue scale before disclosing tests results.

*Outcome Measure.*—Area under the curves (AUC) of the receiver operating characteristic curves.

*Results.*—Among the 328 children included in the study, 54 (16%) were diagnosed with an SBI: 48 urinary tract infections, 4 pneumonias, 1 meningitis and 1 bacteraemia. The AUC were similar for PCT (0.82; 95% CI 0.77 to 0.86), CRP (0.88; 95% CI 0.84 to 0.91), WBC (0.81; 95% CI 0.76 to 0.85) and ANC (0.80; 95% CI 0.75 to 0.84). The only statistically significant difference was between CRP and ANC ($\Delta$ AUC 0.08; 95% CI 0.01 to 0.16). It is important to note that all the surrogate markers were statistically superior to the clinical evaluation that had an AUC of only 0.59 (95% CI 0.54 to 0.65).

*Conclusion.*—The study data demonstrate that CRP, PCT, WBC and ANC had almost similar diagnostic properties and were superior to clinical evaluation in predicting SBI in children aged 1 month to 3 years (Table 3).

▶ This report reminds us that anything we once knew about use of the white blood cell count and other markers of inflammation in the detection of serious bacterial infection in children with fever became outdated with the introduction of the widespread use of the pneumococcal vaccine. This vaccine has significantly

TABLE 3.—Diagnostic Accuracy of PCT, CRP, WBC, ANC and Clinical Evaluation on a VAS to Detect an SBI in Children Aged 1–36 Months Presenting to a Paediatric Emergency Department With Fever Without Source

| Variable Best Cut-Off | Sensitivity (95% CI) | Specificity (95% CI) | Positive Predictive Value (95% CI) | Negative Predictive Value (95% CI) |
|---|---|---|---|---|
| PCT >0.20 ng/ml | 85.2 (74.4 to 92.1) | 69.7 (67.6 to 71.1) | 35.7 (31.2 to 38.6) | 96.0 (93.1 to 97.9) |
| CRP >17.7 mg/l | 94.4 (85.5 to 98.1) | 68.6 (66.9 to 69.3) | 37.2 (33.7 to 38.7) | 98.4 (95.9 to 99.5) |
| WBC >14 100×10$^6$/l | 81.5 (70.3 to 89.3) | 70.8 (68.6 to 72.4) | 35.5 (30.6 to 38.9) | 95.1 (92.1 to 97.2) |
| ANC >5200×10$^6$/l | 87.0 (76.5 to 93.5) | 59.9 (57.8 to 61.1) | 29.9 (26.3 to 32.1) | 95.9 (92.6 to 97.9) |
| VAS >14.8% | 68.5 (56.5 to 78.8) | 38.7 (36.3 to 40.7) | 18.0 (14.9 to 20.7) | 86.2 (80.9 to 90.7) |

ANC, absolute neutrophil count; CRP, C reactive protein; PCT, procalcitonin; SBI, serious bacterial infection; VAS, visual analogue scale; WBC, white blood cells count.

reduced the prevalence of serious bacterial infection and, in particular, of occult bacteremia in children younger than 3 years. Still, we commonly use a total white blood cell count (WBC) and absolute neutrophil count (ANC), hoping to distinguish such children, but these tests have disappointing diagnostic properties. For this reason, other surrogate markers of serious bacterial infection are being used now, including C-reactive protein (CRP) and procalcitonin (PCT), both of which have been shown to have better predictive value for serious bacterial infection than a white blood cell count. Nonetheless, the use of these surrogate markers is not well established in the postpneumococcal vaccination era since their diagnostic properties depend on the prevalence of the disease detected. In addition, it is not known whether a clinical evaluation by a physician is good enough to rule out serious bacterial infection when most of the serious bacterial infections these days are more likely caused by urinary tract infections.

Manzano et al undertook a study to compare the diagnostic properties of PCT, CRP, WBC, and ANC and a clinical evaluation to detect serious bacterial infection in children age 1 month to 36 months presenting to a pediatric emergency department with fever without a source. This study was prospective. Based on multilevel likelihood ratios, the study suggests that CRP, PTC, WBC, and ANC have almost similar diagnostic properties, and each in the aggregate are superior to a clinical evaluation by a seasoned physician in predicting serious bacterial infection in those 1 month to 36 months of age. Also, the more abnormal each of these test results, the higher the probability of having a serious bacterial infection. The authors suggest that by reporting multilevel likelihood ratios, one can show that these markers play an important role in the decision-making process. The table shows the diagnostic accuracy of tests and a clinical evaluation.

This commentary closes with the observation that one cause of serious illness at any age, influenza, is one that carries a greater risk of morbidity and mortality if associated fever is treated with antipyretics. In animal studies, treatment with antipyretics for influenza infection actually increases the risk of death. There are no randomized, placebo-controlled trials currently of antipyretics in human influenza infection, and very few other clinical data are available by which to assess their actual efficacy versus untoward consequences. To learn more about this, see the *Journal of the Royal Society of Medicine* report in 2010.[1]

**J. A. Stockman III, MD**

*Reference*

1. Eyers S, Weatherall M, Shirtcliffe P, et al. The effect on mortality of antipyretics in the treatment of influenza infection: systematic review and meta-analysis. *J R Soc Med.* 2010;103:403-411.

---

## Is a Lumbar Puncture Necessary When Evaluating Febrile Infants (30 to 90 Days of Age) With an Abnormal Urinalysis?

Paquette K, Cheng MP, McGillivray D, et al (McGill Univ, Montréal, Québec, Canada)
*Pediatr Emerg Care* 27:1057-1061, 2011

---

*Objectives.*—Guidelines for the management of febrile infants aged 30 to 90 days presenting to the emergency department (ED) suggest that a lumbar puncture (LP) should be performed routinely if a positive urinalysis is found during initial investigations. The aim of our study was to assess the necessity of routine LPs in infants aged 30 to 90 days presenting to the ED for a fever without source but are found to have a positive urine analysis.

*Methods.*—We retrospectively reviewed the records of all infants aged 30 to 90 days, presenting to the Montreal Children's Hospital ED from October 2001 to August 2005 who underwent an LP for bacterial culture, in addition to urinalysis and blood and urine cultures. Descriptive statistics and their corresponding confidence intervals were used.

*Results.* Overall, 392 infants were identified using the microbiology laboratory database. Fifty-seven patients had an abnormal urinalysis. Of these, 1 infant (71 days old) had an *Escherichia coli* urinary tract infection, bacteremia, and meningitis. This patient, however, was not well on history, and the peripheral white blood cell count was low at $2.9 \times 10^9$/L. Thus, the negative predictive value of an abnormal urinalysis for meningitis was 98.2%.

*Conclusions.*—Routine LPs are not required in infants (30–90 days) presenting to the ED with a fever and a positive urinalysis if they are considered at low risk for serious bacterial infection based on clinical and laboratory criteria. However, we recommend that judicious clinical judgment be used; in doubt, an LP should be performed before empiric antibiotic therapy is begun.

▶ This report addresses the age-old question of whether a lumbar puncture (LP) must be performed as part of the evaluation of febrile infants 1 to 3 months of age. Most pediatricians in practice know that this has been a controversial topic. A number of ways of thinking about the evaluation of febrile infants have appeared in the literature. The approach has been based on various signs and symptoms. The most commonly used approach is based on protocols that have emanated from Rochester, Philadelphia, and Boston. These protocols place febrile neonates into high-risk and low-risk categories for serious bacterial infections (SBIs), largely related to the clinical appearance and baseline laboratory investigation results. The Rochester criteria, for example, note that an infant is at low risk of having an SBI if he or she had a normal pregnancy and birth, was well since birth, appears nontoxic at emergency room presentation in the presence of a completely normal physical examination, and investigations reveal a white blood cell count between 5 and $15 \times 10^9$/L, a differential with bands of less than $1.5 \times 10^9$/L, and a urinalysis with less than 10 white blood cells per high-power field. If an infant is assessed to have a low risk of infection, an LP is not necessary according to the protocol emanating from New York. This recommendation is in opposition to the protocols published from Boston and Philadelphia that deem an LP necessary in all cases. The Rochester criteria, however, suggest that if a urinalysis is positive, the infant must go through a full septic workup including an LP and the use of antibiotics pending culture results.

Paquette et al, from the Children's Hospital in Montreal, designed a study to assess the necessity of performing routine LPs in infants 30 to 90 days of age presenting to the emergency department with fever and found to have a positive urinalysis but who are otherwise well by clinical and laboratory investigation. Their hypothesis was that a lumbar puncture would not be necessary in all such infants. In this study, 392 patients were identified as having a lumbar puncture for fever without an apparent source. Of the 392 infants, 4 were ultimately diagnosed with bacterial meningitis, but of these, only one had an abnormal urinalysis.

The authors of this report suggest that routine LPs may not be required in infants in this age group if the urinalysis is compatible with a urinary tract infection and if they are considered low risk of serious bacterial infection according to the Rochester criteria. The negative predictive value of an abnormal urinalysis alone for meningitis in this report again was 98.2%. The authors are very cautious with their conclusions, recommending that judicious clinical judgment be used and, in the event of uncertainty, a lumbar puncture should be performed prior to empiric antibiotic therapy.

This commentary closes with a thought or two about antibiotics. If you think the widespread use of antibiotics in livestock is a danger to humans, think about the poor vulture. Eating carcasses of livestock treated with antibiotics appears to be wrecking the immune systems of vultures, at least in Spain, according to a new study. Spain is the European strong hold of vultures who have long lived off of dead livestock dumped by farmers at sites called *muladares*. Because research suggests the overuse of antibiotics can suppress the immune system, investigators have examined and now have reported that high antibiotic levels in the birds are associated with severe bacterial and fungal diseases. The investigators climbed trees to reach vulture nests in Central Spain and took blood samples from 71 nestlings of three species and then compared their immune system and blood samples with vultures in Southern and Western Spain where fewer antibiotics are used and the birds feed mainly on wild prey. Both the cellular and the humoral immune systems of the Central Spain vultures were suppressed, some to a remarkable degree. Needless to say, all of us need to be aware of the unexpected effects of widespread antibiotic use in cattle, pigs, etc.[1]

**J. A. Stockman III, MD**

*Reference*

1. Editorial comment. Antibiotics bad for vultures. *Science.* 2009;323:5922.

---

## Diagnosis of Bacteremia in Febrile Neutropenic Episodes in Children With Cancer: Microbiologic and Molecular Approach

Santolaya ME, Farfán MJ, De La Maza V, et al (Hosp L. Calvo Mackenna, Santiago, Chile; et al)
*Pediatr Infect Dis J* 30:957-961, 2011

---

*Background.*—Bacterial isolation using conventional microbiologic techniques rarely surpasses 25% in children with clinical and laboratory findings indicative of an invasive bacterial infection. The aim of this study was to determine the role of real-time polymerase chain reaction (RT-PCR) from whole blood samples compared with automated blood cultures (BC) in detection of relevant microorganisms causing bacteremia in episodes of high-risk febrile neutropenia (HRFN) in children with cancer.

*Methods.*—Children presenting with HRFN at 6 hospitals in Santiago, Chile, were invited to participate. Blood samples were obtained at admission for BC, and at admission and 24 hours for RT-PCR targeting DNA of *Escherichia coli, Staphylococcus aureus,* and *Pseudomonas aeruginosa* causing bacteremia in children with HRFN.

*Results.*—A total of 177 HRFN episodes were evaluated from May 2009 to August 2010, of which 29 (16.3%) had positive BC, 9 (5%) positive for 1 of the 3 selected bacterial species: 5 for *E. coli,* 3 for *S. aureus,* and 1 for *P. aeruginosa.* RT-PCR detected 39 bacteria in 36 episodes (20%): 14 *E. coli,* 20 *S. aureus,* and 5 *P. aeruginosa.* The sensitivity, specificity, and positive and negative predictive values of RT-PCR compared with BC were 56%, 80%, 13%, and 97%. The final clinical diagnosis was compatible with an invasive bacterial infection in 30/36 (83%) RT-PCR-positive episodes.

*Conclusions.*—In our series, RT-PCR significantly improved detection of the most relevant bacteria associated with HRFN episodes. Large number of patients and close clinical monitoring, in addition to improved RT-PCR techniques will be required to fully recommend RT-PCR-based diagnosis for the routine workup of children with cancer, fever, and neutropenia.

▶ All of us have seen febrile neutropenic children, usually in the situation of childhood cancer. Try as we may to isolate bacteria as a cause of serious illness, bacterial isolation using conventional microbiologic techniques rarely exceeds 25% in children with clinical signs and laboratory findings that would otherwise suggest a high risk for invasive bacterial infection. This percentage increases to

60% in children who have overt clinical sepsis and 80% among children who die with a sepsislike syndrome. The rub is that 75% of children with a high-risk febrile neutropenia who do not appear septic will not have an organism detected by currently available conventional microbiologic techniques.

Santolaya et al have added the use of realtime polymerase chain reaction (PCR) to determine the bacterial etiology of febrile neutropenic episodes in children with cancer. The significant majority of all children who have a bacterial cause identified tend to have it as a result of infection with *Escherichia coli*, *Klebsiella pneumoniae*, *Pseudomonas aeruginosa*, coagulase-negative *Staphylococcus*, *Staphylococcus aureus*, and *Viridans* group *Streptococcus*. Of these organisms, the most common species identified are *E coli*, *S aureus*, and *P aeruginosa*. These investigators examined PCR panels against commonly found bacteria, examining whole blood samples of febrile neutropenic cancer patients ranging in age from 4 to 13 years. There were 177 episodes of high-risk febrile neutropenia evaluated. Of the 177 episodes, 16.3% had a positive blood culture. The PCR panel was performed for *E coli*, *S aureus*, and *P aeruginosa*. Five percent of febrile neutropenic episodes had positive blood cultures for these organisms, whereas PCR detected 20% of episodes to have infection with these organisms, increasing the yield for these organisms by more than 4-fold. Interestingly, PCR positivity was highest at 24 hours following admission and the start of antibiotics. One can hypothesize that the increase in findings of positive PCR are the result of increased bacterial DNA in the blood at 24 hours, resulting from lysis of organisms once antibiotics were instituted.

Although the PCR panel used here did not cover all the infectious organisms that can cause problems in febrile neutropenic patients, the study does suggest the possibility that DNA analysis, complemented by traditional bacterial microbiologic studies, would yield higher rates of accurate diagnosis for the causes of infections when they are present.

PCR has been around a long time as part of the triage for bacterial infection. It has not widely caught on because the technology has not been readily implementable in the standard laboratory setting. Hopefully in the future it will be.

This commentary closes with a quiz. You are traveling throughout Indonesia on a holiday. Your 5-year-old daughter is bitten by a Komodo dragon. The bite looks quite superficial. You clean the wound with hydrogen peroxide. Everything looks great. Should you still worry? The answer is yes, you should worry. These creatures are lizards that grow 8 to 10 feet in length, nose to tip of tail. They have razor sharp teeth and tear apart a goat, pig, or other unfortunate animals in a matter of minutes, but they have evolved a more clever way of killing that requires less energy expenditure. They bite the prey once, thereby injecting oral bacteria that induce sepsis. They then wait for the animal to die even if it takes a couple of weeks before inviting dragon friends to feast on the carrion. They never eat flesh that is fresh, only putrefied matter. The bacteria that cause the sepsis have not been investigated. The lesson: Beware the dragon's bite![1]

**J. A. Stockman III, MD**

*Reference*

1. Editorial comment. Of dragons and bacteria. *Pediatr Infect Dis J Newsletter.* February 2012;1.

## Mortality after Fluid Bolus in African Children with Severe Infection

Maitland K, for the FEAST Trial Group (Kenya Med Res Inst (KEMRI)—Wellcome Trust Res Programme, Kilifi; et al)

*N Engl J Med* 364:2483-2495, 2011

*Background.*—The role of fluid resuscitation in the treatment of children with shock and life-threatening infections who live in resource-limited settings is not established.

*Methods.*—We randomly assigned children with severe febrile illness and impaired perfusion to receive boluses of 20 to 40 ml of 5% albumin solution (albumin-bolus group) or 0.9% saline solution (saline-bolus group) per kilogram of body weight or no bolus (control group) at the time of admission to a hospital in Uganda, Kenya, or Tanzania (stratum A); children with severe hypotension were randomly assigned to one of the bolus groups only (stratum B). All children received appropriate antimicrobial treatment, intravenous maintenance fluids, and supportive care, according to guidelines. Children with malnutrition or gastroenteritis were excluded. The primary end point was 48-hour mortality; secondary end points included pulmonary edema, increased intracranial pressure, and mortality or neurologic sequelae at 4 weeks.

*Results.*—The data and safety monitoring committee recommended halting recruitment after 3141 of the projected 3600 children in stratum A were enrolled. Malaria status (57% overall) and clinical severity were similar across groups. The 48-hour mortality was 10.6% (111 of 1050 children), 10.5% (110 of 1047 children), and 7.3% (76 of 1044 children) in the albumin-bolus, saline-bolus, and control groups, respectively (relative risk for saline bolus vs. control, 1.44; 95% confidence interval [CI], 1.09 to 1.90; $P = 0.01$; relative risk for albumin bolus vs. saline bolus, 1.01; 95% CI, 0.78 to 1.29; $P = 0.96$; and relative risk for any bolus vs. control, 1.45; 95% CI, 1.13 to 1.86; $P = 0.003$). The 4-week mortality was 12.2%, 12.0%, and 8.7% in the three groups, respectively ($P = 0.004$ for the comparison of bolus with control). Neurologic sequelae occurred in 2.2%, 1.9%, and 2.0% of the children in the respective groups ($P = 0.92$), and pulmonary edema or increased intracranial pressure occurred in 2.6%, 2.2%, and 1.7% ($P = 0.17$), respectively. In stratum B, 69% of the children (9 of 13) in the albumin-bolus group and 56% (9 of 16) in the saline-bolus group died ($P = 0.45$). The results were consistent across centers and across subgroups according to the severity of shock and status with respect to malaria, coma, sepsis, acidosis, and severe anemia.

*Conclusions.*—Fluid boluses significantly increased 48-hour mortality in critically ill children with impaired perfusion in these resource-limited settings in Africa. (Funded by the Medical Research Council, United Kingdom; FEAST Current Controlled Trials number, ISRCTN69856593.)

▶ Even though this report focuses on the intravenous management of youngsters with serious infections in Africa, there is a lot to be learned about how we might change our management approaches on US shores. Fluid resuscitation remains a fundamental intervention in the treatment of critically ill patients, although there is very little evidence to guide care providers about the best type of resuscitation fluid, the volumes that should be given, and the timing of the administration itself with respect to rates of fluid administration. We do know that complications can result from excessive volumes of fluid given as part of a resuscitation. We also know that the type of resuscitation fluid may adversely affect patients in specific clinical circumstances. As one example, albumin is associated with increased mortality in patients with traumatic brain injury. High-molecular-weight preparations of hydroxyethyl starch are associated with acute renal injury in patients with severe sepsis. At the same time, albumin shows improved outcomes when used in resuscitating children with severe malaria. The information provided in the report by Maitland et al shows results of the Fluid Expansion as Supportive Therapy (FEAST) trial. The trial itself is a randomized controlled study that was conducted in 6 hospitals in Kenya, Tanzania, and Uganda. The trial assessed the benefits and adverse outcomes of bolus-fluid resuscitation with albumin or saline as compared with no bolus fluid in children with febrile medical illness and impaired perfusion. Children with severe hypotension or decompensated shock received boluses of either albumin or saline. The centers where these trials were carried out had no access to intensive care units, and the trial included a comprehensive education program aimed at optimizing early case recognition and treating emergency pediatric life support. The primary outcome was mortality at 48 hours from the time of presentation. The design of the trial has been very carefully reviewed, and one editorial on the results from the trial notes the excellent study design that was used.[1]

The results from this trial are quite interesting. The trial was stopped after the recruitment of 3141 patients when bolus-fluid resuscitation with either albumin or saline was shown to increase the absolute risk of death at 48 hours by 3.3 percentage points and the risk of death, neurologic sequelae, or both at 4 weeks by 4 percentage points. No difference in mortality was observed in patients with decompensated shock, although these patients were few in number and had significantly higher mortality. The excess mortality associated with bolus-fluid resuscitation was consistent across all prespecified subgroups of age, lactate level, base deficit, presence or absence of severe anemia, and status with respect to coma and malaria.

There is no question that the results of the FEAST trial are contrary to clinical opinion and practice, but the results speak for themselves. It is clear that the entrenched practice of fluid-bolus resuscitation in patients with compensated shock remains highly questionable. One can only speculate about the mechanisms by which fluid-bolus resuscitation has adverse biologic effects in these patients. It is suggested that potential mechanisms might include the interruption of genetically determined catecholamine-mediated host defense responses by the rapid increase in plasma volume, which might result in reperfusion injury. Similarly, transient hypervolemia or hyperosmolality might exacerbate capillary leak in patients who are susceptible to intracranial hypertension or pulmonary edema, with fatal consequences.

The important question is how clinicians who work under circumstances very different from those in this trial, that is those of us who work in high-income countries with access to intensive care units, should embrace the results of this study. In the editorial that accompanied this report, it is stated that "it seems clear that the results of this trial indicate that fluid-bolus resuscitation with either crystalloids or colloids in patients with compensated shock who do not have a clinical fluid deficit must be practiced with much greater caution than is now the case and with increased vigilance."[1] These seem like wise words in view of the results and quality of the FEAST report. The quality of the research reported cannot be ignored simply because the study was carried out in sub-Saharan Africa. It will be interesting to see how new treatment guidelines are designed so that none of us are left on our own with trying to readjust how we manage patients who are severely ill.

This commentary closes with an observation related to an anniversary. In case you missed it, 2009 was the centennial of the discovery of Chagas disease, named for Carlos Chagas, MD. The discovery of this disease is a fascinating story. Because of an epidemic of malaria sickening hundreds of railroad workers in Brazil, government officials contacted Oswaldo Cruz, MD, Brazil's famed infectious disease fighter and Director of what is now known as the Oswaldo Cruz Institute, a vaccine and sera production center in Rio de Janeiro. Cruz chose to send a young researcher from the institute, Carlos Chagas, MD, out in the field to investigate a solution to the malaria problem. By age 28, Chagas had already two successful antimalaria campaigns under his belt and successfully dealt with the problem that was occurring with railroad workers. He did find something interesting that fascinated him while doing this work. He came across nocturnal blood-sucking Triatominae insects, also known as kissing bugs because they bite human victims on the face near the lips and eyes. Chagas wanted to know more about the bug's biology and whether they were capable of transmitting any disease. He suspected that these insects might be associated with unexplained cardiac abnormalities he found in many of the railroad workers, regardless of their malaria status. He examined the bugs and found they harbored a new species of trypanosome that, when transmitted in the laboratory to monkeys and other small animals, could be fatal. He named the protozoan parasite *Trypanosoma cruzi* for Cruz, his boss and mentor. Chagas also found an ill cat that was infected with *T cruzi*, but more importantly, in the same household was a young girl with a high fever and additional symptoms: an enlarged spleen, liver, lymph nodes, and facial swelling. A blood sample from the girl revealed the presence of *T cruzi*.

By combining his knowledge of insect-transmitted malaria with a high level of clinical suspicion and shoe-leather epidemiology, Chagas made a unique discovery of a new disease. In a span of just 2 years, he linked Triatomines with a new species of parasite that caused acute and chronic infectious illness. He was honored by the Brazilian Academy of Medicine, which named the new disease for Chagas. It is said that Chagas is the only researcher to describe, solely on his own, a new infectious disease, its pathogen, its vector, its host, and the clinical manifestations and epidemiology related to the disease. It is extremely unlikely that what Chagas achieved more than a century ago will ever be repeated by a single researcher again.[2]

**J. A. Stockman III, MD**

*References*

1. Myburgh JA. Fluid resuscitation in acute illness—time to reappraise the basics. *N Engl J Med.* 2011;364:2543-2544.
2. Voelket R. A century after Chagas disease discovery, hurdles to tackling the infection remain. *JAMA.* 2009;302:1045.

## Alternative Vaccination Schedule Preferences Among Parents of Young Children

Dempsey AF, Schaffer S, Singer D, et al (Univ of Michigan, Ann Arbor)
*Pediatrics* 128:848-856, 2011

*Objective.*—Increasing numbers of parents use alternative vaccination schedules that differ from the recommended childhood vaccination schedule for their children. We sought to describe national patterns of alternative vaccination schedule use and the potential "malleability" of parents' current vaccination schedule choices.

*Methods.*—We performed a cross-sectional, Internet-based survey of a nationally representative sample of parents of children 6 months to 6 years of age. Bivariate and multivariate analyses determined associations between demographic and attitudinal factors and alternative vaccination schedule use.

*Results.*—The response rate was 61% ($N = 748$). Of the 13% of parents who reported following an alternative vaccination schedule, most refused only certain vaccines (53%) and/or delayed some vaccines until the child was older (55%). Only 17% reported refusing all vaccines. In multivariate models, nonblack race and not having a regular health care provider for the child were the only factors significantly associated with higher odds of using an alternative schedule. A large proportion of alternative vaccinators (30%) reported having initially followed the recommended vaccination schedule. Among parents following the recommended vaccination schedule, 28% thought that delaying vaccine doses was safer than the schedule they used, and 22% disagreed that the best vaccination schedule to follow was the one recommended by vaccination experts.

*Conclusions.*—More than 1 of 10 parents of young children currently use an alternative vaccination schedule. In addition, a large proportion of parents currently following the recommended schedule seem to be "at risk" for switching to an alternative schedule.

▶ Surveys of parents show that one-quarter still hold the mistaken belief that vaccines can cause autism in healthy children, and more than 1 in 10 have refused at least 1 recommended vaccine. In California, 10 children died in 2010 during the worst whooping cough outbreak to sweep the state since 1947. In the first half of 2011, the Centers for Disease Control and Prevention (CDC) recorded 10 measles outbreaks—the largest of which occurred in Minnesota County, where many children are unvaccinated because of parent concerns about the safety of the standard MMR vaccine against measles, mumps, and rubella. Data from Kaiser Permanente's Institute for Healthcare Research suggest that unvaccinated children are roughly 23 times more likely to develop whooping cough, 9 times more likely to be infected with chickenpox, and 6.5 times more likely to be hospitalized with pneumonia or pneumococcal disease than vaccinated children from the same communities. These results also show the flaws in the "free rider" argument, which erroneously suggests that unvaccinated children can avoid any real or perceived risks of inoculation, because enough other children will have been vaccinated to protect the untreated child. Herd immunity does not necessarily cover the whole herd. If you are the one youngster in the herd who gets measles, for example, 1 of 20 will come down with pneumonia. One of 1000 will suffer a measles-related encephalitis leading to convulsions and potentially mental retardation, and 1 to 2 of 1000 will die.

The data from Dempsey et al show how pervasive the thinking is on the part of antivaccinationists or even on the part of worried parents. Dempsey's study is one of the first national studies to detail parents' views of alternative vaccination schedules for their young children showing that nearly 1 of 10 parents report using a vaccination schedule other than that recommended by the CDC. An even larger proportion of parents currently following the recommended schedule have attitudes that suggest they may in fact switch to an alternative schedule at some time in the future. Daily and Glanz discuss this topic in a recent issue of *Scientific American*.[1] These commentators note that pediatricians typically first bring up the need for vaccines during the well-baby check up at about 2 months of age. This visit is jam-packed with topics such as growth and development; feeding difficulties; measurements of height, weight, and head circumference; and a full examination and discussion of growth patterns, introduction of solid foods later in infancy, and sleep patterns. Somewhere in that visit is the discussion about the required schedule for recommended inoculations: the first DTaP, polio, the second hepatitis B vaccine, the pneumococcal conjugate vaccine, the HiB vaccine, and finally the rotavirus vaccine. Unfortunately, it is at this point that many questions are unleashed by parents with little actual time left to hold a decent conversation that could last another additional 20 minutes or so. Daily and Glanz suggest that to counter this phenomenon, discussion about vaccinations with medical professionals should begin long before: either during or prior to pregnancy. In their editorial commentary in *Scientific American*, the authors provide a complete and detailed analysis of what can and should be discussed with parents about the "cost" of not vaccinating according to schedule. This commentary is well worth reading, copying, and handing to parents and those who are soon to be parents.

This commentary about vaccines closes with a thought on how quickly one can vaccinate if one is efficient. The record is held by officials in Louisville, Kentucky (population 1.2 million), who found a new way to rapidly inoculate a population. In 2008, the Public Health Department offered free seasonal flu shots at the empty county fairground, a massive complex with good road transportation. The complex had a single entry point with toll booths, which is where they set up 9 inoculation stations. Hundreds of cars were lined up at the appointed hour. Subjects were asked to roll up their sleeves and roll down their windows by the time they hit the toll booth. The plan allowed 16 seconds to administer the injection. At the peak of the vaccination effort, officials had administered 1000 flu shots in just 40 minutes.[2]

**J. A. Stockman III, MD**

*References*

1. Daily MF, Glanz JM. Straight talk about vaccination: parents need better information ideally before a baby is born. *Sci Am.* 2011;118:32-33.
2. Roehr B. Drive-in vaccination allows 16 seconds per shot. *BMJ.* 2009;339:447.

## Temperature of Foods Sent by Parents of Preschool-Aged Children

Almansour FD, Sweitzer SJ, Magness AA, et al (Univ of Texas, Austin; et al)
*Pediatrics* 128:519-523, 2011

*Objective.*—To measure the temperatures of foods in sack lunches of preschool-aged children before consumption at child care centers.

*Methods.*—All parents of 3- to 5-year-old children in full-time child care at 9 central Texas centers were invited to participate in the study. Foods packed by the parents for lunch were individually removed from the sack and immediately measured with noncontact temperature guns 1.5 hours before food was served to the children. Type of food and number of ice packs in the lunch sack were also recorded. Descriptive analyses were conducted by using SPSS 13.0 for Windows.

*Results.*—Lunches, with at least 1 perishable item in each, were assessed from 235 parent-child dyads. Approximately 39% ($n = 276$) of the 705 lunches analyzed had no ice packs, 45.1% ($n = 318$) had 1 ice pack, and 88.2% ($n = 622$) of lunches were at ambient temperatures. Only 1.6% ($n = 22$) of perishable items ($n = 1361$) were in the safe temperature zone. Even with multiple ice packs, the majority of lunch items (> 90%) were at unsafe temperatures.

*Conclusions.*—These results provide initial data on how frequently sack lunches sent by parents of preschool-aged children are kept at unsafe temperatures. Education of parents and the public must be focused on methods of packing lunches that allow the food to remain in the safe temperature zone to prevent foodborne illness.

▶ This report reminds us that keeping foods above 60°C (140°F) or below 4°C (39.2°F) is critical in the prevention of foodborne illness. Foods left in the temperature zone of 4°C (39.2°F) to 60°C (140°F) for more than 2 hours are unsafe to consume and must be discarded because of the production of heat-resistant toxin by a bacteria that can cause foodborne illness. The authors of this report estimate that of the 20 million children younger than 5 years in the United States, approximately 63% are in regular child-care arrangement, and many are required to carry their own lunch to school. About 50% of day-care centers require parents to pack lunches, and this number is expected to increase in future years. This report calls such lunches "sack lunch," defined as a meal brought from home in a container to be consumed. A study in the United Kingdom concluded that on a week-by-week basis, between 52% and 78% of children take a sack lunch to school with them.[1] Sustaining a safe temperature in a sack lunch can be difficult. Even the presence of a cold pack in the sack lunch does not always guarantee lower temperatures.

Almansour et al provide us with valuable information about the risks of sack lunches brought to school. No prior study has documented the temperature of individual items in sack lunches at child-care centers. By examining the temperature of specific foods in sack lunches brought to a child-care center, this study contributes to the sparse knowledge base regarding the prevention of foodborne illness.

These investigators examined the content of sack lunches parents packed for their 3- to 5-year-old children at 9 child-care centers. Sack lunches sent by parents were assessed on 3 random, nonconsecutive days between 9:30 AM and 11:00 AM on site at the child-care centers. Food items were individually removed from the sack lunch, and temperatures were recorded using a temperature gun. These temperatures were recorded about 1.5 hours before the lunches were served to the children. The temperature gun device has a sensitivity of 0.2°C, and the infrared technology prevents cross-contamination between the instrument and the foods. Wrappers were removed from all food items before taking a temperature reading except items that were prepackaged by manufacturers (eg, Lunchables, Kraft Foods, Glenview, IL). Medical-grade gloves were used to ensure that observers had no direct contact with the food. Thermoses were opened to measure the temperature of their fluid content. The number and kind of ice packs in each sack lunch were recorded. An acceptable temperature range was noted if the temperature was less than 4°C (39.2°F) or greater than 60°C (140°F). An unacceptable temperature was noted if the food products were within the 4°C and 60°C range. Seven hundred five lunches were assessed. Although some lunches (11.8%) were stored in refrigerators, the majority (88.2%) were stored at ambient classroom temperature in a storage cube with little air circulation. Ninety-one percent of lunches were packed in thermally insulated plastic bags. Even when refrigeration was available, teachers often failed to use them, leaving lunches at room temperature for an average of 2 hours before refrigeration.

So what did the investigators find? They found that only 1.6% of 1361 perishable food items in the 705 sack lunches registered a safe temperature: 97.4% of meats, 99% of dairy, and 98.5% of vegetables were not in an acceptable temperature range when measured before the children consumed their lunches. Only 0.9% of the 458 items in 83 sack lunches located in refrigerators used by teachers were in an acceptable temperature range. Parents put 1 ice pack in 45.1% of 705 sack lunches, and 39.1% of the sack lunches had no ice packs. Of the 618 perishable items in lunches with 1 ice pack, only 14 food items were in an acceptable temperature range. Only 8.2% of items packed with multiple ice packs (2–4) were in a safe temperature range.

The dismal findings from this report were not the result of poverty on the part of the kids whose sack lunches were examined: 75% of the parents of these youngsters had household incomes over $80 000 a year, and almost 60% had household incomes of over $100 000 a year.

The authors of this report were quick to note that there is no easy solution to address the issue of inadequately stored sack lunches. It is not likely that child-care centers or schools will provide refrigeration for such lunches brought to school. This means that parents need to find better ways to keep perishable items cold, or alternatively perishable items should not be included in such sack lunches.

**J. A. Stockman III, MD**

*Reference*

1. Ofsted. *North Baddesley Junior School Inspection Report*. London, UK: Ofsted; 2008.

---

**Accuracy and Precision of the Signs and Symptoms of Streptococcal Pharyngitis in Children: A Systematic Review**
Shaikh N, Swaminathan N, Hooper EG (Children's Hosp of Pittsburgh of UPMC, PA; Maria Fareri Children's Hosp, Valhalla, NY)
*J Pediatr* 160:487-493, 2012

*Objective.*—To conduct a systematic review to determine whether clinical findings can be used to rule in or to rule out streptococcal pharyngitis in children.

*Study Design.*—Two authors independently searched MEDLINE and EMBASE. We included articles if they contained data on the accuracy of symptoms or signs of streptococcal pharyngitis, individually or combined into prediction rules, in children 3-18 years of age.

*Results.*—Thirty-eight articles with data on individual symptoms and signs and 15 articles with data on prediction rules met all inclusion criteria. In children with sore throat, the presence of a scarlatiniform rash (likelihood ratio [LR], 3.91; 95% CI, 2.00-7.62), palatal petechiae (LR, 2.69; CI, 1.92-3.77), pharyngeal exudates (LR, 1.85; CI, 1.58-2.16), vomiting (LR, 1.79; CI, 1.58-2.16), and tender cervical nodes (LR, 1.72; CI, 1.54-1.93) were moderately useful in identifying those with streptococcal pharyngitis. Nevertheless, no individual symptoms or signs were effective in ruling in or ruling out streptococcal pharyngitis.

*Conclusions.*—Symptoms and signs, either individually or combined into prediction rules, cannot be used to definitively diagnose or rule out streptococcal pharyngitis.

▶ Because streptococcal pharyngitis can lead to both suppurative and nonsuppurative complications, there is a tendency to do more than is possibly necessary to exclude the diagnosis. Indiscriminate testing of all children with sore throats will lead to antimicrobial overuse; apart from increased cost and additional discomfort, this approach is likely to result in overtreatment of carriers of group A streptococcus (defined as individuals with a positive throat culture for group A streptococcus but without an immunologic response to this organism). Accordingly, the question of whether clinical findings can be used to accurately identify high-risk children who can be treated empirically or to identify low-risk children who could be treated without additional testing is an important one.

There are guidelines for the diagnosis of children with streptococcal pharyngitis. Unfortunately, guidelines from different sources tend to differ. Although most guidelines suggest that clinical diagnosis is unreliable (and thus recommend a microbiologic testing for all suspected children), other guidelines recommend using the presence or absence of certain symptoms and signs to guide clinical decision making. The authors of this article decided to evaluate just how good signs and symptoms may be, individually or in combination, to identify children who should be tested for streptococcal pharyngitis. The investigators searched the medical literature to determine the accuracy of the clinical examination in such circumstances by searching MEDLINE for articles published from 1950 through April 2011. This computerized search was supplemented with a manual review of bibliographies of relevant articles meeting inclusion criteria.

The conclusions reached from this review were fairly straightforward. Individual clinical findings and historical symptoms were not found to be particularly useful in either ruling in or ruling out streptococcal pharyngitis. It was clear from this review that in children with sore throat, certain signs and symptoms (scarlatiniform rash, palatal petechiae, pharyngeal exudate, vomiting, and tender cervical nodes) increase the probability of streptococcal pharyngitis to over 50%. However, no finding in isolation had a sufficiently high predictive value to permit a definitive diagnosis (defined as a probability of greater than 50%). Similarly, in a child with a sore throat, individual symptoms and signs cannot be used to exclude streptococcal pharyngitis, based on the findings from this report. It should be noted that these conclusions are predicated on a relatively high prevalence of streptococcal pharyngitis in children aged 3 to 18 years with sore throats. A different conclusion would be required in groups of children who would be expected to have a substantially lower prevalence of streptococcal pharyngitis. Most children with an isolated upper respiratory tract infection do not have sore throats. These children probably have a low risk of having streptococcal pharyngitis and therefore do not require testing. Likewise, routine testing is not required in children aged less than 24 months, in whom the prevalence of streptococcal pharyngitis runs approximately 6%, or in asymptomatic siblings of children with streptococcal pharyngitis, because this is likely to result in overtreatment of carriers.

The data from this report support the current strategies suggested by the American Academy of Pediatrics, the American Heart Association, and the Infectious Disease Society of America, all of which recommend testing (rapid test or throat culture) in suspected cases and avoidance of testing in children with symptoms clearly consistent with a simple viral upper respiratory tract infection. The bottom line is that symptoms and signs, either individually or combined, cannot be built into a prediction model that definitively diagnoses or rules out streptococcal pharyngitis. If a child clearly has a simple cold, do nothing more.

If you are concerned about the signs and symptom complex being caused by streptococcal infection, it is up to you to decide what to do next.

**J. A. Stockman III, MD**

---

### Clinical Factors Associated with Pediatric Autoimmune Neuropsychiatric Disorders Associated with Streptococcal Infections

Murphy TK, Storch EA, Lewin AB, et al (Univ of South Florida, St Petersburg, FL; et al)

*J Pediatr* 160:314-319, 2012

---

*Objective.*—To explore associated clinical factors in children with pediatric autoimmune neuropsychiatric disorders associated with streptococcal infections (PANDAS).

*Study Design.*—Children with tics, obsessive-compulsive disorder, or both (n = 109) were examined with personal and family history, diagnostic interview, physical examination, medical record review, and measurement of baseline levels of streptococcal antibodies.

*Results.*—Significant group differences were found on several variables, such that children in whom PANDAS (versus without PANDAS) were more likely to have had dramatic onset, definite remissions, remission of neuropsychiatric symptoms during antibiotic therapy, a history of tonsillectomies/adenoidectomies, evidence of group A streptococcal infection, and clumsiness.

*Conclusion.*—The identification of clinical features associated with PANDAS should assist in delineating risks for this subtype of obsessive-compulsive disorder/tics.

▶ There is still a great deal of controversy about what constitutes the entity known as PANDAS (pediatric autoimmune neuropsychiatric disorders associated with streptococcal infections). PANDAS refers to the disorder in children who manifest symptoms of obsessive-compulsive disorder (OCD), tic disorders, or both, associated with a distinctive course, a temporal association with group A streptococcal infection, and evidence of concurrent neurologic abnormalities (ie, severe hyperactivity, fine motor skill loss [hand writing deterioration] or adventitious movements such as choreiform movements). It is important to distinguish PANDAS from other presentations of OCD or tics and occasionally from Sydenham chorea. The core feature of PANDAS has been a dramatic onset and a fluctuating course.

We are seeing more and more cases of OCD or tic disorders diagnosed in children prior to onset of puberty these days. This is not unlike the situation for autism spectrum disorder. Unfortunately, the causes of most cases remain ill defined, although much debate has focused on the role of group A streptococcus in causing or precipitating the so-called PANDAS. Murphy et al undertook a study of patients 4 years to 17 years of age with childhood onset of OCD or tic disorders and carried out extensive interviewing, neuropsychiatric testing, streptococcal antibody testing, and review of the medical records in some 109 affected children. Cases were assigned as PANDAS (including requirement of at least one elevated GAS-associated antibody) or non-PANDAS by the criteria used by Susan Swedo who first described the PANDAS entity.[1] The investigators found differences in those with PANDAS and non-PANDAS OCD/tics. Those ultimately diagnosed with PANDAS had a much more dramatic onset, clear-cut remissions, and history of tonsillectomy/adenoidectomy compared with those not fulfilling the requirements for PANDAS. These findings of what one might call "typical" PANDAS do help us in distinguishing this interesting disorder from disorders that might have somewhat similar findings.

**J. A. Stockman III, MD**

*Reference*

1. Swedo SE, Garvey M, Snider L, Hamilton C, Leonard HL. The PANDAS subgroup: recognition and treatment. *CNS Spectr.* 2001;6:419-422.

---

**Bacterial Meningitis in the United States, 1998–2007**
Thigpen MC, for the Emerging Infections Programs Network (Ctrs for Disease Control and Prevention, Atlanta, GA; et al)
*N Engl J Med* 364:2016 2025, 2011

---

*Background.*—The rate of bacterial meningitis declined by 55% in the United States in the early 1990s, when the *Haemophilus influenzae* type b (Hib) conjugate vaccine for infants was introduced. More recent prevention measures such as the pneumococcal conjugate vaccine and universal screening of pregnant women for group B streptococcus (GBS) have further changed the epidemiology of bacterial meningitis.

*Methods.*—We analyzed data on cases of bacterial meningitis reported among residents in eight surveillance areas of the Emerging Infections Programs Network, consisting of approximately 17.4 million persons, during 1998–2007. We defined bacterial meningitis as the presence of *H. influenzae, Streptococcus pneumoniae*, GBS, *Listeria monocytogenes*, or *Neisseria meningitidis* in cerebrospinal fluid or other normally sterile site in association with a clinical diagnosis of meningitis.

*Results.*—We identified 3188 patients with bacterial meningitis; of 3155 patients for whom outcome data were available, 466 (14.8%) died. The incidence of meningitis changed by −31% (95% confidence interval [CI], −33 to −29) during the surveillance period, from 2.00 cases per 100,000 population (95% CI, 1.85 to 2.15) in 1998–1999 to 1.38 cases per 100,000 population (95% CI 1.27 to 1.50) in 2006–2007. The median age of patients increased from 30.3 years in 1998–1999 to 41.9 years in 2006–2007 ($P < 0.001$ by the Wilcoxon rank-sum test). The case fatality rate did not change significantly: it was 15.7% in 1998–1999 and 14.3% in 2006–2007 ($P = 0.50$). Of the 1670 cases reported during 2003–2007, *S. pneumoniae* was the predominant infective species (58.0%), followed by GBS (18.1%), *N. meningitidis* (13.9%), *H. influenzae* (6.7%), and *L.*

*monocytogenes* (3.4%). An estimated 4100 cases and 500 deaths from bacterial meningitis occurred annually in the United States during 2003–2007.

*Conclusions.*—The rates of bacterial meningitis have decreased since 1998, but the disease still often results in death. With the success of pneumococcal and Hib conjugate vaccines in reducing the risk of meningitis among young children, the burden of bacterial meningitis is now borne more by older adults. (Funded by the Emerging Infections Programs, Centers for Disease Control and Prevention.)

▶ The Centers for Disease Control and Prevention (CDC) is terrific at accumulating statistical data on rates of specific types of infections. This report tells us about bacterial meningitis over a decade in the United States (1998–2007). Thirty or more years ago, studies found that 5 pathogens (*Haemophilus influenzae*, *Streptococcus pneumoniae*, *Neisseria meningitidis*, group B *Streptococcus* [GBS], and *Listeria monocytogenes*) cause more than 80% of cases of bacterial meningitis. Between 1986 and 1995, however, the incidence of bacterial meningitis from these 5 pathogens decreased by more than 50%. This was the result of the introduction in 1990 of the *H influenzae* type b conjugate vaccine for infants. This vaccine was followed by the heptavalent protein-polysaccharide pneumococcal conjugate vaccine (PCV7) in 2000. After the latter vaccine's introduction, invasive pneumococcal disease declined by 75% among children younger than 5 years and by 32% among adults 65 years of age or older.

The report abstracted from the CDC used data from their surveillance systems to describe trends in the incidence of bacterial meningitis from 1998 through 2007 and also described the epidemiology of meningitis to provide detailed information serving as a baseline for the evaluation of future interventions. The investigators were able to identify just more than 3000 patients with bacterial meningitis almost all of whom had outcome data available. During this period, the incidence of meningitis declined by almost one-third, and the age of affected patients increased from 30.3 years to 41.9 years. There was no change in the probability that a patient with meningitis would die (15.7%). The CDC noted that 500 patients die of bacterial meningitis annually in the United States, at least in recent years. In children, group B streptococcus accounts for 86.1% of cases of bacterial meningitis for those younger than 2 months of age. *N meningitidis* caused 45.9% of cases among those 11 to 17 years of age. Among the other pediatric age groups, *S pneumoniae* was the most common cause of meningitis. The pediatric case fatality rate ran 6.9% on average. Nearly 10% of this group of patients had underlying immunocompromising or chronic medical conditions. The overall case fatality rate in adults was 16.4%, with *S pneumoniae* being the most common pathogen.

It should be noted that despite significant declines in the incidence of pediatric bacterial meningitis, the incidence among infants younger than 2 months, which is the group at greatest risk for bacterial meningitis, did not decrease. The major causative organism in this vulnerable age group remains group B *Streptococcus* with infection manifested as late-onset disease 7 or more days after birth. Although intrapartum antibiotic prophylaxis has markedly reduced the risk of early-onset infection, this has had little effect on the risk of late-onset disease. The good news is that there has been a 36% decline in the rate of *L monocytogenes* meningitis. In contrast to other causes of bacterial meningitis, almost all listeriosis cases are foodborne, most commonly associated with ready-to-eat meat products. Part of the decline in children may be the result of educational efforts leading to a decreased consumption of high-risk foods, such as cheeses, by pregnant women.

All too often, children are at the bottom of the food chain of investment of dollars in medical care and prevention. At least when it comes to bacterial meningitis, the investment in vaccines against certain bacterial pathogens has really paid off.

**J. A. Stockman III, MD**

---

## German Outbreak of *Escherichia coli* O104:H4 Associated with Sprouts

Buchholz U, Bernard H, Werber D, et al (Robert Koch Inst, Berlin, Germany; et al)
*N Engl J Med* 365:1763-1770, 2011

---

*Background.*—A large outbreak of the hemolytic—uremic syndrome caused by Shiga-toxin producing *Escherichia coli* O104:H4 occurred in Germany in May 2011. The source of infection was undetermined.

*Methods.*—We conducted a matched case—control study and a recipe-based restaurant cohort study, along with environmental, trace-back, and trace-forward investigations, to determine the source of infection.

*Results.*—The case—control study included 26 case subjects with the hemolytic—uremic syndrome and 81 control subjects. The outbreak of illness was associated with sprout consumption in univariable analysis (matched odds ratio, 5.8; 95% confidence interval [CI], 1.2 to 29) and with sprout and cucumber consumption in multivariable analysis. Among case subjects, 25% reported having eaten sprouts, and 88% reported having eaten cucumbers. The recipe-based study among 10 groups of visitors to restaurant K included 152 persons, among whom bloody diarrhea or diarrhea confirmed to be associated with Shiga-toxin—producing *E. coli* developed in 31 (20%). Visitors who were served sprouts were significantly more likely to become ill (relative risk, 14.2; 95% CI, 2.6 to ∞). Sprout consumption explained 100% of cases. Trace-back investigation of sprouts from the distributor that supplied restaurant K led to producer A. All 41 case clusters with known trading connections could be explained by producer A. The outbreak strain could not be identified on seeds from the implicated lot.

*Conclusions.*—Our investigations identified sprouts as the most likely outbreak vehicle, underlining the need to take into account food items that may be overlooked during subjects' recall of consumption.

▶ It all started in May 2011 when a massive epidemic of bloody diarrhea and the hemolytic-uremic syndrome (HUS) caused by the shiga-toxin-producing *Escherichia coli* began. By the time the outbreak ended 2 months later, there were reports of more than 4000 illnesses, 800 cases of HUS, and 50 deaths in Germany and in 15 other countries. Buchholz et al tell us about this outbreak. The outbreak of lethal foodborne disease in Germany turns out to be associated with a single clone of a strain of enterohemorrhagic *E coli* classified as O104:H4. This 2011 strain was quite novel, having genes from very aggressive *E coli*. It is thought that this strain emerged because beta-lactam antibiotics had suppressed competitors for this bacterium. The outbreak was foodborne in contaminated sprouts. The initial investigation pointed to other uncooked salad foods, illustrating the difficulty in identifying vehicles in multisite outbreaks when exposures occurred days earlier and when answers are needed immediately. The chain of transmission appears to have begun in Egypt, with fecal contamination of fenugreek seeds either by human or farm animals during storage or transportation, perhaps as long ago as 2009. These seeds went to a European distributor and from there to farms in several countries. During sprout germination, bacteria multiplied and moved from farms to restaurants to consumers as well outlined by Buchholz et al. The fact that the outbreak began suddenly in early May and ended in early July—just a few weeks—suggests a pattern very consistent with a single point source.

The long median incubation period of 8 days of the epidemic in Germany and related countries is in contrast to other outbreaks of enterohemorrhagic *E coli*, which generally have incubation periods of just 3 to 4 days. This suggests that a relatively small inocula was consumed by most individuals. The outbreak was also unusual in that it had an atypical age distribution affecting adults as frequently as children (most HUS affects children) and also was characterized by a very high death rate in those who developed HUS. HUS developed quite suddenly, about 5 days after onset of diarrhea.

The total magnitude of the numbers of affected individuals overwhelmed the health care system in the European Union. In an editorial by Blaser[1] that accompanied this report, it was noted that most physicians were challenged by questions such as trying to decide whether antibiotics or steroids would help or whether plasma exchange would be of assistance. There were no easy answers. It has been suggested that it is more than likely that the next large outbreak of a similar nature could be just around the corner and could be more global than that seen in northern Europe.

For more on the epidemic profile of the *E coli* outbreak in Germany, see the excellent article that accompanied that of Buchholz by Frank et al.[2] We have certainly heard a lot about *E coli*, particularly as it relates to O157:H7, the particular strain that in the past has caused severe food poisoning linked to Jack in the Box hamburgers, Taco Bell lettuce, and prepackaged spinach. Hopefully, O104:H4 will stay far from US shores. We do know that giving certain antibiotics, including fluoroquinolones such as cipro, can kill those who have been sickened by any strain of shiga-toxin *E coli*. As bacteria are killed by antibiotics, they will release toxins in massive amounts. Fortunately, one particular group of drugs, the carbapenems, seem not to trigger a major toxin release. This is a highly specialized class of drugs given quite infrequently. Travelers with diarrhea who bring antibiotics along with them should be extremely cautious about continuing antibiotics if they develop an episode of bloody diarrhea. To learn more about *E coli* and why it is on the march, see the excellent commentary that appeared in *Scientific American.*[3]

**J. A. Stockman III, MD**

*References*

1. Blaser MJ. Deconstructing a lethal foodborne epidemic. *N Engl J Med*. 2011;365: 1835-1836.
2. Frank C, Werber D, Cramer JP, et al. Epidemic profile of Shiga-toxin-producing *Escherichia coli* O104:H4 outbreak in Germany. *N Engl J Med*. 2011;365: 1771-1780.
3. Gorman C. *E. coli* on the March: toxic strains of a common gut microbe are multiplying. *Sci Am*. August 2011:26.

---

**Management of an acute outbreak of diarrhoea-associated haemolytic uraemic syndrome with early plasma exchange in adults from southern Denmark: an observational study**

Colic E, Dieperink H, Titlestad K, et al (Odense Univ Hosp, Denmark)
*Lancet* 378:1089-1093, 2011

---

*Background.*—Diarrhoea-associated haemolytic uraemic syndrome in adults is a life-threatening, but rare multisystem disorder that is characterised by acute haemolytic anaemia, thrombocytopenia, and renal insufficiency. We aimed to assess the success of management of this disorder with plasma exchange therapy.

*Methods.*—Patients diagnosed with diarrhoea-associated haemolytic uraemic syndrome in southern Denmark were treated with daily plasma exchange by centrifugation and substitution with fresh frozen plasma. Stool culture and serological testing was done to identify the cause of disease, and the success of management with plasma exchange therapy was assessed from change in platelet count, glomerular filtration rate, and lactate dehydrogenase.

*Findings.*—During May 25–28, 2011, five patients with a median age of 62 years (range 44–70) presented with diarrhoea-associated haemolytic uraemic syndrome, which was caused by an unusual Shiga-toxin-producing *Escherichia coli* serotype O104:H4. Strains of *E coli* showed a high resistance to third-generation cephalosporins because the strains had extended-spectrum $\beta$ lactamases. After plasma exchange, median platelet count and glomerular filtration rate increased, median lactate dehydrogenase concentration decreased, and neurological status improved. The time interval from onset of bloody diarrhoea to start of plasma exchange had an inverse correlation with reduction of lactate dehydrogenase concentrations by plasma exchange ($p = 0.02$). All patients were discharged with normal neurological status at 7 days (range 5–8) after starting plasma exchange.

*Interpretation.*—Early plasma exchange might ameliorate the course of diarrhoea-associated haemolytic uraemic syndrome in adults. However, this finding should be verified in randomised controlled trials.

▶ Colic et al describe the management of patients in Germany during the outbreak of *Escherichia coli* infection that occurred in May, June, and July of 2011. Although antimicrobial therapy is not recommended for enterohemorrhagic *E coli* infection, 4 of the 5 patients in the report by Colic et al had been treated with ciprofloxacin or metronidazole at the onset of their gastrointestinal symptoms, which, conceivably, offered resistant *E coli* O104:H4 a selective advantage over the normal intestinal flora. Patients were also treated with daily plasma exchange. The latter was associated with prompt disease recovery. Plasma exchange has rapidly emerged as the front-line therapy for typical hemolytic uremic syndrome (HUS) associated with severe renal insufficiency or brain impairment and also for atypical HUS. Presumably, plasma exchange helps to remove the Shiga toxin.

Thus it is that early plasmapheresis with or without the use of an antibody against the C5 component of the complement system is the cornerstone of management of HUS. The antibody currently being used is eculizumab, which previously has been used successfully to treat children with typical HUS. We do not know as of now whether early treatment with the class of antibiotics known as carbapenems would be helpful during therapy. This class of antibiotics, unlike ciprofloxacin, does not release Shiga toxin in massive amounts.

**J. A. Stockman III, MD**

---

**Treatment of severe neurological deficits with IgG depletion through immunoadsorption in patients with *Escherichia coli* O104:H4-associated haemolytic uraemic syndrome: a prospective trial**

Greinacher A, Friesecke S, Abel P, et al (Ernst-Moritz-Arndt-Universität, Greifswald, Germany; et al)
*Lancet* 378:1166-1173, 2011

---

*Background.*—In May 2011, an outbreak of Shiga toxin-producing enterohaemorrhagic *E coli* O104:H4 in northern Germany led to a high proportion of patients developing post-enteritis haemolytic uraemic syndrome and thrombotic microangiopathy that were unresponsive to therapeutic plasma exchange or complement-blocking antibody (eculizumab). Some patients needed ventilatory support due to severe neurological complications, which arose 1 week after onset of enteritis, suggesting an antibody-mediated mechanism. Therefore, we aimed to assess immunoadsorption as rescue therapy.

*Methods.*—In our prospective non-controlled trial, we enrolled patients with severe neurological symptoms and confirmed recent *E coli* O104:H4 infection without other acute bacterial infection or raised procalcitonin concentrations. We did IgG immunoadsorption processing of 12 L plasma volumes on 2 consecutive days, followed by IgG replacement ($0 \cdot 5$ g/kg intravenous IgG). We calculated a composite neurological symptom score (lowest score was best) every day and assessed changes before and after immunoadsorption.

*Findings.*—We enrolled 12 patients who initially presented with enteritis and subsequent renal failure; 10 (83%) of 12 patients needed renal replacement therapy by a median of $8 \cdot 0$ days (range 5—12). Neurological complications (delirium, stimulus sensitive myoclonus, aphasia, and epileptic seizures in 50% of patients) occurred at a median of $8 \cdot 0$ days (range 5—15) and mandated mechanical ventilation in nine patients. Composite neurological symptom scores increased in the 3 days before immunoadsorption to $3 \cdot 0$ (SD $1 \cdot 1$, $p = 0 \cdot 038$), and improved to $1 \cdot 0$ ($1 \cdot 2$, $p = 0 \cdot 0006$) 3 days after immunoadsorption. In non-intubated patients, improvement was apparent during immunoadsorption (eg, disappearance of aphasia). Five patients who were intubated were weaned within 48 h, two within 4 days, and two patients needed continued ventilation for respiratory problems. All 12 patients survived and ten had complete neurological and renal function recovery.

*Interpretation.*—Antibodies are probably involved in the pathogenesis of severe neurological symptoms in patients with *E coli* O104:H4-induced haemolytic uraemic syndrome. Immunoadsorption can safely be used to rapidly ameliorate these severe neurological complications.

▶ This is the last of the 3 reports dealing with the outbreak of *Escherichia coli* in Germany in 2011. The report by Greinacher et al tells us about how some of the patients who developed this infection were treated. The report describes the clinical presentation and response of neurological symptoms in 12 patients who were managed by IgG immunodepletion through immunoadsorption. It appears that 12 of 63 patients with hemorrhagic enteritis who were treated at Greifswald University at Hannover Medical School Hospitals developed severe neurological complications necessitating management in intensive care units. Patients with these neurological complications did not respond to therapeutic plasma exchange or to the use of eculizumab, an antibody that has been reported to be effective in hemolytic uremic syndrome (HUS) in children. This antibody blocks the action of a particular complement (C5) constituent. The fact that the neurologic complications were delayed into the second week of symptoms following the onset of diarrhea suggested to the investigators that the problem might be immune mediated, prompting the investigators to use IgG immunodepletion as a rescue therapy in this life-threatening situation. Immunoadsorption provides a rapid and efficient method of antibody removal and has been used successfully in diseases associated with autoantibodies.

If you are not familiar with immunodepletion using immunoadsorption technology, this is done by passing blood over immunoglobulin-binding columns, a method that is capable of removing large amounts of immunoglobulin, primarily IgG. In patients so treated, IgG concentrations are restored by the administration of intravenous IgG, thus removing only "bad" antibodies and leaving the patient still immunocompetent. Investigators have shown that IgG immunodepletion by immunoadsorption strikingly improves neurological complications in patients with *E coli* O104:H4—associated HUS. All tolerated immunoadsorption very well, consistent with findings from other reports in which this technique has been used to treat entities such as dilated cardiomyopathy and autoimmune neurological disorders. Immunoadsorption is capable of removing more than 80% of a patient's IgG and therefore is much more efficient than plasma exchange. It is thought that part of the problem affecting the kidneys in hemorrhagic enterocolitis—related HUS is the result of antibodies that have formed against Shiga toxin, which result in deposition of immune complexes. In this series, all 12 patients survived, and 10 had complete neurological and renal function recovery. While a dozen patients do not make a controlled series, the data from this report are compelling, suggesting that immunoadsorption might be the way to go in many patients with HUS resulting from *E coli* enteritis.

While on the topic of infections related to food, recognize that cases of *E coli* enteritis have been linked to unwashed vegetables. England, Wales, and Scotland had 250 cases of *E coli* O157 reported between December 2010 and July 2011. Most cases were mild, but 74 individuals needed hospital treatment and 1 individual died.[1] Also in 2011, the US Food and Drug Administration and the Centers for Disease Control and Prevention (CDC) warned consumers not to eat cantaloupe melons produced in the Rocky Ford region of Colorado by Jensen Farms after an outbreak of listeriosis was traced to the producers. This outbreak involved 22 cases and 4 deaths across 7 states.[2] Also, be aware of the risk of eating oysters contaminated with *Vibrio vulnificus*. The latter is a naturally occurring halophilic (salt-requiring) gram-negative rod-shaped bacterium that is ubiquitous in coastal waters. Infection with these bacteria has a case fatality rate that can exceed 50% and in fact is the leading cause of seafood-related deaths in the United States. The CDC estimates that about 100 cases are being reported annually in the United States that result in about 50 deaths per year. Oysters are among the most common vehicles for *V vulnificus* infections. These are typically found in estuaries, sounds, and bays. Consumption of raw or undercooked oysters has been implicated as the vehicle of transmission in most instances. The highest density of *V vulnificus* has been reported in oysters from the waters of the Gulf of Mexico, which have a higher mean water temperature compared with coastal waters along the eastern seaboard. To read more about *V vulnificus* and oysters, see the report by Daniels et al.[3]

**J. A. Stockman III, MD**

*References*

1. Editorial comment. Cases of *E. coli* linked to unwashed vegetables. *BMJ*. 2011; 343:712.
2. Editorial comment. Melon warning. *Lancet*. 2011;378:922.
3. Daniels NA. Vibrio vulnificus oysters: pearls and perils. *Clin Infect Dis*. 2011;52: 788-792.

### *Salmonella* Typhimurium Infections Associated with Peanut Products

Cavallaro E, for the *Salmonella* Typhimurium Outbreak Investigation Team (Natl Ctr for Emerging and Zoonotic Infectious Diseases, Atlanta, GA; et al)

*N Engl J Med* 365:601-610, 2011

*Background.*—Contaminated food ingredients can affect multiple products, each distributed through various channels and consumed in multiple settings. Beginning in November 2008, we investigated a nationwide outbreak of salmonella infections.

*Methods.*—A case was defined as laboratory-confirmed infection with the outbreak strain of *Salmonella* Typhimurium occurring between September 1, 2008, and April 20, 2009. We conducted two case–control studies, product "trace-back," and environmental investigations.

*Results.*—Among 714 case patients identified in 46 states, 166 (23%) were hospitalized and 9 (1%) died. In study 1, illness was associated with eating any peanut butter (matched odds ratio, 2.5; 95% confidence interval [CI], 1.3 to 5.3), peanut butter–containing products (matched odds ratio, 2.2; 95% CI, 1.1 to 4.7), and frozen chicken products (matched odds ratio, 4.6; 95% CI, 1.7 to 14.7). Investigations of focal clusters and single cases associated with nine institutions identified a single institutional brand of peanut butter (here called brand X) distributed to all facilities. In study 2, illness was associated with eating peanut butter outside the home (matched odds ratio, 3.9; 95% CI, 1.6 to 10.0) and two brands of peanut butter crackers (brand A: matched odds ratio, 17.2; 95% CI, 6.9 to 51.5; brand B: matched odds ratio, 3.6; 95% CI, 1.3 to 9.8). Both cracker brands were made from brand X peanut paste. The outbreak strain was isolated from brand X peanut butter, brand A crackers, and 15 other products. A total of 3918 peanut butter–containing products were recalled between January 10 and April 29, 2009.

*Conclusions.*—Contaminated peanut butter and peanut products caused a nationwide salmonellosis outbreak. Ingredient-driven outbreaks are challenging to detect and may lead to widespread contamination of numerous food products.

▶ It was back in November 2008 that a cluster of 35 *Salmonella enterica* serotyped Typhimurium isolates was detected in 16 states. Later that month, a second cluster of 27 *Salmonella* Typhimurium isolates in 14 states was reported. Cavallaro et al now describe this outbreak in some detail and have identified the sources of contaminated food related to the outbreak. It turns out that the national outbreak of human *Salmonella* Typhimurium infection was linked to the eating of contaminated peanut butter, peanut paste, and roasted peanuts produced at processing facilities in Georgia and Texas.

The human *Salmonella* Typhimurium outbreak in 2008 resulted in one of the largest food recalls in US history and an estimated 1 billion dollar economic loss in peanut sales. Because many people with *Salmonella* infection do not seek medical care or are not tested, it is estimated that 16 times as many cases of illness occurred in 2008 than were actually reported. By the time the outbreak ultimately settled down, many in the United States were skipping the Skippy and throwing out the Jiffy in a jiffy.

So why did the outbreak occur to begin with? *Salmonella* contamination can occur during many stages of peanut butter production. *Salmonella* introduced into the soil through the addition of manure or through irrigation can survive for months to years, contaminating peanuts growing underground. Further contamination can occur during peanut harvesting, transportation, or storage and can also be introduced in the processing facility. In the case of 2008, it is not possible to say where the contamination actually originated. *Salmonella* can survive in low-moisture foods, such as peanut butter, for at least 24 weeks. Therefore, if postprocessing contamination occurs, *Salmonella* may survive in peanut butter for its entire shelf life of 18 to 24 months. Indeed, *Salmonella* has caused long-lasting and highly distributed outbreaks in other low-moisture foods.

If there was any good that came from the *Salmonella* outbreak of several years ago, it is that the outbreak was instrumental in refocusing discussions about gaps in the food safety system in the United States. As a result, the President's Food Safety Working Group was created in March 2009 to identify actions that might improve foodborne disease prevention and strengthen surveillance and regulatory authority. As a result of recommendations by this group, the US Food and Drug Administration (FDA) launched the Reportable Food Registry (RFR), which requires the food industry to alert the FDA within 24 hours after the discovery that a food product has had a reasonable probability of causing adverse health consequences in humans and animals. In the first 6 months after its launch, the RFR received 125 primary reports from industry and regulatory officials for about 25 commodities. Of the latter, 37% were related to *Salmonella* contamination. The Food Safety Modernization Act, signed into law January 4, 2011, represents a positive step toward transforming the food safety system. This law gives the FDA the regulatory authority to mandate food recalls, stop production and distribution of unsafe food, and require prevention-based food safety plans from domestic and foreign food suppliers.

**J. A. Stockman III, MD**

---

**Emergence of a New Pathogenic Ehrlichia Species, Wisconsin and Minnesota, 2009**
Pritt BS, Sloan LM, Hoang Johnson DK, et al (Mayo Clinic, Rochester, MN; Wisconsin Division of Public Health, Madison; et al)
*N Engl J Med* 365:422-429, 2011

---

*Background.*—Ehrlichiosis is a clinically important, emerging zoonosis. Only *Ehrlichia chaffeensis* and *E. ewingii* have been thought to cause ehrlichiosis in humans in the United States. Patients with suspected ehrlichiosis routinely undergo testing to ensure proper diagnosis and to ascertain the cause.

*Methods.*—We used molecular methods, culturing, and serologic testing to diagnose and ascertain the cause of cases of ehrlichiosis.

*Results.*—On testing, four cases of ehrlichiosis in Minnesota or Wisconsin were found not to be from *E. chaffeensis* or *E. ewingii* and instead to be caused by a newly discovered ehrlichia species. All patients had fever, malaise, headache, and lymphopenia; three had thrombocytopenia; and two had elevated liver-enzyme levels. All recovered after receiving doxycycline treatment. At least 17 of 697 *Ixodes scapularis* ticks collected in Minnesota or Wisconsin were positive for the same ehrlichia species on polymerase-chain-reaction testing. Genetic analyses revealed that this new ehrlichia species is closely related to *E. muris*.

*Conclusions.*—We report a new ehrlichia species in Minnesota and Wisconsin and provide supportive clinical, epidemiologic, culture, DNA-sequence, and vector data. Physicians need to be aware of this newly discovered close relative of *E. muris* to ensure appropriate testing, treatment, and regional surveillance. (Funded by the National Institutes of Health and the Centers for Disease Control and Prevention.)

▶ Ehrlichiosis infection does affect children in the United States, and for this reason we should be aware of the types of organisms that cause this problem Ehrlichiosis and anaplasmosis are both tick-borne zoonoses caused by gram-negative bacteria in the family Anaplasmataceae. Patients with ehrlichiosis typically have fever, myalgia, and headache in association with a rash in some cases. Severe disease may result from this infection as the result of gastrointestinal, renal, respiratory, and central nervous system involvement. Some patients die. In the United States, human disease is primarily caused by *Ehrlichia chaffeensis*, which infects monocytes and less commonly by *E ewingii*, which infects granulocytes. Anaplasma phagocytophilum is closely related to Ehrlichiae and causes human granulocytic anaplasmosis. *E ewingii* and *E chaffeensis* are transmitted to humans by the bite of an infected tick, *Amblyomma americanum*, whereas infection related to human granulocytic anaplasmosis is transmitted by the tick, *Ixodes scapularis* and *I pacificus*.

Until the report of Pritt et al appeared, only *E chaffeensis* and *E ewingii* had been thought to cause ehrlichiosis in humans in the United States. Pritt et al have identified, however, a new *Ehrlichia* species (subsequently referred to as *Ehrlichia* species *Wisconsin*) in blood from 4 patients living in Wisconsin or Minnesota by using molecular, culture, and serologic methods. All 4 patients recovered after administration of doxycycline, the antibiotic of choice for the treatment of ehrlichiosis. This identification of a new species of *Ehrlichia* in humans has important clinical and epidemiologic implications. Ehrlichiosis, for example, was not thought to be endemic in Minnesota and Wisconsin and would not have routinely been tested for in patients from these areas of the country. Routine panels testing for ehrlichiosis might have missed this organism because polymerase chain reaction assays may not have detected *Ehrlichia* species *Wisconsin* because of lack of specificity of the primers used.

*Ehrlichia* infections in the United States are commonly transmitted by *A americanum*, but this tick is not thought to extend into Wisconsin and Minnesota. The authors of this report suggest that *I scapularis* is the vector for *Ehrlichia* species *Wisconsin*.

Thus all of us need to be aware of the recent finding of a new *Ehrlichia* species and the need for our microbiologic probes to detect this form. Although the organism has been described only in Minnesota and Wisconsin, chances are that the tick that carries it will likely spread the infection to other parts of the United States.

This commentary closes with a whodunit! A 24-year-old woman delivers a newborn at 39 weeks gestation in a remote cabin in Colorado. There is no medical care at the time of the delivery. She seeks treatment at an emergency room several hours after delivery and gives a history of one week of fever, nausea, headache, stiff neck, and occasional blurred vision. Physical examination reveals an ill-appearing but afebrile woman with hypotension. Physical examination does not give a clue to the diagnosis, nor does routine laboratory testing. The patient's newborn is admitted for observation. The infant has blood cultures obtained which show no growth several days later. At 4 days of age neonatal jaundice develops. At 5 days of age the infant becomes febrile. Various laboratory studies are obtained. Treatment for sepsis is initiated. Blood and serum samples from the mother and her newborn are tested by the Center for Disease Control and Prevention laboratory in Fort Collins, Colorado. The diagnosis of both infant and mother is made solely on the basis of examination of the peripheral blood smear. Your diagnosis? If you diagnosed tick-borne relapsing fever, you would be correct. A thin smear of the newborn and mother's peripheral blood showed the presence of numerous spirochetes. This made a diagnosis of tickborne relapsing fever. This entity is caused by *Borrelia hermsii* and is transmitted by the soft tick, *Ornithodoros hermsi*. This tick is usually associated with nests of chipmunks and other wild rodents. Unlike hard ticks, it can transmit spirochetes through a brief (under 30 minutes duration) and painless nocturnal bite. Humans typically are exposed to these ticks during an overnight stay in rodent-infested dwellings at elevations greater than 2000 feet. Only 12 tickborne relapsing fever cases have been described among pregnant women in the United States. Among these cases, serious maternal complications have been documented. Newborns born to such mothers have more than a 50% likelihood of developing infection. One-third of infected infants have died. This illness should be considered a potential diagnosis among febrile patients who reside in or have traveled to the western United States, especially those inhabiting rustic housing.[1]

**J. A. Stockman III, MD**

*Reference*

1. Editorial comment. Tickborne relapsing fever and a mother and newborn child—Colorado, 2011. *MMWR*. March 16, 2012:174-175.

### Transfusion-Associated Babesiosis in the United States: A Description of Cases

Herwaldt BL, Linden JV, Bosserman E, et al (Ctrs for Disease Control and Prevention, Atlanta, GA; Wadsworth Ctr, Albany, NY; Rhode Island Blood Ctr, Providence)
*Ann Intern Med* 155:509-519, 2011

*Background.*—Babesiosis is a potentially life-threatening disease caused by intraerythrocytic parasites, which usually are tickborne but also are transmissible by transfusion. Tickborne transmission of *Babesia microti* mainly occurs in 7 states in the Northeast and the upper Midwest of the United States. No *Babesia* test for screening blood donors has been licensed.

*Objective.*—To ascertain and summarize data on U.S. transfusion-associated *Babesia* cases identified since the first described case in 1979.

*Design.*—Case series.

*Setting.*—United States.

*Patients.*—Case patients were transfused during 1979–2009 and had posttransfusion *Babesia* infection diagnosed by 2010, without reported evidence that another transmission route was more likely than transfusion. Implicated donors had laboratory evidence of infection. Potential cases were excluded if all pertinent donors tested negative.

*Measurements.*—Distributions of ascertained cases according to *Babesia* species and period and state of transfusion.

*Results.*—159 transfusion-associated *B. microti* cases were included; donors were implicated for 136 (86%). The case patients' median age was 65 years (range, <1 to 94 years). Most cases were associated with red blood cell components; 4 were linked to whole blood–derived platelets. Cases occurred in all 4 seasons and in 22 (of 31) years, but 77% (122 cases) occurred during 2000–2009. Cases occurred in 19 states, but 87% (138 cases) were in the 7 main *B. microti*–endemic states. In addition, 3 *B. duncani* cases were documented in western states.

*Limitation.*—The extent to which cases were not diagnosed, investigated, reported, or ascertained is unknown.

*Conclusion.*—Donor-screening strategies that mitigate the risk for transfusion transmission are needed. Babesiosis should be included in the differential diagnosis of unexplained posttransfusion hemolytic anemia or fever, regardless of the season or U.S. region.

▶ Babesiosis is an infection that affects children and adults. Human babesiosis in the United States is attributable almost exclusively to infection with the intraerythrocytic protozoan parasite *Babesia microti*. The primary mechanism of parasite transmission to humans is via the bite of an infected deer/black-legged tick, *Ixodes scapularis*—the same tick that serves as the vector for Lime borreliosis, human granulocytic anaplasmosis, and several other tick-borne diseases. The first documented case of clinical disease caused by *B microti* was reported on Nantucket Island, Massachusetts, in 1969. Since then, hundreds to thousands of babesiosis cases have been described, and it is now a nationally notifiable disease with reporting being mandatory beginning in January 2011. Endemic areas in the United States are in the Northeast (Connecticut, Massachusetts, New Jersey, New York, Rhode Island) and upper Midwest (Minnesota and Wisconsin). Another species, *B duncani*, is reported on rare occasions in the states of California and Washington.

Infections with *B microti* produce a spectrum of disease, ranging from asymptomatic, self-resolving infections to severe, life-threatening illnesses that are often dictated by the host immune system. Common signs and symptoms of babesiosis included fever, headache, chills, drenching sweats, myalgia, malaise, and hemolytic anemia. More severe cases occur in immunocompromised populations including newborns and infants, elderly people, and those without spleens. Complicated babesiosis can cause respiratory distress, severe hemolysis, disseminated intravascular coagulation, renal dysfunction, hepatic compromise, myocardial infarction, and death.

Herwaldt et al remind us that babesiosis can be transmitted not only by ticks but also by human blood. The first documented case of transfusion-transmitted *Babesia* was reported in Boston in 1979. Since then, the number of transfusion-related cases of *B microti* infection has increased rapidly. Herwaldt et al have compiled an exhaustive list of known cases of transfusion-associated babesiosis from 1979 through 2009. These investigators have identified 159 cases of *B microti* transmission during the 30-year study (plus 3 additional cases attributed to *B duncani*). The investigators also note that these numbers are probably an underestimate. Unfortunately, infection with babesiosis is frequently missed or misdiagnosed. It is often mistaken for malaria given the presence of intraerythrocytic ring forms on blood smear analysis.

Data presented by Herwaldt et al suggest that the number and frequency of transfusion-associated babesiosis cases are increasing rapidly. Seventy-seven percent of the cases reported over a 30-year period were reported in the past 10 years. This precipitous increase is corroborated by recent reports from the US Food and Drug Administration, the American Red Cross, and the New York City Department of Mental Health and Hygiene. This observed increase in cases raises the question of whether the parasite's endemic range is expanding.

Individuals who have been infected with *Babesia* can remain infectious via blood transfusion for long periods of time. *Babesia* parasites can survive in stored blood almost indefinitely. Transmission has been reported with all forms of blood component therapy including frozen blood.

Unfortunately, donor-screening practices do not yet include routine testing for evidence of *Babesia* infection. Currently, a blood screening assay (serologic or nucleic acid) does not exist. Although *Babesia* transmission risk clearly peaks during the summer months (that is, active tick season), it poses a significant risk year-round that will need to be addressed. Also, although 87% of cases compiled by Herwaldt et al were reported in the 7 endemic states noted, transfusion-associated cases of babesiosis are more widespread. For example, transfusion-associated babesiosis has been reported in Florida and Texas. It should be noted that infants and children have been infected via blood transfusion. In the absence of a feasible and approved method for screening the blood supply, it appears that *B microti* has become the infectious agent most frequently transmitted by blood transfusion now in the United States.

While on the topic of unusual organisms, it should be noted that while we all know about cyanosis, were you aware that even bacteria like organisms can be blue? Cyanobacteria are tiny photosynthetic organisms floating in the sea. Binding together into chains and then mats by the millions, they can become a threat. Before long, the bacteria change the color of the sea's surface and even soften the wind-tossed chop. One study of cyanobacteria, also known as blue–green algae, although they are not actually algae, predicted that rising sea temperatures would help the already widespread creatures to expand their territory by more than 10%. These creatures are ubiquitous. They generate enough oxygen into the atmosphere to dictate the current make-up of the gases we breathe. They compete with great success for nutrients such as nitrogen and phosphorus. When cyanobacteria blossom, it is often at the cost of neighboring species such as fish or other phytoplankton. The proliferation may in fact accelerate warming of the atmosphere. Studies are now underway where these organisms are located to measure sea water temperature and the temperature in near by areas to test the prediction that these blue organisms have a significant impact on our atmosphere and global warming.[1]

**J. A. Stockman III, MD**

*Reference*

1. Editorial comment. Blue bacteria in bloom. *Scientific American.* April 2012:91.

---

### A Field Trial to Assess a Blood-Stage Malaria Vaccine

Thera MA, Doumbo OK, Coulibaly D, et al (Univ of Bamako, Mali; et al)
*N Engl J Med* 365:1004-1013, 2011

*Background.*—Blood-stage malaria vaccines are intended to prevent clinical disease. The malaria vaccine FMP2.1/AS02$_A$, a recombinant protein based on apical membrane antigen 1 (AMA1) from the 3D7 strain of *Plasmodium falciparum*, has previously been shown to have immunogenicity and acceptable safety in Malian adults and children.

*Methods.*—In a double-blind, randomized trial, we immunized 400 Malian children with either the malaria vaccine or a control (rabies) vaccine and followed them for 6 months. The primary end point was clinical malaria, defined as fever and at least 2500 parasites per cubic millimeter of blood. A secondary end point was clinical malaria caused by parasites with the AMA1 DNA sequence found in the vaccine strain.

*Results.*—The cumulative incidence of the primary end point was 48.4% in the malaria-vaccine group and 54.4% in the control group; efficacy against the primary end point was 17.4% (hazard ratio for the primary end point, 0.83; 95% confidence interval [CI], 0.63 to 1.09; $P = 0.18$). Efficacy against the first and subsequent episodes of clinical malaria, as defined on the basis of various parasite-density thresholds, was approximately 20%. Efficacy against clinical malaria caused by parasites with AMA1 corresponding to that of the vaccine strain was 64.3% (hazard ratio, 0.36; 95% CI, 0.08

to 0.86; $P = 0.03$). Local reactions and fever after vaccination were more frequent with the malaria vaccine.

*Conclusions.*—On the basis of the primary end point, the malaria vaccine did not provide significant protection against clinical malaria, but on the basis of secondary results, it may have strain-specific efficacy. If this finding is confirmed, AMA1 might be useful in a multicomponent malaria vaccine. (Funded by the National Institute of Allergy and Infectious Diseases and others; ClinicalTrials.gov number, NCT00460525.)

▶ This report contains some important statistics that all of us should become familiar with as pediatric care providers. Musculoskeletal pain is a common symptom in children. Somewhere between 10% and 20% of children of school age will have musculoskeletal pain of some sort. Fewer than 1% of such children will turn out to have a malignancy, but conversely, 40% of children with malignancy, particularly acute lymphoblastic leukemia (ALL), will have musculoskeletal pain as a presenting symptom. Another 20% will have such symptoms mixed in with other findings consistent with ALL.

All too often, children with musculoskeletal pain and ALL present to either an orthopedist or a rheumatologist, and in such cases the referral is either to rule out structural causes of musculoskeletal pain or to exclude juvenile idiopathic arthritis. Fortunately, well-trained pediatric rheumatologists are more than able to look for the clinical findings and laboratory clues that would trigger a suspicion of malignancy. Nocturnal pain is one such sentinel finding for ALL and often for other types of malignancy. Thus pain awakening a patient from sleep is not a good finding. In such cases, pediatric rheumatologists know to look carefully at the complete blood count and peripheral blood smear, the LDH, uric acid levels, and x-rays showing the typical bone findings of leukemia (lytic lesions and/or metaphyseal rarefactions).

The reason it is important for all of us, including our pediatric rheumatology colleagues, to recognize the musculoskeletal findings in ALL relates to the fact that delayed diagnosis can affect survival in an adverse way. Hashkes et al report on just how good pediatric rheumatologists are in quickly making a diagnosis of ALL when the latter is a presenting sign of musculoskeletal pain. Using the pediatric rheumatology disease registry, the authors of this report were able to find 89 patients in the registry who presented with musculoskeletal pain and who ultimately had a diagnosis of ALL. The survival rate in these patients was 95.5%, and the 10-year survival rate was just under 90%. These survival rates are actually higher than the overall survival rates from the literature of all children presenting with leukemia within similar timeframes. These data suggest that such patients may actually have improved survival compared with the general ALL population, a phenomenon that is not easily explained. It should be noted that other studies have also suggested a better than average prognosis in children with ALL presenting with bone abnormalities on radiographic study.[1] It would be interesting to see someone put together the data from the pediatric rheumatology disease registry to correlate survivorship with initial prognostic features other than musculoskeletal pain. Such features could include immunophenotyping, genetic markers, and evidence or not of minimal residual disease after initial induction therapy. These data surely exist in these children's cancer registry databases. This would be an easy undertaking to study this information.

This commentary closes with a reflection on one of the cheapest ways to help control malaria in underdeveloped countries. A persistent question about sustainable development is how to help the world's poorest people. Many have incomes that are so low they lack access to the most basic goods and services: adequate nutrition, safe drinking water, sanitation, and vital health interventions. One strategy is to provide targeted financial help to the poor to meet their basic needs and thereby escape from the poverty trap. It has been suggested that the cost of insuring basic lifesaving health coverage for the world's poor would be around 0.1% of gross national product of the high-income countries.[2] One example of such targeted aid is a mass free distribution of antimalaria bednets to people living in impoverished malarious regions of Africa. Each of these long-lasting insecticide-treated nets costs only about $10 to produce, transport, and distribute to households in rural Africa. Because these nets last for 5 years and two children typically sleep under each net, the cost per child per year is very small. Even at this remarkably low cost, however, some critics have opposed such an approach. They have claimed that free nets would "go missing" in large numbers because of waste by recipients and others in the supply chain who did not properly value them. These critics' preferred solution is a market sale of nets at a discount, on the grounds that even a small price would encourage more efficient use of these nets. The suggestion is that the nets should be sold at $2 to $3 per net. Unfortunately because Africa's rural poor are so destitute, attempts to sell them even at these subsidized lower prices surprisingly have fallen short in actual practice. Recently the Poverty Action Lab at the Massachusetts Institute of Technology carried out a detailed experiment in Western Kenya that compared mass distribution with a partial subsidy approach: even a small charge for bed nets led to a tremendous drop in their adoption. Moreover there was no greater wastage of nets received for free than those purchased at a discount price. The study's conclusion was clear: free distribution is both more effective and more cost effective than cost-sharing.

**J. A. Stockman III, MD**

*References*

1. Dini G, Taccone A, De Bernardi B, Comelli A, Garrè ML, Gandus S. Skeletal changes in acute lymphoblastic leukemia in children. Incidence and prognostic significance. *Radiol Med.* 1983;69:644-649.
2. Sachs JD. Good news on malarial control: The best price for getting antimosquito bednets to the poor proves to be "free." *Scientific American.* August 2009:29.

### First Results of Phase 3 Trial of RTS,S/AS01 Malaria Vaccine in African Children

The RTS,S Clinical Trials Partnership (Univ of Tübingen, Germany; et al)

N Engl J Med 365:1863-1875, 2011

*Background.*—An ongoing phase 3 study of the efficacy, safety, and immunogenicity of candidate malaria vaccine RTS,S/AS01 is being conducted in seven African countries.

*Methods.*—From March 2009 through January 2011, we enrolled 15,460 children in two age categories — 6 to 12 weeks of age and 5 to 17 months of age — for vaccination with either RTS,S/AS01 or a non-malaria comparator vaccine. The primary end point of the analysis was vaccine efficacy against clinical malaria during the 12 months after vaccination in the first 6000 children 5 to 17 months of age at enrollment who received all three doses of vaccine according to protocol. After 250 children had an episode of severe malaria, we evaluated vaccine efficacy against severe malaria in both age categories.

*Results.*—In the 14 months after the first dose of vaccine, the incidence of first episodes of clinical malaria in the first 6000 children in the older age category was 0.32 episodes per person-year in the RTS,S/AS01 group and 0.55 episodes per person-year in the control group, for an efficacy of 50.4% (95% confidence interval [CI], 45.8 to 54.6) in the intention-to-treat population and 55.8% (97.5% CI, 50.6 to 60.4) in the per-protocol population. Vaccine efficacy against severe malaria was 45.1% (95% CI, 23.8 to 60.5) in the intention-to-treat population and 47.3% (95% CI, 22.4 to 64.2) in the per-protocol population. Vaccine efficacy against severe malaria in the combined age categories was 34.8% (95% CI, 16.2 to 49.2) in the per-protocol population during an average follow-up of 11 months. Serious adverse events occurred with a similar frequency in the two study groups. Among children in the older age category, the rate of generalized convulsive seizures after RTS,S/AS01 vaccination was 1.04 per 1000 doses (95% CI, 0.62 to 1.64).

*Conclusions.*—The RTS,S/AS01 vaccine provided protection against both clinical and severe malaria in African children. (Funded by Glaxo-SmithKline Biologicals and the PATH Malaria Vaccine Initiative; RTS,S ClinicalTrials.gov number, NCT00866619.)

▶ The initial results of the phase 3 clinical trial for RTS,S, currently the leading malaria vaccine candidate, seem very positive. The RTS,S Clinical Trials Partnership has provided an interim report of a large, multicenter phase 3 trial of this vaccine. A total of 15 460 children in 2 age categories—6 weeks to 12 weeks and 5 months to 17 months—was enrolled. The report describes vaccine efficacy against *Plasmodium falciparum* malaria in the first 6000 of 8923 children in the older age category, and an evaluation of the fist 250 cases of severe malaria from both age groups. The target population for this vaccine is the young infant who would receive the malaria vaccine together with routine immunizations. Protective efficacy against *P falciparum* malaria was shown to be 55% against all malarial episodes. There was an unexpected finding. There were significantly more cases of meningitis among children receiving RTS,S/AS01 vaccine than among those receiving comparison vaccines. There is no reasonable explanation anyone has found for this finding. Hopefully, this is on the basis of chance and chance alone. There is also an increased risk of febrile reactions or seizures among vaccine recipients, and it will be necessary to study the vaccine more in the future to understand what this finding means.

The road to finding an effective vaccine has been long and hard. This well-conducted multicenter trial showing a 50% reduction in the incidence of malaria among young children is a major accomplishment. The future impact on overall public health of this vaccine, which is likely to be licensed by the end of 2015, is difficult to assess. It is not known, for example, what the duration of protection is. As far as costs are concerned, the manufacturer, GlaxoSmithKline, has consistently said that it will charge just 5% above cost of manufacturing for the vaccine. Time will tell whether this pricing actually holds true. An assessment of an 18-month booster dose will not be available until 2014.

In the war against malaria, researchers may have recruited an unlikely ally: a seaweed found in Fiji. In 2005, investigators at the Georgia Institute of Technology in Atlanta discovered that seaweed, a red alga called *Callophycus serratus*, contains unusual ring-shaped compounds called bromophycolides that are particularly effective at killing certain fungi. In 2009 these investigators found one that also kills the malaria parasite in red blood cells.[1] This group of investigators has elucidated the mechanism by which this occurs. Malarial parasites invade intact red blood cells, where they thrive on hemoglobin. As the parasites break hemoglobin down, they release heme, a pigment that is toxic to the parasite. To protect themselves, the parasites crystallize the heme and store it in a separate chamber. It is now reported that bromophycolides prevent this crystallization, causing heme to accumulate and poison the parasites. Well, a least there is one weed that is good for you.

**J. A. Stockman III, MD**

*Reference*

1. Editorial comment. Seaweed: Malaria's nemesis. *Science.* 2011;331:995.

---

**Children With Retinopathy-negative Cerebral Malaria: A Pathophysiologic Puzzle**
Postels DG, Birbeck GL (Michigan State Univ, East Lansing)
*Pediatr Infect Dis J* 30:953-956, 2011

---

*Background.*—Cerebral malaria, defined as otherwise unexplained coma in a patient with circulating parasitemia, is a common disease in the developing world. The clinical diagnosis lacks specificity and children with other underlying causes of coma might be misdiagnosed as having cerebral malaria. The presence of malarial retinopathy can be used to differentiate children whose comas are caused by *Plasmodium falciparum* and its attendant pathophysiologies from those with other reasons for their abnormal mental status. Children with cerebral malaria who lack malarial retinopathy have not previously been described.

*Methods.*—All patients admitted to Queen Elizabeth Central Hospital in Blantyre, Malawi, during a 12-month period with a clinical diagnosis of cerebral malaria were evaluated for the presence of malarial retinopathy. Thirty-two patients lacked retinopathy findings. Clinical, laboratory, and radiologic information data were collected.

*Results.*—Thirty-two cases of retinopathy-negative cerebral malaria are presented.

*Conclusions.*—Children with retinopathy-negative cerebral malaria share a common clinical phenotype with lower rates of mortality compared with those who have malarial retinopathy. There are at least 4 possible pathophysiologic explanations for this common condition.

▶ It has been said that the eye is the window into the soul, but in the case of cerebral malaria, the eye is the window into the brain. About half a million individuals each year develop cerebral malaria. This occasionally happens even in the United States. Although the malarial organism does not directly invade the cerebral parenchyma, infection does set in motion a cascade of pathophysiologic processes that induce coma and often death. These include sequestration of circulating infected erythrocytes, abnormalities in cytokines, and inducible nitric oxide synthase that increase permeability of the blood brain barrier. Most believe that the principal mechanism causing coma and death is sequestration of infected red blood cells within the brain without actual involvement of brain tissue.

So what does all this brain pathology have to do with the eye? If one examines carefully the retina of the eye of a patient with cerebral malaria (as defined by World Health Organization criteria) one will see an infection-related retinopathy. Retinal abnormalities are 90% sensitive and 95% specific for detecting those with cerebral malaria without having to do further studies. These figures relate largely to infection caused by *Plasmodium falciparum*. Retinopathy-positive patients have eye findings that confirm cerebral malaria's pathophysiologic processes as responsible for their comatose state.

Postels et al report on patients who meet the World Health Organization's criteria defining cerebral malaria but who have no retinal abnormalities. They suggest that there are several possible pathophysiologic explanations for these sets of findings. It is possible that parasitemia in children with retinopathy-negative cerebral malaria is truly incidental, reflecting residence in a high area of malaria transmission. In such a scenario, affected patients should be considered as having an acute febrile encephalopathy (AFE) of unknown origin. In such cases, the absence of retinopathy is not a missed diagnosis; rather the patient's coma is caused by something else, and one had better look for what that cause is or the patient may very well die, as malaria treatment will not affect the course of the illness. If retinopathy-negative cerebral malaria is a variant of AEF in a patient with otherwise asymptomatic circulating malaria organisms, then a search for a causative infectious, postinfectious, or other etiology is absolutely warranted.

Remember that an eye examination should always be part of the evaluation of a patient with malaria.

**J. A. Stockman III, MD**

---

**Feasibility, diagnostic accuracy, and effectiveness of decentralised use of the Xpert MTB/RIF test for diagnosis of tuberculosis and multidrug resistance: a multicentre implementation study**

Boehme CC, Nicol MP, Nabeta P, et al (Foundation for Innovative New Diagnostics (FIND), Geneva, Switzerland; Groote Schuur Hosp, Cape Town, South Africa; et al)

*Lancet* 377:1495-1505, 2011

---

*Background.*—The Xpert MTB/RIF test (Cepheid, Sunnyvale, CA, USA) can detect tuberculosis and its multidrug-resistant form with very high sensitivity and specificity in controlled studies, but no performance data exist from district and subdistrict health facilities in tuberculosis-endemic countries. We aimed to assess operational feasibility, accuracy, and effectiveness of implementation in such settings.

*Methods.*—We assessed adults ($\geq$18 years) with suspected tuberculosis or multidrug-resistant tuberculosis consecutively presenting with cough lasting at least 2 weeks to urban health centres in South Africa, Peru, and India, drug resistance screening facilities in Azerbaijan and the Philippines, and an emergency room in Uganda. Patients were excluded from the main analyses if their second sputum sample was collected more than 1 week after the first sample, or if no valid reference standard or MTB/RIF test was available. We compared one-off direct MTB/RIF testing in nine microscopy laboratories adjacent to study sites with 2–3 sputum smears and 1–3 cultures, dependent on site, and drug-susceptibility testing. We assessed indicators of robustness including indeterminate rate and between-site performance, and compared time to detection, reporting, and treatment, and patient dropouts for the techniques used.

*Findings.*—We enrolled 6648 participants between Aug 11, 2009, and June 26, 2010. One-off MTB/RIF testing detected 933 (90·3%) of 1033 culture-confirmed cases of tuberculosis, compared with 699 (67·1%) of 1041 for microscopy. MTB/RIF test sensitivity was 76·9% in smear-negative, culture-positive patients (296 of 385 samples), and 99·0% specific (2846 of 2876 non-tuberculosis samples). MTB/RIF test sensitivity for rifampicin resistance was 94·4% (236 of 250) and specificity was 98·3% (796 of 810). Unlike microscopy, MTB/RIF test sensitivity was not significantly lower in patients with HIV co-infection. Median time to detection of tuberculosis for the MTB/RIF test was 0 days (IQR 0–1), compared with 1 day (0–1) for microscopy, 30 days (23–43) for solid culture, and 16 days (13–21) for liquid culture. Median time to detection of resistance was 20 days (10–26) for line-probe assay and 106 days

(30—124) for conventional drug-susceptibility testing. Use of the MTB/RIF test reduced median time to treatment for smear-negative tuberculosis from 56 days (39—81) to 5 days (2—8). The indeterminate rate of MTB/RIF testing was 2·4% (126 of 5321 samples) compared with 4·6% (441 of 9690) for cultures.

*Interpretation.*—The MTB/RIF test can effectively be used in low-resource settings to simplify patients' access to early and accurate diagnosis, thereby potentially decreasing morbidity associated with diagnostic delay, dropout and mistreatment.

▶ More and more is being written about rapid diagnostic testing to define the presence of tuberculosis. Even in the United States, tuberculosis remains a problem in some subsets of patients of the population. Globally, some 9.4 million new cases of tuberculosis were seen as recently as 2009. Most of the major burden of worldwide tuberculosis occurs in 22 low-income countries with few financial resources. Laboratory capacity in most of these countries is highly insufficient with few laboratories being able to undertake the challenge of high-quality microbiologic testing and drug sensitivity. It is estimated that worldwide, case detection rates for all cases of tuberculosis run only about 60%. Reduction of diagnostic delay is desirable to decrease morbidity, mortality, and transmission.

Assessment of the feasibility and robustness of the MTB/RIF test is what the report of Boehme et al is all about. This is a real-time polymerase chain reaction (PCR) assay for *Mycobacterium tuberculosis*. It simultaneously detects rifampicin resistance. The assay in field testing has shown excellent performance in comparison with standardized testing for tuberculosis in reference laboratories. Unfortunately, diagnostic tests often do well in initial studies that are done in near ideal settings in reference laboratories but ultimately perform poorly when these assays are tested in settings of intended use. The report of Boehme et al tells us about testing in the latter circumstances.

What we learn from this report is that the MTB/RIF test does have some problems with sensitivity and specificity. It is 90% sensitive. In some respects this is a good-news/bad-news situation. The good news is that it is better than most tests of other types. The bad news is that missing 10% of potentially life-threatening disease is far from ideal. As noted in a commentary related to this report, on average, a positive MTB/RIF test result for rifampicin resistance will have a 37% chance of being a false-positive.[1]

Even if we were able to more rapidly and accurately diagnose tuberculosis, mechanisms do not exist to provide treatment for the millions of patients who will be diagnosed in this fashion. The positive results with the MTB/RIF test are an urgent wake-up call to the international community that a substantial increase in capacity to manage multidrug-resistant tuberculosis at full scale is needed, together with major improvements in the availability of high-quality affordable treatments.

What role, if any, MTB/RIF testing will have in the United States remains to be seen. For now it is designed specifically for use close to point-of-treatment in endemic disease settings and remains the first of a new generation of diagnostic tests that have the potential to bring highly sensitive nucleic acid amplification testing to peripheral sections of the health system. If this form of testing turns out to have better sensitivity and specificity, we could easily see it as a first-line screening test while awaiting bacteriologic confirmation. In 2010, a total of 1181 tuberculosis cases were reported in the United States. The tuberculosis rate among foreign-born individuals here was 11 times greater than among US-born people. It is clear that the goal of eliminating tuberculosis in the United States by 2012 (the challenge at the beginning of the preceding decade) will not be achieved. To read more about trends in tuberculosis in the United States, see the report in the *Centers for Disease Control and Prevention, Weekly Morbidity and Mortality Reports.*[2]

This commentary closes with an observation having to do with tuberculosis. When all else fails, and a patient's tuberculosis is not responding, you might try a therapy that was used in the mid-1800s in England. In 1848, a study was undertaken at the Royal Brompton Hospital to determine whether liver oil would help cure patients of tuberculosis. Five hundred forty-two patients with tuberculosis were treated with cod liver oil at a dose of 3.6 mL, 3 times daily, gradually increased in some cases up to 1.5 ounces per dose. These patients were compared with 535 patients who received standard treatment without cod liver oil. Tuberculosis was arrested in 18% of patients given cod liver oil, compared with just 6% of those in the control group. Deterioration or death was reduced from 33% to 19%. One of the most striking effects of the use of cod liver oil was an increase in the patients' weight. A gain in weight occurred in 70% and a loss in weight in only 21%.

In reviewing the report from 1848, Green et al observed that the likely effect of cod liver oil was its content vitamin D.[3] A role for vitamin D in immune defense against tuberculosis can be explained by how vitamin D enhances immune function. This may be one reason why putting patients with tuberculosis out into the sun as was done many decades ago may have had a positive impact on some patients' health. By the late 1800s, most everyone in England was receiving cod liver oil supplements. Curiously, during this period there was a rapid decline in the prevalence of tuberculosis. The review by Green of the report from 1848 found no mental methodological errors. The century-and-a-half-old report is a testimony to good clinical research and how durable that research can be over time.

**J. A. Stockman III, MD**

*References*

1. Kranzer K. Improving tuberculosis diagnostics and treatment. *Lancet.* 2011;337:1467-1468.
2. Centers for Disease Control and Prevention (CDC). Trends in tuberculosis—United States, 2010. *MMWR Morb Mortal Wkly Rep.* 2011;60:333-337.
3. Green M. Cod liver oil and tuberculosis. *BMJ.* 2011;343:1305-1306.

### The Role of Chest Radiographs and Tuberculin Skin Tests in Tuberculosis Screening of Internationally Adopted Children

George SA, Ko CA, Kirchner HL, et al (Case Western Reserve Univ, Cleveland, OH; Geisinger Med Ctr, Danville, PA; et al)
*Pediatr Infect Dis J* 30:387-391, 2011

*Background.*—Internationally adopted children (IAC) are a growing group of US immigrants who often come from countries with high tuberculosis (TB) burdens. There is limited evidence to support current TB screening guidelines in these high-risk children. Therefore, we have prospectively examined the clinical utility of tuberculin skin testing (TST) and subsequent chest radiograph screening for TB disease in recently immigrated, asymptomatic IAC.

*Methods.*—Within 6 months of immigration to the United States, we collected demographic information and assessed the nutritional status of 566 IAC who presented for routine postadoptive care. Children completed standardized clinical examination and TSTs. Chest radiographs were recommended for children with TST induration ≥5 mm. The association between TST induration and clinical outcome was assessed. The clinical utility of chest radiographs was evaluated.

*Results.*—There was no difference in age, birth country, or nutritional status between IAC with TST induration of 0 to <5 mm and those with 5 to <10 mm; IAC with TST ≥10 mm were older, more chronically malnourished, and more likely to emigrate from Guatemala. Among children with TST ≥5 mm (35%), 4 IAC had chest radiographs which were initially interpreted to be abnormal and consistent with TB; ultimately none were diagnosed with TB.

*Conclusions.*—The 5-mm TST cut point did not capture IAC with risk factors for latent TB infection or progression to TB disease, suggesting that this is not a useful screening threshold. In contrast, a 10-mm cut point identified IAC at risk for TB infection and therefore should be a more useful screening threshold. We question the clinical utility of radiographic screening for pulmonary TB in asymptomatic children.

▶ While there has been a slight decrease over time in the number of reported cases of tuberculosis here in the United States, there has been an annual increase in the rate of infection of approximately 5% in foreign-born persons on our shores. In 2008, the tuberculosis disease rate was 10 times higher in foreign-born persons than in natives. In that same year, more than 17 000 internationally adopted children joined US families. This growing group of US foreign-born people is also advised to complete more rigorous screening after immigration to ensure that those who might have tuberculosis are detected and treated. Historically, international adoption clinics have elected to obtain chest x-rays to rule out pulmonary tuberculosis when tuberculin skin results are ≥5 mm, but <10 mm. Also, treatment for latent tuberculosis is done when tuberculosis skin testing indurations are ≥10 mm. Although conservative, this treatment strategy can result in false-positive chest x-rays that may result in unnecessary treatment and additional evaluation.

The authors of this report undertook a prospective examination of the utility of tuberculosis skin testing and subsequent chest x-ray screening for tuberculosis in recently immigrated asymptomatic internationally adopted children. Within 6 months of immigration into the United States, the authors collected demographic information on hundreds of internationally adopted children. They found that the 5-mm tuberculosis skin test cutoff did not capture internationally adopted children with risk factors for latent tuberculosis infection or progression to tuberculosis disease, suggesting that this is not a useful screening threshold. In contrast, a 10-mm cut point did identify those at risk for tuberculosis infection and therefore would be a more useful screening threshold. They strongly questioned the use of chest x-ray screening for pulmonary tuberculosis in asymptomatic children.

As noted in the commentary of Boehme et al, a new automated molecular test for tuberculosis may enable relatively unskilled health care workers in resource-poor settings to diagnose the disease and accurately detect drug-resistant strains in most cases in less than 2 hours.[1] The test, Xpert MTB/RIF, uses an automated molecular probe for *Mycobacterium tuberculosis* and a real-time polymerase chain reaction that greatly amplifies sections of genes conferring drug resistance, thus improving detection. The equipment needed to do this costs approximately $17 000.[2]

**J. A. Stockman III, MD**

*References*

1. Boehme CC, Nicol MP, Nabeta P, et al. Feasibility, diagnostic accuracy, and effectiveness of decentralised use of the Xpert MTB/RIF test for diagnosis of tuberculosis and multidrug resistance: a multicentre implementation study. *Lancet*. 2011; 377:1495-1505.
2. Zarocostas J. New molecular test can diagnose tuberculosis in less than two hours. *BMJ*. 2010;341:c4897.

---

**Unexplained Deterioration During Antituberculous Therapy in Children and Adolescents: Clinical Presentation and Risk Factors**

Thampi N, Stephens D, Rea E, et al (Univ of Toronto, Ontario, Canada; Toronto Public Health, Ontario, Canada)
*Pediatr Infect Dis J* 31:129-133, 2012

---

*Background.*—Patients may unexpectedly deteriorate clinically and/or radiographically during the course of appropriate treatment for tuberculosis. These events have been extensively studied in human immunodeficiency virus—positive patients; however, there are few data about immunocompetent children and adolescents.

*Methods.*—We studied all human immunodeficiency virus—negative patients treated for tuberculosis at our center between January 2002 and July 2009. Demographics, sites of disease at diagnosis and deterioration, and actions at the time of deterioration were reviewed. Cases were compared with patients who remained well during therapy.

*Results.*—Unexplained deteriorations occurred in 15 of 110 patients (14%), all of whom were receiving directly observed therapy. The median time to deterioration was 80 days (range, 10–181 days). Enlarging intrathoracic lymphadenopathy often leading to severe airway compromise was common (7 of 15 patients). Four patients developed symptoms at sites remote from primary disease, including pericardial and pleural effusions and abdominal masses. Corticosteroid therapy was initiated in 9 patients. Deterioration was associated with multiple sites of disease at diagnosis ($P = 0.02$) and weight-for-age $\leq$25th percentile ($P = 0.03$).

*Conclusions.*—Deteriorations during therapy occur frequently among immunocompetent children and may present months into treatment as clinically significant events. Those with lower weight-for-age percentiles and with multiple sites of disease at initial presentation are more likely to deteriorate. Many patients improve with corticosteroids, supporting an immunopathologic basis for many of these episodes. These deteriorations can be difficult to distinguish from drug resistance, treatment failure, or infection with other pathogens.

▶ It has been known for some time that patients with the human immunodeficiency virus (HIV) who have tuberculosis may get into trouble when they are treated for their HIV infection. Patients may have rapid dissemination of their tuberculosis with worsening radiographic changes. This has been noted in nearly half of tuberculosis-positive HIV-infected individuals once antiretroviral therapy has been undertaken. This paradoxical response has been termed *immune reconstitution inflammatory syndrome*. This syndrome has also been reported on occasion in otherwise immunocompetent individuals who are on antituberculosis therapy. Though sometimes difficult to differentiate from clinical failure, these paradoxical reactions are generally defined as clinical or radiologic worsening of preexisting tuberculosis lesions or the development of new lesions in a patient who initially improves. They are not attributable to the normal course of the disease or drug failure. It is important to recognize and differentiate paradoxical reactions from drug resistance or infection with other organisms for which different management strategies are required.

Thampi et al have attempted to examine the incidence, timing of, and risk factors for the immune reconstitution and inflammatory syndrome in children with tuberculosis by looking at the case records of youngsters being treated for tuberculosis at the Hospital for Sick Children in Toronto. Their study is the largest case study of deterioration and paradoxical reactions in HIV-negative pediatric patients treated for tuberculosis and the first to explore risk factors for deterioration. A total of 112 children and adolescents were identified with clinical or microbiologic diagnosis of tuberculosis during a 7-year period. No patient with HIV infection was included. The average age of the patients was 11.8 years, and all of them had confirmed infection with M tuberculosis. A total of 19 patients (17%) experienced clinical or radiographic deterioration after initiating tuberculosis therapy. Of these, 4 were excluded because there was an identifiable cause of the deterioration. The onset of the syndrome occurred in an average of 80 days from the initiation of primary treatment. The most common variety of deterioration was increased intrathoracic lymphadenopathy with or without parenchymal involvement, followed by extrathoracic lymphadenopathy (including intra-abdominal, inguinal, and cervical) and abdominal viscera, brain, bone, pericardium, and pleural involvement. At particularly high risk were children who initially presented with extrapulmonary lymphadenopathy. These youngsters had a 3-fold increased risk of developing the syndrome.

This report is the largest series reported in an era of optimal antituberculosis therapy to identify and determine the incidence of unexplained deterioration in an immunocompetent pediatric population. The report clearly shows that deteriorations are not infrequent and that the events themselves may be clinically difficult to differentiate from disease progression, relapse, drug fever, or secondary complications. The incidence of unexplained deterioration in this patient population was 14%. The authors chose to use a short course of steroids in this group of youngsters and saw a response in most patients. Others have used the antitumor necrosis factor antibody, infliximab, in steroid refractory cases.

The lesson from this report is that if you are involved with the care of a patient with tuberculosis, be aware that some months into therapy a clinical deterioration may occur and that this may be due to the syndrome described. The chances are this syndrome is a reflection of the body kicking in its own immune system to attempt to eradicate the tuberculosis organism, but in doing so it produces a reaction that is very difficult to tell from worsening of the underlying disease. Thank goodness for our infectious disease colleagues who can help sort all this out.

This commentary closes with a couple of observations about totally drug-resistant tuberculosis. India has one of the world's highest burdens of drug resistance to tuberculosis (around 100 000 people), according to the World Health Organization. The failure of the government to provide treatment for all of these patients is due to the cost—about $4000 (US) per patient, a high cost for India, which spends only $45 per head on health care. Researchers in Mumbai have now identified 12 patients with a virulent strain of tuberculosis that seems to be resistant to all known treatments. The cases of so-called totally drug-resistant tuberculosis (TDR-TB) have been detected within the last year or so. Worldwide, the only other episodes of TDR-TB reported were in Iran in 2009 and Italy in 2007. Patients with TDR-TB are walking the streets of Mumbai given that isolation is not practical because of cost and lack of hospital beds. Several identified patients come from Dharavi, a notorious Mumbai slum with a population of 2.5 million. As of 2012, 3 of the TDR-TB patients died from their tuberculosis. One of the patients had passed on her infection to her daughter. All of us should be aware of this problem because it will clearly crop up on US shores sooner or later.[1]

**J. A. Stockman III, MD**

*Reference*

1. Loewenberg S. India reports cases of totally drug-resistant tuberculosis. *Lancet.* 2012;379:205.

### Preliminary Study of Two Antiviral Agents for Hepatitis C Genotype 1

Lok AS, Gardiner DF, Lawitz E, et al (Univ of Michigan, Ann Arbor; Bristol-Myers Squibb Res and Development, Hopewell, NJ; Alamo Med Res, San Antonio, TX; et al)
*N Engl J Med* 366:216-224, 2012

*Background.*—Patients with chronic hepatitis C virus (HCV) infection who have not had a response to therapy with peginterferon and ribavirin may benefit from the addition of multiple direct-acting antiviral agents to their treatment regimen.

*Methods.*—This open-label, phase 2a study included an exploratory cohort of 21 patients with chronic HCV genotype 1 infection who had not had a response to previous therapy (*i.e.*, had not had $\geq 2$ $\log_{10}$ decline in HCV RNA after $\geq 12$ weeks of treatment with peginterferon and ribavirin). We randomly assigned patients to receive the NS5A replication complex inhibitor daclatasvir (60 mg once daily) and the NS3 protease inhibitor asunaprevir (600 mg twice daily) alone (group A, 11 patients) or in combination with peginterferon alfa-2a and ribavirin (group B, 10 patients) for 24 weeks. The primary end point was the percentage of patients with a sustained virologic response 12 weeks after the end of the treatment period.

*Results.*—A total of 4 patients in group A (36%; 2 of 9 with HCV genotype 1a and 2 of 2 with genotype 1b) had a sustained virologic response at 12 weeks after treatment and also at 24 weeks after treatment. Six patients (all with HCV genotype 1a) had viral breakthrough while receiving therapy, and resistance mutations to both antiviral agents were found in all cases; 1 patient had a viral response at the end of treatment but had a relapse after the treatment period. All 10 patients in group B had a sustained virologic response at 12 weeks after treatment, and 9 had a sustained virologic response at 24 weeks after treatment. Diarrhea was the most common adverse event in both groups. Six patients had transient elevations of alanine aminotransferase levels to more than 3 times the upper limit of the normal range.

*Conclusions.*—This preliminary study involving patients with HCV genotype 1 infection who had not had a response to prior therapy showed that a sustained virologic response can be achieved with two direct-acting antiviral agents only. In addition, a high rate of sustained virologic response was achieved when the two direct-acting antiviral agents were combined with peginterferon alfa-2a and ribavirin. (Funded by Bristol-Myers Squibb; ClinicalTrials.gov number, NCT01012895.)

▶ Hepatitis C (HCV) affects children as well as adults. This report largely deals with the treatment of adults, but be assured that the lessons learned from this report also apply to children. We see in this report that about 180 million people worldwide are currently affected with HCV. This number includes approximately 4.1 million individuals in the United States. HCV infection turns out to be the most common cause of chronic liver disease on US shores. This infection is a leading cause of cirrhosis and hepatocellular carcinoma worldwide. The most common form of hepatitis C results from infection due to genotype 1. The latter is the most common genotype of the 6 major genotypes.

Chronic hepatitis C infection has been managed for about 20 years with the use of nonspecific antiviral agents such as interferon alfa. When first used in the early 1990s, management with interferon alfa resulted in sustained virologic response in very few patients. Over the past 2 decades, however, there have been steady improvements combining pegylated interferon alfa with ribavirin. This combination produces overall rates of sustained virologic response in the upper 50% range. The response when the infection is caused by genotype 1 is in the range of 45% to 50% as opposed to 80% in patients with HCV genotype 2 or 3. The rub with interferon treatment is its numerous side effects including flulike symptoms, cytopenia, autoimmunity, and depression. Ribavirin can induce hemolysis. As good as this combination of agents is in those who respond, their use in the real world is limited by the side effects profile of both agents and the unwillingness of many to stay on long-term therapy. Indeed, the great majority of the 4 million individuals in the United States who are infected with HCV have never been treated, much less cured. Thus there is a need to identify treatment regimens that are effective and shorter, with much better side-effect profiles.

What is new in the treatment of HCV has been the testing of agents that directly act to block viral enzymes that permit the production of mature viral proteins. Specifically investigators have looked at new protease inhibitors, specifically telaprevir and boceprevir, which were specifically designed for treatment of HCV genotype 1. These agents require the addition of peginterferon and ribavirin to help cover resistant strains, but this "add-on" strategy to standard-of-care therapy has, gratifyingly, resulted in superior rates of sustained virologic response both in patients who have not received prior therapy and in those who have.

Lok et al successfully show that the combination of oral HCV protease and protease inhibitors given for 24 weeks will result in sustained virologic response in more than one-third of patients who have not had a response to prior therapy with peginterferon and ribavirin. This is an incredibly important finding because it shows that a sustained virologic response can be achieved without interferon. The concept here has merit: 2 potent agents with complementary resistance profiles, given for a significant period of time, can impose a complete suppression of viral replication and result in virus clearance.

A host of clinical trials are now underway looking at the efficacy of various combinations of oral-acting antiviral agents. It is expected that within the next couple of years, we will see good data from these studies—data that are likely to result in approval of oral antiviral combination agents different from what we are now using.

In an editorial that accompanied this report, Chung noted that "there has never been a more exciting time for patients and providers who grapple with this silent killer."[1]

**J. A. Stockman III, MD**

*Reference*

1. Chung RT. A watershed moment in the treatment of hepatitis C. *N Engl J Med.* 2012;366:273-275.

## Rotavirus Vaccine and Health Care Utilization for Diarrhea in U.S. Children

Cortes JE, Curns AT, Tate JE, et al (Ctrs for Disease Control and Prevention, Atlanta, GA)

*N Engl J Med* 365:1108-1117, 2011

*Background.*—Routine vaccination of U.S. infants with pentavalent rotavirus vaccine (RV5) began in 2006.

*Methods.*—Using MarketScan databases, we assessed RV5 coverage and diarrhea-associated health care use from July 2007 through June 2009 versus July 2001 through June 2006 in children under 5 years of age. We compared the rates of diarrhea-associated health care use in unvaccinated children in the period from January through June (when rotavirus is most prevalent) in 2008 and 2009 with the prevaccine rates to estimate indirect benefits. We estimated national reductions in the number of hospitalizations for diarrhea, and associated costs, by extrapolation.

*Results.*—By December 31, 2008, at least one dose of RV5 had been administered in 73% of children under 1 year of age, 64% of children 1 year of age, and 8% of children 2 to 4 years of age. Among children under 5 years of age, rates of hospitalization for diarrhea in 2001–2006, 2007–2008, and 2008–2009 were 52, 35, and 39 cases per 10,000 person-years, respectively, for relative reductions from 2001–2006 by 33% (95% confidence interval [CI], 31 to 35) in 2007–2008 and by 25% (95% CI, 23 to 27) in 2008–2009; rates of hospitalization specifically coded for rotavirus infection were 14, 4, and 6 cases per 10,000 person-years, respectively, for relative reductions in the rate from 2001–2006 by 75% (95% CI, 72 to 77) in 2007–2008 and by 60% (95% CI, 58 to 63) in 2008–2009. In the January–June periods of 2008 and 2009, the respective relative rate reductions among vaccinated children as compared with unvaccinated children were as follows: hospitalization for diarrhea, 44% (95% CI, 33 to 53) and 58% (95% CI, 52 to 64); rotavirus-coded hospitalization, 89% (95% CI, 79 to 94) and 89% (95% CI, 84 to 93); emergency department visits for diarrhea, 37% (95% CI, 31 to 43) and 48% (95% CI, 44 to 51); and outpatient visits for diarrhea, 9% (95% CI, 6 to 11) and 12% (95% CI, 10 to 15). Indirect benefits (in unvaccinated children) were seen in 2007–2008 but not in 2008–2009. Nationally, for the 2007–2009 period, there was an estimated reduction of 64,855 hospitalizations, saving approximately $278 million in treatment costs.

*Conclusions.*—Since the introduction of rotavirus vaccine, diarrhea-associated health care utilization and medical expenditures for U.S. children have decreased substantially.

▶ This is another report documenting how well the reintroduction of the rotavirus vaccine has positively affected the care of children. Prior to the rotavirus vaccine, it was estimated that as many as 400 000 visits to physicians' offices were the result of infectious diarrhea caused by the rotavirus organism. Add to that some 200 000 emergency room visits and 55 000 hospitalizations, not to mention as many as 60 deaths annually among children 5 years of age or younger in the United States prevaccine, and you can see the magnitude of the problem. In clinical trials of the vaccine, hospitalizations and emergency room visits decreased by more than 90%.

What Cortes et al have done is to examine both direct and indirect vaccine benefits, estimating the national reduction in hospitalizations for diarrhea and associated cost after the introduction of the RV5 vaccine. They examined data from the 2001 to 2009 MarketScan Commercial Claims and Encounters Database. These data are derived from insurance claims and contain d-identified information from various public and private health care plans, including health maintenance organizations, fully or partially capitated health plans, preferred-provider organizations, point-of-service plans, indemnity plans, and consumer-directed health care plans. The survey did not include Medicaid recipients. In the aggregate, the investigators looked at data from approximately 2 million children less than 5 years of age. The results of the analysis show that from 2007 to 2008, overall annual rates of hospitalization for rotavirus-related diarrhea among children less than 5 years of age declined by 75% from a baseline of 14 hospitalizations per 10 000 person-years to 4 per 10 000 person-years. These declines were similar across age groups despite variations in vaccine coverage. Hospitalizations in vaccinated children decreased by 89%. All regions of the United States had significant reductions in rates of hospitalization for diarrhea. The estimated cost savings related to fewer hospitalizations was estimated at about 0.25 billion dollars for 2007 to 2008.

The findings from this report confirm those of other reports of a decline in rotavirus activity in the United States after the introduction of the rotavirus vaccine. If there are shortcomings to this report, it is that data were lacking on uninsured and Medicaid populations. Also, there was no information provided from this report about possible differences based on racial or ethnic group differences as well as no data existing on socioeconomic status of the vaccine recipients.

Finally, it should be noted that a small increase in the risk of intussusception (by 1 to 2 cases per 100 000 vaccinated infants) has been recently reported in association with rotavirus vaccination in Latin America and Australia.[1,2] No such increase in risk was noted in the United States, but if present, this risk would translate into an excess of approximately 50 intussusceptions in a fully vaccinated national birth cohort. Translated into dollars and cents, this would result in a cost burden in the United States of approximately $532 000, showing that this level of risk and its economic impact versus the economic benefits of vaccination clearly favor continuing vaccination of the US population.

**J. A. Stockman III, MD**

*References*

1. Buttery JP, Danchin MH, Lee KJ, et al. Intussusception following rotavirus vaccine administration: post-marketing surveillance in the National Immunization Program in Australia. *Vaccine.* 2011;29:3061-3066.
2. Patel MM, López-Collada VR, Bulhões MM, et al. Intussusception risk and health benefits of rotavirus vaccination in Mexico and Brazil. *N Engl J Med.* 2011;364: 2283-2292.

## Reduction in the Incidence of Influenza A But Not Influenza B Associated With Use of Hand Sanitizer and Cough Hygiene in Schools: A Randomized Controlled Trial

Stebbins S, Cummings DAT, Stark JH, et al (Univ of Pittsburgh, PA; Johns Hopkins Univ, Baltimore, MD; et al)
*Pediatr Infect Dis J* 30:921-926, 2011

*Background.*—Laboratory-based evidence is lacking regarding the efficacy of nonpharmaceutical interventions (NPIs) such as alcohol-based hand sanitizer and respiratory hygiene to reduce the spread of influenza.

*Methods.*—The Pittsburgh Influenza Prevention Project was a cluster-randomized trial conducted in 10 elementary schools in Pittsburgh, PA, during the 2007 to 2008 influenza season. Children in 5 intervention schools received training in hand and respiratory hygiene, and were provided and encouraged to use hand sanitizer regularly. Children in 5 schools acted as controls. Children with influenza-like illness were tested for influenza A and B by reverse-transcriptase polymerase chain reaction.

*Results.*—A total of 3360 children participated in this study. Using reverse-transcriptase polymerase chain reaction, 54 cases of influenza A and 50 cases of influenza B were detected. We found no significant effect of the intervention on the primary study outcome of all laboratory-confirmed influenza cases (incidence rate ratio [IRR]: 0.81; 95% confidence interval [CI]: 0.54, 1.23). However, we did find statistically significant differences in protocol-specified ancillary outcomes. Children in intervention schools had significantly fewer laboratory-confirmed influenza A infections than children in control schools, with an adjusted IRR of 0.48 (95% CI: 0.26, 0.87). Total absent episodes were also significantly lower among the intervention group than among the control group; adjusted IRR 0.74 (95% CI: 0.56, 0.97).

*Conclusions.*—NPIs (respiratory hygiene education and the regular use of hand sanitizer) did not reduce total laboratory-confirmed influenza. However, the interventions did reduce school total absence episodes by 26% and laboratory-confirmed influenza A infections by 52%. Our results suggest that NPIs can be an important adjunct to influenza vaccination programs to reduce the number of influenza A infections among children.

▶ Lots of schools have instituted procedures during flu season in an attempt to reduce the transmission rate of both influenza A and influenza B infection. The school systems in Pittsburgh are a good example of how far some schools have come. The Pittsburgh Influenza Prevention Project (PIPP) has placed in the Pittsburgh school system, school-based nonpharmaceutical interventions (NPIs) that include teaching elementary school children the basic principles of how to reduce transmission of the flu virus. The program in place is called "WHACK the Flu." This particular program was first developed by the Berkeley Public Health Division in California. The intervention in Pittsburgh was modified to add "or sanitize" to the W to read Wash or sanitize your hands often; Home is where you stay when you are sick; Avoid touching your eyes, nose, and mouth; Cover your coughs and sneezes; and Keep your distance from sick people. This program includes instruction in proper handwashing technique and sanitizer use. Hand sanitizer dispensers were ubiquitously placed in the school systems in Pittsburgh. They contain 62% alcohol.

Stebbins et al designed a study to see if the addition of hand sanitizers to the traditional "WHACK the Flu" program would in any way affect the incidence of influenza infection in elementary schools in Pittsburgh. Five schools received very specific training in hand and respiratory hygiene and 5 schools acted as controls. The use of hand sanitizers reduced the cumulative incidence of influenza A by 52% and absenteeism during the intervention period by 26%. No statistically significant reductions in influenza B or total influenza infections were observed. These data indicate that "WHACK the Flu" intervention combined with the regular use of alcohol-based hand sanitizer may indeed help to reduce the spread of influenza A among elementary school children and presumably in anyone using hand sanitizer in the general population.

The real issue is why there was no effect on influenza B infection rates with the use of hand sanitizers. The observation of no effect on influenza B could be attributed to differences in the basic biology and epidemiology of influenza B compared with A or the fact that influenza B infections occurred late in the season, after compliance with the intervention possibly had waned. The influenza B outbreak began just as the preceding influenza A outbreak was peaking in participating schools and throughout the region. Nonetheless, the study found that a set of NPIs can be implemented successfully on a large scale within urban schools to reduce absenteeism in the incidence of influenza A. If you want to "WHACK" influenza in the bud, a little alcohol applied frequently to your hands just might do the trick.

This commentary closes with a little bit of history on swine flu. Before 1918, influenza in humans was well known, but the disease had never been described in pigs. For pig farmers in Iowa, everything changed after the 1918 Cedar Rapids Swine Show, which was held from September 30 to October 5 of that year. Just as the 1918 epidemic spread the human influenza A (H1N1) virus worldwide and killed 40 million to 50 million people, herds of swine were hit with a respiratory illness that closely resembled the clinical syndrome affecting humans. Similarities in the clinical presentations and pathologic features of influenza in human and swine suggested that pandemic human influenza in 1918 was actually adapted to the pig, and the search for the causative agent then began. A breakthrough came in 1931 when Roger Shope, a veterinarian, transmitted the infectious agent of swine influenza from sick pigs, by filtering their virus-containing secretions, to healthy animals. Infectivity of the filtrate was subsequently confirmed by others who used the ferret model of influenza infection to document transmissibility for both human and swine viruses. Shope furthered the notion that the human pandemic strain of influenza A (H1N1) and the infectious agent of swine influenza were closely related by showing that human adult serum could neutralize the swine flu virus. In a mouse model, samples from patients ranging from newborn infants to 76-year-olds were tested for their ability to neutralize a swine influenza virus strain. This work showed that nearly all serum samples from subjects who were at least 12 years of age were able to protect mice from challenge with a virus isolated from pigs in 1930, whereas those from children older than one month but under the age of 12 years had no neutralizing antibody. These experiments suggested that the swine influenza virus or an antigenically similar one had been in circulation in the human population and had originated from the 1918 pandemic strain. Advanced virologic and molecular studies of viral relatedness support Shope's early hypotheses.

To learn more about the emergence of influenza A (H1N1) viruses from a historical perspective, see the superb review article by Zimmer and Burke.[1]

**J. A. Stockman III, MD**

*Reference*

1. Zimmer SM, Burke DS. Historical perspective-emergence of influenza A (H1N1) viruses. *N Engl J Med.* 2009;361:279-285.

### Risk of triple-class virological failure in children with HIV: a retrospective cohort study

The Pursuing Later Treatment Options II (PLATO II) project team for the Collaboration of Observational HIV Epidemiological Research Europe (COHERE) (Med Res Council Clinical Trials Unit, London, UK)
*Lancet* 377:1580-1587, 2011

*Background.*—In adults with HIV treated with antiretroviral drug regimens from within the three original drug classes (nucleoside or nucleotide reverse transcriptase inhibitors [NRTIs], non-NRTIs [NNRTIs], and protease inhibitors), virological failure occurs slowly, suggesting that long-term virological suppression can be achieved in most people, even in areas where access is restricted to drugs from these classes. It is unclear whether this is the case for children, the group who will need to maintain viral suppression for longest. We aimed to determine the rate and predictors of triple-class virological failure to the three original drugs classes in children.

*Methods.*—In the Collaboration of Observational HIV Epidemiological Research Europe, the rate of triple-class virological failure was studied in children infected perinatally with HIV who were aged less than 16 years, starting antiretroviral therapy (ART) with three or more drugs, between 1998 and 2008. We used Kaplan-Meier and Cox regression methods to investigate the risk and predictors of triple-class virological failure after ART initiation.

*Findings.*—Of 1007 children followed up for a median of 4·2 (IQR 2·4—6·5) years, 237 (24%) were triple-class exposed and 105 (10%) had triple-class virological failure, of whom 29 never had a viral-load measurement less than 500 copies per mL. Incidence of triple-class virological failure after ART initiation increased with time, and risk by 5 years after ART initiation was 12·0% (95% CI 9·4—14·6). In multivariate analysis, older age at ART initiation was associated with increased risk of failure ($p = 0·02$). Of 686 children starting ART with NRTIs and either a NNRTI or ritonavir-boosted protease inhibitor, the rate of failure was higher than in adults with heterosexually transmitted HIV (hazard ratio 2·2 [95% CI 1·6—3·0, $p < 0·0001$]).

*Interpretation.*—Findings highlight the challenges of attaining long-term viral suppression in children who will be taking life-long ART. Early identification of children not responding to ART, adherence support, particularly for children and adolescents aged 13 years or older starting ART, and ART simplification strategies are all needed to attain and sustain virological suppression.

▶ Human immunodeficiency virus (HIV) remains a problem for children throughout the world and is still a significant issue in the United States. It is estimated that more than 2 million youngsters are infected with HIV and that 700 die of HIV/acquired immunodeficiency syndrome (AIDS)-related causes every day. Currently, almost all youngsters with HIV infection have been infected through perinatal transmission, which, if left untreated, will result in death usually before the age of 2 years. Generally speaking, the ideal is to institute retroviral therapy in children as soon as possible after a diagnosis is made of HIV infection.

There is a lot to be learned from the PLATO II investigators' report. For young children, whose adherence to antiretroviral therapy depends totally on caregivers, treatment options are extremely limited and often poorly adopted. Of the 22 antiretroviral drugs currently approved by the US Food and Drug Administration, 5 are not approved for use in children, and 6 are not available in pediatric formulations. Additionally, treatment has to be adjusted constantly for body weight, and most pediatric antiretrovirals are formulated as syrups (often in large volumes), which are difficult to administer and store and are extremely unpalatable. Such problems contribute to the explanations of why, in the PLATO II and other studies, children are more prone to virologic failure than adults.

One of the ways of addressing drug compliance in children on antiretroviral therapy would be to press for more widespread use of solid formulations, particularly those including fixed-dose combinations. Currently, only 4 quality assured, triple-drug, fixed-dose combinations are available in solid and dispersible formulations from manufacturers of generic drugs, and less desirable dose formulations continue to dominate this small and fragmented market. The development of new fix-drug formulations is hindered by scarcity of clinical data about the use of certain drugs in children. Tenofovir has not been validated by regulatory authorities for use in patients younger than 12 years. No data about the safety of efavirenz or atazanavir in younger children are available. Some of the newer classes of drugs are not approved for children younger than 16 years.

The rate of virologic failure of the 3 original drug classes used to treat HIV infection in children shows the challenge of maintaining lifelong viral suppression in those who start such treatment much earlier in life. There is truly a need for strategies to promote optimum drug adherence in children and young people to minimize the likelihood of triple-class drug failure and for the development of suitable new drugs and formulations to optimize the treatment of children with drug failure. The authors of this report believe that fixed drug combinations and simplification of treatment strategies could be important ways to maintain therapeutic options.

**J. A. Stockman III, MD**

---

**Long-term outcome and lineage-specific chimerism in 194 patients with Wiskott-Aldrich syndrome treated by hematopoietic cell transplantation in the period 1980-2009: an international collaborative study**

Moratto D, Giliani S, Bonfim C, et al (Univ of Brescia, Italy; Federal Univ of Parana, Curitiba, Brazil; et al)
*Blood* 118:1675-1684, 2011

---

In this retrospective collaborative study, we have analyzed long-term outcome and donor cell engraftment in 194 patients with Wiskott-Aldrich syndrome (WAS) who have been treated by hematopoietic cell transplantation (HCT) in the period 1980-2009. Overall survival was 84.0% and was even higher (89.1% 5-year survival) for those who received HCT since the year 2000, reflecting recent improvement of outcome after transplantation from mismatched family donors and for patients who received HCT from an unrelated donor at older than 5 years. Patients who went to transplantation in better clinical conditions had a lower rate of post-HCT complications. Retrospective analysis of lineage-specific donor cell engraftment showed that stable full donor chimerism was attained by 72.3% of the patients who survived for at least 1 year after HCT. Mixed chimerism was associated with an increased risk of incomplete reconstitution of lymphocyte count and post-HCT autoimmunity, and myeloid donor cell chimerism < 50% was associated with persistent thrombocytopenia. These observations indicate continuous improvement of outcome after HCT for WAS and may have important implications for the development of novel protocols aiming to obtain full correction of the disease and reduce post-HCT complications.

▶ We have learned a lot about the Wiskott-Aldrich syndrome (WAS) since it was first described many decades ago. The syndrome is a severe X-linked disorder characterized by microthrombocytopenia, eczema, and immunodeficiency and is caused by a hemizygous mutation in the WAS gene, which encodes the WAS protein (WASp). This protein is expressed in hematopoietic cells. A functional deficit of the protein is often associated with immunologic defects, including reduced number and function of T lymphocytes, impaired antibody production, defective natural killer cell function, reduced chemokinesis of phagocytes and dendritic cells, functional deficits of regulatory T-cells, and abnormal induction of cell death (apoptosis). Clinicians dealing with WAS have developed a scoring system to describe the variability in the clinical presentation associated with WAS mutation. Patients with the typical WAS phenotype (scored 3 to 5) are highly susceptible to severe bacterial, viral, and opportunistic infections. Many of these patients will develop autoimmune and inflammatory complications, and there is an increased risk of hematologic malignancy, mainly lymphoma and leukemia. Patients with the milder forms of WAS (a score of 1 or 2) may show only an X-linked thrombocytopenia, which is characterized by reduced and delayed occurrence of infection, autoimmunity, and malignancy and prolonged survival. These differences in disease severity correlate, albeit imperfectly, with the amount of residual expression of the WASp. Despite advances in clinical care, patients with classic WAS have a poor prognosis with a median life expectancy of only 15 years, unless hematologic and immune reconstitution is achieved by hematopoietic cell transplantation (HCT).

The authors of the report abstracted tell us about the results of a retrospective collaborative study on 194 patients with WAS who have received HCT. The authors analyzed the clinical outcomes and the effects of clinical status and age at HCT, donor type, lineage-specific chimerism with respect to survival, and complications of HCT. The report tells us a lot about how well these young-sters do with HCT and which youngsters will do better and which will do worse.

Of the 194 patients reported who received a transplant, 82% were alive at the time of the study, with a median follow-up of 76.8 months. The 8-year survival rate was significantly better for patients who had received a transplant after the year 2000. Improved survival was observed for all donor types in the last decade but was particularly significant for recipients of transplants from mismatched related donors whose overall survival increased from 52.2% to 91.7% over the years looked at. Complications were common in the first year after transplant, affecting some 45% of patients, but occurred more rarely in surviving patients thereafter. Primary graft failure or graft rejection was seen in just 7% of patients. Autoimmune manifestations, predominantly cytopenias and endocrinopathies, were observed in 14% of patients.

Over the 30 years of accumulated data in this report, it was clear that for each decade looked at, survivor rates markedly improved for WAS patients who received a transplant. The study confirms that hematopoietic stem cell transplantation is an effective treatment and should be considered not only for patients younger than 5 years, but also for those older than 5 years, especially if the patient is in good clinical shape. Part of the improvement in outcome has been the ability to identify less toxic conditioning regimens prior to transplant. Parents of youngsters with this problem can be reassured that the significant majority of their affected children will likely do well in the long run with hematopoietic stem cell transplantation.

**J. A. Stockman III, MD**

---

**Morbidity and mortality in common variable immune deficiency over 4 decades**

Resnick ES, Moshier EL, Godbold JH, et al (Mount Sinai School of Medicine, NY)
*Blood* 119:1650-1657, 2012

---

The demographics, immunologic parameters, medical complications, and mortality statistics from 473 subjects with common variable immune deficiency followed over 4 decades in New York were analyzed. Median immunoglobulin levels were IgG, 246 mg/dL; IgA, 8 mg/dL; and IgM, 21 mg/dL; 22.6% had an IgG less than 100 mg/dL. Males were diagnosed earlier (median age, 30 years) than females (median age, 33.5 years; $P = .004$). Ninety-four percent of patients had a history of infections; 68% also had noninfectious complications: hematologic or organ-specific autoimmunity, 28.6%; chronic lung disease, 28.5%; bronchiectasis, 11.2%; gastrointestinal inflammatory disease, 15.4%; malabsorption, 5.9%; granulomatous disease, 9.7%; liver diseases and hepatitis, 9.1%; lymphoma, 8.2%; or other cancers, 7.0%. Females had higher baseline serum IgM ($P = .009$) and were more likely to develop lymphoma ($P = .04$); 19.6% of patients died, a significantly shorter survival than age- and sex-matched population controls ($P < .0001$). Reduced survival was associated with age at diagnosis, lower baseline IgG, higher IgM, and fewer peripheral B cells. The risk of death was 11 times higher for patients with noninfectious complications (hazard ratio = 10.95; $P < .0001$). Mortality was associated with lymphoma, any form of hepatitis, functional or structural lung impairment, and gastrointestinal disease with or without malabsorption, but not with bronchiectasis, autoimmunity, other cancers, granulomatous disease, or previous splenectomy (Tables 2-5).

▶ Common variable immunodeficiency is a primary immunodeficiency characterized by low serum levels of immunoglobulins G, A, or M with reduced or absence of specific antibody production. The diagnosis is typically made between the ages of 20 and 40 years, but 20% of affected individuals are less than 20 years of age at presentation. A delay in diagnosis of 6 to 7 years is common. Because of the relative prevalence, 1 in 25 000 to 1 in 50 000, and numbers of medical encounters, primary immunodeficiency is a clinically important immune defect. Most subjects have normal overall numbers of peripheral B cells, but they are depleted of specific types of memory-containing B cells. Although there have been many investigations into the nature of this immune defect since it was first recognized in 1953, the fundamental genetic or other causes of common variable immunodeficiency have remained unclear for the majority of patients. In a few cases, it is linked to an autosomal recessive condition. In other cases it is not.

The standard of care for subjects with common variable immunodeficiency is replacement with immunoglobulin G (IgG) given at frequent intervals for life. This type of replacement reduces the number of bacterial infections and certainly can enhance survival. Unfortunately, this treatment does not seem to protect against or treat the largely noninfectious complications, such as functional and structural lung disease, autoimmunity, granulomatous disease, liver disease and hepatitis, gastrointestinal inflammatory disease, or the development of cancer or lymphoma that are found in varying percentages of patients. These conditions are important because the autoimmune and inflammatory conditions over time can lead to significant morbidity and mortality. It is not clear, however, whether all complications are equally deleterious or whether some of these are relatively benign with no increased risk to survival over long periods.

**TABLE 2.**—Selected Complications

| Associated Condition | No. | % of Cohort (n = 473) |
|---|---|---|
| Infections only (no complications) | 151 | 31.9 |
| Chronic lung disease (functional/structural) | 135 | 28.5 |
| Bronchiectasis | 53 | 11.2 |
| **Autoimmunity** | 134 | 28.6 |
| ITP | 67 | 14.2 |
| AIHA | 33 | 7 |
| Evans syndrome | 20 | 4.2 |
| Rheumatoid arthritis | 15 | 3.2 |
| Anti-IgA antibody | 7 | 1.5 |
| Alopecia | 5 | 1.1 |
| Neutropenia, pernicious anemia, anticardiolipin antibody, antiphospholipid syndrome, diabetes mellitus, juvenile rheumatoid arthritis, uveitis, multiple sclerosis, systemic lupus erythematosis, autoimmune thyroid disease, lichen planus, vasculitis, vitiligo, psoriasis | < 5 | < 1 |
| **Gastrointestinal disease** | 73 | 15.4 |
| Malabsorption | 28 | 5.9 |
| Inflammatory bowel disease (Crohn disease, ulcerative colitis, ulcerative proctitis) | 20 | 4.2 |
| Chronic diarrhea | 9 | 1.9 |
| Idiopathic mucosal inflammation | 6 | 1.3 |
| Nodular lymphoid hyperplasia | 5 | 1.1 |
| Gastrointestinal bleeding, irritable bowel syndrome, partial gastrectomy, diverticulitis, esophagitis | 1 | < 1 |
| Liver disease/hepatitis | 43 | 9.1 |
| Hepatitis C | 9 | 1.9 |
| Liver granuloma | 8 | 1.7 |
| Idiopathic liver disease | 8 | 1.7 |
| Non-A, non-B hepatitis* | 6 | 1.3 |
| Chronic hepatitis of unknown origin | 5 | 1.1 |
| Primary biliary cirrhosis | 3 | < 1 |
| Nodular regenerative hyperplasia | 2 | < 1 |
| Hepatitis B, cirrhosis of unknown etiology | 1 | < 1 |

*Diagnosed before availability of the hepatitis C PCR.

The report of Resnick et al examines the outcomes of a cohort of 473 subjects affected by common variable immunodeficiency. The subjects were followed at a single institution over 4 decades. The report tells us about the demographic and immunologic markers associated with the complications of common variable immunodeficiency. Tables 2-5 illustrate the frequency of the complications seen in affected individuals. Of 411 subjects with complete follow-up (87% of the group), 19.6% had died. The median age of death was 44 years for women and 42 years for men, not significantly different. The predominant causes of death included respiratory failure from chronic lung disease, lymphoid or other malignancy, and overwhelming infection. The risk of death over the time period studied was nearly 11 times greater for patients compared with controls. Interestingly, not all complications were associated with reduced survival. Patients with gastrointestinal disease, liver disease, and hepatitis, lymphoma, chronic lung disease, and malabsorption had reduced survival compared with patients without these particular complications. Patients with autoimmune conditions, absent the previously listed complications, did not have significantly reduced survival over a 4-decade period. Subjects with higher

TABLE 3.—Granulomatous Disease by Location

| Tissue Location | No. (n = 46) |
|---|---|
| Lung | 20 |
| Multiple locations (ie, liver, lung, and spleen) | 7 |
| Lymph node | 6 |
| Liver | 4 |
| Skin | 3 |
| Spleen | 2 |
| Bone marrow | 1 |
| Brain | 1 |
| Neck tissue | 1 |
| Operative site | 1 |

TABLE 4.—Lymphoma and Selected Outcomes

| Lymphoma Type | No. (n = 39) | Outcome |
|---|---|---|
| Non-Hodgkin lymphoma, B-cell type, not further classified | 23 | 11 died of lymphoma, 12 alive |
| Diffuse large B-cell lymphoma | 3 | 2 died of lymphoma, 1 also had severe lung disease, 1 alive |
| Hodgkin disease | 4 | 3 developed B-cell lymphoma years after treatment for Hodgkin disease, 2 of these died of lymphoma, 2 alive |
| MALT | 5 | 3 no treatment, 2 chemotherapy, 5 alive |
| Marginal zone Lymphoma/monoclonal B lymphocytosis | 1 | No treatment given, 1 alive |
| Monoclonal B lymphocytosis | 1 | No treatment given, 1 alive |
| Diffuse poorly differentiated lymphoma with IgM-k macroglobulinemia | 1 | 1 died of lymphoma |
| T cell-rich B cell EBV + lymphoma | 1 | 1 died of lymphoma |

TABLE 5.—Other Cancers and Selected Outcomes

| Malignancy Type | No. (n = 33) | Outcome |
|---|---|---|
| Breast cancer | 9 | 1 died of breast cancer, 2 died of other causes, 6 alive |
| Gastric cancer | 3 | 2 died of gastric cancer, 1 alive |
| Melanome | 3 | 1 died of other causes, 2 alive |
| Malignancy of unknown primary | 3 | 3 alive |
| Colon cancer | 2 | 1 died of colon cancer, 1 died of other causes |
| Lung cancer | 2 | 2 died of lung cancer |
| Oral cancer | 2 | 1 died of oral cancer, 1 alive |
| Skin cancer | 2 | 2 alive |
| Hepatic carcinoid tumor | 1 | 1 died of carcinoid tumor |
| Colon, prostate cancer | 1 | 1 alive |
| Prostate, skin cancer | 1 | 1 alive |
| Thyroid cancer | 1 | 1 alive |
| Vaginal Cancer | 1 | 1 alive |
| Ovarian cancer | 1 | 1 died of ovarian cancer |
| Esophageal cancer | 1 | 1 died of esophageal cancer |

levels of IgA or IgG and higher percentages of peripheral blood B cells were found to have significantly better survival.

Although the genetic causes of common variable immunodeficiency are likely to be multiple and most remain to be elucidated, these data show that the overall survival of patients has improved somewhat over time. Fifty percent of the surviving subjects in this report are students working, retired but healthy, or otherwise pursuing normal activities of daily living. It is obvious that the majority of patients are carrying out normal lives on replacement IgG therapy. Unfortunately, a subset of patients will have significant complications and will die prematurely. Additional biomarkers are needed to provide clues to these clinical outcomes. It is possible that some patients need much higher doses of intravenous IgG. The authors of this report are to be congratulated on their diligence in carrying on a study spanning a 40-year period. In a sense, this is a one-of-a-kind report.

While on the topic of infectious diseases, one of the most significant problems in this regard 100 years ago was the presence of dead horses in the streets of New York City. These resulted in a significant health risk at that time. The Health Department in New York City, which had the task of removing dead horses, reported that during 6 working day periods in the hot July of 1911, 171 horses died each day—a total of 1026 horses in less than one week. These horses at that time represented over $0.5 million dollars, a sum entirely wiped out in a single week. When this was reported back then, it was estimated that this amount of money could pay for a sufficient number of electric vehicles to do all the work done by the horses and to do it more efficiently and economically.[1]

**J. A. Stockman, III, MD**

*Reference*

1. Editorial comment. Horses and Heat. *Scientific American*. September 2011:95.

# 11 Miscellaneous

## Correction of Cerebrospinal Fluid Protein for the Presence of Red Blood Cells in Children with a Traumatic Lumbar Puncture
Nigrovic LE, Shah SS, Neuman MI (Children's Hosp Boston and Harvard Med School, MA; Univ of Pennsylvania School of Medicine, Philadelphia)
*J Pediatr* 159:158-159, 2011

We sought to determine the relationship between cerebrospinal fluid (CSF) protein and CSF red blood cells in children with traumatic lumbar punctures. For every 1000 cell increase in CSF red blood cells per mm$^3$, CSF protein increases by 1.1 mg/dL (95% CI, 0.9-1.1 mg/dL) (Fig).

▶ Most of us have been reading about how to correct cerebrospinal fluid chemistries for the presence of blood since we were residents, and for some of us that was well back into the last millennium. Various formulas have appeared from time to time that have been touted to have improved the accuracy of such calculations. It is especially important to know how to do this if one is caring for children, because as many as 30% of lumbar punctures (LPs) done in pediatrics have some

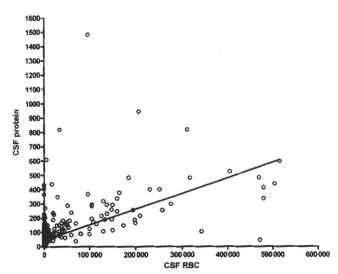

FIGURE.—Scatter plot of CSF RBC (cells/mm$^3$) versus CSF protein level (mg/dl; n = 1298). (Reprinted from Journal of Pediatrics, Nigrovic LE, Shah SS, Neuman MI. Correction of Cerebrospinal Fluid Protein for the Presence of Red Blood Cells in Children with a Traumatic Lumbar Puncture. *J Pediatr.* 2011;159:158-159. Copyright 2011, with permission from Elsevier.)

red blood cells (RBCs) observed in the cerebrospinal fluid (CSF). The presence of peripheral blood complicates the interpretation of CSF white blood cell (WBC) count as well as CSF protein, but rarely does it interfere with CSF glucose determinations. Nigrovic et al examined the CSF of almost 1500 patients who had CSF cell counts and chemistry analyses performed. Patients with bacterial meningitis, aseptic meningitis, herpes simplex virus encephalitis, and lyme meningitis as well as other neurologic conditions were excluded. One hundred eighty-nine CSF samples were found to have blood in them and were felt to represent a traumatic LP.

The findings from this report are clearly articulated in the Fig. One can draw a linear regression line representing the increasing CSF protein that is seen with increasing numbers of CSF RBCs. Overall, CSF protein increases by 1.1 mg/dL for every 1000 increase in CSF RBCs. It does not get much simpler than this. Although this study did not specifically examine the relationship between CSF RBCs and CSF WBCs, one can correct CSF WBC count or CSF RBC count. For every 500 RBC, one would expect to see 1 WBC.

**J. A. Stockman III, MD**

---

### Visualizing Veins With Near-Infrared Light to Facilitate Blood Withdrawal in Children

Cuper NJ, Verdaasdonk RM, de Roode R, et al (Univ Med Ctr, Utrecht, Netherlands; VU Univ Med Ctr, Amsterdam, Netherlands)
*Clin Pediatr* 50:508-512, 2011

---

*Introduction.*—This study aims to evaluate for the first time the value of visualizing veins by a prototype of a near-infrared (NIR) vascular imaging system for venipuncture in children.

*Methods.*—An observational feasibility study of venipunctures in children (0-6 years) attending the clinical laboratory of a pediatric university hospital during a period of 2 months without (n = 80) and subsequently during a period of 1 month with a prototype of an NIR vascular imaging system (n = 45) was conducted. Failure rate (ie, more than 1 puncture) and time of needle manipulation were determined.

*Results.*—With the NIR vascular imaging system, failure rate decreased from 10/80 to 1/45 (P = .05) and time decreased from 2 seconds (1-10) to 1 second (1-4, P = .07).

*Conclusion.*—This study showed promising results on the value of an NIR vascular imaging system in facilitating venipunctures (Fig 1).

▶ The report of Cuper et al provides us with information showing that a very simple instrument, a near-infrared light source, can be a great aid when starting an intravenous line. Most of us learned years ago that transillumination with a simple flashlight sometimes could help locate blood vessels that are not readily visible. The rub with a standard flashlight, however, is that the light does not penetrate particularly deeply. The advantage of a near-infrared light

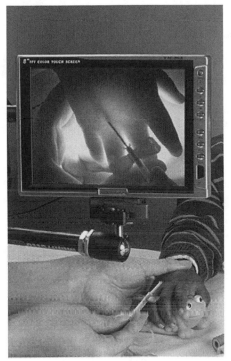

FIGURE 1.—Picture of the prototype of near-infrared vascular imaging system in use. The light emitting diode is placed underneath the puncture site; the camera and monitor are located directly above the puncture site. (Reprinted from Cuper NJ, Verdaasdonk RM, de Roode R, et al. Visualizing Veins With Near-Infrared Light to Facilitate Blood Withdrawal in Children. *Clin Pediatr.* 2011;50:508-512. © 2011 by Clinical Pediatrics. Reprinted by Permission of SAGE Publications.)

is that it can penetrate up to several centimeters into tissue thanks to a combination of reduced scattering and absorption compared with visible light. It is minimally absorbed by melanin in the epidermis, even in dark-skinned children. Better yet, it is absorbed by blood, which enables discrimination between blood vessels and surrounding tissues.

In this report, we see exactly how a near-infrared light source can be used. The near-infrared vascular imaging system uses a compact infrared-sensitive camera with visual grading analysis level resolution (640 × 480). Visible light is discarded by a filter blocking all light less than 800 nm. The camera is mounted on an articulated arm in combination with a compact 8-in liquid crystal display (LCD) monitor. High-power, near-infrared, light-emitting diodes (LEDs) of 850 nm are used to transilluminate the puncture site from underneath, through the hand or arm. A safety limiter is set to the power source to prevent heating of the skin. The transilluminated near-infrared light is scattered by the tissue and provides a diffuse background of light, while subsurface blood vessels become visible as dark lines on the LCD monitor. Such vascular imaging is able to visualize veins in the hand as well as in the wrist in children and adults. In younger children, it is also possible to visualize veins in the elbow or foot. Thus, the use of such an instrument gives one the x-ray vision of Superman in detecting blood vessels.

Fig 1 demonstrates the use of this near-infrared vascular imaging system in use. The system permits our visual senses to accomplish what they normally are incapable of sensing. On an unrelated topic dealing with blood vessels, please be aware that interventional cardiologists in the United States are more and more often imaging coronary blood vessels, not via the femoral artery, but rather the radial artery. Data show that access through the radial artery in the wrist is as effective in older children and adults as through the femoral artery and reduces the risk of bleeding complications. Of 7021 patients, 1.7% of those assigned to have coronary angiography with radial access had a major vascular complication compared with 3.7% of patients with femoral access.

**J. A. Stockman III, MD**

---

### The health risks and benefits of cycling in urban environments compared with car use: health impact assessment study

Rojas-Rueda D, de Nazelle A, Tainio M, et al (Ctr for Res in Environmental Epidemiology, Barcelona, Spain; Polish Academy of Sciences, Newelska, Warsaw, Poland)
*BMJ* 343:d4521, 2011

*Objective.*—To estimate the risks and benefits to health of travel by bicycle, using a bicycle sharing scheme, compared with travel by car in an urban environment.

*Design.*—Health impact assessment study.

*Setting.*—Public bicycle sharing initiative, Bicing, in Barcelona, Spain.

*Participants.*—181 982 Bicing subscribers.

*Main Outcomes Measures.*—The primary outcome measure was all cause mortality for the three domains of physical activity, air pollution (exposure to particulate matter <2.5 μm), and road traffic incidents. The secondary outcome was change in levels of carbon dioxide emissions.

*Results.*—Compared with car users the estimated annual change in mortality of the Barcelona residents using Bicing (n = 181 982) was 0.03 deaths from road traffic incidents and 0.13 deaths from air pollution. As a result of physical activity, 12.46 deaths were avoided (benefit:risk ratio 77). The annual number of deaths avoided was 12.28. As a result of journeys by Bicing, annual carbon dioxide emissions were reduced by an estimated 9 062 344 kg.

*Conclusions.*—Public bicycle sharing initiatives such as Bicing in Barcelona have greater benefits than risks to health and reduce carbon dioxide emissions.

▶ In 2010, the *British Medical Journal* published a systematic review that looked at whether community interventions promoting bicycling were successful.[1] The authors concluded that such schemes had the potential to get people on their bikes—but what are the actual benefits to health? Rojas-Rueda et al have attempted to answer this latter question in the context of a bike-sharing scheme, "Bicing," a phenomenon studied in Barcelona, Spain.

Rojas-Rueda et al estimated that as a result of the physical activity involved in using bicycles, 12.46 deaths would be avoided per year—a large benefit compared with the risks from inhalation of air pollutants and road traffic incidents—and that the scheme also reduced carbon dioxide emissions. The reliability of the conclusions is somewhat limited by the assumptions made in the model, but in sensitivity analyses the authors found a net benefit for Bicing users in all the scenarios they tested. The work undertaken is part of the European-wide project Transportation Air Pollution and Physical Activities, an integrated health risk assessment program of climate change and urban policies that has partners in Barcelona, Basel, Copenhagen, Paris, Prague, and Warsaw. One of the principal funders of this project is the Coca-Cola Corporation.

If you want an interesting read, pull out the September 2011 copy of *Scientific American*, which has much of its content focused on how we should rethink how we live in cities of the future. William Rees, Professor at the University of British Columbia and originator of the "ecological footprint" concept, suggests that we should completely rethink our definition of "the city" and see cities as complete human ecosystems recognizing that the complementary (and arguably more important) productive component of the urban human ecosystem is its resource hinterland, an area typically hundreds of times larger than the city itself and increasingly scattered all over the planet. In short, the city's true ecological footprint dwarfs the tiny consumptive urban center. The big footprint is essential to the survival of the urban core and yet it is typically ignored or taken for granted, or so says Dr Rees.

This commentary closes with a thought or two another type of recreational injury, having to do with kites. Kite strings can in fact cause serious injuries, including electrocution when wet and caught in power lines. Kites are banned during festive seasons in parts of Asia, where important events are often celebrated by kite flying. A motorcycle rider was recently injured, sustaining a fractured humerus and a lacerated internal jugular vein, when a kite string flowed across the road. He survived to tell the tale, but the authors of this case report say that such injuries are generally underrepresented in the medical literature and the hazards should be more heavily publicized.[2]

**J. A. Stockman III, MD**

*References*

1. Yang L, Sahlqvist S, McMinn A, Griffin SJ, Ogilvie D. Interventions to promote cycling: systematic review. *BMJ*. 2010;341:c5293.
2. Singla SL, Marwah S, Kamal H. Kite string injury—A trap for the unwary. *Injury*. 2009;40:277-278.

## Grandparents Driving Grandchildren: An Evaluation of Child Passenger Safety and Injuries

Henretig FM, Durbin DR, Kallan MJ, et al (Children's Hosp of Philadelphia, PA; Univ of Pennsylvania School of Medicine, Philadelphia)

*Pediatrics* 128:289-295, 2011

*Objectives.*—To compare restraint-use practices and injuries among children in crashes with grandparent versus parent drivers.

*Methods.*—This was a cross-sectional study of motor vehicle crashes that occurred from January 15, 2003, to November 30, 2007, involving children aged 15 years or younger, with cases identified via insurance claims and data collected via follow-up telephone surveys. We calculated the relative risk of significant child-passenger injury for grandparent-driven versus parent-driven vehicles. Logistic regression modeling estimated odds ratios (ORs) and 95% confidence intervals (CIs), adjusting for several child occupant, driver, vehicle, and crash characteristics.

*Results.*—Children driven by grandparents comprised 9.5% of the sample but resulted in only 6.6% of the total injuries. Injuries were reported for 1302 children, for an overall injury rate of 1.02 (95% CI: 0.90—1.17) per 100 child occupants. These represented 161 weighted injuries (0.70% injury rate) with grandparent drivers and 2293 injuries (1.05% injury rate) with parent drivers. Although nearly all children were reported to have been restrained, children in crashes with grandparent drivers used optimal restraint slightly less often. Despite this, children in grandparent-driven crashes were at one-half the risk of injuries as those in parent-driven crashes (OR: 0.50 [95% CI: 0.33—0.75]) after adjustment.

*Conclusions.*—Grandchildren seem to be safer in crashes when driven by grandparents than by their parents, but safety could be enhanced if grandparents followed current child-restraint guidelines. Additional elucidation of safe grandparent driving practices when carrying their grandchildren may inform future child-occupant driving education guidelines for all drivers.

▶ Until this report appeared, I had seen virtually nothing written about whether grandparents were more safe or less safe drivers of their grandchildren compared with children's parents. The report contains a number of interesting statistics. For example, based on data from the National Highway Traffic Safety Administration, almost one-half of adults who drive with a passenger aged under 9 years live outside the child's home.[1] The frequency of such trips is less likely than that for in-home drivers, but up to 33% of nonresidential drivers will make trips with children a few days per month, 14% a few days per week, and 5% almost every day. Of such nonresidential adult drivers, 42% are a child's grandparents, representing a significant pool of drivers with child-age passengers.

One might think, as did the authors of this report hypothesized, that older drivers (ie, grandparents) when taking their children about in a car would pose a greater risk of safety to a youngster. This in part would be based on the fact that older drivers have a higher accident rate, tend to travel in older and less crash-worthy vehicles, and are less compliant with current best-practices with respect to appropriate use of child restraints and rear seating. The investigators of this report tested the hypothesis that grandparents are a greater risk to their grandchildren than their parents are when driving.

The authors of this report collected data as part of the Partners for Child Passenger Safety Study, which was conducted from June 1998 through November 2007. The primary purpose of the analysis was to compute the odds of child-occupant injury in crashes involving grandparent drivers versus those involving parent drivers. During the study period, data were collected on 11 859 children representing 240 897 child occupants in motor vehicle crashes. Grandparents comprised 9.5% of the drivers with the remainder being parent drivers. Grandparents were older (obviously) with an average age of 58 years versus 36 years for parents. Nearly all children were reported to have been restrained at the time of an auto crash (98% for grandparents and 98.7% for parent drivers). However, child occupants in the grandparent-driven vehicles more often were not restrained according to best-practice recommendations (25.5% vs 19.3%). A small minority of children were seated in the front seat in both groups, but this difference did not reach statistical significance.

Despite the fact that grandparents do not comply with current best practice recommendations for optimal child restraint as often as parents, children in crashes with grandparents were at one half the risk of injury compared with children in crashes with parent drivers. One can speculate about why this is so. Perhaps grandparents are more nervous about the task of driving with the "precious cargo" of their grandchildren and establish more cautious driving habits to offset these challenges. Such adaptations might mitigate child injury after crashes when compared with parent drivers, even with very comparable gross measures of crash severity.

Being a grandparent myself, if we are doing something right with respect to child occupant injury prevention, maybe society as a whole can learn from us and apply this insight to driver-education targeted to all drivers of children.

This commentary ends with some data on the relationship between road fatalities and speed limits in the United States. Analyses of road fatalities provide yet more evidence that speed kills. Federal speed limit controls were altered in 1978 and again in 1995 allowing individual states to set their own limits. All states in fact raised their limits, but at different times and to different extents. Overall there has been a 3% increase in fatalities since 1995, with the largest increases in those states and on those roads where speed limits were raised the most.[2]

**J. A. Stockman III, MD**

*References*

1. National Highway Traffic Safety Administration (NHTSA). *Traffic safety facts: 2007 data: Children.* Washington, DC: US Department of Transportation; 2009. Report DOT HS 810 987.
2. Yakovlev PA, Inden M. Mind the weather: A panel data analysis of time-invariant factors and traffic fatalities. *Am J Public Health.* 2009;99:1626-1631.

## National Profile of Children with Down Syndrome: Disease Burden, Access to Care, and Family Impact

McGrath RJ, Stransky ML, Cooley WC, et al (Univ of New Hampshire, Durham; Dartmouth Med School, Hanover, NH)
*J Pediatr* 159:535-540, 2011

*Objective.*—To measure the co-morbidities associated with Down syndrome compared with those in other children with special health care needs (CSHCN). Additionally, to examine reported access to care, family impact, and unmet needs for children with Down syndrome compared with other CSHCN.

*Study Design.*—An analysis was conducted on the nationally representative 2005 to 2006 National Survey of Children with Special Health Care Needs. Bivariate analyses compared children with Down syndrome with all other CSHCN. Multivariate analyses examined the role of demographic, socioeconomic, and medical factors on measures of care receipt and family impact.

*Results.*—An estimated 98 000 CSHCN have Down syndrome nationally. Compared with other CSHCN, children with Down syndrome had a greater number of co-morbid conditions, were more likely to have unmet needs, faced greater family impacts, and were less likely to have access to a medical home. These differences become more pronounced for children without insurance and from low socioeconomic status families.

*Conclusions.*—Children with Down syndrome disproportionately face greater disease burden, more negatively pronounced family impacts, and greater unmet needs than other CSHCN. Promoting medical homes at the practice level and use of those services by children with Down syndrome and other CSHCN may help mitigate these family impacts.

▶ McGrath et al estimate that there are approximately 98 000 individuals with Down syndrome within the group of children with special health care needs in the United States as determined in 2005 to 2006. Compared with other children with special health care needs, children with Down syndrome appear to be significantly less likely to have private medical insurance, 47% less likely to have a medical home, and twice as likely to have unmet needs for care and family support services. It is also noted that children with Down syndrome require more care coordination and face serious health care disparities related to medical complexity, relative lack of health insurance, and decreased likelihood of having a medical home. These data are consistent with that of Goldman et al who have noted that in the state of Tennessee, the mortality rate for infants with Down syndrome is 8.3 times the state's overall infant mortality rate with excess morbidity being related to heart and respiratory conditions.[1]

In the same issue of the *Journal of Pediatrics* that contained the report of McGrath et al, Geelhoed et al provided information about the health care cost of children and adolescents with Down syndrome in Australia.[2] The data from Australia indicate that the cost of care for children with Down syndrome runs 4.2-fold higher for 0- to 4-year-olds, 3.8-fold for 5- to 14-year-olds, and 1.7-fold for 15- to 24-year-olds. Forty-five percent of youngsters with

Down syndrome cared for in Australia had congenital heart disease. Across all age groups, the mean annual cost of medical care for youngsters with Down syndrome ran $4209, significantly in excess of the care cost for otherwise unaffected youngsters.

In an editorial that accompanied this report, McCabe et al remind us that the lack of coordination of comorbid conditions for medically at-risk children with Down syndrome will continue to have preventable dire consequences and that these gaps in services must be addressed.[3]

**J. A. Stockman III, MD**

*References*

1. Goldman SE, Urbano RC, Hodapp RM. Determining the amount, timing and causes of mortality among infants with Down syndrome. *J Intellect Disabil Res.* 2011;55:85-94.
2. Geelhoed EA, Bebbington A, Bower C, Deshpande A, Leonard H. Direct health care costs of children and adolescents with Down syndrome. *J Pediatr.* 2011; 159:541-545.
3. McCabe LL, Hickey F, McCabe ER. Down syndrome: addressing the gaps. *J Pediatr.* 2011;159:525-526.

---

**Induced abortion: incidence and trends worldwide from 1995 to 2008**
Sedgh G, Singh S, Shah IH, et al (Guttmacher Inst, NY; World Health Organization, Geneva, Switzerland)
*Lancet* 379:625-632, 2012

---

*Background.*—Data of abortion incidence and trends are needed to monitor progress toward improvement of maternal health and access to family planning. To date, estimates of safe and unsafe abortion worldwide have only been made for 1995 and 2003.

*Methods.*—We used the standard WHO definition of unsafe abortions. Safe abortion estimates were based largely on official statistics and nationally representative surveys. Unsafe abortion estimates were based primarily on information from published studies, hospital records, and surveys of women. We used additional sources and systematic approaches to make corrections and projections as needed where data were misreported, incomplete, or from earlier years. We assessed trends in abortion incidence using rates developed for 1995, 2003, and 2008 with the same methodology. We used linear regression models to explore the association of the legal status of abortion with the abortion rate across subregions of the world in 2008.

*Findings.*—The global abortion rate was stable between 2003 and 2008, with rates of 29 and 28 abortions per 1000 women aged 15—44 years, respectively, following a period of decline from 35 abortions per 1000 women in 1995. The average annual percent change in the rate was nearly 2·4% between 1995 and 2003 and 0·3% between 2003 and 2008. Worldwide, 49% of abortions were unsafe in 2008, compared to 44% in 1995. About one in five pregnancies ended in abortion in 2008. The abortion rate was lower in subregions where more women live under liberal abortion laws ($p < 0.05$).

*Interpretation.*—The substantial decline in the abortion rate observed earlier has stalled, and the proportion of all abortions that are unsafe has increased. Restrictive abortion laws are not associated with lower abortion rates. Measures to reduce the incidence of unintended pregnancy and unsafe abortion, including investments in family planning services and safe abortion care, are crucial steps toward achieving the Millennium Development Goals.

▶ Whether a person supports a woman's decision to have an abortion or believes otherwise, the information from this report should be understood by all. This article coincides with the anniversary of the *Roe v Wade* US Supreme Court decision that effectively legalized abortion in all 50 states. In the nearly 3 decades that have followed this landmark decision, there has been no end to the controversy surrounding abortion. These authors present an article on global abortion rates that will generate debate once again. The article documents stagnation in global abortion rates between 2003 and 2008 (29 and 28 abortions per 1000 women aged 15—44 years, respectively), effectively ending the nearly decade-long decline that preceded 2003, suggesting a recent growth in the number of women seeking abortion, possibly because of an unmet need for contraception. The report also showed that the share of abortions worldwide that were unsafe has risen, from 44% in 1995 to 49% in 2008, showing little progress in tackling this preventable source of maternal mortality.

There are some findings in this article worthy of additional comment. For example, the authors point out a potential weakness in some arguments in favor of restriction of abortion services. First, legal restrictions on abortion have not led to decreased use of the procedure in most places; in fact, there may be an inverse relation. The lowest rate of abortion reported (12 per 1000 women aged 15—44 years) is seen in Western European countries, where laws are among the least restrictive. In recognition of this finding, the government of Mexico City voted in 2007 to legalize abortion for the first 12 weeks of pregnancy. For the rest of the country, abortion remains illegal. It does appear that women who wished to terminate unwanted pregnancies will seek abortion at any cost, even when it is illegal or involves a risk to the woman's life.

My commentary began with the observation that no matter what a person's opinion is regarding abortion, the data from this report should be carefully reviewed. The article takes little position on this topic, but it does provide information of which we should all be aware.

**J. A. Stockman III, MD**

## Adults With Chronic Health Conditions Originating in Childhood: Inpatient Experience in Children's Hospitals

Goodman DM, Hall M, Levin A, et al (Univ Feinberg School of Medicine and Children's Memorial Hosp, Chicago, IL; Children's Hosp of Pittsburgh of UPMC, PA; et al)
*Pediatrics* 128:5-13, 2011

*Objective.*—To describe the rate of increase of the population of adults seeking care as inpatients in children's hospitals over time.

*Patients and Methods.*—We analyzed data from January 1, 1999, to December 31, 2008, from patients hospitalized at 30 academic children's hospitals, including growth rates according to age group (pediatric: aged <18 years; transitional: aged 18–21 years; or adult: aged >21 years) and disease.

*Results.*—There were 3 343 194 hospital discharges for 2 143 696 patients. Transitional patients represented 2.0%, and adults represented 0.8%, totaling 59 974 patients older than 18 years. The number of unique patients, admissions, patient-days, and charges increased in all age groups over the study period and are projected to continue to increase. Resource use was disproportionately higher in the older ages. The growth of transitional patients exceeded that of others, with 6.9% average annual increase in discharges, 7.6% in patient-days, and 15% in charges. Chronic conditions occurred in 87% of adults compared with 48% of pediatric patients. Compared with pediatric patients, the rates of increase of inpatient-days increased significantly for transitional age patients with cystic fibrosis, malignant neoplasms, and epilepsy, and for adults with cerebral palsy. Annual growth rates of charges increased for transitional and adult patients for all diagnoses except cystic fibrosis and sickle cell disease.

*Conclusions.*—The population of adults with diseases originating in childhood who are hospitalized at children's hospitals is increasing, with varying disease-specific changes over time. Our findings underscore the need for proactive identification of strategies to care for adult survivors of pediatric diseases.

▶ As children and adolescents have survived serious chronic illnesses in childhood, the population of young adults with these disorders has increased rapidly. In 2002, a consensus statement coauthored by the American Academy of Pediatrics, the American Academy of Family Physicians, and the American College of Physicians—American Society of Internal Medicine was published stating the importance of supporting and facilitating the transition of adolescents with special health care needs into adulthood.[1] This statement represented the shared perspectives of health care professionals, families, youth, researchers, and policy makers and established a foundational guidance for health care processes that include health care planning and information exchange, for professional education and certification and for insurance and payment reform. Unfortunately, a recent national survey has revealed that pediatricians remain poorly informed about the conclusions of the consensus statement and that most pediatric practices neither initiate transition planning early in adolescence nor offer transition-support services. Both have been found to be critical for ensuring a smooth transition to an adult health care model.[2]

Goodman et al expand our knowledge about transition of care by examining more than 3 million hospital discharges of pediatric-age individuals (<18 years), transitional age individuals (aged 18–21 years), or adults (aged >21 years) admitted to children's hospitals in the United States. It was clear that the growth of transitional-age patients exceeded that of all other discharges with a 6.9% annual increase in discharges, a 7.6% in patient days, and a 15% in overall hospital charges. These admissions were largely for young adults with chronic conditions. Chronic conditions occurred in 87% of adults compared with just 48% of pediatric admissions to children's hospitals.

Without question, children's hospitals are caring for increasing numbers of patients outside of the traditional pediatric age range. This increase of patients aged 18 to 21 years exceeds that for pediatric patients. Projections suggest that both transitional and adult inpatient populations will continue to grow. Transitional-age patients with cystic fibrosis and congenital heart disease comprise a fair percentage of young adults who are still admitted to children's hospitals. Other diagnostic categories that make up a significant percentage of young adults in children's hospitals include malignant neoplasm, sickle cell disease, cerebral palsy, and epilepsy with recurrent seizures.

The consensus statement on transition of care from adolescence to adulthood concludes that a well-timed, well-planned, and well-executed transition from child- to adult-oriented health care, ideally occurring between the ages of 18 and 21, enables youth to optimize their ability to assume adult roles and activities. Such transition planning should be a standard part of the provision of care for all youth and young adults, and every patient should have an individualized transition plan regardless of his or her specific health care needs. All primary care physicians, nurse practitioners, and physician assistants, as well as medical subspecialists, are encouraged to adopt the recommendations of the American Academy of Pediatrics, the American Academy of Family Physicians, and the American College of Physicians—American Society of Internal Medicine.

This commentary closes with a question having to do with longevity. Is there any correlation between perceived age (versus actual age) and longevity? How would you design a study to address this? By way of background, perceived age—usually the estimated age of a person—is an integral part of assessment of patients. It is influenced negatively by exposure to the sun, smoking, and low body mass index and positively by high social status, low depression score, and being married, although the strengths of these associations vary by sex. Investigators in Denmark, Germany, the Netherlands and the United States tackled this ponderous question by looking at the survival of twins who had their ages estimated by visual appearance of their face, estimates that were done by trained observers. A total of 1826 twins (840 men and 986 women) had a passport-type photograph taken. The photograph was taken in 2001 and these twins were then followed to determine their survival rates. The twins were already at an older age; over the interval period of time, 33% of the men and 26% of the women had died. The bottom line was clear: The likelihood that the older-looking twin of the pair died first increased with increasing discordance in perceived age within the pair; that is, the bigger the difference in perceived age within the pair, the more likely that the older-looking twin would die first. Interestingly, perceived age, controlled for chronological age and sex, also correlated significantly with physical and cognitive functioning as well as with lymphocyte telomere length. Please note that this report was done on individuals who had already reached the age of 70, so perhaps if you are a bit younger, but look a bit older, you still have a chance to modify your future.[3]

**J. A. Stockman III, MD**

*References*

1. American Academy of Pediatrics; American Academy of Family Physicians; American College of Physicians-American Society of Internal Medicine. A consensus statement on health care transitions for young adults with special health care needs. *Pediatrics.* 2002;110:1304-1306.
2. AAP Department of Research. Survey: transition services lacking for teens with special needs. *AAP News.* 2009;30:12.
3. Christensen K, Thinggaard M, McGue M, et al. Perceived age as clinically useful biomarker of aging. *BMJ.* 2009;339:1433-1434.

---

### Yoga for Chronic Low Back Pain: A Randomized Trial

Tilbrook HE, Cox H, Hewitt CE, et al (Univ of York, Heslington, UK; Univ of Manchester, UK; Yoga in York, UK; et al)
*Ann Intern Med* 155:569-578, 2011

---

*Background.*—Previous studies indicate that yoga may be an effective treatment for chronic or recurrent low back pain.

*Objective.*—To compare the effectiveness of yoga and usual care for chronic or recurrent low back pain.

*Design.*—Parallel-group, randomized, controlled trial using computer-generated randomization conducted from April 2007 to March 2010. Outcomes were assessed by postal questionnaire. (International Standard Randomised Controlled Trial Number Register: ISRCTN 81079604).

*Setting.*—13 non–National Health Service premises in the United Kingdom.

*Patients.*—313 adults with chronic or recurrent low back pain.

*Intervention.*—Yoga ($n = 156$) or usual care ($n = 157$). All participants received a back pain education booklet. The intervention group was offered a 12-class, gradually progressing yoga program delivered by 12 teachers over 3 months.

*Measurements.*—Scores on the Roland—Morris Disability Questionnaire (RMDQ) at 3 (primary outcome), 6, and 12 (secondary outcomes) months; pain, pain self-efficacy, and general health measures at 3, 6, and 12 months (secondary outcomes).

*Results.*—93 (60%) patients offered yoga attended at least 3 of the first 6 sessions and at least 3 other sessions. The yoga group had better back function at 3, 6, and 12 months than the usual care group. The adjusted mean RMDQ score was 2.17 points (95% CI, 1.03 to 3.31 points) lower in the yoga group at 3 months, 1.48 points (CI, 0.33 to 2.62 points) lower at 6 months, and 1.57 points (CI, 0.42 to 2.71 points) lower at 12 months. The yoga and usual care groups had similar back pain and general health scores at 3, 6, and 12 months, and the yoga group had higher pain self-efficacy scores at 3 and 6 months but not at 12 months. Two of the 157 usual care participants and 12 of the 156 yoga participants reported adverse events, mostly increased pain.

*Limitation.*—There were missing data for the primary outcome (yoga group, $n = 21$; usual care group, $n = 18$) and differential missing data (more in the yoga group) for secondary outcomes.

*Conclusion.*—Offering a 12-week yoga program to adults with chronic or recurrent low back pain led to greater improvements in back function than did usual care.

▶ Yoga is not just for personal relaxation. It is being used increasingly as part of the management of both psychological and physical disorders. Its use in the latter regard is not restricted to adults. Increasingly those in the older pediatric population are seeking the therapeutic benefits of yoga. Tilbrook et al tell us a little bit about the value of yoga for management of low back pain.

Back pain is common in both teens and adults. Yoga may offer an alternative approach to the treatment of low back pain. Some have also noted that the benefits of yoga may be greater than those of exercise alone because yoga offers a combination of physical exercise with mental focus. Recently, a literature review based on published evidence has suggested that yoga may be an effective treatment of chronic low back pain. Tilbrook et al have taken this one step further, conducting a trial to determine whether offering a 12-week yoga program to adults (mostly young adults) with chronic or recurrent low back pain would lead to greater improvements in back function than usual care. Individuals as young as 18 years were included in this report. Subjects with chronic or recurrent low back pain were randomly assigned to a 12-session, 3-month yoga program or usual care. This trial found that offering a 12-week yoga program to young adults with chronic or recurrent low back pain did lead to greater improvement in back function than usual care. The improvement in back function was observed across the 12-month follow-up period but was much more pronounced at 3 months, immediately after the intervention. Although there was no evidence of actual pain reduction at 12 months, confidence in performing normal activities despite pain improved more in the yoga group than in the usual care group. Yoga seemed to be a safe form of activity with only a few participants reporting adverse effects that were possibly or probably related to yoga. It should be noted that just 60% of participants strictly adhered to the yoga program and its requirements.

This report represents a large randomized trial with long-term follow-up. Other interventions for low back pain have included both exercise and manipulation as well as cognitive behavioral treatment. Comparing the findings of the report abstracted with these other interventions suggests that yoga may improve back function more than exercise and manipulation or cognitive behavioral treatment. The bottom line is that yoga is a safe and somewhat effective activity that one can recommend with some degree of confidence to an adolescent/young adult population suffering from low back pain.[1]

If you are not familiar with the derivation of the word yoga, the Sanskrit word *yoga* has the literal meaning of "yoke," from a root *yuj* meaning to join, to unite, or to attach. As a term for a system of abstract meditation or mental abstraction, it was introduced into society in the second century BC but uncovered statues from earlier periods suggest that meditation of the type that we now call yoga may go back long before even that period of time.

All in all, based on the theory of the report of Tilbrook et al, put yoga into your practice and remember the words of the most famous yogi (Berra, that is): "In theory, there is no difference between theory and practice. In practice there is."

This commentary dealt with a clinical trial of yoga and closes with a remark or two about other clinical trials. A recent investigation shows that the design of more than 90% of around 2000 randomized controlled trials published in Chinese medical journals was flawed. Researchers have searched the China national infrastructure electronic database for reports of randomized controlled trials on 20 common diseases published between 1994 and 2005. The authors of 2235 of these trials were then interviewed about the methods they used to randomize participants. Only 207 of these studies used accepted randomized methods. The study's leader, Taixing Wu of the Chinese Cochrane Center at Sichuan University, overlooked the study. The review was published in the open access online journal *Trials*.[2]

**J. A. Stockman III, MD**

*References*

1. Sherman KJ, Cherkin DC, Erro J, Miglioretti DL, Deyo RA. Comparing yoga, exercise, and a self-care book for chronic low back pain: a randomized, controlled trial. *Ann Intern Med*. 2005;143:849-856.
2. Wu T, Li Y, Bian Z, Liu G, Moher D. Randomized trials published in some Chinese journals: How many are randomized? *Trials*. 2009;10:46.

---

**Exercise and Genetic Rescue of SCA1 via the Transcriptional Repressor Capicua**

Fryer JD, Yu P, Kang H, et al (Baylor College of Medicine, Houston, TX; et al)

*Science* 334:690-693, 2011

---

Spinocerebellar ataxia type 1 (SCA1) is a fatal neurodegenerative disease caused by expansion of a translated CAG repeat in Ataxin-1 (ATXN1). To determine the long-term effects of exercise, we implemented a mild exercise regimen in a mouse model of SCA1 and found a considerable improvement in survival accompanied by up-regulation of epidermal growth factor and consequential down-regulation of Capicua, which is an ATXN1 interactor. Offspring of Capicua mutant mice bred to SCA1 mice showed significant improvement of all disease phenotypes. Although polyglutamine-expanded Atxn1 caused some loss of Capicua function, further reduction of Capicua levels—either genetically or by exercise—mitigated the disease phenotypes by dampening the toxic gain of function. Thus, exercise might have long-term beneficial effects in other ataxias and neurodegenerative diseases.

▶ The report of Fryer et al is heavy-duty reading, but if you are into exercise or even if you are one who believes that you are born with a finite number of heartbeats that should not be wasted on exercise, the report is well worth your reading. Modern medicine has demonstrated the virtues of healthy diet and routine exercise for cardiovascular health, preventing diabetes, and lowering cholesterol, but a role for exercise in combating neurodegenerative diseases is less well understood. The report of Fryer et al presents compelling evidence suggesting that exercise might have a long-lasting beneficial effect on slowing neurodegenerative degree progression.

Though various neurodegenerative disorders have distinct clinical presentations, many of these, such as Alzheimer and Parkinson disease, are characterized in a similar fashion by the accumulation of insoluble protein aggregates in neurons. Thus, therapies that combat the deleterious effects of protein aggregation in one disease might turn out to be applicable to multiple other neurodegenerative diseases. Spinocerebellar ataxia type 1 (SCA1) is one of a group of 9 autosomal dominant hereditary neurodegenerative disorders caused by proteins that contain tracts of several uninterrupted glutamine residues. These disorders can and do affect children. Like other spinocerebellar ataxias, the hallmark pathology of SCA1 is the atrophy and loss of Purkinje neurons from the cerebellar cortex. This manifests itself as deficits in motor coordination that affect gaze, speech, gait, and balance.

The report of Fryer et al looks at an animal model of SCA1 and its causes. The animal model is the mouse, which can be genetically engineered to harbor the gene that reflects SCA1. Fryer et al showed that a modest exercise regimen substantially extended the lifespan of mice with this neurodegenerative disorder. They showed that SCAI-affected mice who exercised had increased concentrations of epidermal growth factor in brain tissue which persisted long after exercise. The heavy duty reading aspect of the article has to do with the explanation of why exercise actually pulls off this neat trick.

Given the encouraging results with exercise and SCA1, it will be of immediate interest to test the effects of exercise on other neurodegenerative disorders, for which effective treatments have been elusive and are desperately needed. For more on this topic, see the excellent editorial by Gitler.[1]

**J. A. Stockman III, MD**

*Reference*

1. Gitler AD. Neuroscience. Another reason to exercise. *Science*. 2011;334:606-607.

## A Mosaic Activating Mutation in *AKT1* Associated with the Proteus Syndrome

Lindhurst MJ, Sapp JC, Teer JK, et al (Natl Human Genome Res Inst, Bethesda, MD; et al)
*N Engl J Med* 365:611-619, 2011

*Background.*—The Proteus syndrome is characterized by the overgrowth of skin, connective tissue, brain, and other tissues. It has been hypothesized that the syndrome is caused by somatic mosaicism for a mutation that is lethal in the nonmosaic state.

*Methods.*—We performed exome sequencing of DNA from biopsy samples obtained from patients with the Proteus syndrome and compared the resultant DNA sequences with those of unaffected tissues obtained from the same patients. We confirmed and extended an observed association, using a custom restriction-enzyme assay to analyze the DNA in 158 samples from 29 patients with the Proteus syndrome. We then assayed activation of the AKT protein in affected tissues, using phosphorylation-specific antibodies on Western blots.

*Results.*—Of 29 patients with the Proteus syndrome, 26 had a somatic activating mutation (c.49G→A, p.Glu17Lys) in the oncogene *AKT1*, encoding the AKT1 kinase, an enzyme known to mediate processes such as cell proliferation and apoptosis. Tissues and cell lines from patients with the Proteus syndrome harbored admixtures of mutant alleles that ranged from 1% to approximately 50%. Mutant cell lines showed greater AKT phosphorylation than did control cell lines. A pair of single-cell clones that were established from the same starting culture and differed with respect to their mutation status had different levels of AKT phosphorylation.

*Conclusions.*—The Proteus syndrome is caused by a somatic activating mutation in *AKT1*, proving the hypothesis of somatic mosaicism and implicating activation of the PI3K—AKT pathway in the characteristic clinical findings of overgrowth and tumor susceptibility in this disorder. (Funded by the Intramural Research Program of the National Human Genome Research Institute.) (Fig 1).

▶ Proteus syndrome is associated with the development of hamartomata, which are localized outgrowths of a single tissue or a combination of tissues, indigenous to the affected body part or organ, usually growing at the same rate as the normal components and causing little pain or functional impairment. They are a key element of proteus syndrome, the cause of which has been identified by Lindhurst et al.

By way of background, proteus syndrome was first described in a 7-year-old boy with macrodactyly, hemihypertrophy of the right side of the body, depigmented skin patches over the trunk, and connective-tissue nevi over the dorsa of both hands, left foot, back of the elbows and axillae. The term "proteus" was applied to this syndrome because of the protean nature of the findings, and of course the name is based on the Greek mythological figure who assumed many shapes and forms. It is believed that Joseph Merrick, an

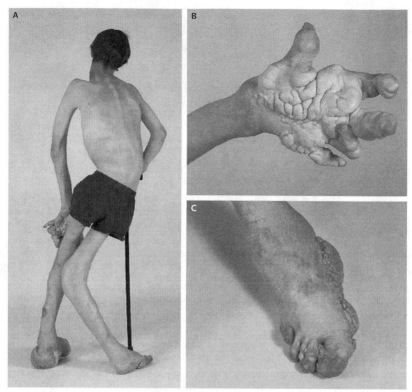

**FIGURE 1.**—Clinical Manifestations of the Proteus Syndrome in a 12-Year-Old Boy. Panel A shows severe orthopedic manifestations, including scoliosis, overgrowth with a resultant discrepancy in leg length, and valgus deformity and distortion of the skeleton, in Patient 53. Panels B and C show the characteristic cerebriform connective-tissue nevus and overgrowth and distortion of the hands and feet. Cutaneous vascular anomalies are present on the dorsum of the foot. (Reprinted from Lindhurst MJ, Sapp JC, Teer JK, et al. A Mosaic Activating Mutation in *AKT1* Associated with the Proteus Syndrome. *N Engl J Med.* 2011;365:611-619. © 2011 Massachusetts Medical Society.)

Englishman who lived in the late 19th century and became the subject of the film and play *The Elephant Man*, had proteus syndrome. It has been thought that proteus syndrome is caused by a somatic mutation that is lethal when constitutive. It is an uncommon syndrome with an incidence of less than 1 case per 1 million population and has not been reported to recur in a family. Some somatic or mosaic disorders such as the McCune-Albright syndrome are caused by single gene mutations, whereas other disorders such as certain cancers are caused by multiple mutations. A mosaic disorder is one in which cells within the same person have a different composition from one another.

Lindhurst et al have identified the cause of proteus syndrome. The identification of somatic mutations can be approached by sequencing the exons in the genomes of affected and unaffected tissues from patients with disorders of interest. Lindhurst et al used exome sequencing to identify a somatic mutation in patients with the proteus syndrome.

Just a few years ago, the DNA sequencing necessary to undertake the kind of effort that Lindhurst et al did would have been unaffordable. Through exome sequencing, they have generated billions of base pairs of sequence data. They were able to identify a small set of causal variants in a genome of more than 3 billion base pairs. Such sequencing and analytic techniques are improving. It is likely that the genetic causes of virtually all Mendelian or single-gene disorders will be identified. Thus, as the capacity to obtain and analyze DNA sequences continues to increase, solutions to riddles such as Proteus syndrome may become truly commonplace. Such technology will ultimately contribute to understandings about common conditions such as heart disease, cancer, and diabetes.

**J. A. Stockman III, MD**

---

## Prospective Evaluation of Residents On Call: Before and After Duty-Hour Reduction

Bismilla Z, Breakey VR, Swales J, et al (Hosp for Sick Children, Toronto, Ontario, Canada)
*Pediatrics* 127:1080-1087, 2011

---

*Background.*—On July 1, 2009, in Ontario the maximum period of continuous duty that residents were permitted to work was reduced from 28 to 24 hours. We evaluated the effect of regulation on residents in 3 eras: 2 before (2005 and early 2009) and 1 after (late 2009) the duty-hour reduction.

*Methods.*—On-call pediatric residents on pediatric medicine rotations prospectively recorded the numbers of patients (assigned and admitted) and the durations of direct patient care, documentation, staff supervision, and education attended. Sleep was measured with actigraphy.

*Results.*—The 51 residents worked 180 duty periods, were assigned a median of 6 (interquartile range: 4–12) daytime patients and 24 (interquartile range: 19–30) overnight patients. Residents reported spending means of 239 minutes providing direct patient care, 235 minutes documenting, and 243 minutes sleeping and receiving 73 minutes of staff supervision and 52 minutes of education. From early 2009 to after duty-hour reduction, residents provided 47 fewer (19.6%) minutes of direct patient care ($P = .056$) and received 44 fewer minutes (60.3%) of supervision ($P = .0005$) but spent similar times documenting, receiving education, and sleeping. In early 2009, residents provided 73 more minutes (30.5%) of direct patient care ($P = .0016$), spent 63 more minutes (26.8%) documenting, and slept 105 fewer minutes (43.0%) ($P = .0062$) than in 2005.

*Discussion.*—After duty-hour reduction in 2009, we found reduced supervision and direct patient care. Comparison of the 2 periods before duty-hour reduction showed less sleep and longer patient contact in early 2009, which suggests that changes occurred without regulation.

▶ This report about resident work hours emanates from Canada. Duty-hours worked by physician trainees are being reduced in jurisdictions that include Europe, Canada, and the United States. There is a lot to be learned from what is happening in Canada in this regard. The report of Bismilla et al looks at 3 training eras. The first era extended from May to August 2005, the second from May to June 2009, and the third from July to September 2009. In the 2 earlier eras, a 28-hour on-call duty period was in place, with duty periods beginning at 8:00 AM and ending at noon the following day. The third era took place after the implementation of new duty regulations that reduced the on-call duty period to 24 hours plus a minimum time for handover. In each of these eras, analyses were performed of the duration of direct patient care by residents, documentation time, staff supervision time, and time invested in education. Sleep was directly measured by actigraphy.

The results of this study showed that with no change in regulation between 2005 and 2009, comparing 2005 and 2009 regulations, residents slept 42.7% fewer minutes, spent 30.5% more time in direct patient care, and spent 26.8% more time documenting their care than did residents in 2005, despite working under the same regulations. These findings suggest that the nature of on-call activities may have been influenced by other factors that were not measured and were unrelated to work hour requirements. Such factors could include cultural changes, patient expectations, and complexity of patient disorders. When the duty-hour restrictions of 2009 were put into place, it was observed that the immediate effect of the 2 to 3 hours of duty-hour reduction included 20% fewer minutes of direct patient care, 60.1% fewer minutes of supervision by a staff physician, and reductions in the numbers of new patients admitted and discharged. The duration of participation in educational programs attended by residents did not change over any of these eras. Acute sleep deprivation, defined as less than 4 hours of sleep, occurred during 58% of duty periods.

The findings of this report do question the assumptions about the effect of duty-hour reduction on attendance at educational sessions and demonstrate significant absolute and proportional reductions in the amount of supervision and direct patient care. There seems to be no benefit to sleep duration as a result of the duty-hour restrictions. It is very clear that simply reducing work hours does not have a linearly positive impact on resident training, at least in Canada.

While on the topic of resident work hours, MacGregor et al found that surgical residents do not always record their work hours accurately and that most (52%) seem to intentionally under-report work hours.[1] It seems clear that in certain disciplines, duty-hour restrictions have created an ethical dilemma for residents and that many residents feel compelled to exceed work hour regulations in order to carry out their duties as they see them and to report those hours falsely.[2]

This commentary closes with a question. What do parents and family members prefer to be called by their pediatrician and is there any science behind this query? Indeed, a report has looked at the question of how best parents and families should be greeted by care providers.[3] It appears that 83% of adults want to be greeted by their doctor first with a handshake (just 8% of parents and family members did not like a handshake). Unfortunately, only 70% of residents and just 65% of attending physicians greet a patient/family with a handshake. Also, most parents (87%) want to be addressed by name (13% by first name, 53% by last name, and 21% by both). Unfortunately, residents greet parents by name in a scant 14% of incidences (1% by first name, 13% by last name, and none by both names). Attending physicians did not do any better. Curiously, physicians incorrectly addressed the mother by the child's last name in 9% of encounters. In this same report, all parents or caretakers when asked wanted a physician to introduce herself or himself, most with last name. In 84% of encounters, residents introduced themselves compared with 93% of attending physicians. Residents used their last name in two-thirds of these encounters and attending physicians in 86%. This report by Amer and Fisher examined 100 visits in which the child's mother was the parent in 81. When I was a house officer, it was in the days when attending physicians tended to be more voyeurs than physician on record. On many occasions, one could hear such physicians greet a parent with use of the term "mother." Parents want to be called more than "mother" and "father." Times have changed, but not all that much, at least according to the data of Amer and Fisher.

While on the topic of the use of names, when I was Chair of the Department of Pediatrics at Northwestern University Medical School (now called the Feinberg School of Medicine), there was a closing graduation ceremony for senior residents. This was associated with a great deal of pomp and circumstance and a speech given by the chair. I would always close that speech with the same comment, letting the residents know that they were now free, having graduated, to call me by my first name: Sir.

**J. A. Stockman III, MD**

*References*

1. MacGregor JM, Sticca R. General surgery residents' views on work hours regulations. *J Surg Educ.* 2010;67:376-380.
2. Carpenter RO, Austin MT, Tarpley JL, Griffin MR, Lomis KD. Work-hour restrictions as an ethical dilemma for residents. *Am J Surg.* 2006;191:527-532.
3. Amer A, Fischer H. "Don't call me mom": How parents want to be greeted by their pediatrician. *Clin Pediatr.* 2009;48:720-722.

---

**Ethnicity and academic performance in UK trained doctors and medical students: systematic review and meta-analysis**
Woolf K, Potts HWW, McManus IC (UCL Division of Med Education, UK, UCL Division of Population Health, UK)
*BMJ* 342:d901, 2011

---

*Objective.*—To determine whether the ethnicity of UK trained doctors and medical students is related to their academic performance.

*Design.*—Systematic review and meta-analysis.

*Data Sources.*—Online databases PubMed, Scopus, and ERIC; Google and Google Scholar; personal knowledge; backwards and forwards citations; specific searches of medical education journals and medical education conference abstracts.

*Study Selection.*—The included quantitative reports measured the performance of medical students or UK trained doctors from different ethnic groups in undergraduate or postgraduate assessments. Exclusions were non-UK assessments, only non-UK trained candidates, only self reported assessment data, only dropouts or another non-academic variable, obvious sampling bias, or insufficient details of ethnicity or outcomes. Results 23 reports comparing the academic performance of medical students and doctors from different ethnic groups were included. Meta-analyses of effects from 22 reports ($n = 23,742$) indicated candidates of "non-white" ethnicity underperformed compared with white candidates (Cohen's d $= -0.42$, 95% confidence interval $-0.50$ to $-0.34$; $P < 0.001$). Effects in the same direction and of similar magnitude were found in meta-analyses of undergraduate assessments only, postgraduate assessments only, machine marked written assessments only, practical clinical assessments only, assessments with pass/fail outcomes only, assessments with continuous outcomes only, and in a meta-analysis of white v Asian candidates only. Heterogeneity was present in all meta-analyses.

*Conclusion.*—Ethnic differences in academic performance are widespread across different medical schools, different types of exam, and in undergraduates and postgraduates. They have persisted for many years and cannot be dismissed as atypical or local problems. We need to recognise this as an issue that probably affects all of UK medical and higher education. More detailed information to track the problem as well as further research into its causes is required. Such actions are necessary to ensure a fair and just method of training and of assessing current and future doctors.

▶ There is no comprehensive study performed in the United States that is comparable to that reported by Woolf et al from Great Britain. The systematic review by Woolf et al tackles a sensitive subject and comes to a controversial conclusion. The authors reviewed 23 quantitative studies that evaluated the performance of nearly 28 000 United Kingdom—trained medical students and doctors, with both summative and formative assessments (including machine-marked examinations), and found that candidates from nonwhite ethnic groups did significantly less well than white candidates. The full article, which may be found on BMJ.com, is very detailed, showing how the authors did 7 separate meta-analyses and took into account adjustments for confounding factors such as sex, first language, previous examination performance, and socioeconomic status. The association persisted despite limitations that included considerable heterogeneity in the primary studies and a mainly white versus nonwhite classification. An editorial that accompanied this report stated that the *BMJ* reviewers, editorial advisors, and editors all agreed that the findings were robust.

In the United States we are moving quickly into a better standard of evaluation of our trainees based on competency assessments, milestones, and what is known as *entrustable professional activities*. These new tools allow evaluators to decide whether an individual is performing to broadly accepted standards and in a manner that places much less emphasis on time and place in training. The Milestone Project, for example, has created tools for residency program directors to compare one resident with all other residents in terms of the acquisition of the 6 general competencies embraced now within graduate medical education. With these tools we can accelerate the training of quick learners and allow more focus on the deficiencies that any one resident may have.

It will be interesting to see if these newer approaches to both medical student education and resident training can assist those who have not had a fair start in life, for whatever reason. It is unacceptable that ethnicity should be a factor in determining the progress of students who enter medical school or to qualify doctors who sit for professional examinations. Solutions to the educational conundrum will be found through critically appraising assessment methods, curriculums, the way we engage with students in an increasingly multicultural society, and the role models that we provide.

For more on ethnicity and academic performance, see the editorial in the *British Medical Journal.*[1]

**J. A. Stockman III, MD**

*Reference*

1. Esmail A. Ethnicity and academic performance in the UK. *BMJ.* 2011;342:d709.

---

## "July Effect": Impact of the Academic Year-End Changeover on Patient Outcomes: A Systematic Review

Young JQ, Ranji SR, Wachter RM, et al (Univ of California, San Francisco)
*Ann Intern Med* 155:309-315, 2011

---

*Background.*—It is commonly believed that the quality of health care decreases during trainee changeovers at the end of the academic year.

*Purpose.*—To systematically review studies describing the effects of trainee changeover on patient outcomes.

*Data Sources.*—Electronic literature search of PubMed, Educational Research Information Center (ERIC), EMBASE, and the Cochrane Library for English-language studies published between 1989 and July 2010.

*Study Selection.*—Title and abstract review followed by full-text review to identify studies that assessed the effect of the changeover on patient outcomes and that used a control group or period as a comparator.

*Data Extraction.*—Using a standardized form, 2 authors independently abstracted data on outcomes, study setting and design, and statistical methods. Differences between reviewers were reconciled by consensus. Studies were then categorized according to methodological quality, sample size, and outcomes reported.

*Data Synthesis.*—Of the 39 included studies, 27 (69%) reported mortality, 19 (49%) reported efficiency (length of stay, duration of procedure, hospital charges), 23 (59%) reported morbidity, and 6 (15%) reported medical error outcomes; all studies focused on inpatient settings. Most studies were conducted in the United States. Thirteen (33%) were of higher quality. Studies with higherquality designs and larger sample sizes more often showed increased mortality and decreased efficiency at time of changeover. Studies examining morbidity and medical error outcomes were of lower quality and produced inconsistent results.

*Limitations.*—The review was limited to English-language reports. No study focused on the effect of changeovers in ambulatory care settings. The definition of changeover, resident role in patient care, and supervision structure varied considerably among studies. Most studies did not control for time trends or level of supervision or use methods appropriate for hierarchical data.

*Conclusion.*—Mortality increases and efficiency decreases in hospitals because of year-end changeovers, although heterogeneity in the existing literature does not permit firm conclusions about the degree of risk posed, how changeover affects morbidity and rates of medical errors, or whether particular models are more or less problematic.

▶ It is not a secret that most care providers themselves would prefer not to be admitted to a hospital on or about July 1 if that hospital is an academic medical center with a residency teaching program. The systematic review by Young et al adds evidence to the long-held suspicion of this belief that the quality of care in teaching hospitals decreases at the start of the academic year. Prior studies have offered inconclusive findings. Now we have the evidence. The "July Effect" is real, and the findings from this report are sobering.

Young et al suggest there are a number of reasons for the decline in quality of care seen during transitions of interns and residents. The authors identified clinical inexperience, inadequate supervision of trainees functioning in new clinical roles, and loss of "systems knowledge" because of team turnover and departure of the experienced and loss of "systems-literate" clinicians. Young et al also offer us solutions, such as enhancing supervision, reducing the tempo of the uptake of clinical responsibilities in the first weeks of service, avoiding overnight responsibilities during that period, coupling experienced providers with inexperienced ones in a buddy system, and implementing certain other interventions (eg, staggering the start dates of trainees over the year). Better orientation to the medical microsystem would also be ideal.

There is a lot of information appearing these days related to competency-based assessments of residents in training. If one had a longitudinal assessment mechanism that went from medical school training into residency and into the postresidency period, one could be better assured that individuals are ready for whatever the next steps are in their career. More dollars should be invested in such competency-based training and assessment.

**J. A. Stockman III, MD**

## Quality of Life, Burnout, Educational Debt, and Medical Knowledge Among Internal Medicine Residents
West CP, Shanafelt TD, Kolars JC (Mayo Clinic, Rochester, MN; Univ of Michigan Med School, Ann Arbor)
*JAMA* 306:952-960, 2011

*Context.*—Physician distress is common and has been associated with negative effects on patient care. However, factors associated with resident distress and well-being have not been well described at a national level.

*Objectives.*—To measure well-being in a national sample of internal medicine residents and to evaluate relationships with demographics, educational debt, and medical knowledge.

*Design, Setting, and Participants.*—Study of internal medicine residents using data collected on 2008 and 2009 Internal Medicine In-Training Examination (IM-ITE) scores and the 2008 IM-ITE survey. Participants were 16 394 residents, representing 74.1% of all eligible US internal medicine residents in the 2008-2009 academic year. This total included 7743 US medical graduates and 8571 international medical graduates.

*Main Outcome Measures.*—Quality of life (QOL) and symptoms of burnout were assessed, as were year of training, sex, medical school location, educational debt, and IM-ITE score reported as percentage of correct responses.

*Results.*—Quality of life was rated "as bad as it can be" or "somewhat bad" by 2402 of 16 187 responding residents (14.8%). Overall burnout and high levels of emotional exhaustion and depersonalization were reported by 8343 of 16 192 (51.5%), 7394 of 16 154 (45.8%), and 4541 of 15 737 (28.9%) responding residents, respectively. In multivariable models, burnout was less common among international medical graduates than among US medical graduates (45.1% vs 58.7%; odds ratio, 0.70 [99% CI, 0.63-0.77]; P<.001). Greater educational debt was associated with the presence of at least 1 symptom of burnout (61.5% vs 43.7%; odds ratio, 1.72 [99% CI, 1.49-1.99]; P<.001 for debt >$200 000 relative to no debt). Residents reporting QOL "as bad as it can be" and emotional exhaustion symptoms daily had mean IM-ITE scores 2.7 points (99% CI, 1.2-4.3; P<.001) and 4.2 points (99% CI, 2.5-5.9; P<.001) lower than those with QOL "as good as it can be" and no emotional exhaustion symptoms, respectively. Residents reporting debt greater than $200 000 had mean IM-ITE scores 5.0 points (99% CI, 4.4-5.6; P<.001) lower than those with no debt. These differences were similar in magnitude to the 4.1-point (99% CI, 3.9-4.3) and 2.6-point (99% CI, 2.4-2.8) mean differences associated with progressing from first to second and second to third years of training, respectively.

*Conclusions.*—In this national study of internal medicine residents, suboptimal QOL and symptoms of burnout were common. Symptoms of burnout were associated with higher debt and were less frequent among international medical graduates. Low QOL, emotional exhaustion, and educational debt were associated with lower IM-ITE scores.

▶ West et al have examined medical knowledge on an in-training examination among US internal medicine residents as one marker of professional success, but also looked at burnout and quality of life as meaningful outcomes and as predictors of success. Included in their findings was that educational debt was a predictor of burnout and a lower quality of life. Moreover, they also found that educational debt, lower quality of life, and burnout were predictors of lower examination scores. The residents evaluated entered training after duty hour limit restrictions were put into place in 2003; thus, the results suggest that stress remains common despite the fewer hours worked in recent years.

Interestingly, one of the curious findings in this report was that international medical school graduates (IMGs) were markedly less likely than US graduates (AMGs) to report high levels of emotional exhaustion or depersonalization. This suggests different experiences of burnout between the AMGs and IMGs. The authors of this report suggest an explanation for this is that IMGs training in US residency programs represent a subset of international graduates who are more resilient and less prone to burnout owing to their successful navigation through the complex and highly competitive selection process for US residency as foreign graduates. This lower burnout rate is true despite similar debt burdens when analyzed for the latter. It should be noted, however, that the authors did find an association of increased debt with lower test scores in both AMGs and IMGs. For example, among IMGs, the difference in the internal medicine in-training examination scores between those with no debt and those with more than $200 000 debt was 8 points. Men appear to have steeper declines in test scores with higher debt levels than do women. It is unclear why there is a difference in these resident groups, but the differences are sufficiently large to merit some additional critical thinking on this topic.

If there is one conclusion we should draw from this report, it is that work hours are hardly the only stressor for residents in training. Family issues and debt along with personal satisfaction with one's work are just as important as anything else. The figure in the original article shows how dramatic the impact of educational debt on examination scores is.

This commentary closes with an observation having to do with differences in subspecialties of medicine. It has been suggested that anesthesiologists are brainy while orthopedic surgeons are less so but are otherwise possessive of great strength. Is this true? Subramanian et al have studied this issue by examining the IQ and strength of 36 male orthopedic surgeons and 40 male anesthesiologists.[1] Intelligence was tested using a Mensa quiz. Strength was assessed by testing handgrip. In the final analysis, intelligence did not vary significantly from a normal distribution for either anesthesiologists or orthopedic surgeons, although orthopedists did score higher on the Mensa quiz. Strength was on the side of orthopedists who were definitely stronger. Thus it is that the stereotypical image of male orthopedic surgeons as being strong but not so smart is not justified in comparison with her male anesthesiologist counterparts.

Anesthesiologist's might exercise some degree of caution at making fun of orthopedic surgeons, as they may find themselves on the receiving end of a sharp and quick-witted retort from their intellectually sharper friends or may be greeted with a crushing handshake at their next encounter.

**J. A. Stockman III, MD**

*Reference*

1. Subramanian P, Kantharuban V, Subramanian V, Willis-Owen SA, Willis-Owen CA. As strong as an ox and almost twice as clever? Multicentre prospective comparative study. *BMJ*. 2011;343:1328-1329.

## Factors Associated With American Board of Medical Specialties Member Board Certification Among US Medical School Graduates

Jeffe DB, Andriole DA (Washington Univ School of Medicine, St Louis, MO)
*JAMA* 306:961-970, 2011

*Context.*—Certification by an American Board of Medical Specialties (ABMS) member board is emerging as a measure of physician quality.

*Objective.*—To identify demographic and educational factors associated with ABMS member board certification of US medical school graduates.

*Design, Setting, and Participants.*—Retrospective study of a national cohort of 1997-2000 US medical school graduates, grouped by specialty choice at graduation and followed up through March 2, 2009. In separate multivariable logistic regression models for each specialty category, factors associated with ABMS member board certification were identified.

*Main Outcome Measure.*—ABMS member board certification.

*Results.*—Of 42 440 graduates in the study sample, 37 054 (87.3%) were board certified. Graduates in all specialty categories with first-attempt passing scores in the highest tertile (vs first-attempt failing scores) on US Medical Licensing Examination Step 2 Clinical Knowledge were more likely to be board certified; adjusted odds ratios (AORs) varied by specialty category, with the lowest odds for emergency medicine (87.4% vs 73.6%; AOR, 1.82; 95% CI, 1.03-3.20) and highest odds for radiology (98.1% vs 74.9%; AOR, 13.19; 95% CI, 5.55-31.32). In each specialty category except family medicine, graduates self-identified as underrepresented racial/ethnic minorities (vs white) were less likely to be board certified, ranging from 83.5% vs 95.6% in the pediatrics category (AOR, 0.44; 95% CI, 0.33-0.58) to 71.5% vs 83.7% in the other nongeneralist specialties category (AOR, 0.79; 95% CI, 0.64-0.96). With each $50 000 unit increase in debt (vs no debt), graduates choosing obstetrics/gynecology were less likely to be board certified (AOR, 0.89; 95% CI, 0.83-0.96), and graduates choosing family medicine were more likely to be board certified (AOR, 1.13; 95% CI, 1.01-1.26).

*Conclusion.*—Demographic and educational factors were associated with board certification among US medical school graduates in every specialty category examined; findings varied among specialty categories.

▶ This report reminds us that better outcomes have been observed for patients under the care of board-certified physicians compared with non–board-certified physicians. The American Board of Medical Specialties (ABMS) Member Board certification and higher scores on certifying examinations have also been associated with a lower risk of physician disciplinary action, whereas lack of board certification has been associated with higher risk of such disciplinary actions, including license revocation, suspension, probation, and public reprimand.[1]

ABMS Member Board certification has emerged as a de facto requirement for the full participation of physicians in the US health care system. Non–board-certified physicians compose an increasingly marginalized group. Such certification is used by health maintenance organizations, hospitals, and insurance plans in evaluating physicians who wish to obtain privileges or join provider organizations; by medical school promotion committees and evaluating physician faculty members for promotion and tenure; and by the Accreditation Council for Graduate Medical Education as criteria for selection of physicians to serve as graduate medical education program directors and residency review committee members. Given the relative importance of such certification, Jeffe and Andriole have explored in a retrospective national cohort of graduating medical students, demographic and educational factors associated with ABMS Member Board certification of US medical school graduates. The study found that for the period of 1997 to 2000, US medical school graduates achieved board certification at a rate of approximately 87%. Certain variables were found to be associated with a lesser likelihood of becoming board certified. Older graduates in each specialty studied were less likely to be board certified. This is not a new finding. Failure to become certified was the result of a greater likelihood of failing the certifying examinations offered by the boards evaluated. This suggests that older graduates may experience greater difficulties in their graduate medical education process. While early studies suggested that women had a lower certification rate than men, such differences are no longer seen. In every specialty category except family medicine, underrepresented minorities were less likely than whites to be board certified, as were Asian/Pacific Islander graduates in the surgery/surgical specialties category. There was no consistent relationship between higher debt and board certification among specialty categories.

This report also found that successful first attempts on the Step 1 and Step 2 Clinical Knowledge examinations were associated with a much higher greater likelihood of board certification. There were also two graduate medical education variables related to a lower likelihood of board certification. Withdrawal/dismissal from a program during graduate medical education was associated with a markedly lower likelihood of board certification among graduates in all specialty groups, raising the possibility that, as a group, graduates who withdraw or who are dismissed from training may represent a particularly poorly performing group of graduates. A leave of absence during graduate medical education also is weakly associated with a lesser probability of board certification, but this finding was not uniform across all specialty categories.

This report did not examine whether any of the characteristics associated with non—board certification were the result of failure on board examinations versus not applying or being accepted for examination by a certifying board. Lack of board certification within the study's period of analysis does not necessarily mean that a graduate will never become board certified. Longer follow-up might show that some graduates become board certified. This may be especially true among graduates in those specialty categories with relatively longer graduate medical education requirements that mandate clinical practice and an oral examination for certification.

All certifying boards of the ABMS have placed a time limit on individuals to become certified from the completion of residency. On average, this is running about 7 years. This means that if one is not certified within that 7-year period, an individual will have to show a certifying board that they are still up to date with the type of skills that they exited residency training with. For most certifying boards, this means that such candidates will have to go back into training for a period of time should they ever wish to be board certified.

This commentary closes with the observation that Norwegian doctors appear to be one of the most healthy groups of individuals in the world. In a 40-year review of national health records, these physicians had lower mortality rates for all causes of death apart from suicide than the general population in that country, although they had a higher mortality than other nonphysician graduates unadjusted for suicide rates. Physicians' higher rate of suicide was thought to account for the mortality differences between doctors and other university graduates.[2] Maybe there's something to be learned by studying our Scandinavian colleagues.

**J. A. Stockman III, MD**

*References*

1. Kohatsu ND, Gould D, Ross LK, Fox PJ. Characteristics associated with physician discipline: a case-control study. *Arch Intern Med.* 2004;164:653-658.
2. Aasland OG, Hem E, Haldorsen T, Ekeberg Ø. Mortality among Norwegian doctors 1960-2000. *BMC Public Health.* 2011;11:173.

---

**Factors associated with variability in the assessment of UK doctors' professionalism: analysis of survey results**
Campbell JL, Roberts M, Wright C, et al (Peninsula College of Medicine and Dentistry, Exeter, UK; et al)
*BMJ* 343:d6212, 2011

---

*Objectives.*—To investigate potential sources of systematic bias arising in the assessment of doctors' professionalism.

*Design.*—Linear regression modelling of cross sectional questionnaire survey data.

*Setting.*—11 clinical practices in England and Wales.

*Participants.*—1065 non-training grade doctors from various clinical specialties and settings, 17 031 of their colleagues, and 30 333 of their patients.

*Main Outcome Measures.*—Two measures of a doctor's professional performance using patient and colleague questionnaires from the United Kingdom's General Medical Council (GMC). We selected potential predictor variables from the characteristics of the doctors and of their patient and colleague assessors.

*Results.*—After we adjusted for characteristics of the doctor as well as characteristics of the patient sample, less favourable scores from patient feedback were independently predicted by doctors having obtained their primary medical degree from any non-European country; doctors practising as a psychiatrist; lower proportions of white patients providing feedback; lower proportions of patients rating their consultation as being very important; and lower proportions of patients reporting that they were seeing their usual doctor. Lower scores from colleague feedback were independently predicted by doctors having obtained their primary medical degree from countries outside the UK and South Asia; currently employed in a locum capacity; working as a general practitioner or psychiatrist; being employed in a staff grade, associate specialist, or other equivalent role; and with a lower proportion of colleagues reporting they had daily or weekly professional contact with the doctor. In fully adjusted models, the doctor's age, sex, and ethnic group were not independent predictors of patient or colleague feedback. Neither the age or sex profiles of the patient or colleague samples were independent predictors of doctors' feedback scores, and nor was the ethnic group of colleague samples.

*Conclusions.*—Caution is necessary when considering patient and colleague feedback regarding doctors' professionalism. Multisource feedback undertaken for revalidation using the GMC patient and colleague questionnaires should, at least initially, be principally formative in nature.

▶ This report emanates from the United Kingdom where beginning in 2012, physicians licensed will have to show they are up to date and fit to practice via a process known as revalidation, not widely dissimilar to the maintenance of certification processes seen in the United States. What Campbell et al have done is examine factors that can be associated with variability in patient and peer assessments of a physician's professionalism. These investigators were looking for potential biases that might influence such patient and peer evaluations. Campbell et al have been part of a team that has studied biases related to the characteristics of patients and colleagues who are assessing physicians. More than 1000 physicians beyond training from 11 different clinical settings in England and Wales took part in the study. They were assessed by 17 000 of their colleagues and 30 000 of their patients.

So what did this study show? Campbell et al did find some possible systematic biases that appear to be built into peer and patient surveys that seem to influence the results, perhaps based on inherent prejudices some have. Independent predictors of less favorable feedback regarding a physician's professionalism included not having been trained in England and being a psychiatrist. Such less favorable feedback came from patients. With respect to colleagues, less favorable feedback, largely related to whether a colleague had not trained in the United Kingdom, was a locum tenens physician, or was a general practitioner or psychiatrist. A physician's age, sex, and ethnicity were not independent predictors of patient or colleague feedback.

It does appear that peer and patient surveys may manifest systemic bias, at least in the United Kingdom, when it comes to assessment of a physician's professionalism. It would be interesting to see if this exact study could be performed in the United States to determine whether such feedback as part of maintenance of certification suffers from the same or similar biases.

In the United States, we have been hearing more and more about how various states' licensing bodies are dealing with unprofessionalism. There is a great deal to be learned from other countries, however, regarding their experiences with unprofessionalism. Recently, Wakeford reported on how the British General Medical Council (GMC) has dealt with physicians being struck from the British medical register, the equivalent of having one's license revoked in the United

States.[1] For the period 1858 through 1991, the first 133 years of the GMC's existence, 584 doctors were taken off the British Medical Registry. In 1991 there was a complete revision of the way physicians were reviewed. The data from 1991 to present were reviewed by Wakeford. Analyzing the information from 227 457 potentially practicing physicians in Great Britain, it was noted that 790 doctors were removed from the GMC Registry. Proportionately, men were many more times as likely to be erased or suspended as women. Hospital specialists were erased or suspended at about half the rate of general physicians. Non-UK graduates as a group were significantly more likely to be erased or suspended as those with UK qualifications, specifically 2 times more likely. Physicians in Great Britain from foreign countries including France, Bangladesh, The Netherlands, and Australia were 5 times more likely to be struck from the registry as physicians trained in the United Kingdom itself. It might be of some surprise that of the top 20 countries other than the United Kingdom that represented physicians struck from the registry, half are in the European Union.

**J. A. Stockman III, MD**

*Reference*

1. Wakeford R. Who gets struck off? *BMJ*. 2011,343.1325-1327.

---

**An analysis of successful litigation claims in children in England**
Raine JE (Whittington Hosp, London, UK)
*Arch Dis Child* 96:838-840, 2011

---

*Objective.*—To analyse the number of successful claims against the National Health Service (NHS) involving children, the nature and outcome of incidents leading to litigation and the costs of claims.

*Method.*—Under the Freedom of Information Act, details were sought of claims involving children made to the National Health Service Litigation Authority (NHSLA) from 1 April 2005 to 31 March 2010 together with the claim status on 30 September 2010. Closed cases involving financial compensation were analysed in relation to the nature of the incident, outcome and total cost of litigation.

*Results.*—195 closed cases were examined. The commonest causes of litigation were medication or vaccination errors (10), delayed septicaemia diagnosis (8), delayed meningitis diagnosis (7), delayed unspecified sepsis diagnosis (7), extravasation (7), delayed anorectal abnormality diagnosis (6), delayed cardiological diagnosis (6), delayed appendicitis diagnosis (6), epilepsy misdiagnosis (6), psychological/psychiatric effects on parent(s) following a medical error (4), delayed fracture diagnosis (4), gastrostomy related errors (3) and delayed testicular torsion diagnosis (3). The commonest outcomes were death (74), unnecessary pain (35), unnecessary operation (16), brain damage (12), scarring (12), psychiatric/psychological morbidity in parent(s) and/or child (10) and amputation (5). Total costs of litigation ranged from £600 to £3 044 943 (mean £127 975).

*Conclusion.*—Delayed diagnosis of severe sepsis is the commonest adverse incident leading to successful litigation and the commonest adverse outcome is death. The cost to the NHS is considerable. A better understanding of the causes of common errors in paediatrics should inform training and help to decrease these adverse events (Tables 1-3).

▶ The *Archives of Diseases of Childhood* has had a number of reports in recent years about medical malpractice and medical errors. The report of Raine provides data from the National Health Service Litigation Authority telling about the commonest events that result in litigation, their causes and consequences, as well as cost to the British National Health Service. The authority is the body that handles claims made against the National Health Service. It receives a number of claims related to children each year. For a recent 5-year period, there were 469 closed cases as the result of claims of medical errors. Some 42% of these resulted in payment of damages to the claimant, including 7 cases of children with brain damage. Tables 1-3 show the causes of the incidence and the results and injuries sustained.

In data from the Physician Insurers Association of America, the 5 most common events that lead to claims against pediatric care providers are brain damage to infants, meningitis, routine infant or child health check, neonatal

---

TABLE 1.—Incidents Leading to Successful Litigation, 1 April 2005 to 31 March 2010

|  | Number | % |
|---|---|---|
| Medication/vaccination error | 10 | 5.1 |
| Delayed/failed diagnosis of septicaemia | 8 | 4.1 |
| Delayed/failed diagnosis of meningitis | 7 | 3.6 |
| Extravasation | 7 | 3.6 |
| Delayed/failed diagnosis of unspecified sepsis | 6 | 3.1 |
| Delayed diagnosis of anorectal abnormality | 6 | 3.1 |
| Delayed/failed cardiological diagnosis | 6 | 3.1 |
| Delayed diagnosis of appendicitis | 6 | 3.1 |
| Misdiagnosis of epilepsy | 6 | 3.1 |
| Psychological/psychiatric effects on the parent(s) or child following a medical error | 4 | 2.1 |
| Delayed diagnosis of a fracture | 4 | 2.1 |
| Gastrostomy related errors | 3 | 1.5 |
| Delayed diagnosis of testicular torsion | 3 | 1.5 |
| Cold light injury | 3 | 1.5 |
| Pressure sores | 3 | 1.5 |
| Delayed renal diagnosis | 3 | 1.5 |
| Delayed/failed diagnosis of a respiratory infection | 3 | 1.5 |
| Inadequate nursing monitoring | 3 | 1.5 |
| Foreign body left in situ | 2 | 1.0 |
| Delayed diagnosis of a bowel perforation | 2 | 1.0 |
| Delayed diagnosis of a brain tumour | 2 | 1.0 |
| Delayed diagnosis of a tumour recurrence | 2 | 1.0 |
| Delayed diagnosis of intussusception | 2 | 1.0 |
| Burn/bruising due to a saturation probe | 2 | 1.0 |
| Failure to act on abnormal results | 2 | 1.0 |
| Partial amputation of a finger while removing a dressing | 2 | 1.0 |
| Delayed diagnosis of a shunt blockage | 2 | 1.0 |
| Delayed diagnosis of Turner's syndrome | 2 | 1.0 |
| Miscellaneous | 84 | 43.1 |

TABLE 2.—Causes of Incidents Leading to Successful Litigation, 1 April 2005 to 31 March 2010

|  | Number | % |
| --- | --- | --- |
| Delayed/failed diagnosis | 91 | 46.7 |
| Delayed/failed treatment | 25 | 12.8 |
| Inadequate nursing care | 15 | 7.7 |
| Medication/vaccination error | 12 | 6.2 |
| Infusion problems | 10 | 5.1 |
| Failure to recognise a complication | 9 | 4.6 |
| Operative problem | 6 | 3.1 |
| Failure to act on results | 5 | 2.6 |
| Procedure error | 5 | 2.6 |
| Failure to perform tests | 4 | 2.1 |
| Lack of facilities/equipment | 3 | 1.5 |
| Unclear cause | 3 | 1.5 |
| Communication error with parents | 1 | 0.5 |
| Delayed/failed resuscitation | 1 | 0.5 |
| Delayed transfer to paediatric intensive care unit | 1 | 0.5 |
| Cross infection | 1 | 0.5 |
| Accidental fracture in neonatal intensive care unit | 1 | 0.5 |
| Overdose of platelets | 1 | 0.5 |
| Failure of sterilisation | 1 | 0.5 |

TABLE 3.—The Results of Injuries Sustained Due to the Incidents that Led to Successful Litigation, 1 April 2005 to 31 March 2010

|  | Number | % |
| --- | --- | --- |
| Death | 74 | 37.9 |
| Unnecessary pain | 35 | 17.9 |
| Unnecessary surgery | 16 | 8.2 |
| Brain damage/developmental delay | 12 | 6.2 |
| Scarring | 12 | 6.2 |
| Psychiatric/psychological morbidity in the parent(s) and/or child | 10 | 5.1 |
| Amputation | 5 | 2.6 |
| Damage to peripheral nervous system | 3 | 1.5 |
| Visual problems | 3 | 1.5 |
| Pressure sores | 3 | 1.5 |
| Cardiological conditions | 2 | 1.0 |
| Perforated appendix | 2 | 1.0 |
| Infection | 2 | 1.0 |
| Respiratory disorder | 2 | 1.0 |
| Fracture | 2 | 1.0 |
| Renal damage | 2 | 1.0 |
| Unnecessary medical treatment | 2 | 1.0 |
| Bowel damage | 2 | 1.0 |
| Infertility | 1 | 0.5 |
| Anaphylactic shock | 1 | 0.5 |
| Short stature | 1 | 0.5 |
| Feeding difficulties | 1 | 0.5 |
| Bladder damage | 1 | 0.5 |
| Unclear | 1 | 0.5 |

respiratory problems, and appendicitis. Nearly half (43%) of the incidents resulting in claims occur in the office setting, out of hospital.[1] In a survey of pediatric malpractice in France, the most common reasons for claims are meningitis, dehydration, malignancy, pneumonia, and appendicitis.[2] The causes of medical errors in all studies to date mostly related to a delay or failure to diagnose and treat. Fortunately, most medical errors do not result in harm. However, in the British study, for adverse events that led to successful claims against the National Health Service, the most common result of an error was death.

Needless to say, information provided by the United Kingdom's experience with medical errors will inform the training of physicians and nurses and in doing so will help avoid the reoccurrence of errors and improve the safety of medical and nursing practice.

**J. A. Stockman III, MD**

*References*

1. Carroll AE, Buddenbaum JL. Malpractice claims involving pediatricians: epidemiology and etiology. *Pediatrics.* 2007;120:10-17.
2. Najaf-Zadeh A, Dubos F, Pruvost I, et al. Epidemiology and aetiology of paediatric malpractice claims in France. *Arch Dis Child.* 2011;96:127-130.

---

## Malpractice Risk According to Physician Specialty

Jena AB, Seabury S, Lakdawalla D, et al (Massachusetts General Hosp, Boston; RAND, Santa Monica, CA; Univ of Southern California, Los Angeles, CA; et al)
*N Engl J Med* 365:629-636, 2011

---

*Background.*—Data are lacking on the proportion of physicians who face malpractice claims in a year, the size of those claims, and the cumulative career malpractice risk according to specialty.

*Methods.*—We analyzed malpractice data from 1991 through 2005 for all physicians who were covered by a large professional liability insurer with a nationwide client base (40,916 physicians and 233,738 physician-years of coverage). For 25 specialties, we reported the proportion of physicians who had malpractice claims in a year, the proportion of claims leading to an indemnity payment (compensation paid to a plaintiff), and the size of indemnity payments. We estimated the cumulative risk of ever being sued among physicians in high- and low-risk specialties.

*Results.*—Each year during the study period, 7.4% of all physicians had a malpractice claim, with 1.6% having a claim leading to a payment (i.e., 78% of all claims did not result in payments to claimants). The proportion of physicians facing a claim each year ranged from 19.1% in neurosurgery, 18.9% in thoracic—cardiovascular surgery, and 15.3% in general surgery to 5.2% in family medicine, 3.1% in pediatrics, and 2.6% in psychiatry. The mean indemnity payment was $274,887, and the median was $111,749. Mean payments ranged from $117,832 for dermatology to $520,923 for pediatrics. It was estimated that by the age of 65 years, 75% of physicians in low-risk specialties had faced a malpractice claim, as compared with 99% of physicians in high-risk specialties.

*Conclusions.*—There is substantial variation in the likelihood of malpractice suits and the size of indemnity payments across specialties. The cumulative risk of facing a malpractice claim is high in all specialties, although most claims do not lead to payments to plaintiffs. (Funded by the RAND Institute for Civil Justice and the National Institute on Aging.) (Figs 1, 3 and 4).

▶ Despite the fact there has been tremendous interest in reform malpractice, the data on the actual prevalence of malpractice claims in the United States are fairly sketchy. For example, although the National Practitioner Data Bank includes most cases in the United States in which a plaintiff was paid on behalf a licensed health care provider, it does not report the specialties of physicians nor does it record information on cases that do not result in a payment. Jena et al have added enormously to our understanding about the magnitude of malpractice claims against physicians by exploring physician-level data on malpractice claims from a large, physician-owned professional liability insurer that provides coverage to physicians in every state and the District of Columbia It should be noted that while the data included physicians from all 50 states, California was overrepresented in the database, accounting for almost 40% of

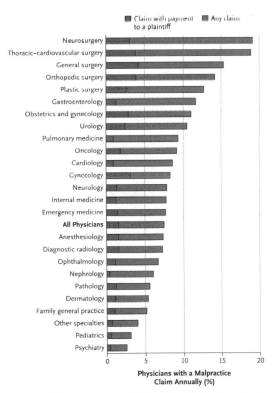

FIGURE 1.—Proportion of Physicians Facing a Malpractice Claim Annually, According to Specialty. (Reprinted from Jena AB, Seabury S, Lakdawalla D, et al. Malpractice Risk According to Physician Specialty. *N Engl J Med.* 2011;365:629-636. © 2011 Massachusetts Medical Society.)

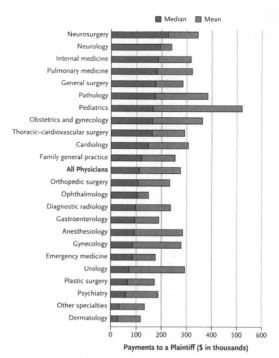

FIGURE 3.—Amount of Malpractice Payments, According to Specialty. Payments are shown in 2008 dollars. Specialties that had fewer than 30 payments (i.e., oncology and nephrology) are not listed. (Reprinted from Jena AB, Seabury S, Lakdawalla D, et al. Malpractice Risk According to Physician Specialty. *N Engl J Med.* 2011;365:629-636. © 2011 Massachusetts Medical Society.)

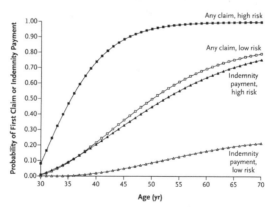

FIGURE 4.—Cumulative Career Probability of Facing a Malpractice Claim or Indemnity Payment, According to Risk of Specialty and Age of Physician. Cumulative probabilities were estimated from a multi-variate linear regression model with adjustment for physician random effects, physician specialty, state of practice, and county demographic characteristics. (Reprinted from Jena AB, Seabury S, Lakdawalla D, et al. Malpractice Risk According to Physician Specialty. *N Engl J Med.* 2011;365:629-636. © 2011 Massa-chusetts Medical Society.)

all physicians. The investigators corrected for this oversampling by weighting each physician in the database by the relative number of physicians who are not employed by the federal government reported in the Area Resource File of the Department of Health and Human Services. With such waiting, the share of physicians in California was reduced to 12.2%, which matches the overall average for the country as a whole. The ages of the physicians whose data were included in this report varied between 30 and 70 years with the youngest specialty age being emergency medicine at an average age of 43 years and the oldest being gynecology with an average age of 53 years.

So what did these investigators find? It was determined that across all specialties, 7.4% of physicians annually will have a malpractice claim filed against them, whereas 1.6% will make an indemnity payment (Fig 1). There was a wide range of probability of facing such a claim, ranging annually from almost 20% in neurosurgery and thoracic cardiovascular surgery to 15% in general surgery, but just 5.2% in family medicine, 3.1% in pediatrics, and 2.6% in psychiatry. Roughly 5% of physicians in low-risk specialties and 33% in high-risk specialties were projected to make their first indemnity payment by age 45 years; by the age of 65 years, the risk had increased to 19% and 71%, respectively. Roughly 55% of physicians in internal medicine and its subspecialties were projected to face a malpractice claim by 45 years and 89% by 65 years. In contrast, 80% of physicians in surgical specialties (including general surgery) and 74% of physicians in obstetrics and gynecology were projected to face a claim by 45 years. Projections suggest that nearly all physicians in high-risk specialties will face at least 1 claim during their career (Fig 4).

The authors of this report note that the perceived threat of malpractice among physicians may boil down to 3 factors, the risk of a claim, the probability of a claim leading to a payment, and the size of payment.

While pediatrics is the second least likely specialty (only psychiatry is lower) in which a practitioner will have any claim filed against them, it leads all specialties with the highest mean payments to plaintiffs by a large margin with over $500 000 outlaid per paid claim (Fig 3). This is almost 25% higher than the paid claims against neurosurgeons.

It should be noted that the situation with medical malpractice is substantially different in the military, where no matter how gross the negligence or how severe the resulting injury, active-duty service personnel are prevented from suing for malpractice by a judicial rule known as the Feres Doctrine. This rule, which has attracted long-standing criticism, recently assumed new salience as the Supreme Court considered whether to hear a case calling for reconsideration of the doctrine as it relates to medical malpractice. The court opted not to accept the case, leaving the controversy unresolved. Some commentators, including veteran groups, advocate repealing the Feres Doctrine, shifting military claims to a civil liabilities system. The rub is that replacing the Feres Doctrine with a civil liabilities system is simply replacing what some consider one injustice with an even greater injustice. In an editorial on this topic by Mangalmurti et al, it was noted that problems with the military's administrative compensation system are myriad but are fairly tractable when compared with those of the private tort system.[1]

**J. A. Stockman III, MD**

*Reference*

1. Mangalmurti SS, Murtagh L, Mello MM. Medical malpractice in the military. *N Engl J Med.* 2011;365:664-670.

---

### Private Practice Rates Among Pediatric Subspecialists
Freed GL, the American Board of Pediatrics Research Advisory (Univ of Michigan, Ann Arbor; et al)
*Pediatrics* 128:673-676, 2011

---

*Objective.*—Historically, most pediatric subspecialists have conducted their clinical work in academic health centers. However, increases in the absolute numbers of pediatric subspecialists in past decades, combined with greater concentrations of children in urban and suburban settings, might result in more opportunities for pediatric subspecialists to enter private practice. Our goal was to assess the proportions of subspecialists in private practice.

*Methods.*—We surveyed a stratified, random, national sample of 1696 subspecialists from 5 subspecialties and assessed the ownership of their current clinical practice settings.

*Results.*—The response rate was 77%. Two-thirds of respondents (65% [$n = 705$]) reported that they work in academic hospitals or outpatient clinics. Compared with other subspecialists, greater proportions of neonatologists (38% [$n = 92$]) and critical care physicians (19% [$n = 44$]) reported that they work in community hospitals. Larger proportions of cardiologists (27% [$n = 58$]) and gastroenterologists (24% [$n = 47$]) reported that they work in private outpatient practices.

*Conclusions.*—There were significant proportions of pediatric subspecialists in private practice in most of the 5 subspecialties studied. Ensuring children's access to pediatric subspecialists likely will require a robust workforce in both academic and private clinical settings. Ongoing studies of the career trajectories of pediatric subspecialists with respect to their venues of practice will be essential for future workforce planning (Table 2).

▶ This report has remarkable relevance for some rapidly occurring changes that are coming into play with respect to the pediatric subspecialty workforce. Because of the profound interest in primary care in the early to mid and late 1990s, a sharp decline occurred in interest in pediatric subspecialty training. Indeed, as we entered the past decade, a serious shortage of pediatric subspecialists, particularly in certain disciplines, was rapidly emerging. Fortunately, the United States, being what it is, the free market responded and we have seen more than a doubling in the numbers of individuals entering first-year fellowship subspecialty training. There are still significant shortages in areas such as child neurology, pediatric rheumatology, adolescent medicine, and several other subspecialty disciplines. Traditionally, pediatric subspecialists have functioned largely within academic health care systems, adding to our body of knowledge in both clinical and research areas. This

TABLE 2.—Ownership of Primary Practice Setting ($N = 1083$)

| | Overall | Cardiologists $(N = 218)$ | Critical Care $(N = 231)$ | Gastroenterologists $(N = 198)$ | Hematologists-Oncologists $(N = 197)$ | Neonatologists $(N = 239)$ |
|---|---|---|---|---|---|---|
| | | | | Proportion, % (*n*) | | |
| Academic hospital/ outpatient clinic | 65 (705) | 64 (140) | 71 (163) | 67 (132) | 77 (152) | 49 (118) |
| Community hospital | 16 (170) | 5 (10) | 19 (44) | 4 (7) | 9 (17) | 38 (92) |
| Private outpatient practice | 12 (129) | 27 (58) | 0 (1) | 24 (47) | 10 (19) | 2 (4) |
| Other | 5 (49) | 2 (4) | 9 (21) | 2 (3) | 2 (3) | 8 (18) |
| Managed care organization | 2 (25) | 3 (6) | 0 (1) | 4 (8) | 2 (4) | 3 (6) |
| Public health clinic/community health center | 0 (5) | 0 (0) | 0 (1) | 1 (1) | 1 (2) | 0 (1) |

is very different from the circumstance in adult medicine, where most adult subspecialists work in the private sector. The reason pediatricians have largely congregated within academic health care systems is that the prevalence of many pediatric conditions requiring subspecialty care is relatively low and sparsely distributed, lacking large numbers of patients in any single geographic community. Certain disciplines, of course, differ in this respect. The push toward increasing the availability of neonatologists at level II nurseries has resulted in many in this discipline entering community practice.

So what has happened to the geographic distribution of pediatric subspecialists coming out of training in the past decade? That is what Freed et al have attempted to address in their report, which analyzes data from a national sample of more than 1600 pediatric subspecialists across 5 disciplines. The study did observe that neonatology is the most populated pediatric subspecialty and has the highest proportion of providers in nonacademic settings. Hematology-oncology is the subspecialty with the largest proportion of providers practicing in academic centers. This is intuitively obvious, given the relative rarity of childhood cancers and the need for highly sophisticated infrastructural support services that are exceedingly expensive to develop in community settings. For details on the distribution of subspecialists in the academic hospital setting versus the community practice setting, see Table 2.

With the increasing survival times of patients with chronic diseases, it seems plausible to believe that the population of patients in the United States with subspecialty problems will continue to increase. Whether this will result in a further diffusion of subspecialists into nonacademic positions or not remains to be seen. As of now, it is only the field of neonatology in which the majority of subspecialists practice outside of academic health care centers.

This commentary closes with an observation having to do with the US workforce and starting salaries. It appears that neurologic surgeons in the United States who have just completed their training in residencies or fellowships earn more than any other newly qualified doctors in their first year. The median salary in the first year for all neurological surgeons joining a new practice (which would include more experienced surgeons) was $605 000.[1] Other specialties paying high salaries in the first year after residency were invasive cardiology (median of $300 000), invasive and interventional cardiology ($350 000), hematology—oncology ($325 000), maternal—fetal medicine ($300 000), general orthopedic surgery ($375 000), hip and joint orthopedic surgery ($306 000), sports medicine orthopedic surgery ($300 000), diagnostic and interventional radiology ($350 000), diagnostic interventional radiology ($370 000) and vascular surgery ($300 000). In contrast, the newly qualified specialist doctors earning the lowest salaries in 2008 were those in pediatrics ($125 000) and general and ambulatory internal medicine ($150 000 and $130 000, respectively). During their first year in practice, men received higher salaries than women in almost all specialties except ambulatory internal medicine, nephrology, anatomical and clinical pathology, and neonatal medicine. Salaries for graduates of US medical schools and graduates from abroad who were practicing in the United States were virtually identical. The survey that provides this information was conducted by the Medical Group Management Association in collaboration with the National Association of Physician Recruiters. Data were collected in 2009. The management association sent questionnaires to independent recruiters and hospital and medical center recruiters.

**J. A. Stockman III, MD**

*Reference*

1. Tanne JH. US surgeons earn nearly $0.5 million in their first year. *BMJ.* 2009; 339:12.

# 12 Musculoskeletal

**Moderate to Vigorous Physical Activity and Sedentary Time and Cardiometabolic Risk Factors in Children and Adolescents**
Ekelund U, for the International Children's Accelerometry Database (ICAD) Collaborators (Inst of Metabolic Science, Cambridge, UK; et al)
*JAMA* 307:704-712, 2012

*Context.*—Sparse data exist on the combined associations between physical activity and sedentary time with cardiometabolic risk factors in healthy children.

*Objective.*—To examine the independent and combined associations between objectively measured time in moderate- to vigorous-intensity physical activity (MVPA) and sedentary time with cardiometabolic risk factors.

*Design, Setting, and Participants.*—Pooled data from 14 studies between 1998 and 2009 comprising 20 871 children (aged 4-18 years) from the International Children's Accelerometry Database. Time spent in MVPA and sedentary time were measured using accelerometry after reanalyzing raw data. The independent associations between time in MVPA and sedentary time, with outcomes, were examined using meta-analysis. Participants were stratified by tertiles of MVPA and sedentary time.

*Main Outcome Measures.*—Waist circumference, systolic blood pressure, fasting triglycerides, high-density lipoprotein cholesterol, and insulin.

*Results.*—Times (mean [SD] min/d) accumulated by children in MVPA and being sedentary were 30 (21) and 354 (96), respectively. Time in MVPA was significantly associated with all cardiometabolic outcomes independent of sex, age, monitor wear time, time spent sedentary, and waist circumference (when not the outcome). Sedentary time was not associated with any outcome independent of time in MVPA. In the combined analyses, higher levels of MVPA were associated with better cardiometabolic risk factors across tertiles of sedentary time. The differences in outcomes between higher and lower MVPA were greater with lower sedentary time. Mean differences in waist circumference between the bottom and top tertiles of MVPA were 5.6 cm (95% CI, 4.8-6.4 cm) for high sedentary time and 3.6 cm (95% CI, 2.8-4.3 cm) for low sedentary time. Mean differences in systolic blood pressure for high and low sedentary time were 0.7 mm Hg (95% CI, −0.07 to 1.6) and 2.5 mm Hg (95% CI, 1.7-3.3), and for high-density lipoprotein cholesterol, differences were −2.6 mg/dL (95% CI, −1.4 to −3.9) and −4.5 mg/dL (95% CI, −3.3 to −5.6), respectively. Geometric mean differences for insulin and triglycerides showed similar variation. Those in the top tertile of MVPA accumulated more than 35 minutes per day in this intensity level compared with fewer than 18 minutes per day for those in the bottom tertile. In prospective analyses (N = 6413 at 2.1 years' follow-up), MVPA and sedentary time were not associated with waist circumference at follow-up, but a higher waist circumference at baseline was associated with higher amounts of sedentary time at follow-up.

*Conclusion.*—Higher MVPA time by children and adolescents was associated with better cardiometabolic risk factors regardless of the amount of sedentary time.

▶ The general consensus is that the amount of exercise children and adolescents need each day should accumulate to at least 60 minutes of moderate- to vigorous-intensity physical activity. By and large the amount of physical activity experienced by this age group is inversely related to adiposity and cardiometabolic risk factors. In and of itself, a higher level of time spent sedentary is associated with adiposity and an adverse cardiometabolic risk factor profile.

The authors of this report have examined the associations between moderate- to vigorous-intensity physical activity and time spent sedentary with established cardiometabolic risk factors in more than 2000 children and adolescents aged 4 to 18 years using a meta-analysis approach combining data from multiple cohorts in which physical activity and sedentary time have been measured objectively by accelerometry. The intent was to integrate both moderate- to vigorous-intensity physical activity and sedentary time taken together with cardiometabolic risk factors. Is it possible that children who exercise a lot but who also spend a lot of time on the couch would not be better off than children who do not exercise at all? Does being sedentary offset the benefits of being physically active at other times? These were the questions that were addressed. Waist circumference, systolic blood pressure, fasting triglycerides, high-density lipoprotein cholesterol, and insulin were measured in this study population. On average, the time accumulated by children in moderate- to vigorous-intensity physical activity was 30 minutes a day. Time sedentary was 354 minutes. There was sufficient variation in these times to address the objectives of the study.

The study showed that the time spent in vigorous physical activity was associated with multiple cardiometabolic risk factors independent of time spent sedentary and other confounding factors. In contrast, time spent sedentary was unrelated to these risk factors after adjusting for time spent in vigorous physical activity. Neither time spent in vigorous physical activity nor time spent sedentary predicted a higher waist circumference in prospective analysis.

These results have implications for public health policy and physical activity counseling. Children should be encouraged to increase their participation in physical activity of at least moderate intensity rather than reducing their overall sedentary time as this appears more important in relation to cardiometabolic health. However, the measure in this report of sedentary time takes into account the accumulated time spent sedentary rather than any specific behavior such as TV watching. The bottom line is that higher levels of time in moderate to vigorous physical activity appears to be associated with better cardiometabolic risk factors regardless of the amount of time spent sedentary in this population.

This commentary closes with an observation on a "new" clinical disorder, EED, an abbreviation for "exercise deficit disorder." This was recently described in a report from the United States.[1] EED is used to describe a condition characterized by reduced levels of moderate to vigorous physical activity that is inconsistent with long-term health and well-being. In a commentary that accompanied the report describing this new disorder, Meadow countered with a statement: "The larger question to ask is what is gained by taking a conventional wisdom—everyone should get enough exercise and get a good night's sleep—by making absence of either into a disorder? It seems to be taking pediatrics in the way of psychiatry, medicalizing everything with a sort of pseudo-scientific objectivity and by doing so, legitimizing it."[2]

There does seem to be a great deal of medicalization of social problems these days. Given that, we will likely hear much more about the entity EED.

This commentary closes with an observation having to do with exercise. Few would contest that exercise is a healthy habit, even though I admittedly abhor the habit. Still, the mechanisms behind exercise's many benefits remain quite murky. Recent studies now suggest that exercise triggers autophagy. The latter is the "self-eating" process by which cells recycle used or flawed organelles, membranes, or other internal structures. Autophagy recycling helps cells meet energy demands. Studies have shown that exercise induces autophagy in muscles. With this process, a double membrane encircles target materials inside a cell, forming a sphere that then spills its contents into another compartment, the lysosome, where enzymes chop them up so the cell can reuse all the material again. Organisms from yeast to humans maintain a background level of this process and also boost it under stress. Exercise is one such stress. Researchers have shown that running mice for short periods on a treadmill sharply elevates such a process in many organs of the body. It appears that exercise training leads to more and more autophagy, giving a new meaning to "eat her heart out!"[3]

**J. A. Stockman III, MD**

*References*

1. Faigenbaum AD, Stracciolini A, Myer GD. Exercise deficit disorder in youth: a hidden truth. *Acta Paediatr.* 2011;100:1423-1425.
2. Meadow W. Editor's comments. *Acta Paediatr.* 2011;100:1425.
3. Garber K. Explaining exercise: Cellular "self eating" may account for some health benefits of exercise. *Science.* 2012;335:281.

**Growing Pains: A Study of 30 Cases and a Review of the Literature**
Pavone V, Lionetti E, Gargano V, et al (Univ of Catania, Italy)
*J Pediatr Orthop* 31:606-609, 2011

*Background.*—Data from the literature regarding the clinical profile of growing pains are limited. The purpose of this study was to define the clinical features, familial history, laboratory findings, and therapeutic outcome of growing pains in children.

*Methods.*—Thirty children (18 male and 12 female; 3 to 14 y of age) who presented with growing pains between January 2006 and December 2007 were enrolled and prospectively followed up for 1 year. The inclusion criterion was lower extremity pain, which was recurrent and lasted for >3 months. The exclusion criteria were any abnormal systemic or local symptoms and signs, joint involvement, and limp or limitation of activity. Laboratory tests, including complete blood count, erythrocyte sedimentation rate, and serum calcium and phosphorus levels, were performed in all children.

*Results.*—The study group had pain during the night and afternoon in 43.3% and 56.7% of cases, respectively. Both lower limbs were involved in 80% of cases, causing awakening and crying episodes in 40% and 37% of cases, respectively. The frequency of pain was as follows: daily, 5%; weekly, 45%; monthly, 35%; and every 3 months, 15%. The pains were relieved by massaging the affected site in 95% of cases and by analgesics in 5% of children. A family history of growing pains was positive in 20% of patients. All patients had laboratory tests within normal values.

*Conclusion.*—Growing pain is a frequent noninflammatory syndrome consisting of intermittent, often annoying, pains that affect the lower extremities of children. Clinical diagnosis is easy if precise inclusion and exclusion criteria in the history and physical examinations are strictly followed. Patience and family reassurance is mandatory.

*Level of Evidence.*—This is a Level I prospective study.

▶ Any article that includes the term "growing pains" in the title is likely to find a place among my selects. The term goes back to the early 1800s after the first description of it by the French physician Marcel Duchamp.[1] If you Google the words "growing pains," you will find that there actually has been a lot written about the entity in the medical and not-so-medical literature. Needless to say, growing pains remains a largely misunderstood diagnosis. Studies have suggested that the prevalence of growing pains varies from a low of 6% to almost 50%.[2] With such a wide variation, you can be sure that there are no firm agreements about what growing pains really are and that the etiology still remains uncertain. What Pavone et al have done is to design a study to gain a better understanding of the characteristics of growing pains in children by describing the clinical features, family history, laboratory findings, spectrum, and therapeutic outcomes of 30 patients with growing pains seen in the Department of Pediatrics at the University of Catania in Italy.

Over the period January 2006 through December 2007, the Department of Orthopedics at the University of Catania looked at all patients presenting with growing pains diagnosed as the presence of lower extremity pains that are recurrent but intermittent and lasting for more than 3 months. Exclusion criteria included the presence of any abnormal systemic or local symptoms and signs including fever and malaise; localizing signs including tenderness, swelling, erythema, and warmth; joint involvement including swelling, pain, erythema, and warmth; and limp or limitation of activity. All children underwent a full laboratory examination including a complete blood count, erythrocyte sedimentation rate, creatine kinase, serum calcium and phosphorus levels, alkaline phosphatase activity, rheumatoid factor titer, and, when indicated, x-rays. The children were followed up 1 year later.

In this series of 30 children, growing pains presented with a frequency ranging from daily to every 3 months. In all cases, the growing pains were located in the lower extremities, appeared at night or in the afternoon, and were associated in 20% of cases with physical activity. The mean age of onset of growing pains in this series was approximately 8 years, confirming data elsewhere in the literature. This suggests that there is little evidence that growing pains are actually associated with rapid growth, which has been suspected previously as one etiology. There was no specific etiology determined.

Growing pains are real and can be very distressing. They are distressing to the patient and families and to care providers when the latter cannot give a firm basis for diagnosis. Laboratory studies add nothing to the diagnosis. The natural history, however, is that it is a benign diagnosis and will disappear, although it may take several years. In a study by Uziel et al, the 5-year follow-up of children with growing pains shows that growing pains resolve in more than 50% of cases within a 5-year period of time and improve in nearly all other patients with less frequent episodes, less analgesic use, and fewer school absences related to pain.[3]

In most cases practitioners will be left to their own devices in making a diagnosis of growing pains, the most common cause of childhood musculoskeletal pain and a type of noninflammatory pain syndrome. Growing pains mainly affect children between 4 and 14 years of age. They are usually nonarticular and in most children are located in the shins, calves, thighs, or popliteal fossa. The pain usually appears late in the day or at night, often awakening the child. The duration of growing pains ranges from minutes to hours. The intensity of growing pains can be mild or very severe. A tip-off is that by morning, the child is almost always pain free. There are no objective signs of inflammation on physical examination, and to this day, no clear mechanism has been identified that explains growing pains, but there is an increasing body of evidence indicating that several factors, individually or in combination, might be responsible for this phenomenon, including mechanical factors such as joint hypermobility and flat feet, decreased pain threshold in some children, reduced bone strength, and emotional factors involving the patient's family and other social stressors.

This commentary ends with a historical note dealing with a certain portion of a musculoskeletal system. In December 2008, a newspaper in France featured a page one exclusive: "Sarah's leg be found!" The story in fact referred to the rediscovery in the basement of the Faculty of Medicine in Bordeaux of the right leg of actress Sarah Bernhardt, amputated by a Bordeaux surgeon in 1915. Sarah Bernhardt, of course, is probably the most famous theatrical actress of all times. Despite the proclamation that her leg had been found, historians noted that the specimen in formalin was a left leg, amputated below the knee, whereas Sarah Bernhardt's amputated leg had undergone an above-knee removal for an excruciating painful traumatic arthritis of the joint. The problem seems to have begun when she played as Tosca, in Victorien Sardou's play of that name which later became a Puccini opera, and leapt in the final scene from the ramparts of Castel S'Angelo. As the pain in Bernhardt's knee worsened in mid-1914, she consulted a number of physicians who were unwilling to do an amputation simply to relieve arthritic pain. She finally convinced a surgeon to carry out the procedure on February 22, 1915. Pathological analysis of the amputated leg showed tuberculosis of the joint as the cause of the arthritis. Based on physical examination and chest x-ray, no other sign of tuberculosis was present.

Following the surgery, Bernhardt continued to perform, but faced with the reality of a cumbersome wooden leg, she opted instead for a gilded litter with horizontal shafts, in the style of Louis XV, carried by two porters. Occasionally she used a wheelchair. She died in 1923, performing almost to her last breath. Over 30 000 people filed past her coffin to pay respects. She is buried in Père-Lachaise Cemetery in Paris, beneath the single word Bernhardt...minus a right leg, its whereabouts still unknown.[4]

**J. A. Stockman III, MD**

*References*

1. Duchamp M. Maladies de la croissance. In: Levrault FG, ed. *Memories de Medicine Practique*. Paris, France: Jean-Frederic Lobstein; 1823.
2. De Inocencio J. Epidemiology of musculoskeletal pain in primary care. *Arch Dis Child*. 2004;89:431-434.
3. Uziel Y, Chapnick G, Jaber L, Nemet D, Hashkes PJ. Five-year outcome of children with "growing pains": correlations with pain threshold. *J Pediatr*. 2010; 156:838-840.
4. de Costa C, Miller F. The art of medicine: Sarah Bernhardt's missing leg. *Lancet*. 2009;374:284-285.

---

**Transient Creatine Phosphokinase Elevations in Children: A Single-Center Experience**

Perreault S, Birca A, Piper D, et al (Sainte-Justine Hosp, Montreal, Quebec, Canada)

*J Pediatr* 159:682-685, 2011

*Objectives.*—To determine the etiologies and evolution of rhabdomyolysis in children.

*Study Design.*—We performed a retrospective study of patients with rhabdomyolysis who were seen in our tertiary care university-affiliated pediatric hospital. Patients in outpatient clinics, seen in the emergency department, or admitted from 2001 to 2002 were selected. With a standardized case report form, we collected predetermined data from each patient's chart.

*Results.*—A total of 130 patients with rhabdomyolysis were included in the study (male, 56%; mean age, 7.5 ± 5.9 years). The median elevation of creatine phosphokinase was 2207 IU/L (range, 1003 to 811 428 IU/L). The most frequent diagnoses were viral myositis (29, 22.3%), trauma (24, 18.4%), surgery (24, 18.4%), hypoxia (12, 9.2%), and drug reaction (8, 6.2%). Metabolic myopathy was found only in one patient (0.8%). In 17 patients (13.1%), no definite diagnosis could be made.

*Conclusions.*—Etiologies of rhabdomyolysis in children are varied and differ from those reported in adults. In most patients, rhabdomyolysis is

TABLE 1.—Etiologies of Rhabdomyolysis

|  | Number of Patients |
|---|---|
| Viral myositis | 29 (22.3%) |
| Trauma | 24 (18.4%) |
| Surgery | 24 (18.4%) |
| Hypoxia | 12 (9.2%) |
| Drug reaction | 8 (6.2%) |
| Burns | 4 (3.1%) |
| Sepsis | 4 (3.1%) |
| Compartment syndrome | 2 (1.5%) |
| Metabolic myopathy | 1 (0.8%) |
| Metabolic disturbance | 1 (0.8%) |
| Malignant hyperthermia | 1 (0.8%) |
| Seizure | 1 (0.8%) |
| Electrocution | 1 (0.8%) |
| Drug abuse | 1 (0.8%) |
| Unknown | 17 (13.1%) |
| Total | 130 (100%) |

TABLE 2.—Rhabdomyolysis Related to Drug Reaction

|  | Number of Patients |
|---|---|
| Corticosteroid | 2 |
| NSAID intoxication | 1 |
| Propofol | 1 |
| Antilipemic agent | 1 |
| Anticholinergic syndrome | 1 |
| Serotonin syndrome | 1 |
| Neuroleptic malignant syndrome | 1 |
| Total | 8 |

*NSAID*, nonsteroidal anti-inflammatory drug.

benign and without recurrence. In our series, rhabdomyolysis was the initial symptom of a metabolic myopathy in only one patient (Tables 1 and 2).

▶ There is no question that serum creatine phosphokinase (CK) is the best marker for detecting and monitoring skeletal muscle damage and diseases of muscle. CK catalyzes the transfer of energy from phosphate to adenosine diphosphate to form adenosine triphosphate (ATP). The ATP formed is used by myofibrils during muscle contraction. If a muscle is injured in any way, CK will leak into the blood and urine and can be readily measured.

Perreault et al undertook a study to determine the etiology and natural history of rhabdomyolysis in children. Rhabdomyolysis is defined as an acute and transitory elevation of CK greater than 1000 IU/L. In this study, transitory elevation was defined as a return to a CK level in the normal range within a 1-month period. In carrying out their study, the investigators identified all patients with elevated CK levels presenting to the Department of Pediatrics, Sainte Justine Hospital, Montreal, Quebec, Canada. The patients presented between January

2001 and December 2002. Some 130 patients were the source of the data from this report; 86.9% of patients had a clearly identified diagnosis (Tables 1 and 2). Far and away, viral myositis was the most frequent diagnosis. All such patients had fever, myalgia, and signs or symptoms of infection. A distinct minority of patients with presumed viral myositis had a specific virus identified. Trauma was another significant cause of CK elevation. Surgical procedures commonly cause CK elevations. Of the 130 patients with rhabdomyolysis, acute renal failure developed in 20%.

One of the things we learn from this report from Montreal is that rhabdomyolysis is not rare in the pediatric population. The various etiologies of rhabdomyolysis vary significantly and certainly differ from those reported in adults. Fortunately, in the majority of cases, rhabdomyolysis is benign and will not reoccur. Acute renal failure caused solely by rhabdomyolysis seems to be infrequent. Rhabdomyolysis is rarely caused by a metabolic myopathy, one of the things we are trained to think of as an uncommon but important cause of rhabdomyolysis.

**J. A. Stockman III, MD**

## Clinical Status and Cardiovascular Risk Profile of Adults with a History of Juvenile Dermatomyositis

Eimer MJ, Brickman WJ, Seshadri R, et al (Univ of Chicago, IL; Children's Memorial Hosp, Chicago, IL; et al)
*J Pediatr* 159:795-801, 2011

*Objective.*—A pilot study of adults who had onset of juvenile dermatomyositis (JDM) in childhood, before current therapeutic approaches, to characterize JDM symptoms and subclinical cardiovascular disease.

*Study Design.*—Eight adults who had JDM assessed for disease activity and 8 healthy adults (cardiovascular disease controls) were tested for carotid intima media thickness and brachial arterial reactivity. Adults who had JDM and 16 age-, sex-, and body mass index-matched healthy metabolic controls were evaluated for body composition, blood pressure, fasting glucose, lipids, insulin resistance, leptin, adiponectin, proinflammatory oxidized high-density lipoprotein (HDL), and nail-fold capillary end row loops.

*Results.*—Adults with a history of JDM, median age 38 years (24-44 years) enrolled a median 29 years (9-38 years) after disease onset, had elevated disease activity scores, skin (7/8), muscle (4/8), and creatine phosphokinase (2/8). Compared with cardiovascular disease controls, adults who had JDM were younger, had lower body mass index and HDL cholesterol ($P = .002$), and increased intima media thickness ($P = .015$) and their brachial arterial reactivity suggested impairment of endothelial cell function. Compared with metabolic controls, adults who had JDM had higher systolic and diastolic blood pressure, $P = .048$, $P = .002$, respectively; lower adiponectin ($P = .03$); less upper arm fat ($P = .008$); HDL associated with end row loops loss ($r = -0.838$, $P = .009$); and increased proinflammatory oxidized HDL ($P = .0037$).

*Conclusion.*—Adults who had JDM, 29 years after disease onset, had progressive disease and increased cardiovascular risk factors.

▶ The hallmark of juvenile dermatomyositis (JDM) is systemic microvascular injury to arterioles and capillaries reflected in an increase in the number of abnormal nail fold capillary loops. JDM is characterized by symmetric proximal muscle weakness, a typical rash, and objective evidence of inflammation in muscles. The pathophysiology of JDM involves genetic susceptibility, environmental factors, and infectious triggers with associated activation of complement and cellular and humoral immune systems. Cardiovascular involvement has rarely been documented in JDM, but when it does occur, it most commonly includes cardiac arrhythmias or myocardial infarction.

Eimer et al report on the oldest patients in their institution who had been diagnosed with JDM in childhood. They studied these adults and compared them with healthy peers for cardiovascular risk factors. The average age of adults who survived childhood JDM was 38 years. These adults had a remarkable increase in cardiovascular risk factors, including increased intima media thickness, resulting in death.

Seems a shame, but it is true that children with JDM who live into adulthood will face a host of cardiovascular risk factors in addition to other complications of their dermatomyositis.

**J. A. Stockman III, MD**

---

**Whole-Body Vibration Therapy for Osteoporosis: State of the Science**
Wysocki A, Butler M, Shamliyan T, et al (Minnesota Evidence-based Practice Ctr, Minneapolis)
*Ann Intern Med* 155:680-686, 2011

---

Clinical guidelines for osteoporosis recommend dietary and pharmacologic interventions and weight-bearing exercise to prevent bone fractures. These interventions sometimes have low adherence and can cause adverse effects. A proposed alternative or adjunctive treatment is whole-body vibration therapy (WBV), in which energy produced by a forced oscillation is transferred to an individual from a mechanical vibration platform. Whole-body vibration platforms are not approved by the U.S. Food and Drug Administration for medical purposes. This review provides a broad overview of important issues related to WBV therapy for prevention and treatment of osteoporosis. Relying on key informants and a search of the gray and published literature from January 2000 to August 2011, the investigators found that the designs of WBV platforms and protocols for their use vary widely. The optimal target population for the therapy is not defined. Although WBV has some theoretical advantages, key informants have voiced several concerns, including uncertain safety and potential consumer confusion between low-intensity vibration platforms intended for osteoporosis therapy and high-intensity platforms intended for exercise. Finally, the scant literature did not establish whether WBV therapy leads to clinically important increases in bone mineral density or reduces risk for fracture (Figs 1 and 2).

▶ The use of whole-body vibration therapy as part of the management of osteoporosis is rapidly spreading among the adult community. The reason for including this topic is that there are anecdotal reports appearing these days about children with bone density problems who are also being treated with whole-body vibration therapy.

Whole-body vibration was introduced during the last decade as a promising new antiosteoporotic therapy because significant improvements in bone formation rate, bone mineral density, trabecular structure, and cortical thickness were found in animal models. Although commercially available whole-body vibration devices have been marketed to and used by patients, the beneficial effects of

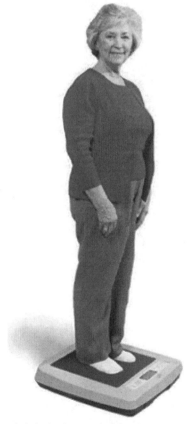

FIGURE 1.—Low-intensity whole-body vibration platform. The Juvent 1000 platform. Photograph courtesy of Juvent, Dynamic Motion Therapy, Somerset, New Jersey. (Reprinted from Wysocki A, Butler M, Shamliyan T, et al. Whole-Body Vibration Therapy for Osteoporosis: State of the Science. *Ann Intern Med.* 2011;155:680-686, with permission from the American College of Physicians.)

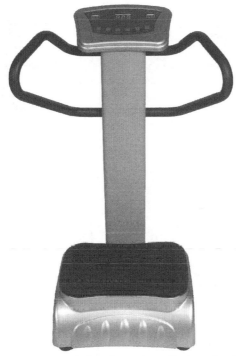

FIGURE 2.—Whole-body vibration platform that produces side-alternating vibration. The Osci Health platform. Image courtesy of Health Mark, Acworth, Georgia. (Reprinted from Wysocki A, Butler M, Shamliyan T, et al. Whole-Body Vibration Therapy for Osteoporosis: State of the Science. *Ann Intern Med.* 2011;155:680-686, with permission from the American College of Physicians.)

such therapy on fracture risk and bone mineral density have in fact not been established, and recent randomized, controlled trials in postmenopausal women have found conflicting results. Therapy involves standing on a motor driven, oscillating platform that produces vertical accelerations, which are transmitted from the feet to the weight-bearing muscles and bones. Transmission of vibrations through the body depends on the intensity of vibration, knee-joint angle, distance of the skeletal site from the oscillating plate, and possibly muscle and soft tissue dampening.

Hypothesized mechanisms by which whole-body vibration might exert osteogenic effects include changes in the flow of bone fluid caused by direct bone stimulation and transduction of mechanical signals or indirect bone stimulation through skeletal muscle activation, possibly by means of the stretch reflex. Vibration therapy has also been suggested to be beneficial in those who have lost muscle mass and who have reduced mobility because it might mimic the mechanical signals typically generated by muscle contractions or such low-density activities as walking.

Wysocki et al undertook a meta-analysis of the research literature to determine the possible benefits of whole-body vibration therapy for osteoporosis. The report abstracted was commissioned as a technical brief by the Agency for Healthcare Research and Quality Effective Health Care Program. The study involved searches of several databases going back some 12 years. The study examined data related to low-intensity, whole-body vibration platforms (Fig 1) and whole-body vibration platforms that produce side-alternating vibration (Fig 2). Unfortunately, for those with or at increased risk for osteoporosis who may have bought one of these instruments, the data from the report showed scant evidence on the benefits (or harms) of whole-body vibration therapy for the prevention and treatment of osteoporosis. The investigators suggest that such treatment should be considered investigational. In the same issue of the *Annals of Internal Medicine*, there appeared a report by Slatkovska et al that actually looked at 202 healthy postmenopausal women with low bone density scores who were treated with 12 months of whole-body vibration therapy.[1] Whole-body vibration therapy did not alter bone mineral density or bone structure in this cohort of women who received calcium and vitamin D supplementation.

Thus, the news is not good for whole-body vibration therapy, at least in adults. Keep your eyes open for studies about this form of therapy in children. Chances are it will not work in them either. Also, be aware of an interesting unrelated syndrome known as the "phantom vibration syndrome" commonly seen among medical staff. In a report that appeared in the *British Medical Journal*, 115 of 169 MDs reported having experienced phantom vibrations from electronic devices they carried.[2] In a commentary that accompanied this report, it was noted that just as the Holy Roman Empire was not holy, Roman, or an empire, phantom vibration syndrome does not involve a phantom nor is it technically a syndrome. The sensations are best characterized as tactile hallucinations in which the brain perceives a sensation that is actually not present. Why doctors believe their pagers and phones are going off remains a mystery. In most cases, the problem was solved by simply moving the device from one pocket to another. Perhaps shutting the darned things off would also help as well.

This commentary closes with an observation on walking speed. In adult men 70 years of age or more, the speed of one's walking correlates directly with one's mortality. Walking speed is a commonly used objective measure of physical capability in older people, predicting survival. Stanaway et al measured the walking speed of 1705 men aged 70 years or more.[3] The investigators used a stopwatch to record the time taken by a man to walk 6 meters. The men were then followed up by telephone at 4-month intervals over a number of years. The men studied came from many different countries. The mean walking speed was 0.88 m/s. Older men who walked at speeds greater than 0.82 m/s were 1.23 times less likely to encounter death. In addition, no man walking at speeds of 1.36 m/s (3 miles per hour) or higher were caught by death over a 5-year period. There were no differences noted in the study subjects' geographic location, sex, or ethnic backgrounds.

Thus it is that one can easily outpace the grim reaper if one moves along at the speed of about 3 mph. Interestingly, the preferred walking speed of the grim reaper while collecting souls is relatively constant irrespective of people's geographical location, sex, and ethnic background.

**J. A. Stockman III, MD**

*References*

1. Slatkovska L, Alibhai SM, Beyene J, Hu H, Demaras A, Cheung AM. Effect of 12 months of whole-body vibration therapy on bone density and structure in post-menopausal women: a randomized trial. *Ann Intern Med.* 2011;155:668-679.
2. Rothberg MB, Arora A, Hermann J, Kleppel R, St Marie P, Visintainer P. Phantom vibration syndrome among medical staff: a cross sectional survey. *BMJ.* 2010;341: c6914.
3. Stanaway F, Gnjidic D, Blyth FM, et al. How fast does the grim reaper walk? *BMJ.* 2011;343:1282-1283.

## Epidemiology of Bowling-Related Injuries Presenting to US Emergency Departments, 1990-2008

Kerr ZY, Collins CL, Comstock RD (The Ohio State Univ, Columbus; The Res Inst at Nationwide Children's Hosp, Columbus, OH)
*Clin Pediatr* 50:738-746, 2011

*Objective.*—To examine bowling-related injuries presenting to US emergency departments (EDs) from 1990 to 2008.

*Methods.*—Bowling-related injury data were analyzed from the US Consumer Product Safety Commission's National Electronic Injury Surveillance System.

*Results.*—From 1990 to 2008, 8754 bowling injuries presented to US EDs, correlating to an estimated 375 468 injuries nationwide. Common body parts injured were the finger (19.0%), trunk (15.8%), and ankle/foot/toe (14.9%). Common diagnoses were sprain/strain (42.7%) and soft-tissue injury (20.3%). Children <7 years old had a higher proportion of finger injuries (49.2%) and injuries from dropping the ball (42.8%) than individuals ≥7 years old (15.9%, injury proportion ratio [IPR] = 3.09, 95% confidence interval [CI] = 2.76-3.45, $P < .001$; and 15.9%, IPR = 2.69, 95% CI = 2.32-3.12, $P < .001$, respectively). Seniors ≥65 years old sustained a greater proportion of injuries related to falling/slipping/tripping (72.4%) than individuals <65 years old (38.3%; IPR = 1.89, 95% CI = 1.74-2.05, $P < .001$).

*Conclusions.*—Bowling injuries vary by age and gender. Further research on such differences is needed to drive the development of targeted, evidence-based injury prevention strategies.

▶ There is not much written about bowling-related injuries. If one scans the literature on such injuries, one sees case reports of "bowler's tendonitis" (medial epicondylitis) and "bowler's thumb." Those are fairly expected injuries in addition to those resulting from dropping a bowling ball on one's foot, slipping, and falling. In adults, herniated discs related to bowling have been reported.

So why are bowling injuries of any significance to the pediatrician? Although the number of 10-pin bowling centers has decreased in the United States over the past several decades, as has the number of frequent bowlers (defined as bowling ≥25 days a year), participation by the occasional bowler, including children, has increased. This is also true of college-age students. With the number of recreational and younger bowlers increasing, there are potentially a cohort of individuals out there who are more inexperienced and unconditioned and at greater risk for injury.

Kerr et al examined information obtained from the US Consumer Product Safety Commission's National Electronic Injury Surveillance System. There is a code in the database for bowling injuries (code 1206). Using the data from these sources, the investigators documented that the number of bowling-related injuries reported range from a low of 16195 in 2004 to a high of 21794 in 1991. Adults (aged 19—64 years) had the highest number of injuries, followed by youngsters 7 to 18 years of age (a ratio of approximately 4:1). Children younger than 7 years of age had about half as many injuries reported as those 7 to 18 years. The body regions most frequently injured include the finger (19%), trunk (15.8%), and ankle/foot/toe (14.9%). The most common diagnoses are sprain/strain (42.7%) and soft tissue (20.3%). No cases of bowler's thumb were reported. The most common mechanism of injury is a fall/slip/trip (41.7%) followed by a dropped ball (19.7%). Of those injured while releasing the ball, almost half got a finger/thumb stuck in the ball. Six fatalities related to bowling were documented in individuals ranging in age from 32 years to 80 years. The most common cause of death was cardiac arrest, presumably brought on by excitement/stress/overexertion. Alcohol as a related cause for injury was infrequent.

The authors of this report suggest that bowling injuries can be minimized by proper conditioning before going out and picking up a bowling ball. Bowlers, whether frequent or occasional participants, should engage in conditioning activities to help withstand the physical stresses of bowling. Exercise routines for the back, trunk, and legs, as well as warm ups prior to bowling, will also help maintain balance and reduce strain. Proper use of equipment is extremely important. When picking up the ball, one should grab the ball from the sides, not the front or back, to avoid an approaching ball that could smash hands and fingers. Bowling shoes should be slick enough to allow them to slide across the lane. Lanes should be periodically wiped and cleaned and moisture avoided on the lane.

If you are not familiar with bowler's thumb, look up the report by Ostrovskiy et al.[1]

This commentary closes with a reflection on a sport frequently associated with orthopedic complications, that is rugby. Unfortunately rugby is increasingly getting a bad reputation, as is true of football (the European version, aka soccer), with players exaggerating the degree of the potential impact of an injury, perhaps thinking it might result in a penalty to the opposing team. Recently a rugby match doctor was accused of cutting a player's lip with a scalpel to conceal the use of fake blood. She was suspended by the General Medical Council in Great Britain pending an investigation. The physician was an accident and emergency consultant who was a match doctor for Harlequins Rugby Team at its Heineken Cup match with Leinster in April 2009. A player told the European Rugby Cup Appeal Committee that the physician cut his lip after the match at his request to conceal his use of a fake blood capsule during the match. He had left the match with apparent blood streaming from his mouth to allow a specialist goal kicker to take his place. The player was found guilty of misconduct and banned from playing for 12 months. The British General Medical Council suspended the physician's license for 18 months and indicated that a fitness to practice hearing would be required prior to reentry into practice. It is obvious that some people go to great lengths to see their favorite team win. There is no record of whether the specialist kicker was able to achieve a goal.[2]

**J. A. Stockman III, MD**

*References*

1. Ostrovskiy D, Wilbourn A. Acute bowler's thumb. *Neurology.* 2004;63:938.
2. Dyer C. Doctor is suspended by GMC after being accused of covering up fake rugby injury. *BMJ.* 2009;339:712-713.

---

**Management of Uncomplicated Nail Bed Lacerations Presenting to a Children's Emergency Department**
Al-Qadhi S, Chan KJ, Fong G, et al (Univ of Toronto, Ontario, Canada; AMD Inc, Ontario, Canada)
*Pediatr Emerg Care* 27:379-383, 2011

*Objective.*—This study examined the mechanisms of injury and the pattern of care for children who presented to the emergency department with uncomplicated nail bed lacerations.

*Methods.*—A retrospective chart review was conducted from January 2004 to December 2007 for all children younger than 18 years who presented to a tertiary children's hospital with an uncomplicated nail bed laceration.

*Results.*—There were 84 cases of uncomplicated nail bed injuries for more than a 4-year period. Sixty percent of the subjects were males. The mean age was 5.3 (SD, 4.1) years. Most injuries occurred at home (58%), and the most common mechanism of injury was a door (67%). Approximately 40% of patients were treated by emergency physicians. There was no significant difference in acute and chronic complications or in the length of stay in the emergency department, between patients treated by emergency physicians and by plastic surgeons.

*Conclusions.*—Most nail bed injuries in children occur at home, and the door seems to be the major mechanism of injury. Approximately 57% of these are children younger than 5 years. Only 42% of uncomplicated nail bed lacerations are treated by emergency physicians, yet there is no significant difference in outcomes between plastic surgeons and emergency physicians. Our study suggests that there is a role in public education for primary prevention, and with proper training, pediatric emergency physicians can treat uncomplicated nail bed lacerations (Fig 1).

▶ This report from the Hospital for Sick Children in Canada describes the largest cohort of children with nail bed injuries reported in the literature and

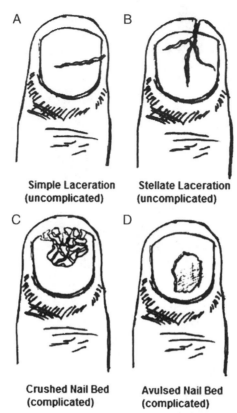

**FIGURE 1.**—Classification of nail bed injuries. (Reprinted from Al-Qadhi S, Chan KJ, Fong G, et al. Management of uncomplicated nail bed lacerations presenting to a children's emergency department. *Pediatr Emerg Care.* 2011;27:379-383.)

the only one performed in the environment of the emergency room. Historically, despite the frequency of nail bed injuries, emergency physicians frequently misdiagnose and underestimate the severity of damage. Nail bed injury accounts for some 15% to 25% of fingertip injuries and can result in significant functional and aesthetic problems if the injury is left to heal by secondary intention. Primary repair of injured nail bed by removal of the nail plate has been the standard of care for nail bed injuries. Such primary repair is desirable not only because it prevents long-term sequelae in 90% of cases, but the repair turns out to be less costly than performing reconstructive secondary surgery that may result in unsatisfactory outcomes.

The report of Al-Qadhi et al. tells us about 84 cases of uncomplicated nail bed injuries seen in the emergency room at Toronto Children's Hospital over a 4-year period. Fig 1 illustrates the difference between a complicated and uncomplicated nail bed injury. The report suggests that uncomplicated nail bed injuries can be adequately cared for by emergency department physicians without the need for calling in a plastic surgeon. Consulting a plastic surgeon when not needed results in significant delays in the ultimate repair and increased cost. The authors of this report suggest that education and training of simple nail bed repair should be provided to all pediatric emergency medicine physicians and trainees.

This commentary closes with a quiz related to nail bed lacerations. Of the 10 fingers and toes that most of us have, which finger in particular is the most likely to be injured? If you answered the middle finger of the right hand, you would be absolutely correct. Forty-one percent of nail bed injuries occur on the middle finger of the right hand. The next sites in terms of frequency are the ring finger of the left hand (23%), the index finger of the left hand (19%), the little finger of the right hand (16%), and the thumb of the left hand (13%). If the math does not add up to 100%, go Fig 1.

**J. A. Stockman III, MD**

---

**Bedside Ultrasound in the Diagnosis of Pediatric Clavicle Fractures**
Chien M, Bulloch B, Garcia-Filion P, et al (Phoenix Children's Hosp, AZ)
*Pediatr Emerg Care* 27:1038-1041, 2011

---

*Objective.*—The objective of the study was to determine the diagnostic accuracy of pediatric emergency physicians in diagnosing clavicle fractures by bedside ultrasound (US).

*Methods.*—This was a prospective study of pediatric emergency department (ED) patients with suspected clavicle fractures conducted in a tertiary-care, freestanding pediatric hospital. A convenience sample of patients younger than 17 years underwent bedside US for detection of clavicle fracture by pediatric emergency physicians with limited US training. Ultrasound findings were compared with standard radiographs, which were considered the criterion standard. Pain scores using the validated color analog scale (0-10) were determined before and during US. Total length of stay in the ED, time to US, and time to radiograph were recorded.

*Results.*—Fifty-eight patients were enrolled, of which 39 (67%) had fracture determined by radiograph. Ultrasound interpretation gave a sensitivity of 89.7% (95% confidence interval [CI], 75.8%−97.1%) and specificity of 89.5% (95% CI, 66.9%−98.7%). Positive and negative predictive values were 94.6% (95% CI, 81.8%−99.3%) and 81.0% (95% CI, 58.1%−94.5%), respectively. Positive and negative likelihood ratios were 8.33 and 0.11, respectively. Pain scores averaged 4.7 before US and 5.2 during US ($P = 0.204$). There was a statistically significant difference between mean time to US (76 minutes) and mean time to radiograph (107 minutes) ($P < 0.001$).

*Conclusions.*—Pediatric emergency physicians with minimal formal training can accurately diagnose clavicle fractures by US. In addition, US itself is not associated with an increase in pain and may reduce length of stay in the ED (Fig 1B).

▶ The clavicle remains the most commonly fractured bone in children. Such fractures represent approximately 5% of all fractures presenting to emergency

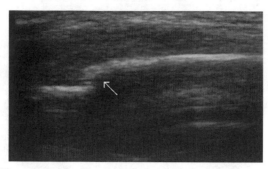

FIGURE 1B.—Ultrasound image of fractured (B) clavicle. Arrows point to region of normal clavicle and region of discontinuity. (Reprinted from Chien M, Bulloch B, Garcia-Filion P, et al. Bedside Ultrasound in the Diagnosis of Pediatric Clavicle Fractures. *Pediatr Emerg Care.* 2011;27:1038-1041.)

departments in the United States. These fractures can be readily diagnosed clinically, but current standard of care is to confirm the diagnosis with an x-ray. Given the concerns that exist these days about the long-term consequences of even a simple x-ray on the risk of subsequent malignancies, it seems reasonable to entertain alternative confirmatory methods to diagnose clavicular fractures. Bedside ultrasound has been used more and more frequently in emergency rooms in the past 10 years to 20 years. Numerous applications for ultrasound have been documented in the literature. What Chien et al have done is to design a study to determine whether ultrasound can accurately diagnose clavicular fractures.

The study design reported here was undertaken in the emergency department of Phoenix Children's Hospital, an emergency room that sees approximately 65 000 visits per year. This is a teaching hospital. Patients under age 17 years with a suspected clavicular fracture were examined with both ultrasound and standard radiographs; 58 patients were enrolled, and 67% had a fracture as determined by x-ray. Ultrasound was highly sensitive (89.7%) and highly specific (89.5%).

The findings from this report are consistent with studies that have shown the capability of emergency room physicians to diagnose long bone fractures in adult trauma patients with 93% sensitivity and 83% specificity using ultrasound.[1] Also, a recent study similarly designed and conducted almost simultaneously with the study from Phoenix showed 95% sensitivity and 96% specificity, 95% positive predictive value, and a 96% negative predictive value in detecting pediatric clavicle fractures using ultrasound.[2] Of 100 patients enrolled in the latter study, the investigators reported 2 false-positive cases and two false-negative cases of missed hairline fractures. The main difference between the latter report and the one performed in Phoenix is that all but 3 of the ultrasound examinations showing the highest level of sensitivity and specificity were performed by a single physician with experience in both adult and pediatric ultrasound.

So what we learn from this Arizona study is that emergency physicians with minimal training in bedside ultrasound can accurately diagnose clavicle fractures with a high degree of accuracy and without causing pain to the patient. Unlike other studies examining the use of bedside ultrasound, these investigators suggest that their study is generalizable to any emergency setting because 12 emergency physicians, mostly with minimal to no experience were involved in performing the examinations. Overall, the results suggest that given a specificity of nearly 90%, if ultrasound is positive for fracture and the patient has no clinical deficits or gross deformity, a confirmatory x-ray may be unnecessary. The rare false-positive result would entail only supportive care, which would essentially be of no harm. Similarly, an x-ray would also be unnecessary given a false-negative study because this would likely indicate only a minor greenstick fracture requiring no additional therapy. Both scenarios could avoid radiation exposure from radiography. Treatment in either case would be the same with a sling or figure-of-eight brace for 2 to 3 weeks. In the management of clavicle fractures, only the rare fracture with neurovascular or mediastinal injury associated with severely angulated or displaced fractures needs orthopedic consultation. Only in these rare circumstance could one imagine obtaining x-rays—or so say the authors of this report. Unfortunately, medicolegal issues still influence the need for a confirmatory x-ray. Ultrasound may, however, provide an expensive and practical alternative.

This commentary ends with a musculoskeletal-type question. Are children more likely to break their limbs falling off play equipment onto sand or onto wood fiber? Investigators in Toronto suggest that fewer limbs are broken falling onto sand than onto engineered wood fiber, this according to a cluster random- ized trial. Primary schools that were randomly allocated to a new sandy surface reported 1.9 arm fractures per 100 000 student months, compared with 9.4 for schools allocated a new surface of wood fiber. The analysis examined only the incidence of arm fractures. Despite the data derived from this report, the schools in Toronto seem to prefer the wood fiber with more than half of those allocated sand switching to wood fiber, perhaps because school officials thought the sand would be messier, tracked into buildings and attract attention of cats and dogs. In any event, the explanation favoring sand is that the latter, with its low friction properties, allows falling limbs to slide and sink rather than to bend and break.[3]

**J. A. Stockman III, MD**

*References*

1. Marshburn TH, Legome E, Sargsyan A, et al. Goal-directed ultrasound in the detection of long-bone fractures. *J Trauma.* 2004;57:329-332.
2. Cross KP, Warkentine FH, Kim IK, et al. Bedside ultrasound diagnosis of clavicle fractures in the pediatric emergency department. *Acad Emerg Med.* 2010;17: 687-693.
3. Editorial comment. Sand is safer playground surface than wood fiber. *BMJ.* 2010; 340:18.

## Meniscus Tears in the Young Athlete: Results of Arthroscopic Repair

Vanderhave KL, Moravek JE Jr, Sekiya JK, et al (Univ of Michigan, Ann Arbor)
*J Pediatr Orthop* 31:496-500, 2011

*Background.*—The purpose of this study was to evaluate the results of arthroscopic repair of the meniscus in children and young athletes.

*Methods.*—Arthroscopic meniscus repairs performed on 49 knees in 31 male and 14 female patients <18 years old were reviewed. All repairs were done using an inside-out technique, and 31 patients required concomitant anterior cruciate ligament (ACL) reconstruction. Age at time of injury, time to surgery, and the extent, type, and location of meniscus tear were noted. All patients underwent postoperative rehabilitation and clinical evaluation. The level of activity at follow-up and postoperative outcomes scores was determined. Analysis included $t$ tests, Wilcoxon tests, $\chi^2$ tests, and Fisher exact tests, with a level of significance of $P \geq 0.05$.

*Results.*—Excellent clinical outcomes were noted in 43 of 45 patients, with mean length of follow-up of 27 months. Between the groups with and without ACL tears, there were no significant differences in mean age at the time of injury or surgery, or in the distribution of open versus closed physes, medial versus lateral repairs, or level-of-activity at follow-up. However, patients with ACL reconstruction had significantly longer return-to-activity times (mean 8.23 mo vs. 5.56 mo) and significantly lower Tegner scores (mean 6.8 vs. 8.0) than patients without simultaneous reconstruction.

*Conclusions.*—The clinical results after arthroscopic meniscus repair in the adolescent were excellent, despite long average time from injury to surgery and a high number of tears in poorly vascularized areas. Meniscal tears in skeletally immature athletes may have greater reparative potential, with and without simultaneous ligament reconstruction. Attempts at repair regardless of time from injury or location of tear should be strongly considered in this age group.

*Level of Evidence.*—Level III retrospective cohort series.

▶ There is no question that we have seen an increasing incidence of intra-articular knee injuries in the young athlete. Many of these result in meniscus tears that will need to be repaired, usually arthroscopically. To date, few studies have specifically addressed outcomes after meniscus repair in the adolescent population. Vanderhave et al designed a study to determine the clinical outcomes and return to sports after arthroscopic meniscus repair in adolescents (age range 9 to 17 years, mean age 13.2 years).

In this report, magnetic resonance imaging scans were obtained to determine the nature of the intra-articular knee injury in the young athlete with a painful knee. The repair was undertaken arthroscopically. At the time of the meniscal repair, patients with anterior cruciate ligament (ACL) deficiency underwent arthroscopically assisted anterior cruciate ligament reconstruction. Following surgery, no squatting or pivoting was allowed for 4 months. Sports were permitted at 4 months for those who had only a meniscus tear and 6 months for those who had a meniscus tear plus an anterior cruciate ligament repair. In this series, 43 of 45 (95.6%) patients were considered clinically healed 2 years after arthroscopic meniscus repair. Repair technique may have played a key role in the clinical success noted in this series since the results were much better than those reported in prior studies. All patients underwent meniscus repair using the inside-out technique with a vertical mattress suture. The approach used in this series was very uniform. In this series, nearly two-thirds of patients with a meniscus tear also had an associated ACL tear. Patients who undergo meniscal repair concurrent with an ACL reconstruction may constitute a distinct subset of patients when compared with meniscal repair alone. In this series, concomitant ACL reconstruction did not worsen the outcome. The majority of all patients were able to return to their preinjury level of activity.

The real issue with these youngsters is what their knees will look like 5, 10, and 30 years later. There are data to suggest that over time knees that have been damaged in adolescence do not necessarily hold up all that well over many decades. At least on the short haul, the outlook is okay.

While on the topic of things orthopedic, if you want to look at an interesting Website, go to the Website of the National Institute of Advanced Industrial Science and Technology and search under human foot morphology. You will learn more than you ever wanted about the human foot. Did you know, for example, that the human foot stops growing at a younger age than overall growth in height? The human foot tends to stop growing at about 14 years of age in boys and 13 years of age in girls. Another conspicuous change in feet is the increase in toe angles with age. The big toe gradually rotates laterally with age. Toe shape gradually narrows, probably because of wearing shoes. Lastly, the most accurate way to measure foot length is to determine the distance between the pterion (the rear most point of the heel) and the tip of the longest toe measured in a straight line axis. Normally the greatest dimension is achieved by connecting the pterion and the tip of the second toe. The width of the foot is actually best measured by determining foot circumference as measured with a tape so the tape passes over the largest circumference, measured usually at the metatarsal tibial at the "ball of the foot." It is possible to have a "not so wide" foot, but a pretty fat one, and this in fact would require a wider shoe, thus the advantage of measuring foot circumference as opposed to actual width.

This commentary closes with a thought or two about falls, these related to nonfatal fall-related injuries associated with cats and dogs in the United States. Recently, the Centers for Disease Control (CDC) published national data on the numbers and types of injuries related to humans tripping over their dogs and cats.[1] In the United States, approximately 43 million households own dogs and people in 37.5 million households own cats; nearly 64% of households with pets have more than one pet. There are on average an estimated 86 000 fall injuries each year associated with cats and dogs for an average annual injury rate of almost 30 per 100 000 population. Nearly 88% of these injuries are associated with dogs, and among people injured, females were more than 2 times more likely to be injured than males. The young and old are the age groups most likely to trip over a pet. Indeed the highest rates of injuries occur among people 75 years of age and older with the most common resulting diagnosis being that of a fracture.

Unfortunately the CDC does not tell us about human-induced injury to their pets by such falls. You know it is not the dog's fault every time a human gets injured. With regards to cats, however, that is a different story.

**J. A. Stockman III, MD**

*Reference*

1. Centers for Disease Control and Prevention (CDC). Nonfatal fall-related injuries associated with dogs and cats—United States, 2001-2006. *MMWR Morb Mortal Wkly Rep.* 2009;58:277-281.

## Classification of Legg-Calvé-Perthes Disease

Kuo KN, Wu K-W, Smith PA, et al (Taipei Med Univ, Taiwan; Natl Taiwan Univ Hosp, Taipei; Shriners Hosp for Children, Chicago, IL; et al)
*J Pediatr Orthop* 31:S168-S173, 2011

Although the etiology of Perthes disease remains unknown 100 years after its first description, there are many articles that describe the disease course, final outcome, and results of treatment. A system of classification of the extent and severity of the disease is essential to understanding variability of Perthes, and along with the age of the patient when first affected, is useful in predicting long-term outcomes. Published reports of treatment strategies and their success depend on effective classification of the disease severity and radiographic result at final follow-up concerning head sphericity, congruency with the acetabulum, and arthritis. This article reviews published articles that contain classification systems and details presently used systems that are helpful in understanding and in treating Perthes.

▶ The year 2010 represented 100 years since the simultaneous publications by Arthur Legg from the United States, Jacque Calvé in France, and George Perthes in Germany of the disorder that is now known by the eponym of their names. Each of these individuals postulated different disease etiologies. Legg presented a series of limping patients with flattened femoral heads, which he believed was due to trauma. In contrast, Calvé reported on 10 patients with noninflammatory hip pain and a flattened femoral head that he felt was caused by abnormal osteogenesis. Perthes reported on 6 patients with hip pain and felt that the disorder was due to an inflammatory condition. It was only in the 1920s that necrosis was documented to be part of Legg-Calvé-Perthes disease. The theory then developed that this was due to a vascular insult.

The report of Kuo et al reminds us of how little we know about the true cause of Legg-Calvé-Perthes disease and how unstandardized the classification of the disease has been over the last 100 years. Part of the problem related to this inconsistency is the lack of constant positioning of the legs when x-rays are taken. Absent a consistent classification system, it is difficult to tell what therapeutic maneuvers really are the most effective in terms of management.

Much is changing with our understanding of the cause and management of Legg-Calvé-Perthes disease. Much new information is being provided by magnetic resonance imaging studies in comparison with plain films, the latter being the basis of most classification systems. To read more about Legg-Calvé-Perthes disease, read the supplement to the *Journal of Pediatric Orthopaedics* that appeared in September 2011. The supplement was entirely devoted to this interesting but enigmatic disorder.

Also, does knuckle cracking in any way increase one's risk of arthritis? The answer to this profound question comes from a report that appeared in the journal *Arthritis and Rheumatism.*[1] The author noted that during his childhood various parties, his mother, several aunts, and his mother-in-law informed him that cracking his knuckles would lead to arthritis of the fingers. To test the accuracy of this hypothesis he undertook a study. For 50 years, the author cracked the knuckles of his left hand at least twice a day, leaving those of his right hand as a control. The knuckles on the left were cracked at least 36 500 times, while those on the right were cracked rarely and spontaneously. At the end of the 50 years hands were compared for evidence of arthritis. The findings showed that there was no arthritis in either hand, and no apparent differences between the 2 hands. While a larger study group would have been ideal to confirm this result, the preliminary investigation suggests a lack of correlation between knuckle cracking and the development of arthritis of the fingers. A search of the literature by the author revealed only 1 previous paper on the subject that also came to the same conclusion.

The results of this single investigator participant study call into question whether other parental beliefs, such as importance of eating spinach or sitting too close to the TV causing nearsightedness, are also flawed. Further investigation in this regard is warranted. It should be noted that this study was done entirely at the author's expense, with no grants from any governmental or pharmaceutical sources. It was undertaken in California, the leading state of many things unusual, and proudly so.

**J. A. Stockman III, MD**

*Reference*

1. Unger DL. Does knuckle cracking lead to arthritis of the fingers? *Arthritis Rheum.* 1998;41:949-950.

---

**General Ultrasound Screening Reduces the Rate of First Operative Procedures for Developmental Dysplasia of the Hip: A Case-Control Study**
von Kries R, Ihme N, Altenhofen L, et al (Ludwig-Maximilians Univ, Munich, Germany; Univ Aachen, Germany; Central Res Inst of Ambulatory Health Care in Germany, Cologne; et al)
*J Pediatr* 160:271-275, 2012

---

*Objectives.*—To assess the effectiveness of general ultrasound screening to prevent first operative procedures of the hip.

*Study Design.*—We conducted a case-control study in a population in which general ultrasound screening supplementing clinical screening is recommended and offered free of charge for all children. Participation in ultrasound screening before week 7 as recommended in Germany was the exposure of interest. Case ascertainment was based on active surveillance in orthopedic hospitals. The case definition was: first operative procedure for developmental dysplasia of the hip (closed reduction, open reduction, or osteotomy) in children >9 weeks old and <5 years old and born between 1996 and 2001. Control subjects from the same birth cohorts were recruited in telephone surveys.

*Results.*—Cases of first operative procedures for developmental dysplasia of the hip (n = 446) were compared with 1173 control subjects for ultrasound screening. Effectiveness of ultrasound screening to prevent first operative procedures for developmental dysplasia of the hip was estimated as 52% (95% CI, 32-67). Effectiveness did not vary substantially for closed and open reductions and osteotomy.

*Conclusions.*—General ultrasound screening reduces the rate of operative procedures for developmental dysplasia of the hip; the impact on developmental dysplasia of the hip. Treatment rates and avascular necrosis need further assessment to balance the benefit against potential overtreatment and adverse effects.

▶ This study demonstrates a practical approach to estimating the relative risks of surgery for developmental dysplasia of the hip in children who were screened with ultrasound examination and in those who were not screened and found that ultrasound screening decreases the need for surgery. Thus the debate regarding the value of using ultrasound in the screen for developmental dysplasia of the hip will continue until measures for treatment are accurately collected and presented. In this report, cases of first operative procedures for developmental dysplasia of the hip were compared with more than 1000 control subjects for ultrasound screening. It was obvious that ultrasound screening prevented the need for operative procedures for developmental dysplasia of the hip in as many as half of the patients enrolled in the study.

There will be much more written about this topic. The reason for this is that there are fewer and fewer surgeries being performed for this congenital disorder. Thus it will take a long time before the picture is totally clear about the role of ultrasound screening in the newborn period.

This commentary closes with the observation that some implanted devices related to orthopedic surgery can make one squeak. The next time you think you hear a squeak as someone walks past, you may be picking up the phenomenon of ceramic-on-ceramic total hip arthroplasty. It appears to be unique to total hip replacements with hard-on-hard surfaces. The implications are yet to be ascertained, but such surfaces apparently offer advantages in terms of wear reduction, which is useful for young and active patients. Recipients of such artificial joints should be warned in advance of the possible squeaking they and others around them might hear.[1]

**J. A. Stockman III, MD**

*Reference*

1. Jarrett CA, Ranawat AS, Bruzzone M, Blum YC, Rodriguez JA, Ranawat CS. The squeaking hip: a phenomenon of ceramic-on-ceramic total hip arthroplasty. *J Bone Joint Surg Am*. 2009;91:1344-1349.

# 13 Neurology and Psychiatry

**Intracranial Hemorrhage after Blunt Head Trauma in Children with Bleeding Disorders**
Lee LK, the Traumatic Brain Injury Study Group for the Pediatric Emergency Care Applied Research Network (PECARN) (Harvard Med School, Boston, MA; et al)
*J Pediatr* 158.1003-1008, 2011

*Objective.*—To determine computerized tomography (CT) use and prevalence of traumatic intracranial hemorrhage (ICH) in children with and without congenital and acquired bleeding disorders.

*Study Design.*—We compared CT use and ICH prevalence in children with and without bleeding disorders in a multicenter cohort study of 43 904 children <18 years old with blunt head trauma evaluated in 25 emergency departments.

*Results.*—A total of 230 children had bleeding disorders; all had Glasgow Coma Scale (GCS) scores of 14 to 15. These children had higher CT rates than children without bleeding disorders and GCS scores of 14 to 15 (risk ratio, 2.29; 95% CI, 2.15 to 2.44). Of the children who underwent imaging with CT, 2 of 186 children with bleeding disorders had ICH (1.1%; 95% CI, 0.1 to 3.8), compared with 655 of 14 969 children without bleeding disorders (4.4%; 95% CI, 4.1-4.7; rate ratio, 0.25; 95% CI, 0.06 to 0.98). Both children with bleeding disorders and ICHs had symptoms; none of the children required neurosurgery.

*Conclusion.*—In children with head trauma, CTs are obtained twice as often in children with bleeding disorders, although ICHs occurred in only 1.1%, and these patients had symptoms. Routine CT imaging after head trauma may not be required in children without symptoms who have congenital and acquired bleeding disorders.

▶ I have never seen a study quite like this that examines the problem of blunt head trauma resulting in bleeding in patients with a variety of bleeding disorders. The investigators looked at patients with hemophilia (mild, moderate, and severe), von Willebrand disease, autoimmune thrombocytopenia, functional platelet disorders, bleeding disorders related to anticoagulation therapy, and a variety of other miscellaneous bleeding disorders. More than 43 000 patients with nontrivial blunt head trauma were enrolled during the 28-month study period. The study represented a multi-institutional commitment to the evaluation of such patients. Of these patients, 230 had a history of congenital or acquired bleeding disorders, including 129 patients (56.1% of the overall group) with hemophilia. After hemophilia, von Willebrand disease and thrombocytopenia comprise the next largest categories of bleeding disorders. Of the children with thrombocytopenia, 18 (54%) had idiopathic thrombocytopenic purpura.

The study showed that 1% of patients with blunt head trauma who had a bleeding disorder had evidence of an intracranial hemorrhage. This suggested that CT imaging might not be routinely needed in the evaluation of children with bleeding disorders after blunt head trauma, particularly in those without signs and symptoms suggestive of intracranial hemorrhage.

It should be noted that intracranial hemorrhage is the leading cause of mortality from bleeding in this population of patients with factor VIII and factor IX deficiency. Current recommendations for the management of head trauma in children with severe hemophilia are to initiate treatment with factor replacement as soon as possible after the traumatic event. It is entirely possible that this significant decrease in mortality rate and the actual incidence of intracranial hemorrhage can be attributed to the wide availability of factor concentrates for replacement. It is not entirely clear what one should do with the information from this report. The 2 patients in this large series who had intracranial hemorrhages had either severe factor VIII deficiency (a patient involved in a motorcycle crash) or were receiving warfarin therapy (a 6-year-old who was receiving anticoagulant therapy for a congenital cardiac condition and who fell 3 to 5 feet. Both of these patients had clinical findings that would have required a computed tomography (CT) scan even without a history of a bleeding disorder.

Is it likely that someone with a known bleeding disorder who has blunt head trauma will not get a CT scan as a result of the findings from this report even if the child has no clinical findings? Not likely. No one would like to miss such a problem in a child. Nonetheless, the data from this report are reassuring that in an overwhelming variety of instances, children with bleeding disorders with blunt head trauma will do well if seen immediately and if replacement therapy is given quickly.

If one reads the adult literature, one has a sense that neurologic cases tend to dominate the literature. Some have suggested that this is the result of neurophobia—the fear of neurology—a well-described entity in medical students. Neurology cases represent more than a quarter of all *Lancet* case reports: 29% of 523 cases during the period 1996 to 2002 and 26% of 360 cases during 2003 to 2008. Such a predominance has been attributed to the trepidation and interest that neurological syndromes generate among physicians and the continued inability to demystify the field of neurology to non-neurologists. To determine whether neurologic cases are disproportionate to disease burden, Thomas and Thomas set about to determine this by comparing the pattern of cases from the *BMJ* case reports with the burden of neurologic disability in the United Kingdom, hypothesizing that a more eloquent explanation for the neurologic case dominance is not neurophobia, but rather that the cases are simply more entertaining.[1] It is entirely possible that clinical neurology is not a dark mystery, but rather a popular thriller. To test this assertion, the authors also examined cases where the motivation is to entertain rather than to educate examining the television drama, *House, MD*. For those who are allergic to medical drama, *House, MD* stars Hugh Laurie as the maverick Gregory House. He is a diagnostician with an acerbic charm who solves mysteries loosely based on real medicine. The character resembles Sherlock Holmes: a drug-using misanthrope and music loving genius. Back in 2008, *House, MD* was the most viewed television series worldwide.

It turns out that in comparison to actual disease prevalence, neurologic cases are overrepresented in the *British Medical Journal* as well as in the *Lancet*, and they are also probably overrepresented in many adult medical journals in the United States. The same is true of *House, MD*, where 27.5% of whodunit cases were neurologic in origin with gastroenterology cases a distant second at 5.5%.

There is no question that neurology is poorly understood by many and mystery can be compelling. With sufficient knowledge, you ultimately can have the satisfaction of predicting correctly where the lesion must be to cause the symptoms. It is no surprise therefore that the public has such an appetite for such cases as Oliver Sacks' *The Man Who Mistook his Wife for a Hat*. There has never been much demand for *The Man Who Passed Frequent Bloody Stools*. Watching *House* cure someone with lower motorneuron disease is much more emotionally resonating than seeing someone treat a glue ear or piles.

**J. A. Stockman III, MD**

*Reference*

1. Thomas R, Thomas N. House calls. *BMJ*. 2009;339:1416-1419.

## Neuron Number and Size in Prefrontal Cortex of Children With Autism

Courchesne E, Mouton PR, Calhoun ME, et al (Univ of California San Diego, La Jolla; Univ of South Florida School of Medicine, Tampa, FL; Sinq Systems Inc, Silver Spring, MD)
*JAMA* 306:2001-2010, 2011

*Context.*—Autism often involves early brain overgrowth, including the prefrontal cortex (PFC). Although prefrontal abnormality has been theorized to underlie some autistic symptoms, the cellular defects that cause abnormal overgrowth remain unknown.

*Objective.*—To investigate whether early brain overgrowth in children with autism involves excess neuron numbers in the PFC.

*Design, Setting, and Cases.*—Postmortem prefrontal tissue from 7 autistic and 6 control male children aged 2 to 16 years was examined by expert anatomists who were blinded to diagnostic status. Number and size of neurons were quantified using stereological methods within the dorsolateral (DL-PFC) and mesial (M-PFC) subdivisions of the PFC. Cases were from the eastern and southeastern United States and died between 2000 and 2006.

*Main Outcome Measures.*—Mean neuron number and size in the DL-PFC and M-PFC were compared between autistic and control postmortem cases. Correlations of neuron number with deviation in brain weight from normative values for age were also performed.

*Results.*—Children with autism had 67% more neurons in the PFC (mean, 1.94 billion; 95% CI, 1.57-2.31) compared with control children (1.16 billion; 95% CI, 0.90-1.42; $P = .002$), including 79% more in DL-PFC (1.57 billion; 95% CI, 1.20-1.94 in autism cases vs 0.88 billion; 95% CI, 0.66-1.10 in controls; $P = .003$) and 29% more in M-PFC (0.36 billion; 95% CI, 0.33-0.40 in autism cases vs 0.28 billion; 95% CI, 0.23-0.34 in controls; $P = .009$). Brain weight in the autistic cases differed from normative mean weight for age by a mean of 17.6% (95% CI, 10.2%-25.0%; $P = .001$), while brains in controls differed by a mean of 0.2% (95% CI, −8.7% to 9.1%; $P = .96$). Plots of counts by weight showed autistic children had both greater total prefrontal neuron counts and brain weight for age than control children.

*Conclusion.*—In this small preliminary study, brain overgrowth in males with autism involved an abnormal excess number of neurons in the PFC.

▶ This report represents a small preliminary study of the brains of 7 autistic children to determine whether they had more neurons in the prefrontal regions of their brains. Overgrowth and neural dysfunction have been long suspected to be one of the characteristics of autism. Overgrowth and neural dysfunction are evident at young ages. In the first magnetic resonance imaging (MRI) report of early brain overgrowth in autism from a decade ago, it was theorized that excess numbers of neurons could be an underlying cause of the disorder, perhaps as a result of prenatal dysregulation of proliferation, apoptosis, or both. The only way for sure, however, is to actually count the number of neurons on a pathologic specimen in affected youngsters. Obviously this can only be done postmortem.

Courchesne et al received permission to study the brains of 7 autistic children who died of unrelated causes between the ages of 2 and 16 years. These specimens are stored at the National Institutes of Health. Their brains, along with carefully matched age controls, were examined. In addition to the finding of a mean 67% greater number of prefrontal neurons, the autistic group also had a larger brain weight average. The number of neurons counted exceeded the expected number even when adjusted for brain weight. In fact, if one attempted to calculate what the brain enlargement would have been adjusted for number of neurons, the brains of autistic children should have been about 30% larger than a control group. The observed increase in size was 17.6%. Thus, the size of the autistic brain, overlarge though it is, might actually underestimate the pathology of excess neuron numbers.

So what is going on with the brains of children with autism? One can only speculate. The authors of this report suggest that the defect is in apoptotic mechanisms. These mechanisms are ones that normally allow involution and destruction of cells in a normal fashion. Apoptotic mechanisms during the third trimester and early postnatal life normally remove subplate neurons, which comprise about half of the neurons produced in the second trimester. A failure of that key early developmental process could create a pathologic excess of cortical neurons. A failure of apoptosis might additionally indicate abnormal development of the brain subplate itself, which plays a critical role in the maturation of inhibitory functions of the brain. Reduced inhibitory functioning and defects of functional and structural connectivity are characteristics of autism, but the causes to date have remained elusive.

The number of brains of autistic children evaluated as part of this study was not large enough to examine brain—behavior relationships. It would be necessary to study many more children to attempt to establish a relationship between neuron counts and symptom severity or intellectual disability. Such a study is extremely unlikely to ever be carried out because the pathologic specimens at the National Institutes of Health characterize the total number of brains that were available for such studies. Nonetheless, this was an important study and is the first direct quantitative test confirming the theory that a pathologic overabundance of neurons in critical brain regions is present at a young age in autism. Because cortical neurons are generated prenatally not postnatally, the pathologic overabundance of neurons indicates a very early developmental disturbance. Thus, the findings from this report have tremendous significance for understanding the etiologic and neurodevelopmental origins of autism.

If you want to read more about genetic testing for autism, see the excellent commentary on this topic by Waters.[1] Known genetic mutations are associated with fewer than 20% of autism spectrum disorder cases. Duplications or deletions of small segments of DNA known as small-copy variants have been found. At least half a dozen clinical laboratories have developed tests to look for microarrays in these variants.

This commentary closes with an observation having to do with the psyche of Doberman pinschers. High-energy Doberman pinschers are a breed particularly susceptible to developing compulsive behaviors, such as incessant licking of flanks or sucking on blankets. Investigators have studied Dobermans and have discovered a really robust psychiatric gene. By way of background, canine compulsive disorder (CCD)—analogous to human obsessive-compulsive disorder (OCD)—is seen in 2% to 5% of dogs. A genome-wide association study of 94 Dobermans with CCD which compared information with 73 healthy controls observed a mutation in neural cadherin-2, a gene involved in the central nervous system development on chromosome 7. Sixty percent of the highest-risk dogs had the mutation, almost 3 times the rate in unaffected dogs. Canine psychiatrists believe that this report gives us a specific target to look at for OCD in humans.[2]

**J. A. Stockman III, MD**

*References*

1. Waters H. Autism, authenticated. *Nat Med.* 2011;17:1336-1338.
2. Editorial comment. Doggie OCD. *Science.* 2010;327:397.

### Cardiac Screening Prior to Stimulant Treatment of ADHD: A Survey of US-Based Pediatricians

Leslie LK, Rodday AM, Saunders TS, et al (Tufts Med Ctr, Boston, MA)
*Pediatrics* 129:222-230, 2012

*Objectives.*—To determine pediatricians' attitudes, barriers, and practices regarding cardiac screening before initiating treatment with stimulants for attention-deficit/hyperactivity disorder.

*Methods.*—A survey of 1600 randomly selected, practicing US pediatricians with American Academy of Pediatrics membership was conducted. Multivariate models were created for 3 screening practices: (1) performing an in-depth cardiac history and physical (H & P) examination, (2) discussing potential stimulant-related cardiac risks, and (3) ordering an electrocardiogram (ECG).

*Results.*—Of 817 respondents (51%), 525 (64%) met eligibility criteria. Regarding attitudes, pediatricians agreed that both the risk for sudden cardiac death (SCD) (24%) and legal liability (30%) were sufficiently high to warrant cardiac assessment; 75% agreed that physicians were responsible for informing families about SCD risk. When identifying cardiac disorders, few (18%) recognized performing an in-depth cardiac H & P as a barrier; in contrast, 71% recognized interpreting a pediatric ECG as a barrier. When asked about cardiac screening practices before initiating stimulant treatment for a recent patient, 93% completed a routine H & P, 48% completed an in-depth cardiac H & P, and 15% ordered an ECG. Almost half (46%) reported discussing stimulant-related cardiac risks. Multivariate modeling indicated that ≥1 of these screening practices were associated with physicians' attitudes about SCD risk, legal liability, their responsibility to inform about risk, their ability to perform an in-depth cardiac H & P, and family concerns about risk.

*Conclusions.*—Variable pediatrician attitudes and cardiac screening practices reflect the limited evidence base and conflicting guidelines regarding cardiac screening. Barriers to identifying cardiac disorders influence practice.

▶ The report of Leslie et al tells us about a survey of 1600 practicing pediatricians in the United States. The survey was undertaken to determine what evaluations pediatricians undertake, if any at all, prior to prescribing attention deficit hyperactivity disorder (ADHD)—related drugs. The pediatricians were selected randomly from the registry of Fellows of the American Academy of Pediatrics. Data from the survey showed that 14.7% of pediatricians order an electrocardiogram prior to starting such drugs. Most do so because they say it is standard practice in their setting. Relatively few order an electrocardiogram (ECG) because of clinical indications. Only about 20% review the results of the ECG themselves. Most ECGs are read by a cardiologist. Needless to say, the cost involved with these approaches is quite high. The real issue is whether anything more than a simple history and physical examination is needed as opposed to a more extended cardiovascular assessment prior to writing a prescription for ADHD-type drugs.

Few medications have received as much public scrutiny as those used for ADHD. The most serious concerns have centered on cardiovascular risk. The most commonly used ADHD medications—psychostimulants and atomoxetine—can cause an increase in blood pressure and heart rate, which some studies have been linked with serious cardiovascular events. These concerns received extensive attention in 2006, when the US Food and Drug Administration (FDA) Advisory Committee proposed placing a black box warning concerning sudden death on psychostimulants in response to adverse event reports. Subsequent epidemiologic studies quantifying this risk generally did not support an association, but concerns have lingered nonetheless.

The most important new information concerning ADHD drugs and cardiovascular risk has appeared recently in *JAMA*. Habel at al compared approximately 150 000 adults prescribed ADHD medication with approximately 300 000 nonusers and found no evidence of a link between ADHD medications and myocardial infarction, sudden cardiac death, or stroke.[1] This study is the most comprehensive assessment to date of the cardiovascular safety of ADHD medications. Although the study did not enroll children, the same group also has reported a similar lack of a significant association between serious cardiovascular events and the use of ADHD medications in children and younger adults.[2] Even when looking at the statistics with a worst case scenario, it was shown that the increase in cardiovascular events was just 0.17 serious cardiovascular events per 1000 person-years, which translates to 1 event associated with ADHD medications occurring for every 5900 person-years of treatment. Such absolute risk estimates allow clinicians to form their own opinion of the clinical importance of these worst case scenarios. It is clear that this study provides no evidence to support the ordering of routine ECGs prior to starting treatment with ADHD drugs. This study does not obviate the need to do a careful history and physical examination, however. The findings from this report do support the most recent decision by the FDA in 2006 not to place a black box warning of serious cardiovascular events on ADHD medications for all children and adults.

Thus, current data seemed to indicate that a history and physical examination alone should suffice prior to starting ADHD medications in children who have no known structural or rhythm cardiac abnormalities. Obviously, you will need to make that decision yourself based on information currently in the medical literature, but the prevailing evidence should be comforting to you and to the families of these children and adolescents.

This commentary closes with the observation that walking for 40 minutes 3 times a week will increase brain volume and memory. A randomized study reports that the 60 healthy older adults who participated in anaerobic training for a year increased their hippocampal volume by 2%, whereas a control group had a 1.4% loss of volume, consistent with normal aging.[3] The 2% increase reversed the usual age-related loss in brain volume by one to two years, and it led to improvements and spatial memory. Aerobic exercise therefore may boost levels of brain-derived neurotrophic factor. At least in the elderly, maybe exercise is good for you!

**J. A. Stockman III, MD**

*References*

1. Habel LA, Cooper WO, Sox CM, et al. ADHD medications and risk of serious cardiovascular events in young and middle-aged adults. *JAMA*. 2011;306: 2673-2683.
2. Cooper WO, Habel LA, Sox CM. ADHD drugs and serious cardiovascular events in children and young adults. *N Engl J Med*. 2011;365:1896-1904.
3. Editorial comment. Exercise-induced increases in brain volume. *BMJ*. 2011; 342:390.

## Risk of Febrile Seizures and Epilepsy After Vaccination With Diphtheria, Tetanus, Acellular Pertussis, Inactivated Poliovirus, and *Haemophilus Influenzae* Type b

Sun Y, Christensen J, Hviid A, et al (Aarhus Univ, Denmark; Aarhus Univ Hosp, Denmark; Statens Serum Institut, Copenhagen, Denmark; et al)
*JAMA* 307:823-831, 2012

*Context.*—Vaccination with whole-cell pertussis vaccine carries an increased risk of febrile seizures, but whether this risk applies to the acellular pertussis vaccine is not known. In Denmark, acellular pertussis vaccine has been included in the combined diphtheria-tetanus toxoids–acellular pertussis–inactivated poliovirus–*Haemophilus influenzae* type b (DTaP-IPV-Hib) vaccine since September 2002.

*Objective.*—To estimate the risk of febrile seizures and epilepsy after DTaP-IPV-Hib vaccination given at 3, 5, and 12 months.

*Design, Setting, and Participants.*—A population-based cohort study of 378 834 children who were born in Denmark between January 1, 2003, and December 31, 2008, and followed up through December 31, 2009; and a self-controlled case series (SCCS) study based on children with febrile seizures during follow-up of the cohort.

*Main Outcome Measures.*—Hazard ratio (HR) of febrile seizures within 0 to 7 days (0, 1-3, and 4-7 days) after each vaccination and HR of epilepsy after first vaccination in the cohort study. Relative incidence of febrile seizures within 0 to 7 days (0, 1-3, and 4-7 days) after each vaccination in the SCCS study.

*Results.*—A total of 7811 children were diagnosed with febrile seizures before 18 months, of whom 17 were diagnosed within 0 to 7 days after the first (incidence rate, 0.8 per 100 000 person-days), 32 children after the second (1.3 per 100 000 person-days), and 201 children after the third (8.5 per 100 000 person-days) vaccinations. Overall, children did not have higher risks of febrile seizures during the 0 to 7 days after the 3 vaccinations vs a reference cohort of children who were not within 0 to 7 days of vaccination. However, a higher risk of febrile seizures was found on the day of the first (HR, 6.02; 95% CI, 2.86-12.65) and on the day of the second (HR, 3.94; 95% CI, 2.18-7.10), but not on the day of the third vaccination (HR, 1.07; 95% CI, 0.73-1.57) vs the reference cohort. On the day of vaccination, 9 children were diagnosed with febrile seizures after the first (5.5 per 100 000 person-days), 12 children after the second (5.7 per 100 000 person-days), and 27 children after the third (13.1 per 100 000 person-days) vaccinations. The relative incidences from the SCCS study design were similar to the cohort study design. Within 7 years of follow-up, 131 unvaccinated children and 2117 vaccinated children were diagnosed with epilepsy, 813 diagnosed between 3 and 15 months (2.4 per 1000 person-years) and 1304 diagnosed later in life (1.3 per 1000 person-years). After vaccination, children had a lower risk of epilepsy between 3 and 15 months (HR, 0.63; 95% CI, 0.50-0.79) and a similar risk for epilepsy later in life (HR, 1.01; 95% CI, 0.66-1.56) vs unvaccinated children.

*Conclusions.*—DTaP-IPV-Hib vaccination was associated with an increased risk of febrile seizures on the day of the first 2 vaccinations given at 3 and 5 months, although the absolute risk was small. Vaccination with DTaP-IPV-Hib was not associated with an increased risk of epilepsy.

▶ The data from this report can be used to help parents make informed decisions about vaccinations and vaccine complications. When the pertussis vaccine became available many years ago, it was associated with a number of complications. This, of course, was the whole-cell variety of pertussis vaccine. This vaccine was associated with serious neurological illness characterized by seizures and intellectual impairment. Recent studies indicate that this type of vaccination only triggers an earlier onset of severe epileptic encephalopathy in children with sodium channel gene mutations. The acellular pertussis vaccine has replaced the whole-cell pertussis vaccine in most countries. The efficacy of the acellular vaccine is comparable to the whole-cell vaccine and has substantially fewer adverse effects, including fever. Previous randomized controlled trials did not reveal differences in the risks of seizures after acellular pertussis vaccination compared with whole-cell vaccine, but such trials were not of sufficient size to detect rare adverse events. A study from the United Kingdom suggested a 2-fold higher risk of seizures on the day of diphtheria-tetanus toxoid-acellular pertussis inactivated polio virus-*Haemophilus influenzae* b vaccination.[1] The estimates from these reports did not reach statistical significance, and it is clear that there was difficulty distinguishing between afebrile and febrile seizures in these prior studies. This led to the more comprehensive study abstracted here, which attempted to examine the risk of febrile seizures and epilepsy following the administration of the acellular combined vaccine.

Some 379 834 children in Denmark were part of this study. All received the combined diphtheria-tetanus toxoid-acellular pertussis-inactivated polio virus-*H influenzae* type b vaccine. The enrolled children were carefully followed to determine the prevalence of febrile seizures as well as the incidence of onset of true epilepsy. The investigators found that the relative risks of febrile seizures were increased on the day of the first and second vaccine administrations but that the absolute risks were low at fewer than 4 per 100 000 vaccine administrations. The overall risk of febrile seizures was not increased 1 to 7 days after the vaccination. The risks of recurrent febrile seizures or subsequent epilepsy were not increased for children whose first febrile seizure occurred within 0 to

7 days postvaccination. The risk of epilepsy was not higher among vaccinated versus unvaccinated children. The study had almost complete follow-up of all children born in Denmark during the 6-year period due to nationwide registries. It is unclear why the risk of febrile seizure increased after the first 2 vaccinations but not after the third. There may be competing risk factors for febrile seizures during a period in which the incidence of febrile seizures is high and the relative importance of a single risk factor like vaccination may be lower.

The transient increased risk of febrile seizures on the day of vaccination was followed up by a slightly lower risk in the days following vaccination. This suggests that the vaccination may have induced febrile seizures that would have occurred a few days later anyway or that recently vaccinated children constitute a select group of relatively healthy children. It is unclear why vaccinated children in this report showed a decreased risk of epilepsy between 3 and 15 months. It may be due to unmeasured confounding factors.

It is unfortunate that public awareness of possible adverse effects following whole-cell pertussis vaccination has caused a reduction in immunization rates and outbreaks of whooping cough in several countries. The vaccine studied in this report has a pattern of adverse events similar to that of diphtheria and tetanus vaccines given as isolated vaccines. The estimates for risk of febrile seizures did not change when pneumococcal vaccine is given at the same time. Parents should be told that although the relative risk of febrile seizures on the day of vaccination is increased, the absolute risk of febrile seizures is low, and the prognosis of febrile seizures occurring shortly after vaccination is similar to the prognosis of febrile seizures occurring absent vaccination. Parents also need to know that this study documented that the vaccine under discussion was not associated with an increased risk of epilepsy.

This commentary closes with the observation that intramuscular midazolam is as effective and safe as lorazepam administered intravenously. The intramuscular route was used by emergency medical services teams as part of the treatment of children and adults with status epilepticus in a recent study.[2] In patients whose seizures ceased before arrival to the emergency department, the median time to active treatment was just 1.2 minutes in the intramuscular treated group and 4.8 minutes in the intravenous treated group. The implications of this report are obvious. Although sometimes it is quite difficult to start an IV in someone who is having a seizure, one cannot always give an intramuscular injection.

**J. A. Stockman III, MD**

*References*

1. Andrews N, Stowe J, Wise L, Miller E. Post licensure comparison of combination acellular pertussis vaccine in the United Kingdom. *Vaccine.* 2010;28:7215-7220.
2. Silbergleit R, Durkalski V, Lowenstein D, et al. Intramuscular versus intravenous therapy for prehospital status epilepticus. *N Engl J Med.* 2012;366:591-600.

## Newer-Generation Antiepileptic Drugs and the Risk of Major Birth Defects

Mølgaard-Nielsen D, Hviid A (Statens Serum Institut, Copenhagen, Denmark)
*JAMA* 305:1996-2002, 2011

*Context.*—Epilepsy during pregnancy is a therapeutic challenge. Since the 1990s, the number of licensed antiepileptic drugs has substantially increased, but safety data on first-trimester use of newer-generation antiepileptic drugs and birth defects are limited.

*Objective.*—To study the association between fetal exposure to newer-generation antiepileptic drugs during the first trimester of pregnancy and the risk of major birth defects.

*Design, Setting, and Participants.*—Population-based cohort study of 837 795 live-born infants in Denmark from January 1, 1996, through September 30, 2008. Individual-level information on dispensed antiepileptic drugs to mothers, birth defect diagnoses, and potential confounders were ascertained from nationwide health registries.

*Main Outcome Measures.*—Prevalence odds ratios (PORs) of any major birth defect diagnosed within the first year of life by fetal exposure to antiepileptic drugs.

*Results.*—Of the 1532 infants exposed to lamotrigine, oxcarbazepine, topiramate, gabapentin, or levetiracetam during the first trimester, 49 were diagnosed with a major birth defect compared with 19 911 of the 836 263 who were not exposed to an antiepileptic drug (3.2% vs 2.4%, respectively; adjusted POR [APOR], 0.99; 95% confidence interval [CI], 0.72-1.36). A major birth defect was diagnosed in 38 of 1019 infants (3.7%) exposed to lamotrigine during the first trimester (APOR, 1.18; 95% CI, 0.83-1.68), in 11 of 393 infants (2.8%) exposed to oxcarbazepine (APOR, 0.86; 95% CI, 0.46-1.59), and in 5 of 108 infants (4.6%) exposed to topiramate (APOR, 1.44; 95% CI, 0.58-3.58). Gabapentin (n = 59) and levetiracetam (n = 58) exposure during the first trimester was uncommon, with only 1 (1.7%) and 0 infants diagnosed with birth defects, respectively.

*Conclusion.*—Among live-born infants in Denmark, first-trimester exposure to lamotrigine, oxcarbazepine, topiramate, gabapentin, or levetiracetam compared with no exposure was not associated with an increased risk of major birth defects.

▶ The use of antiepileptic drugs is spreading like wildfire. While once applied to the management of epilepsy, this class of drugs is now used to treat such diverse entities as bipolar mood disorders, migraine, and neuropathic pain syndrome. Most use of antiepileptics, however, is for the management of seizure disorders. As far as pregnancy is concerned, it is well known that older-generation antiepileptic drugs such as phenobarbital, phenytoin, valproate, and carbamazepine, when used during pregnancy, can be associated with a several-fold increased risk of birth defects. In the last 15 years, newer-generation antiepileptic drugs have offered alternatives to pregnant women, but there is only sparse information on the teratogenic effects of these newly licensed grouping of agents.

What Mølgaard-Nielsen and Hviid have done is look at the risks associated with relatively recently introduced antiepileptic drugs when applied to the management of seizure disorders in pregnant women. They examined the teratogenic effects of lamotrigine, oxcarbazepine, topiramate, gabapentin, and levetiracetam. What they found was that 3.2% of pregnant women exposed to this class of agents delivered a baby with a major birth defect versus 2.4% of control women who were not receiving any antiepileptic agents. Their study examined 1532 infants exposed to the 5 agents mentioned. The study should be considered statistically bulletproof in that 800 000 pregnancies (all in Denmark) were looked at to determine the risk of these antiepileptics. The bottom line is that these Danish investigators found no association between the use of newer-generation antiepileptics during the first trimester of pregnancy and the risk of major birth defects. This study is the largest analytic cohort study on this topic and provides comprehensive safety information on a class of drugs commonly used during pregnancy. In particular, the use of lamotrigine and oxcarbazepine during the first trimester was not found to be associated with moderate or greater risks of major birth defects, unlike older generation antiepileptic drugs, but the study could not exclude a minor excess in the risk of major birth defects or risk of specific birth defects. It would take many more women studied to tease out such findings. Topiramate, gabapentin, and levetiracetam do not appear to be major teratogens, but the study could not specifically exclude minor to moderate risk of birth defects with these 3 agents, which are much less commonly used than lamotrigine and oxcarbazepine.

While on the topic of pregnancy and epilepsy, it is clear that reproductive capability is a worry for women with epilepsy. An Indian cohort study followed up 375 women with epilepsy who were anticipating pregnancy but had not yet conceived. These women were followed for 1 to 10 years. Nearly 40% remained infertile, and of the rest, most became pregnant within the first 2 years of follow-up. Infertility was associated with age, lower education, and the number of epilepsy drugs taken. Phenobarbital exposure was associated with a significant risk of infertility, but valproate and other drugs had no clear individual link.[1] It is not entirely clear from this report whether many of these women, either because of their epilepsy or concerns about birth defects, may have elected not to become pregnant in the long run.

This commentary closes with an unrelated subject having to do with a neurologic condition. A mysterious illness affecting mostly children called the "nodding syndrome" is spreading across a wide part of some countries in Africa, stumping investigators from the CDC who have failed so far to determine what is causing the disease that gives people, young and old, epilepticlike seizures and impairs their cognition. In Northern Uganda, roughly 1000 cases were diagnosed between August and December 2011.[2] There is no known cure for the disease. The nodding syndrome has been given its name because those affected nod their heads when food is put in front of them. It is presumed that the nodding syndrome is due to an infection, most likely onchocerciasis. It appears that malnutrition contributes to the disorder as well.

**J. A. Stockman III, MD**

*References*

1. Sukumaran SC, Sarma PS, Thomas SV. Polytherapy increases the risk of infertility in women with epilepsy. *Neurology.* 2010;75:1351-1355.
2. Centers for Disease Control and Prevention (CDC). Nodding syndrome – South Sudan, 2011. *MMWR Morb Mortal Wkly Rep.* 2012;61:52-53.

---

**The long-term outcome of adult epilepsy surgery, patterns of seizure remission, and relapse: a cohort study**
de Tisi J, Bell GS, Peacock JL, et al (Univ College London Inst of Neurology, UK; King's College London, UK)
*Lancet* 378:1388 1395, 2011

---

*Background.*—Surgery is increasingly used as treatment for refractory focal epilepsy; however, few rigorous reports of long term outcome exist. We did this study to identify long-term outcome of epilepsy surgery in adults by establishing patterns of seizure remission and relapse after surgery.

*Methods* —We report long-term outcome of surgery for epilepsy in 615 adults (497 anterior temporal resections, 40 temporal lesionectomies, 40 extratemporal lesionectomies, 20 extratemporal resections, 11 hemispherectomies, and seven palliative procedures [corpus callosotomy, subpial transection]), with prospective annual follow-up for a median of 8 years (range 1—19). We used Kaplan-Meier survival analysis to estimate time to first seizure, and investigated patterns of seizure outcome.

*Findings.*—We used survival methods to estimate that 52% (95% CI 48—56) of patients remained seizure free (apart from simple partial seizures [SPS]) at 5 years after surgery, and 47% (42—51) at 10 years. Patients who had extratemporal resections were more likely to have seizure recurrence than were those who had anterior temporal resections (hazard ratio [HR] 2·0, 1·1—3·6; p=0·02); whereas for those having lesionectomies, no difference from anterior lobe resection was recorded. Those with SPS in the first 2 years after temporal lobe surgery had a greater chance of subsequent seizures with impaired awareness than did those with no SPS (2·4, 1·5—3·9). Relapse was less likely the longer a person was seizure free and, conversely, remission was less likely the longer seizures continued. In 18 (19%) of 93 people, late remission was associated with introduction of a previously untried antiepileptic drug. 104 of 365 (28%) seizure-free individuals had discontinued drugs at latest follow-up.

*Interpretation.*—Neurosurgical treatment is appealing for selected people with refractory focal epilepsy. Our data provide realistic expectations and indicate the scope for further improvements in presurgical assessment and surgical treatment of people with chronic epilepsy.

▶ There are modest data in the pediatric literature about the benefits of epilepsy surgery. For this reason, it is worthwhile looking at reports that deal largely with adults but do include some in the pediatric age group. The report of de Tisi et al represents the latter type of investigation. This report includes, for example, teen-agers. The report is the largest and longest prospective study of epilepsy surgery outcome for almost 20 years of follow-up. The study is novel in its prospective analysis of seizure freedom at successive annual reviews in individual patients, unlike other studies that review seizure freedom only at last follow-up. The patients largely consisted of individuals who had temporal lobe surgery, typical of most adult epilepsy surgery. de Tisi et al report the percentage of patients remaining free of nonsimple partial seizure to be 63% at 2 years, 52% at 5 years, and 47% at 10 years. The initial and longer period of seizure absence is the strongest indicator of good long-term outcome.

de Tisi et al have also found that the identification of simple partial seizures within 2 years of surgery is a significant risk factor for long-term seizure recurrence. This finding has implications for decisions to discontinue antiepileptic drugs in patients with only simple partial seizures. The outcome in patients not rendered immediately seizure free or suffering a short-lived relapse also allows for optimism, with 15% of the total cohort in this category eventually gaining remission.

Surgical management of medically refractory focal epilepsy has seen a resur-gence in both pediatric and adult patients in the last 2 decades. Advances in structural and functional neuroimaging and invasive electroencephalography have increased success in identifying the seizure focus. Functional magnetic resonance imaging, tractography, and cortical mapping have allowed for safe resection. The report of de Tisi et al adds to our understanding about epilepsy surgery, providing valuable information about predictive factors, prognosis, management, and causation. Epilepsy surgery should not be undertaken in centers that are not well versed in the full range of preoperative and postoper-ative diagnostic and management capabilities.

**J. A. Stockman III, MD**

---

### Early Surgical Therapy for Drug-Resistant Temporal Lobe Epilepsy: A Randomized Trial

Engel J Jr, for the Early Randomized Surgical Epilepsy Trial (ERSET) Study Group (Univ of California, Los Angeles; et al)
*JAMA* 307:922-930, 2012

---

*Context.*—Despite reported success, surgery for pharmacoresistant seizures is often seen as a last resort. Patients are typically referred for surgery after 20 years of seizures, often too late to avoid significant disability and premature death.

*Objective.*—We sought to determine whether surgery soon after failure of 2 antiepileptic drug (AED) trials is superior to continued medical management in controlling seizures and improving quality of life (QOL).

*Design, Setting, and Participants.*—The Early Randomized Surgical Epilepsy Trial (ERSET) is a multicenter, controlled, parallel-group clinical trial performed at 16 US epilepsy surgery centers. The 38 participants (18 men and 20 women; aged ≥12 years) had mesial temporal lobe epilepsy (MTLE) and disabling seizures for no more than 2 consecutive years following adequate trials of 2 brand-name AEDs. Eligibility for anteromesial temporal resection (AMTR) was based on a standardized presurgical evaluation protocol. Participants were randomized to continued AED treatment or AMTR 2003-2007, and observed for 2 years. Planned enrollment was 200, but the trial was halted prematurely due to slow accrual.

*Intervention.*—Receipt of continued AED treatment (n = 23) or a standardized AMTR plus AED treatment (n = 15). In the medical group, 7 participants underwent AMTR prior to the end of follow-up and 1 participant in the surgical group never received surgery.

*Main Outcome Measures.*—The primary outcome variable was freedom from disabling seizures during year 2 of follow-up. Secondary outcome variables were health-related QOL (measured primarily by the 2-year change in the Quality of Life in Epilepsy 89 [QOLIE-89] overall T-score), cognitive function, and social adaptation.

*Results.*—Zero of 23 participants in the medical group and 11 of 15 in the surgical group were seizure free during year 2 of follow-up (odds ratio = ∞; 95% CI, 11.8 to ∞; $P < .001$). In an intention-to-treat analysis, the mean improvement in QOLIE-89 overall T-score was higher in the surgical group than in the medical group but this difference was not statistically significant (12.6 vs 4.0 points; treatment effect = 8.5; 95% CI, −1.0 to 18.1; $P = .08$). When data obtained after surgery from participants in the medical group were excluded, the effect of surgery on QOL was significant (12.8 vs 2.8 points; treatment effect = 9.9; 95% CI, 2.2 to 17.7; $P = .01$). Memory decline (assessed using the Rey Auditory Verbal Learning Test) occurred in 4 participants (36%) after surgery, consistent with rates seen in the literature; but the sample was too small to permit definitive conclusions about treatment group differences in cognitive outcomes. Adverse events included a transient neurologic deficit attributed to a magnetic resonance imaging—identified postoperative stroke in a participant who had surgery and 3 cases of status epilepticus in the medical group.

*Conclusions.*—Among patients with newly intractable disabling MTLE, resective surgery plus AED treatment resulted in a lower probability of seizures during year 2 of follow-up than continued AED treatment alone. Given the premature termination of the trial, the results should be interpreted with appropriate caution.

*Trial Registration.*—clinicaltrials.gov Identifier: NCT 00040326.

▶ Patients with drug-resistant epilepsy are generally referred for surgery after years of seizures, often too late to avoid significant disability. To assess the effect of early surgical therapy on seizure control, investigators who were part of the Early Randomized Surgical Epilepsy Trial Study Group randomly assigned 38 patients with mesial temporal lobe epilepsy refractory to antiepileptic drug therapy for no more than 2 consecutive years to receive mesial temporal lobe resection and continued antiepileptic drug treatment or continued drug treatment alone. The report abstracted showed that the patients who underwent resection therapy had a lower risk of seizures during 2 years of follow-up. It should be noted that this series of patients included adolescents.

The Early Randomized Surgical Epilepsy Trial was designed as a prospective study evaluating the efficacy of surgical treatment for patients with refractory epilepsy. The original intent of the trial was to enroll 200 patients. The trial was terminated on recommendation of a Data and Safety Monitoring Board after just 38 patients had been randomized. This recommendation was based on the slow pace of enrollment, although the monitoring board apparently had access to unblinded primary outcome data for study participants who had completed the second year of follow-up. The difference in outcomes of treated patients versus controls was striking. None of the 23 patients in the medical therapy group were seizure-free during the second year of follow-up whereas 73% in the surgical resection group were seizure-free. An adverse effect on memory was statistically significant in the surgical group. Scores on immediate and delayed recall testing at 24 months were lower, and a higher percentage of surgically treated patients showed decline (36% versus 0%) at 12 months. There was no significant difference between treatment groups in terms of employment status.

In an editorial that accompanied this report, it was commented that results of trials that are terminated very early should be interpreted with caution.[1] The trial, as noted, was stopped because it was difficult to enroll patients. Obviously, patients and their physicians are hesitant to recommend surgery early in the course of refractory epilepsy. Despite this limitation, there are several clinically important messages from this study. First, the early surgical approach for patients with refractory epilepsy was far superior to medical treatment when comparing seizure-free status and quality of life. Second, the surgical treatment of mesial temporal lobe epilepsy may lead to specific memory deficits. It is also well known that this form of epilepsy in and of itself can cause a progressive decline in memory. What is not known is whether the surgically induced memory decline is equal to, greater than, or less than memory decline that might occur during the long-term medical management of such patients. A final conclusion is that freedom from seizures and improved quality of life do not necessarily predict return to work. Employment activities did not seem to show group differences even though measures of social engagement showed a positive effect with surgery.

This study tells us about the critical importance of early diagnosis of mesial temporal lobe epilepsy. This is a disorder with well-recognized premonitory symptoms that include déjà vu, rising epigastric distress, experiential and hallucinatory phenomena, altered awareness, and automatism. These patients also have well-recognized radiographic imaging abnormalities, such as hippocampal atrophy, sclerosis, or both, and a reasonably predictable long-term course. All these findings suggest this particular form of temporal lobe epilepsy may be particularly amenable to surgery.

**J. A. Stockman III, MD**

*Reference*

1. Schomer DL, Lewis RJ. Stopping seizures early and the surgical epilepsy trial that stopped even earlier. *JAMA.* 2012;307:966-968.

### The Tuberous Sclerosis 2000 Study: presentation initial assessments and implications for diagnosis and management

Yates JRW, The Tuberous Sclerosis 2000 Study Group (Univ of Cambridge, UK; et al)
*Arch Dis Child* 96:1020-1025, 2011

*Aims.*—The Tuberous Sclerosis 2000 Study is the first comprehensive longitudinal study of tuberous sclerosis (TS) and aims to identify factors that determine prognosis. Mode of presentation and findings at initial assessments are reported here.

*Methods.*—Children aged 0—16 years newly diagnosed with TS in the UK were evaluated.

*Results.*—125 children with TS were studied. 114 (91%) met clinical criteria for a definite diagnosis and the remaining 11 (9%) had pathogenic *TSC1* or *TSC2* mutations. In families with a definite clinical diagnosis, the detection rate for pathogenic mutations was 89%. 21 cases (17%) were identified prenatally, usually with abnormalities found at routine antenatal ultrasound examination. 30 cases (24%) presented before developing seizures and in 10 of these without a definite diagnosis at onset of seizures, genetic testing could have confirmed TS. 77 cases (62%) presented with seizures. Median age at recruitment assessment was 2.7 years (range: 4 weeks—18 years). Dermatological features of TS were present in 81%. The detection rate of TS abnormalities was 20/107 (19%) for renal ultrasound including three cases with polycystic kidney disease, 51/88 (58%) for echocardiography, 29/35 (83%) for cranial CT and 95/104 (91%) for cranial MRI. 91% of cases had epilepsy and 65% had intellectual disability (IQ < 70).

*Conclusions.*—Genetic testing can be valuable in confirming the diagnosis. Increasing numbers of cases present prenatally or in early infancy, before onset of seizures, raising important questions about whether these children should have EEG monitoring and concerning the criteria for starting anticonvulsant therapy (Boxes 1 and 2, Table 2).

▶ The report of Yates et al is an excellent overview of the presentation and diagnosis of tuberous sclerosis. The latter can be difficult in the young child because characteristic skin lesions may not yet fulfill the clinical criteria for a definitive diagnosis. Most children with tuberous sclerosis will present with seizures in infancy or early childhood, and these can contribute to cognitive impairment. Early diagnosis and treatment to deal with seizures may improve cognitive outcome. Box 1 illustrates the major features of tuberous sclerosis presenting in childhood, and Box 2 gives a suggested series of evaluations for newly suspected tuberous sclerosis.

Yates et al report on the mode of presentation and findings at the initial assessment of youngsters with tuberous sclerosis based on a study that was designed and monitored by a National Coordinating Committee of Health Professionals in Great Britain. The data derived from this study covered children age 0 to 16 years and showed that in the majority of cases (62%) the initial presentation of

---

**Box 1: Major features of tuberous sclerosis (Modified from Roach *et al*[3])**

Two major features: definite diagnosis
One major feature: possible diagnosis

▶ Facial angiofibromas or forehead plaque
▶ Ungual fibroma, non-traumatic
▶ Hypomelanotic macules, three or more
▶ Shagreen patch
▶ Multiple retinal nodular hamartomas
▶ Cortical tuber*
▶ Subependymal nodule
▶ Subependymal giant cell astrocytoma
▶ Cardiac rhabdomyoma, single or multiple
▶ Renal angiomyolipoma *or* pulmonary lymphangiomyomatosis[†]

*When cerebral cortical dysplasia and cerebral white matter migration tracts occur together, they should be counted as one rather than two features of tuberous sclerosis.
†When both lymphangiomyomatosis and renal angiomyolipomas are present, other features of tuberous sclerosis should be present before a definite diagnosis is assigned.
*Editor's Note*: Please refer to original journal article for full references.
Reproduced from Archive of Disease in childhood, Yates JRW; Tuberculous Sclerosis 2000 Study Group. The Tuberculous Sclerosis 2000 Study: Presentation initial assessment and implications for diagnosis and management. *Arch Dis Child.* 2011;96:1020-1025, with permission from BMJ Publishing Group Ltd.

---

**Box 2: Recommended evaluations for the study**

▶ Echocardiography in children under 5 years of age as part of the diagnostic work-up
▶ ECG as a baseline investigation to exclude cardiac conduction defects and arrhythmias
▶ Renal ultrasound scan at diagnosis for detection of polycystic kidney disease associated with contiguous gene deletions of the *TSC2* and *PKD1* genes
▶ Follow-up renal ultrasound scans at age 5, 8, 12 and 16 years as appropriate
▶ EEG for the evaluation of seizures
▶ Cranial MRI scan at age 2 years or older if not already done as part of the diagnostic work-up
▶ Genotyping

Reproduced from Archive of Disease in childhood, Yates JRW; Tuberculous Sclerosis 2000 Study Group. The Tuberculous Sclerosis 2000 Study: Presentation initial assessment and implications for diagnosis and management. *Arch Dis Child.* 2011;96:1020-1025, with permission from BMJ Publishing Group Ltd.

---

tuberous sclerosis involved the onset of seizures in infancy or very early childhood. The mean age at presentation with seizures was 6 months (range, birth to 10 years) and the median time from presentation to diagnosis was 2 months (range, 0 to 14.9 years). Table 2 summarizes the findings at examination. The table allows one to estimate the accumulated frequency with which various organs become affected by various manifestations of the disorder.

It is clear from this report that the diagnosis of tuberous sclerosis can indeed be challenging, particularly in young children. This therefore highlights the necessity not only of thinking about the disease, but then confirming it with genetic testing. The condition is caused by mutation of the TSC1 or TSC2 gene. Rare patients with deletions of TSC2 that encompass the adjacent PKD1 gene present with severe early-onset polycystic disease manifestations of tuberous sclerosis. Genetic testing identifies mutations in most children with tuberous sclerosis. It

TABLE 2.—Findings on Examination and Results of Investigations

| Evaluation/Finding | Number of Cases Evaluated and Number (%) with Specified Finding* | | |
| --- | --- | --- | --- |
| | 0–4 years | 5–18 Years | Whole Sample |
| General examination | 92* | 35* | 124* |
| Facial angiofibromas | 15 (16%) | 10 (29%) | 24 (19%) |
| Forehead or scalp plaque | 12 (13%) | 3 (9%) | 15 (12%) |
| Hypopigmented macules, ≥3 | 57 (62%) | 25 (71%) | 80 (65%) |
| Shagreen patch | 21 (23%) | 9 (26%) | 30 (24%) |
| Ungual fibroma | 1 (1%) | 2 (6%) | 3 (2%) |
| Any of above | 65 (71%) | 26 (74%) | 89 (72%) |
| Hypopigmented macules, 1–2 | 16 (17%) | 2 (6%) | 17 (14%) |
| Any of above | 75 (82%) | 28 (80%) | 100 (81%) |
| Eye examination | 26 | 4 | 30 |
| Retinal hamartoma | 10 (38%) | 2 (50%) | 12 (40%) |
| ECG | 30 | 7 | 37 |
| Abnormal† | 6 (20%) | 0 | 6 (16%) |
| Echocardiography | 77 | 11 | 88 |
| Cardiac rhabdomyoma(s) | 47 (61%) | 4 (36%) | 51 (58%) |
| Renal ultrasound scan | 86* | 24* | 107* |
| PKD | 3 (3%) | 0 | 3 (3%) |
| Renal cysts, not PKD | 7 (8%) | 0 | 7 (7%) |
| Angiomyolipomas | 8 (9%)‡ | 6 (25%) | 13 (12%)‡ |
| Any of above | 15 (17%) | 6 (25%) | 20 (19%) |
| Cranial CT scan§ | 28 | 7 | 35 |
| Cortical tuber | 11 (39%) | 3 (43%) | 14 (40%) |
| Subependymal nodule | 19 (68%) | 5 (71%) | 24 (69%) |
| SEGA | 0 | 0 | 0 |
| Any of above | 24 (86%) | 5 (71%) | 29 (83%) |
| Cranial MRI scan¶ | 89* | 19* | 104* |
| Cortical tuber | 81 (91%) | 16 (84%) | 93 (89%) |
| Subependymal nodule | 68 (76%) | 12 (63%) | 76 (73%) |
| SEGA | 1 (1%) | 4 (21%) | 5 (5%) |
| Any of above | 82 (92%) | 17 (89%) | 95 (91%) |

PKD, polycystic kidney disease; SEGA, subependymal giant cell astrocytoma.

*For cases repeatedly evaluated, number with specified finding on at least one occasion (so finding may have been absent when the same evaluation was carried out at a younger age). Where subjects were evaluated in both age intervals, the number in the last column is not equal to the sum of the first two columns.

†Arrhythmias and in one case left ventricular hypertrophy.

‡Does not include two cases with scans in early infancy reported as showing multiple echogenic lesions but with subsequent normal scans.

§Only 11% of CT scans were available for review so these data are largely based on reported findings.

¶78% of MRI scans were independently reviewed for the study.

should be more widely used for confirming the diagnosis, particularly in young children.

Read this report in detail. You will learn a lot about the presentation of tuberous sclerosis. For example, I was not aware that more than 60% of children younger than 5 years will be found to have cardiac rhabdomyomas or that MRI scans will show subependymal nodules or cortical tubers in more than 90% of children scanned. While these are findings all of us know about, the frequency with which these findings are present are newly revealed by this report.

**J. A. Stockman III, MD**

## Cancer Risk Among Patients With Myotonic Muscular Dystrophy

Gadalla SM, Lund M, Pfeiffer RM, et al (Natl Cancer Inst, Bethesda, Maryland; Statens Serum Institut, Denmark; et al)
*JAMA* 306:2480-2486, 2011

*Context.*—Myotonic muscular dystrophy (MMD) is an autosomal-dominant multisystem neuromuscular disorder characterized by unstable nucleotide repeat expansions. Case reports have suggested that MMD patients may be at increased risk of malignancy, putative risks that have never been quantified.

*Objective.*—To quantitatively evaluate cancer risk in patients with MMD, overall and by sex and age.

*Design, Setting, and Participants.*—We identified 1658 patients with an MMD discharge diagnosis in the Swedish Hospital Discharge Register or Danish National Patient Registry between 1977 and 2008. We linked these patients to their corresponding cancer registry. Patients were followed up from date of first MMD-related inpatient or outpatient contact to first cancer diagnosis, death, emigration, or completion of cancer registration.

*Main Outcome Measures.*—Risks of all cancers combined and by anatomic site, stratified by sex and age.

*Results.*—One hundred four patients with an inpatient or outpatient discharge diagnosis of MMD developed cancer during postdischarge follow-up. This corresponds to an observed cancer rate of 73.4 per 10 000 person-years in MMD vs an expected rate of 36.9 per 10 000 person-years in the general Swedish and Danish populations combined (standardized incidence ratio [SIR], 2.0; 95% CI, 1.6-2.4). Specifically, we observed significant excess risks of cancers of the endometrium (n = 11; observed rate, 16.1/10 000 person-years; SIR, 7.6; 95% CI, 4.0-13.2), brain (n = 7; observed rate, 4.9/10 000 person-years; SIR, 5.3; 95% CI, 2.3-10.4), ovary (n = 7; observed rate, 10.3/10 000 person-years; SIR, 5.2; 95% CI, 2.3-10.2), and colon (n = 10; observed rate, 7.1/10 000 person-years; SIR, 2.9; 95% CI, 1.5-5.1). Cancer risks were similar in women and men after excluding genital organ tumors (SIR, 1.9; 95% CI, 1.4-2.5, vs SIR, 1.8; 95% CI, 1.3-2.5, respectively; *P* = .81 for heterogeneity; observed rates, 64.5 and 47.7 per 10 000 person-years in women and men, respectively). The same pattern of cancer excess was observed first in the Swedish and then in the Danish cohorts, which were studied sequentially and initially analyzed independently.

*Conclusion.*—Patients with MMD identified from the Swedish and Danish patient registries were at increased risk of cancer both overall and for selected anatomic sites.

▶ As one might suspect, children are affected with myotonic muscular dystrophy (MMD) as well as adults because MMD is an autosomal-dominant disorder. The disorder has 2 subtypes. Type 1 MMD is caused by unstable trinucleotide repeat expansion in a region of the dystrophia myotonica-protein kinase gene. Type 2 MMD is a tetra-nucleotide repeat expansion in what is known as the zinc finger

9 gene. Although MMD is the most common adult muscle dystrophy with an estimated prevalence of 1 in 8000, type 1 MMD displays a more severe phenotype that can present at any age and does result in premature death in mid-adulthood. Both forms of MMD result in myotonia and progressive skeletal muscle weakness and wasting. There are other manifestations, however, including cardiac conduction defects, insulin resistance, testicular atrophy, respiratory insufficiency, cognitive impairment, and premature cataract formation.

Based on cases that have been occasionally reported in the literature, it has been suggested that MMD patients might be at increased risk for the formation of benign and malignant tumors. Pilomatricoma, a rare benign calcifying cutaneous neoplasm derived from hair matrix cells, is the most commonly reported tumor. Multiple skin basal cell carcinomas have been seen as an MMD phenotypic variant. The authors of this report further explored whether MMD phenotype carries a broader cancer risk by conducting a population-based study of MMD patients using the nationwide Swedish and Danish registries that have yielded so much other data on the epidemiology of various diseases.

The Swedish and Danish cancer registries have identified all cancers detected in Sweden and Denmark since 1958 and 1943, respectively. In these 2 countries, registry completeness and diagnostic accuracy exceed 95%. What we learn from these registries is that MMD patients do have an elevated risk of cancer primarily due to malignancies of the endometrium, brain, ovary, and colon. These risks run as much as 6 fold higher than in the general population depending on the specific tumor type.

Several biological mechanisms for the apparent increased risk seen in MMD patients have been proposed, including possible RNA-mediated alterations in tumor suppressor genes or oncogene expression, modification of the coding features of proteins, upregulation of signaling pathways, or a combination of these. Further research is needed to explore whether the observed associations are similar in both type 1 and type 2 MMD and to determine whether cancer risk correlates with disease severity, lifespan, or both. These findings have implications in the clinical management of MMD patients including, at a minimum, the implementation of appropriate validated routine population cancer screening strategies for these patients, particularly for colon cancer. While it seems that children with this disorder are unlikely to develop cancer until early adulthood, the families of affected children should be given a heads up about the problem and certainly should be aware of the consequences to further pregnancies related to this autosomal dominant disorder.

This commentary closes with a thought on the management of Parkinson disease. It appears that chewing gum may be an effective strategy for the management of salivary secretions in Parkinson disease. The disease is associated with impairment of swallowing, which can in turn lead to drooling. A pilot study has shown that chewing gum increases the frequency and decreases the latency of swallowing of patients with Parkinson disease who have no substantial problems in swallowing while eating. The positive effects appear to continue for longer than 5 minutes after the gum is spat out.[1]

**J. A. Stockman III, MD**

*Reference*

1. South AR, Somers SM, Joy MS. Gum chewing improves swallow frequency and latency in Parkinson patients: a preliminary study. *Neurology*. 2010;74: 1198-1202.

---

**Paternal Depressive Symptoms and Child Behavioral or Emotional Problems in the United States**
Weitzman M, Rosenthal DG, Liu Y-H (New York Univ School of Medicine)
*Pediatrics* 128:1126-1134, 2011

---

*Background.*—The negative effects of maternal mental health problems on child health are well documented. In contrast, there is a profound paucity of information about paternal mental health's association with child health.

*Objective.*—To investigate the association of paternal mental health problems and depressive symptoms and children's emotional or behavioral problems.

*Methods.*—We analyzed Medical Expenditure Panel Survey data, which included a representative sample of US children ($N = 21\,993$) aged 5 to 17 years and their mothers and fathers. The main outcome measure was child emotional or behavioral problems assessed by using the Columbia Impairment Scale.

*Results.*—Paternal depressive symptoms, as assessed using the Patient Health Questionnaire—2, and mental health problems, more generally, assessed by using the Short-Form 12 Scale, were independently associated with increased rates of child emotional or behavioral problems even after controlling for numerous potential confounders including maternal depressive symptoms and other mental health problems. The adjusted odds ratio (aOR) for emotional or behavioral problems among children of fathers with depressive symptoms was 1.72 (95% confidence interval [CI]: 1.33—2.23) and the aOR associated with abnormal paternal scores on the mental component scale of the Short-Form 12 was 1.33 (95% CI: 1.10—1.62) for those within 1 SD below average and 1.48 (95% CI: 1.20—1.84) for those >1 SD below average.

*Conclusions.*—To the best of our knowledge, this is the first study to use a representative US sample to demonstrate that living with fathers with depressive symptoms and other mental health problems is independently associated with increased rates of emotional or behavioral problems of children.

▶ With so much written about maternal depression, it is good to see information about what the impact is of a father having depressive symptoms and the outcome of such symptoms on child behavioral or emotional problems. The limited amount of research on paternal depression has largely focused on post-partum paternal depression, suggesting an association between postpartum paternal depression and poor childhood outcomes. Unfortunately, studies investigating paternal mental health outside the newborn period have tended to use small and often atypical sample sizes from which it is difficult if not impossible to generalize the conclusions to the population at large. The literature has suggested that because mothers spend substantially more time interacting with their offspring than do fathers, it is likely that maternal mental health problems would be associated with higher rates of children's emotional or behavioral problems than paternal mental health problems. The report of Weitzman et al tells about findings from large, nationally representative samples of the US population evaluating several hypotheses, including that children of fathers with mental health problems and depressive symptoms would in fact have higher rates of emotional and behavioral problems; that the rates of such problems are lower among children with fathers who have mental health problems than among children with mothers who have these problems; and last, that rates of emotional or behavioral problems are highest among children who have both mothers and fathers with mental health problems and depressive symptoms.

Weitzman et al explored their hypotheses using data from the Medical Expenditure Panel Survey, 2004—2008. The survey is a nationally representative survey of the US civilian, noninstitutionalized population and is one sponsored by the Agency for Health Care Research and Quality and the National Center for Health Statistics; it has been conducted annually since 1996. The study looked for generally accepted markers of maternal and paternal mental health including the presence or absence of depression. The study looked at a sample of approximately 22 000 children. Their mothers and fathers were representative of the entire US population. The study found that living with fathers with depressive symptoms and other mental health problems is clearly associated with increased rates of emotional or behavioral problems among school-age children and adolescents. The findings also indicate that the risk of child emotional or behavioral problems is much greater if mother, rather than father, has such problems. Strikingly, an increase in child emotional or behavioral problems was noted when both parents have such problems, with 25% of children living in such homes having behavioral or emotional difficulty (Fig 1 in the original article).

A recent article in the *JAMA* examined the health services organizational implications of the intergenerational transmission of depression from parents to their offspring, highlighting the idea that successful treatment of maternal depression helps alleviate depressive symptoms in their children but also suggests that child mental health benefits might also flow from successfully treating depressed fathers.[1] The study of Weitzman et al clearly shows that paternal depressive symptoms and other mental health problems are unequivocally associated with children's emotional or behavioral problems and act synergistically in a negative way if a mother also has similar categories of problems. It is not all that often that fathers come in for well-baby visits with their offspring, so we need to figure out ways to determine how to facilitate identifying fathers with mental health problems as well as developing better referral systems to deal with such problems. The report of Weitzman et al is an important one, and the data from this report should be understood by all pediatric care providers.

This commentary closes with an observation about depression. Children with depressed mothers show psychiatric and behavioral problems that will improve once the mother's depression is treated as reported in a recent study.[2] A study in the *American Journal of Psychiatry* has looked at what happens during the first year of life after a mother's remission from depression. Children were assessed at 3-month intervals. During the first year of remission, the children of early remitters showed significant improvement in all outcomes. Behavioral problems decreased for children of both early and late remitting mothers but increased in those with nonremitting mothers. Childhood functioning improved only in children whose mothers remitted early.

**J. A. Stockman III, MD**

*References*

1. Weissman MM, Olfson M. Translating intergenerational research on depression into clinical practice. *JAMA*. 2009;302:2695-2696.
2. Wickramarathe P, Gameroff MJ, Pilowsky DJ, et al. Children of depressed mothers 1 year after remission of maternal depression: findings from the STAR*D-Child study. *Am J Psychiatry*. 2011;168:593-602.

---

## Maternal Postnatal Depression and the Development of Depression in Offspring Up to 16 Years of Age

Murray L, Arteche A, Fearon P, et al (Univ of Reading, UK; et al)
*J Am Acad Child Adolesc Psychiatry* 50:460-470, 2011

---

*Objective.*—The aim of this study was to determine the developmental risk pathway to depression by 16 years in offspring of postnatally depressed mothers.

*Method.*—This was a prospective longitudinal study of offspring of postnatally depressed and nondepressed mothers; child and family assessments were made from infancy to 16 years. A total of 702 mothers were screened, and probable cases interviewed. In all, 58 depressed mothers (95% of identified cases) and 42 nondepressed controls were recruited. A total of 93% were assessed through to 16-year follow-up. The main study outcome was offspring lifetime clinical depression (major depression episode and dysthymia) by 16 years, assessed via interview at 8, 13, and 16 years. It was analysed in relation to postnatal depression, repeated measures of child vulnerability (insecure infant attachment and lower childhood resilience), and family adversity.

*Results.*—Children of index mothers were more likely than controls to experience depression by 16 years (41.5% versus 12.5%; odds ratio = 4.99; 95% confidence interval = 1.68–14.70). Lower childhood resilience predicted adolescent depression, and insecure infant attachment influenced adolescent depression via lower resilience (model $R^2 = 31\%$). Family adversity added further to offspring risk (expanded model $R^2 = 43\%$).

*Conclusions.*—Offspring of postnatally depressed mothers are at increased risk for depression by 16 years of age. This may be partially explained by within child vulnerability established in infancy and the early years, and by exposure to family adversity. Routine screening for postnatal depression, and parenting support for postnatally depressed mothers, might reduce offspring developmental risks for clinical depression in childhood and adolescence.

▶ Depression is a very common problem. It has been said that at least one-third of people will experience a major depressive episode at least once during their lifetime.[1] Unfortunately, for some, the experience is persistent. This is especially true when the onset of depression first occurs during school age years, as this is particularly associated with poorer outcome in terms of severity, chronicity, and recurrence.

The report of Murray et al tells us about the association between maternal depression and the development of depression in children. The investigators prospectively identified 58 depressed mothers and 42 nondepressed controls. Offspring were followed up to 16 years of age. Offspring lifetime clinical depression (major depressive episode and dysthymia) by 16 years was assessed via interview at 8, 13, and 16 years. A total of 41.5% of the offspring of depressed mothers experienced depression themselves during childhood by 16 years of age compared with 12.5% of children of nondepressed mothers.

The findings from this study are consistent with others that have found a substantially increased risk for depression in children of depressed mothers. A marker of this problem is insecure attachment to the mother in infancy. Marital conflict only compounds the problem. Even absent depression, many children of depressed mothers experienced levels of anxiety that were not seen in controls.

On a related note, were you aware that living in high altitude is an independent risk factor for suicide? It indeed is, according to a report from the *American Journal of Psychiatry*.[2] Previous studies have suggested that gun ownership and low population density might be accountable for a raised risk of suicide in the mountains of the western United States, but a new study now indicates that altitude alone may be a factor. These observations may be related to the effects of metabolic stress associated with mild hypoxia in people with mood disorders. If that is so, such a pathophysiologic cause of depression should be easily verified by suitable investigations.

No wonder people get depressed when they fly on planes, which are only pressurized to about 6500 feet. Maybe that is why we occasionally read reports of people who go berserk on commercial airliners. For more on the topic of parent depression and childhood depressive/anxiety symptoms, see the interesting report by Lewis et al.[3]

This commentary closes with information about lawsuits involving Paxil. A Philadelphia jury found that the antidepressant paroxetine (marketed as Paxil in the United States and Seroxat in the United Kingdom) caused heart defects in a child whose mother took the drug while pregnant. The jury awarded the family $2.5 million. The child was the first of about 600 US lawsuits that claimed that Paxil caused birth defects in infants born to mothers who took the drug while pregnant. GlaxoSmithKline, the drug manufacturer, disagrees with the verdict and has appealed, saying that birth defects occur in 3% to 5% of all live births and that any linkage with Paxil is impossible to document. The jury found that GlaxoSmithKline officials "negligently failed to warn" the doctor treating the child's mother about Paxil's risk and concluded the drug was a "factual cause" of the child's heart defects.[4]

**J. A. Stockman III, MD**

*References*

1. Andrews G, Poulton R, Skoog I. Lifetime risk of depression: restricted to a minority or waiting for most. *Br J Psychiatr.* 2005;187:495-496.
2. Kim N, Mickelson JB, Brenner BE, Haws CA, Yurgelun-Todd DA, Renshaw PF. Altitude, gun ownership, rural areas, and suicide. *Am J Psychiatry.* 2011;168: 49-54. http://dx.doi.org/10.1176/appi.ajp.2010.10020289.
3. Lewis G, Rice F, Harold GT, Collishaw S, Thapar A. Investigating environmental links between parent depression and child depressive/anxiety symptoms using an assisted conception design. *J Am Acad Child Adolesc Psychiatr.* 2011;50:451-459.
4. Tanne JH. GlaxoSmithKline is told to pay family $2.5 million after jury finds Paroxetine caused son's heart defects. *BMJ.* 2009;339:942-943.

---

**Treatment-Resistant Depressed Youth Show a Higher Response Rate if Treatment Ends During Summer School Break**

Shamseddeen W, Clarke G, Wagner KD, et al (Rosalind Franklin Univ of Medicine and Sciences, North Chicago, IL; Kaiser Permanente Ctr for Health Res, Portland, OR; The Univ of Texas Med Branch, Galveston; et al)

*J Am Acad Child Adolesc Psychiatry* 50:1140-1148, 2011

---

*Objective.*—There is little work on the effect of school on response to treatment of depression, with available research suggesting that children and adolescents with school difficulties are less likely to respond to fluoxetine compared with those with no school difficulties.

*Method.*—Depressed adolescents in the Treatment of Resistant Depression in Adolescents study, who had not responded to a previous adequate selective serotonin reuptake inhibitor (SSRI) trial, were randomly assigned to one of the following: another SSRI, venlafaxine, another SSRI + cognitive behavior therapy (CBT), or venlafaxine + CBT. Participants were classified into four groups depending on whether their enrollment in the study and end of treatment was during school or summer vacation.

*Results.*—Controlling for baseline differences, adolescents ending their 12-week treatment during summer vacation had odds 1.7 times (95% confidence interval = 1.02-2.8, $p = .04$) greater to have an adequate response as those ending their treatment while being in school. In addition, adequate depression response was associated with fewer school problems at week 12 (scores <5 versus scores ≥5: odds ratio = 3.3, 95% confidence interval = 1.9-5.8, $p < .001$). There was a significant interaction between school difficulties and timing of treatment, with the lowest rates of response being among adolescents having school difficulties and ending their treatment during the active school year.

*Conclusion.*—School problems are relevant to treatment response in depressed adolescents and should be incorporated into the treatment plan. These findings also suggest that the time of the year might need to be taken into consideration for analysis of clinical trials in school-aged youth.

*Clinical Trial Registration Information.*—Treatment of SSRI-Resistant Depression in Adolescents (TORDIA); http://www.clinicaltrials.gov; NCT00018902.

▶ The Treatment of Resistant Depression in Adolescents (TORDIA) study is a multisite randomized treatment study funded by the National Institute of Mental Health of adolescent depression. TORDIA, from 2000 through 2006, enrolled 334 participants who had major depression as defined by DSM-IV criteria. These patients had depression despite traditional treatment with a selective serotonin reuptake inhibitor (SSRI) for at least 8 weeks. TORDIA is currently providing much useful information, including shedding light on variables that may significantly influence treatment response.

Shamseddeen et al using information from TORDIA noted that adolescents who completed their antidepressant treatment when school was "out" (for the summer) had a more positive response than subjects who completed their antidepressant treatment amid the school year. Indeed, 59% of those on summer vacation responded to treatment with another antidepressant (+cognitive-behavioral therapy) compared with 41% who completed treatment during the school year. The implication is that school stress may substantially affect treatment response and should be factored into treatment planning. As you might suspect, however, the TORDIA trial was not designed to quantify the effects of various school variables on treatment response or the potential of seasonal variation in the ability to respond to antidepressants. That said, treatment-resistant students appear less likely to respond to antidepressants while experiencing the stress of being in school compared with those on summer vacation.

The findings from TORDIA do have implications for clinicians. The TORDIA data suggest that we should be working very carefully with a patient's school staff to identify particular stressors that might in fact make a patient more treatment resistant during the school year. Collaborative efforts with the school staff therefore are potentially very important in terms of increasing the likelihood of a positive outcome with SSRIs. All too often, schools are not involved for privacy reasons.

I live in the part of a state where year-round schools are becoming increasingly more common. Kids in such schools do attend class year-round but have significant blocks of time off during the school year. It would be interesting to see in such schools what the rates are of depression because kids in year-round schools have a "popoff valve" (called frequent breaks) in comparison with kids in traditional schools who have only an extended break during the summer. Comparing year-round schools with traditional schools would make a very interesting investigation.

This commentary closes with a query and an observation on a recently described form of social phobia. Are you familiar with the term gelatophobia? Though it sounds like an ailment involving Italian ice cream, scientists worldwide now recognize gelatophobia as a distinct social phobia. The term means a debilitating fear of being laughed at. Most people fear being laughed at to some degree and do their best to avoid embarrassment. One thing, however, that sets gelatophobes apart is their inability to distinguish ridicule from playful teasing. For them, all laughter is aggressive and a harmless joke may come across as a mean spirited insult. Such individuals do not understand the positive side of humor and do not experience it in a warm way, but rather as a means to put others down. Investigators from the University of Zurich have done extensive investigations into the problem of gelatophobia. They have interviewed more than 23 000 people in 73 countries and found gelatophobia is present to some degree in every nation, infecting somewhere between 2% and 30% of the population. In the United States, the incidence is about 11%. They observed that gelatophobes report a much higher intensity of being laughed at. Studies using cartoons to illustrate people laughing at various situations show that those with a fear of being laughed at are more likely to assume that the laughter is directed at them. Other studies using laugh tracks show that gelatophobes have problems distinguishing a happy har-de-har from a scornful snicker. While most people feel joy and surprise at playful teasing, gelatophobes feel the same anger, shame, and fear that they would feel during ridicule. The study of 20 000 people from around the world that included 73 countries showed that the most resistant individuals (the fewest gelatophobes) are found in the Nordic countries, Denmark, and the United States, whereas the highest percentage of gelatophobes tend to be found in Southeast Asia in countries such as Thailand, Cambodia, Indonesia, Hong Kong, and Japan.[1]

**J. A. Stockman III, MD**

*Reference*

1. Gaidos S. When humor humiliates: for gelatophobes, even good-natured laughter can sound a lot like ridicule. *Science News*. August 1, 2009:19-22.

---

**Length of Stay of Pediatric Mental Health Emergency Department Visits in the United States**

Case SD, Case BG, Olfson M, et al (Warren Alpert Med School of Brown Univ; East Providence, RI; Columbia Univ, NY; et al)
*J Am Acad Child Adolesc Psychiatry* 50:1110-1119, 2011

---

*Objective.*—To compare pediatric mental health emergency department visits to other pediatric emergency department visits, focusing on length of stay.

*Method.*—We analyzed data from the National Hospital Ambulatory Medical Care Survey, a nationally representative sample of US emergency department visits from 2001 to 2008, for patients aged ≤18 years (n = 73,015). Visits with a principal diagnosis of a mental disorder (n = 1,476) were compared to visits (n = 71,539) with regard to patient and hospital characteristics, treatment, and length of stay. Predictors of prolonged mental health visits were identified.

*Results.*—Mental health visits were more likely than other visits to arrive by ambulance (21.8% versus 6.3%, $p < .001$), to be triaged to rapid evaluation (27.9% versus 14.9%, $p < .001$), and to be admitted (16.4% versus 7.6%, $p < .001$) or transferred (15.7% versus 1.5%, $p < .001$). The median length of stay for mental health visits (169 minutes) significantly exceeded that of other visits (108 minutes). The odds of extended stay beyond 4 hours for mental health visits was almost twice that for other visits (adjusted odds ratio 1.9, 95% CI = 1.5−2.4) and was not explained by observed differences in evaluation, treatment, or disposition. Among mental health visits, advancing calendar year of study, intentional self-injury, age 6−3 years, Northeastern, Southern, and metropolitan hospital location, use of laboratory studies, and patient transfer all predicted extended stays.

*Conclusions.*—Compared with other pediatric emergency visits, mental health visits are longer, are more frequently triaged to urgent evaluation, and more likely to result in patient admission or transfer, thereby placing distinctive burdens on US emergency departments.

▶ The number of pediatric mental health emergency department visits in the United States has been increasing. One reason for this, and only one reason, is that after a series of school shooting events, many school systems have implemented protocols requiring emergency psychiatric evaluation of children and adolescents displaying suicidal or homicidal ideation/behavior or severe aggression in the school setting. Emergency departments ideally could provide high-quality evaluation and treatment planning for a range of young patients accessing mental health services in psychiatric crises. Instead, children and families encounter a system poorly equipped to safely and effectively evaluate and manage their child's or teenager's mental health problem. All too often, young patients are treated in medical or adult psychiatry settings that lack round-the-clock access to child and adolescent psychiatric clinicians. Many of these young people require immediate clinical intervention, and there is little capacity to provide care to such acutely ill children and adolescents in the outpatient clinic system. Often, the only option for these patients is admission to an inpatient unit.

The report of Case et al documents the significant burden that pediatric mental health visits place on emergency departments in the United States. The increase in these types of visits seen in the 1990s has persisted. As one would expect, pediatric emergency mental health visits report longer lengths of stay in the emergency department and higher rates of admission than other pediatric medical visits. This study found that more than 30% of children and adolescents evaluated emergently were admitted or transferred for inpatient psychiatric care.

This report probes solutions to the problems described. Specialized, dedicated child and adolescent psychiatry emergency programs with brief stabilization facilities are feasible in larger-volume settings (2000 emergency psychiatric visits per year) but do require considerable capital investment and institutional commitment to develop and implement. New York State at New York Presbyterian Hospital decreased inpatient psychiatric admissions in Manhattan from 35% to fewer than 10% but was closed when volume and reimbursement did not support program cost. The second dedicated Children's Comprehensive Psychiatry

Emergency Program in New York State at Bellevue Hospital Center serves Bellevue Hospital and several other public hospitals in New York City without child and adolescent inpatient services. Only 20% of children and adolescents evaluated in the Bellevue Children's Comprehensive Psychiatry Emergency Program are admitted to inpatient psychiatry units. Thus, there are models for the delivery of intensive and ongoing care for young people in psychiatric crisis that can provide expert evaluation and diversion from longer-stay inpatient admissions. A specialized team providing in-home and community services makes more sense in smaller-volume settings (less than 1000 visits per year). Large-volume settings may support specialized brief stabilization units. These types of programs become increasingly important as the child and adolescent inpatient care system continues to downsize, and young patients face longer and longer waits in the outpatient setting.

To read more about the problem of psychiatric emergency services for children and adolescents, see the editorial by Havens.[1]

**J. A. Stockman III, MD**

*Reference*

1. Havens JF. Making psychiatric emergency services work better for children and families. *J Am Acad Child Adolesc Psychiatry.* 2011;50:1093-1094.

---

### Suicidal Behavior Differs Among Early and Late Adolescents Treated With Antidepressant Agents

Hysinger EB, Callahan ST, Caples TL, et al (Vanderbilt School of Medicine, Nashville, TN)

*Pediatrics* 128:447-454, 2011

---

*Objective.*—To identify circumstances and characteristics of suicidal behavior among early (aged 10—14 years) and late (aged 15—18 years) adolescents from a cohort of youth who were prescribed antidepressant medication.

*Methods.*—In-depth reviews of all available medical records were performed for 250 randomly chosen confirmed episodes of suicidal behavior identified as part of a large retrospective cohort study of antidepressant users and suicidal behavior. Study data were obtained from Tennessee Medicaid records and death certificates from January 1, 1995, to December 31, 2006. Medical records and autopsy reports for cases identified from electronic data were adjudicated by 2 investigators blinded to exposure status and classified by using a validated scale.

*Results.*—Of the 250 cases reviewed, 65.6% were female and 26.4% were aged 10 to 14 years. Medication ingestion was the most frequent method of suicidal behavior for both early and late adolescents; however, early adolescents were significantly more likely to use hanging as a method of suicide. Nearly one-half of the adolescents had previously attempted suicide. Early adolescents were significantly more likely to have a history

TABLE 2.—Substances Ingested During Confirmed Episodes of Suicidal Behavior Among Early and Late Adolescents Who Were Treated With Antidepressant Medications

| | Total ($N = 213$), % | Early Adolescents ($n = 54$), % | Late Adolescents ($n = 159$), % | $P^a$ |
|---|---|---|---|---|
| Selective serotonin reuptake inhibitor | 31.9 | 33.3 | 31.4 | NS |
| Tricyclic antidepressant agent | 14.1 | 13.0 | 14.5 | NS |
| Antipsychotic agent | 13.1 | 24.1 | 9.4 | .01 |
| Benzodiazepine | 13.1 | 9.3 | 14.5 | NS |
| Antihistamine | 12.2 | 16.7 | 10.6 | NS |
| Acetaminophen | 11.7 | 9.3 | 12.6 | NS |
| Nonsteroidal anti-inflammatory drug | 10.3 | 0.0 | 13.8 | .003 |
| Mood stabilizer | 9.9 | 7.4 | 10.6 | NS |
| Psychostimulants | 5.6 | 5.6 | 5.7 | NS |
| Antibiotics | 4.7 | 5.6 | 4.4 | NS |
| Trazodone | 4.7 | 1.9 | 5.7 | NS |
| Other medications | 33.3 | 29.8 | 34.7 | NS |
| Nonmedicinal chemicals | 4.7 | 11.1 | 2.5 | .02 |

Sum of columns exceeds 100% because of multisubstance ingestions.
[a]Comparison using $\chi^2$ and Fisher's exact tests as appropriate

of sexual abuse and significantly less likely to have a history of substance abuse. Early adolescents were also significantly more likely than older adolescents to have a history of a psychotic disorder and to report hallucinations before the suicide attempt.

*Conclusion.*—Suicidal behavior among early and late adolescents prescribed antidepressant medication differed in terms of methods used, previous psychiatric history, and proximal symptoms (Table 2).

▶ Suicide is the 11th leading cause of death in the United States and the third leading cause among people aged 15 to 34 years, accounting for 9418 deaths in this age group in 2007, according to data from the Centers for Disease Control and Prevention (CDC).[1] The report of Hysinger et al reminds us that adolescents treated with antidepressant agents are an important risk group for suicidal behavior because of the association between depression and suicide and recent concerns that some antidepressant agents may actually increase suicide risk for young people. The article is important because it provides information about the methods of suicide and attempted suicide in those who are at such increased risk because of the recent administration of antidepressants. This information is crucial for care providers so that they can understand the circumstances and characteristics of suicidal behavior in this population. The investigators who were part of this study identified 250 confirmed episodes of suicidal behavior in pediatric patients ranging in age from 10 to 18 years. Nearly two-thirds of this group were female. The most common method of suicide or attempted suicide behavior was ingestion, used by 85.2% of adolescents. Hanging was 5 times more common among early adolescents than late adolescents (10.6% vs 2.2%). About one-half of adolescents had a history of previous suicide attempt, and some 15% had 2 or more previous suicide attempts. Early adolescents were nearly twice as likely to report a previous history of sexual abuse (29% vs 16%). Interpersonal conflict, usually with a parent or family member, was the documented precipitant in most occurrences of suicidal behavior. As one might suspect, romantic relationships were significantly more likely to be documented as precipitant for late adolescence than for early adolescence. Table 2 shows the substances ingested along with the differences observed in the substances used between early adolescence and late adolescence.

While on the topic of suicides, the CDC recently highlighted a relatively new method of suicide, chemical suicide in an automobile. Chemical suicide became an increasingly popular method of killing oneself in Japan in the past decade or so. This has spread to the United States.[2] Chemical suicide refers to the mixing of chemicals to produce toxic gases. The chemicals involved are usually simple household cleaning chemicals. These suicides tend to occur inside the cabin of an automobile because this permits a high concentration of gas in an enclosed space. In addition to household cleaners (not otherwise specified in the CDC report), the following chemicals were used in reported incidents: ammonium hydroxide, aluminum sulfide, calcium hypochlorite, calcium sulfide, germanium oxide, hydrochloric acid, potassium ferrocyanide, sodium hypochlorite, sulfur, sulfuric acid, and trichloroethylene. Youngsters under age 18 have been reported to have killed themselves inside an automobile using mixtures of chemicals. The toxic gases most commonly formed by combining chemicals found in household cleaners are hydrogen sulfide and hydrogen cyanide. Hydrogen sulfide is a colorless, toxic gas. Its odor is often described as that of rotten eggs, but even a short exposure can cause olfactory fatigue (ie, a temporary inability to smell the gas). At low doses, exposure to hydrogen sulfite can cause eye and respiratory irritation, headache, dizziness, loss of appetite, and upset stomach. Brief exposures to high concentrations ($> 500$ ppm) of hydrogen sulfite can cause loss of consciousness and death. Hydrogen cyanide is a bluish-white liquid or a colorless gas with a faint odor of bitter almonds and a bitter, burning taste. It can cause death in a very short period of time.

It is wise to become aware of the potential of suicide by chemical poisoning inside an automobile to be sure first responders know about the risks associated with such suicides. First responders have taken ill when opening the doors of such vehicles. Mouth-to-mouth resuscitation of suicide victims must be avoided. Usually one can quickly suspect such a chemical suicide by looking inside the cabin of the car before entering it. There will be a bucket placed on a seat wherein the chemicals were mixed. If one sees this, a HazMat team should be called before any attempt to enter a vehicle. Unfortunately, the recipe for such suicide can be easily found on the Internet.

This commentary closes with a couple of queries. Is it fact or fiction that suicides increase over holidays? Is it fact or fiction that more suicides occur in winter months than in summer months? Chances are you will get the answers to these queries wrong. A study in the United States of suicides over a 35-year period shows that there is no increase before, during, or after holidays. In fact, people might actually experience increased emotional and social support during holidays. In the United States, rates of psychiatric visits decrease before Christmas and increase again afterwards. A small study of adolescents has shown a peak in suicide attempts at the end of the school year, possibly reflecting a decrease in social support. Data from Ireland on suicides during an 8-year period in the 1990s also failed to connect suicides with holidays. While Irish women were no more likely to commit suicide on holidays than any other days, Irish men were actually significantly less likely to do so.

Further debunking myths about suicide, people are not more likely to commit suicide during the dark winter months. Around the world, suicides peak in summer months and are actually lowest in the winter. In Finland, suicides peak in autumn and are lowest in the winter. A 30-year study of suicides in Hungary showed the highest rates of suicide occur in the summer with the lowest rates of suicide in the winter. Studies of suicide rates from India also show peaks in April and May. Studies from the United States reflect this pattern, with lower rates in November and December.

None of these reports suggest that suicides do not happen at all over holidays. The epidemiologic evidence just does not support that holidays are a time of increased risk.[3]

**J. A. Stockman III, MD**

*References*

1. Centers for Disease Control and Prevention (CDC). Injury prevention & control: data & statistics (WISQARSTM): Welcome to WISQARSTM. http://www.cdc.gov/injury/wisqars/index.html. Accessed July 31, 2012.
2. Centers for Disease Control and Prevention (CDC). Chemical suicides in automobiles—six states, 2006–2010. *MMWR Morb Mortal Wkly Rep.* 2011;60:1189-1192.
3. Vreeman R, Carroll A. Seasonal medical myths that lack convincing evidence. *BMJ.* 2008;337:1442-1443.

## Childhood Onset Schizophrenia: High Rate of Visual Hallucinations

David CN, Greenstein D, Clasen L, et al (Natl Inst of Mental Health, Bethesda, MD)

*J Am Acad Child Adolesc Psychiatry* 50:681-686, 2011

*Objective.*—To document high rates and clinical correlates of nonauditory hallucinations in childhood onset schizophrenia (COS).

*Method.*—Within a sample of 117 pediatric patients (mean age 13.6 years), diagnosed with COS, the presence of auditory, visual, somatic/tactile, and olfactory hallucinations was examined using the Scale for the Assessment of Positive Symptoms (SAPS). We also compared hallucination modality membership (presence/absence) groups on gender, socioeconomic status, ethnicity, age of onset (of psychosis), Full Scale IQ, Verbal IQ, and clinical severity (Children's Global Assessment Scale [CGAS] and Scale for the Assessment of Negative Symptoms [SANS]).

*Results.*—A total of 111 COS patients (94.9%) had auditory and 94 patients (80.3%) had visual hallucinations. Somatic/tactile (60.7%) and olfactory (29.9%) hallucinations occurred almost exclusively in patients who also had visual hallucinations. Children who had visual hallucinations had lower IQ, earlier age of onset, and more severe illness relative to children who did not have visual hallucinations.

*Conclusions.*—In this study, we observed that patients with COS have high rates of hallucinations across all modalities. An increased rate of visual hallucinations is associated with greater clinical impairment and greater compromise in overall brain functioning. Somatic and olfactory hallucinations reflect an additive rather than alternative symptom pattern.

▶ Most of us are familiar with the fact that children with schizophrenia frequently have auditory hallucinations. In fact, auditory hallucinations are important diagnostic criteria for pediatric age patents. What has not been well understood, however, is the actual prevalence of visual hallucinations in this population of patients. We learn from the report of David et al about the latter. These investigators report on the National Institute of Mental Health Childhood Onset Schizophrenia (COS) study that has been ongoing since 1990. The database related to this study has accumulated information on approximately 3000 cases of children diagnosed with schizophrenia. Of these cases, more than 300 were invited to the National Institutes of Health campus for more specific testing. A subset of these children, approximately 200, was admitted for inpatient observation, which included a 2- to 3-week drug-free observation period. As one might suspect, during this drug-free period, one could also look at the natural course of childhood schizophrenia. Appropriate parent waivers were obtained for this study.

The COS study reported auditory hallucinations in approximately 95% of cases of childhood schizophrenia. Eighty percent also reported visual hallucinations. Sixty-eight percent reported somatic/tactile forms of hallucinations. Approximately 30% had olfactory hallucinations. These figures represent generally higher rates of hallucinations compared with adult schizophrenia counterparts across all hallucination subtypes and higher than most previous reports for childhood onset patients. In general, those with visual hallucinations almost all have auditory hallucinations (only 1 child in this report did not). Ethnicity, gender, and socioeconomic status were not significantly different in patients with visual hallucinations. IQ, however, did influence the presence of this form of hallucination. Those who had visual hallucinations had, on average, an IQ 10 points lower than their non–visual hallucination peers. Also, there were surprisingly high rates for tactile and olfactory hallucinations in the group of youngsters with visual hallucinations, and these occurred almost exclusively in those who had such hallucinations. Thus, visual, olfactory and tactile hallucinations appear to be a general marker of increased severity of psychosis.

Although childhood-onset schizophrenia is rare, it does occur. Fortunately, most children experiencing hallucinations do not progress to full-blown childhood schizophrenia. It will be important to see how the National Institutes of Mental Health COS study evolves. Currently, investigators are evaluating children entering this study with functional neuroimaging techniques. Perhaps we will learn more about the mechanisms that cause brain disconnectivity at such a young age.

This commentary closes with some remarks about hash—the smoking kind, not the kind you eat. It appears that the risk of psychosis is much greater with the more potent skunk form of cannabis than with traditional hash. A case-controlled study found that people who smoke skunk or sinsemilla are almost 7 times as likely to have psychotic illnesses such as schizophrenia than people who use ordinary cannabis.[1] The skunk variety of pot contains between 12% and 18% delta-9-tetra-hydrocannabinol (THC) and less than 1.5% cannabidiol whereas traditional cannabis has an average THC level of 3.4% and a similar amount of cannabidiol. Unfortunately, skunk is displacing traditional cannabis preparations in many countries because it gives a quick hit. Unfortunately, all too many who smoke hash develop psychiatric illnesses such as schizophrenia as a consequence.

**J. A. Stockman III, MD**

*Reference*

1. Di Forte M, Morgan C, Dazzan P, et al. High-potency cannabis and the risk of psychosis. *Br J Psychiatry.* 2009;195:488-491.

# 14 Newborn

**Effect of age on decisions about the numbers of embryos to transfer in assisted conception: a prospective study**
Lawlor DA, Nelson SM (Univ of Bristol, UK; Univ of Glasgow, UK)
*Lancet* 379:521-527, 2012

*Background.*—Elective single-embryo transfer has been proposed as a strategy to reduce the risk of multiple birth and adverse pregnancy outcomes after in-vitro fertilisation (IVF). Whether this approach should be restricted to young women is unclear.

*Methods.*—In a prospective study of UK Human Fertilisation and Embryology Authority data, we investigated whether perinatal livebirth outcomes varied by the number of embryos transferred in relation to maternal age. We compared rates of livebirth, multiple births, low birthweight (< 2·5 kg), preterm birth (< 37 weeks), and severe preterm birth (< 33 weeks) in women younger than 40 years and those aged 40 years or older. We used logistic and binomial regression methods to assess, respectively, relative risk and absolute differences in risk.

*Findings.*—We assessed 124 148 IVF cycles overall, which yielded 33 514 livebirths. The odds ratios of livebirth were higher in women aged 40 years or older than in those younger than 40 years when two embryos were transferred compared with one embryo (3·12, 95% CI 2·56–3·77 *vs* 2·33, 2·20–2·46; *p* — 0·0006 for interaction), but the absolute difference in risk of livebirth was smaller (0·090, 0·080 0·099 for women ≥ 40 years *vs* 0·156, 0·148–0·163 for those < 40 years; *p* < 0·0001). The odds ratios and absolute risk differences for multiple birth, preterm birth, and low birthweight were all smaller in older than in younger women (analyses were done in 32 732 cycles in which a livebirth had resulted and data on gestational age and birthweight were complete). Livebirth rates did not increase with transfer of three embryos, but the risk of adverse perinatal outcomes did increase.

*Interpretation.*—Transfer of three or more embryos at any age should be avoided. The decision to transfer one or two embryos should be based on prognostic indicators, such as age.

▶ This report was undertaken to address the risks of assisted contraception in relation to maternal age. The background to the study is interesting. Despite recommendations by several authorities to limit the number of embryos transferred as part of assisted contraception, 40% of treatment cycles in the United States and 21% in Europe involve transfer of at least 3 embryos, and 20% to

30% of pregnancies associated with in vitro fertilization result in twins or higher-order multiple gestations. In view of both maternal and neonatal risks and the associated socioeconomic cost of multiple pregnancies, increased use of the elective single-embryo transfer has been proposed. This has been adopted as a policy by some countries such as Sweden and Belgium. In other countries such as the United Kingdom, legislation restricts the number of embryos transferred to 2 in women younger than 40 years and 3 to an older woman. In the United States, however, restrictive legislation has been resisted in favor of clinicians having the freedom to assess prognosis to individualize the number of embryos transferred. Interestingly, patient preferences have little effect on such legislation and guidance, as illustrated by most surveys that suggest most patients and their partners who undergo assisted contraception would prefer twin to singleton pregnancies.

These authors have addressed the risks of assisted contraception in relation to maternal age by looking at women aged 40 years or older and have shown that the birthrate was lower than in women younger than 40 years, irrespective of the number of embryos transferred. In both age groups, however, the live birthrate was higher after transfer of 2 embryos compared with 1. In the older age group, multiple pregnancies occurred less often than in the younger age group. Adverse perinatal outcomes, including multiple and preterm births and low birth weight, were seen more frequently after transfer of multiple embryos than after 1. The authors firmly conclude the transfer of 3 embryos is not warranted. This important article provides strong arguments in favor of restricting the transfer of embryos to a maximum of 2 per cycle, irrespective of the maternal age.

In countries where there is a limit of only 2 embryos transferred in assisted contraception, different approaches have been used. In Sweden, state regulations allow for transfer of only 1 embryo, except in exceptional circumstances. Since these regulations were adopted, 1 embryo has been transferred in 70% of all cycles and, accordingly, the number of multiple births has decreased from 25% to 5%. In Belgium, the government agreed to reimburse the cost of 6 treatment cycles in exchange for a reduction in the number of embryos transferred to 1 embryo in the first 2 cycles as a general rule. The reduction in multiple births in Belgium now corresponds to that of Sweden. Data from the European programs that monitor in vitro fertilization show large differences between countries in the rates of multiple births after assisted contraception. The rates largely paralleled the cost to the patients: couples who have to cover all costs themselves generally accept the risk of a multiple pregnancy to improve the likelihood of contraception.

We all know that preterm deliveries that result from multiple pregnancies after assisted contraception have a significant financial impact on our health care system. In the United States, the annual cost is estimated to be about $1 billion. In Europe, twins account for 20% of all live births after assisted contraception, but in the United States, the corresponding proportion is 30%.

The conclusions of this article are fairly clear. There seems to be no reason to transfer 3 embryos as part of assisted contraception. The final decision of whether to transfer 1 or 2 embryos should be based on a cooperative approach between embryologists and clinicians, although patients with medical or obstetric complications to twin pregnancies should receive no more than 1 embryo, regardless of age or other prognostic factors. Pediatricians are on the receiving end of pregnancies that begin with assisted contraception. It is important for us to follow the literature related to this topic. This study helps us greatly in this regard.

This commentary closes with a question. Why is there such a shortage of sperm donors in Great Britain? It turns out that there are a number of reasons for this shortage in the British Isles. The number of men volunteering to donate sperm in the United Kingdom has fallen after a change in the law in 2005 that removed donor anonymity. In 2006, after the law was instituted, just 307 donors were registered, 60% as many some 15 years previously. Also in the United Kingdom, a constant supply of new donors is needed because the rules in the United Kingdom limit the number of families that can be created with each donor's sperm to 10. This is despite the lack of any evidence backing the 10-family rule, which is in place to avoid the risk of half-siblings producing offspring together. The Netherlands, by the way, has a limit of 25 sperm donations. It should also be noted that in Great Britain sperm donors are not accepted after age 40, presumably because of studies suggesting more damage to the DNA of sperm donors who are over that age. Sperm donors, by the way, are paid approximately $25.00 for their donation, a payment stated to cover travel expenses rather than payment for the donation itself. Some say the most efficient way to address the problem in Great Britain is simply to raise the limit on the number of families that can be created with each donor's sperm. By analogy, this is not much of a problem in the state where I live, a state, it is said, where the roads have branches, but the family trees do not.[1]

**J. A. Stockman III, MD**

*Reference*

1. Dyer C. Experts suggest ways to tackle shortage of sperm donors. *BMJ.* 2009; 339:11.

---

## Causes of Death Among Stillbirths

The Stillbirth Collaborative Research Network Writing Group (Univ of Texas Med Branch at Galveston; Brown Univ School of Medicine, Providence, RI; Univ of Texas Health Science Ctr at San Antonio; et al)
*JAMA* 306:2459-2468, 2011

---

*Context.*—Stillbirth affects 1 in 160 pregnancies in the United States, equal to the number of infant deaths each year. Rates are higher than those of other developed countries and have stagnated over the past decade. There is significant racial disparity in the rate of stillbirth that is unexplained.

*Objective.*—To ascertain the causes of stillbirth in a population that is diverse by race/ethnicity and geography.

*Design, Setting, and Participants.*—A population-based study from March 2006 to September 2008 with surveillance for all stillbirths at 20 weeks or later in 59 tertiary care and community hospitals in 5 catchment areas defined by state and county boundaries to ensure access to at least 90% of all deliveries. Termination of a live fetus was excluded. Standardized evaluations were performed at delivery.

*Main Outcome Measures.*—Medical history, fetal postmortem and placental pathology, karyotype, other laboratory tests, systematic assignment of causes of death.

*Results.*—Of 663 women with stillbirth enrolled, 500 women consented to complete postmortem examinations of 512 neonates. A probable cause of death was found in 312 stillbirths (60.9%; 95% CI, 56.5%-65.2%) and possible or probable cause in 390 (76.2%; 95% CI, 72.2%-79.8%). The most common causes were obstetric conditions (150 [29.3%; 95% CI, 25.4%-33.5%]), placental abnormalities (121 [23.6%; 95% CI, 20.1%-27.6%]), fetal genetic/structural abnormalities (70 [13.7%; 95% CI, 10.9%-17.0%]), infection (66 [12.9%; 95% CI, 10.2%-16.2%]), umbilical cord abnormalities (53 [10.4%; 95% CI, 7.9%-13.4%]), hypertensive disorders (47 [9.2%; 95% CI, 6.9%-12.1%]), and other maternal medical conditions (40 [7.8%; 95% CI, 5.7%-10.6%]). A higher proportion of stillbirths in non-Hispanic black women compared with non-Hispanic white and Hispanic ones was associated with obstetric complications (43.5% [50] vs 23.7% [85]; difference, 19.8%; 95% CI, 9.7%-29.9%; $P < .001$) and infections (25.2% [29] vs 7.8% [28]; difference, 17.4%; 95% CI, 9.0%-25.8%; $P < .001$). Stillbirths occurring intrapartum and early in gestation were more common in non-Hispanic black women. Sources most likely to provide positive information regarding cause of death were placental histology (268 [52.3%; 95% CI, 47.9%-56.7%]), perinatal postmortem examination (161 [31.4%; 95% CI, 27.5%-35.7%]), and karyotype (32 of 357 with definitive results [9%; 95% CI, 6.3%-12.5%]).

*Conclusions.*—A systematic evaluation led to a probable or possible cause in the majority of stillbirths. Obstetric conditions and placental abnormalities were the most common causes of stillbirth, although the distribution differed by race/ethnicity (Table 3).

▶ Stillbirth is a major problem throughout the world, affecting approximately 4 million pregnancies each year. In the United States, about 1 in 60 pregnancies results in a stillbirth. The math shows that about 26 000 stillbirths occur annually. Although the overall number of stillbirths throughout the world and the United States has decreased in the last 20 years, the stillbirth rate in the United States is higher than in many other developed countries. Data from this report show that from 1990 to 2003, the stillbirth rate declined slowly by an average of 1.4% per year, whereas the overall infant mortality rate declined twice as fast by an average of 2.8% per year. Unfortunately, in the last 10 years, the stillbirth rate has run at 6.2 stillbirths per 1000 births, 59% higher than the Healthy People 2010 target of 4.1 fetal deaths per 1000 births. There is a profound racial disparity in the prevalence of stillbirth. The rate, for example, for non-Hispanic black women is 2.3-fold higher than that of non-Hispanic white women, whereas the rate for Hispanic women is 14% higher than for non-Hispanic white women.

TABLE 3.—Probable and Possible Causes of Death by Timing of Stillbirth in Relation to Labor and Gestational Age[a]

| Cause of Death | Total | Timing of Stillbirth[c] | | Gestational Age, wk[b] | | | | | |
| | | Antepartum | Intrapartum | 18-19 | 20-23 | 24-27 | 28-31 | 32-36 | ≥37 |
| --- | --- | --- | --- | --- | --- | --- | --- | --- | --- |
| | | | | | No. (%) | | | | |
| Obstetric complications | 150 (29.3) | 63 (14.8) | 87 (100.0) | 7 (70.0) | 82 (51.3) | 17 (19.1) | 15 (20.8) | 17 (17.5) | 12 (14.3) |
| Placental disease | 121 (23.6) | 111 (26.1) | 10 (11.5) | 4 (40.0) | 20 (12.5) | 32 (36.0) | 18 (25.0) | 26 (26.8) | 21 (25.0) |
| Fetal genetic/structural | 70 (13.7) | 66 (15.5) | 4 (4.6) | 0 | 22 (13.8) | 10 (11.2) | 10 (13.9) | 17 (17.5) | 11 (13.1) |
| Infection | 66 (12.9) | 43 (10.1) | 23 (26.4) | 2 (20.0) | 35 (21.9) | 7 (7.9) | 4 (5.6) | 8 (8.2) | 10 (11.9) |
| Umbilical cord abnormalities | 53 (10.4) | 46 (10.8) | 7 (8.0) | 1 (10.0) | 13 (8.1) | 10 (11.2) | 4 (5.6) | 13 (13.4) | 12 (14.3) |
| Hypertensive disorders | 47 (9.2) | 40 (9.4) | 7 (8.0) | 1 (10.0) | 6 (3.8) | 14 (15.7) | 12 (16.7) | 10 (10.3) | 4 (4.8) |
| Maternal medical complications | 40 (7.8) | 37 (8.7) | 3 (3.4) | 0 | 11 (6.9) | 9 (10.1) | 3 (4.2) | 8 (8.2) | 9 (10.7) |
| Other | 16 (3.1) | 16 (3.8) | 0 | 0 | 4 (2.5) | 3 (3.4) | 4 (5.6) | 3 (3.1) | 2 (2.4) |
| Any cause | 390 (76.2) | 333 (71.3) | 87 (100.0) | 9 (90) | 136 (85.0) | 62 (69.7) | 52 (72.2) | 71 (73.2) | 60 (71.4) |
| Total No. | 512 | 425 | 87 | 10 | 160 | 89 | 72 | 97 | 84 |

[a]Some stillbirths had more than 1 probable or possible cause.
[b]Different proportions by gestational age are noted for placental disease (nominal P = .001), infection (nominal P = .002), hypertensive disorder (nominal P = .004), and obstetric complications (nominal P < .001).
[c]A higher proportion of causes of antepartum stillbirths were placental disease (nominal P = .003) and fetal abnormalities (nominal P = .007) and a lower proportion were infection (nominal P < .001) and obstetric complications (nominal P < .001) compared with intrapartum stillbirths.

The authors of this report are part of the Stillbirth Collaborative Research Network that was initiated by the Eunice Kennedy Shriver National Institute of Child Health and Human Development (NICHD). The Network was created to address this major health issue. The Network collaborative has designed and conducted a multicenter population-based case-controlled study of stillbirths and live births. The report abstracted tells us about the causes of death among stillbirths according to gestational age at delivery and race/ethnicity. Of 663 women with stillbirth enrolled between March 2006 and September 2008, 500 consented to complete postmortem examinations of their 512 neonates. A probable cause of death was found in 312 stillbirths. Table 3 shows the probable and possible causes of death by timing of stillbirth in relation to labor and gestational age. Obstetrical and placental problems lead the causes. Less common causes include fetal genetics/structural entities, infection, umbilical cord abnormalities, maternal hypertensive disorders, and other maternal medical complications.

This report represents the largest US population-based cohort of stillbirths evaluated to ascertain a probable or possible cause of death. A probable cause of death was found in 61% of cases, and a possible or probable cause was found in more than 76% of cases. The causes were differentially distributed across gestational and racial/ethnic groups. The data support the performing of perinatal postmortem examination, placental histology, and karyotype in all cases because the majority of stillbirths (66%) had at least 1 positive result out of these 3 components of evaluation. Although other diagnostic tests have lower yield, their utility should be considered in specific clinical scenarios according to cost and availability. It should be noted that placental disease remains the leading cause of antepartum stillbirths (26%). Umbilical cord abnormalities account for 10% of possible or probable cause of death, which is considerably higher in this report than in previous studies. A nuchal cord alone should not be considered a cause of death without corroborating evidence from postmortem examination.

This report does not give us further insights as to why the US stillbirth rate remains unacceptably high. A further reduction in stillbirth rates will require thorough investigation into the cause of death. The development of interventions to prevent stillbirths should consider the observed differential distribution of causes of death as gestational age advances, as well as variation by race/ethnicity. The excessive rate of stillbirth in non-Hispanic black women is mostly due to obstetric complications, infection, or both resulting in stillbirth most often at less than 24 weeks' gestation.

See the report that follows, which tells us that multiple risk factors that had been known at the time of pregnancy confirmation are associated with stillbirth but only account for a small proportion of actual stillbirths.[1]

This commentary closes with a fast fact. Twins accounted for just 2% of births in the United States in 1915, but the proportion has risen since the 1970s and 1980s to nearly 3.5%. Figures from the US Department of Health and Human Services show that most of the rise is due to greater numbers of older mothers, who are more likely to have twins This rise appears to be the result of greater use of infertility treatments.[2]

**J. A. Stockman III, MD**

*References*

1. Stillbirth Collaborative Research Network Writing Group. Association between stillbirth and risk factors known at pregnancy confirmation. *JAMA*. 2011;306: 2469-2479.
2. Editorial comment. Twins multiply in the US. *BMJ*. 2012;344:e291.

## Association Between Stillbirth and Risk Factors Known at Pregnancy Confirmation

The Stillbirth Collaborative Research Network Writing Group (Univ of Texas Med Branch at Galveston; Brown Univ School of Medicine, Providence, RI; Univ of Texas Health Science Ctr at San Antonio; et al)
*JAMA* 306:2469-2479, 2011

*Context.* Stillbirths account for almost half of US deaths from 20 weeks' gestation to 1 year of life. Most large studies of risk factors for stillbirth use vital statistics with limited data.

*Objective.*—To determine the relation between stillbirths and risk factors that could be ascertained at the start of pregnancy, particularly the contribution of these factors to racial disparities.

*Design, Setting, and Participants.*—Multisite population-based case-control study conducted between March 2006 and September 2008. Fifty-nine US tertiary care and community hospitals, with access to at least 90% of deliveries within 5 catchment areas defined by state and county lines, enrolled residents with deliveries of 1 or more stillborn fetuses and a representative sample of deliveries of only live-born infants, oversampled for those at less than 32 weeks' gestation and those of African descent.

*Main Outcome Measure.*—Stillbirth.

*Results.*—Analysis included 614 case and 1816 control deliveries. In multivariate analyses, the following factors were independently associated with stillbirth: non-Hispanic black race/ethnicity (23.1% stillbirths, 11.2% live births) (vs non-Hispanic whites; adjusted odds ratio [AOR], 2.12 [95% CI, 1.41-3.20]); previous stillbirth (6.7% stillbirths, 1.4% live births); nulliparity with (10.5% stillbirths, 5.2% live births) and without (34.0% stillbirths, 29.7% live births) previous losses at fewer than 20 weeks' gestation (vs multiparity without stillbirth or previous losses; AOR, 5.91 [95% CI, 3.18-11.00]; AOR, 3.13 [95% CI, 2.06-4.75]; and AOR, 1.98 [95% CI, 1.51-2.60], respectively); diabetes (5.6% stillbirths, 1.6% live births) (vs no diabetes; AOR, 2.50 [95% CI, 1.39-4.48]); maternal age 40 years or older (4.5% stillbirths, 2.1% live births) (vs age 20-34 years; AOR, 2.41 [95% CI, 1.24-4.70]); maternal AB blood type (4.9% stillbirths, 3.0% live births) (vs type O; AOR, 1.96 [95% CI, 1.16-3.30]); history of drug addiction (4.5% stillbirths, 2.1% live births) (vs never use; AOR, 2.08 [95% CI, 1.12-3.88]); smoking during the 3 months prior to pregnancy (<10 cigarettes/d, 10.0% stillbirths, 6.5% live births) (vs none; AOR, 1.55 [95% CI, 1.02-2.35]); obesity/overweight (15.5% stillbirths, 12.4%

live births) (vs normal weight; AOR, 1.72 [95% CI, 1.22-2.43]); not living with a partner (25.4% stillbirths, 15.3% live births) (vs married; AOR, 1.62 [95% CI, 1.15-2.27]); and plurality (6.4% stillbirths, 1.9% live births) (vs singleton; AOR, 4.59 [95% CI, 2.63-8.00]). The generalized $R^2$ was 0.19, explaining little of the variance.

*Conclusion.*—Multiple risk factors that would have been known at the time of pregnancy confirmation were associated with stillbirth but accounted for only a small amount of the variance in this outcome.

▶ This report complements the previous one[1] from the collaborative group coordinated by the Eunice Kennedy Shriver National Institute of Child Health and Human Development. The report tells us about the relation between still-births and risk factors that could be ascertained at the start of pregnancy, partic-ularly the contribution of these factors related to racial disparities. The bottom line is that factors known at the start of pregnancy explain little of the overall burden of stillbirth. Further research is needed to identify pregnancies at highest risk overall and for specific causes. Fetal death during labor before 24 weeks' gestation is a consequence of extreme prematurity because interventions on behalf of the fetus are not indicated before viability. Black women, whose rate of preterm birth is double that of women from other racial/ethnic back-grounds, comprise a majority of this group. Stillbirth and preterm are often considered as separate entities, but this is strong evidence that the 2 are more closely linked than has been previously recognized. Additional evidence of common origins of stillbirth and preterm birth comes from the collaborative analyses of the risk of prior pregnancy outcome for future stillbirth. A history of one stillbirth increases the subsequent risk of stillbirth by almost 6-fold.

As the collaborative work highlights, pregnancies involving fetal death before the limit of viability, including those before 20 weeks' gestation, share impor-tant commonalities with pregnancies resulting in early preterm birth. As such, the reports from the collaborative will not only further the understanding of still-birth, but should encourage the need to reframe thinking about how to address the problem of spontaneous preterm birth and the associated racial/ethnic disparities. To read more about the problem of stillbirth and pregnancy-related complications, see the excellent editorial by Iams and Lynch.[2]

This commentary closes with an observation having to do with home births. Birth certificate data show that in recent years, pregnant women in the United States increasingly agree with the adage that there is no place like home. From 2004 through 2008, home births in the United States increased by 20%, accord-ing to a recent report. The 28 357 home births represented 0.67% of all US births in 2008, the highest proportion of home births since 1990.[3]

**J. A. Stockman III, MD**

*References*

1. Stillbirth Collaborative Research Network Writing Group. Causes of death among stillbirths. *JAMA.* 2011;306:2459-2468.
2. Iams JD, Lynch CD. Stillbirth and lessons for pregnancy care. *JAMA.* 2011;306:2506-2507.
3. Editorial comment. Home births up by 20%. *JAMA.* 2011;305:2401.

## Noninvasive Fetal Sex Determination Using Cell-Free Fetal DNA: A Systematic Review and Meta-analysis

Devaney SA, Palomaki GE, Scott JA, et al (Johns Hopkins Univ, Washington, DC; Alpert Med School of Brown Univ, Providence, RI; et al)
*JAMA* 306:627-636, 2011

*Context.*—Noninvasive prenatal determination of fetal sex using cell-free fetal DNA provides an alternative to invasive techniques for some heritable disorders. In some countries this testing has transitioned to clinical care, despite the absence of a formal assessment of performance.

*Objective.*—To document overall test performance of noninvasive fetal sex determination using cell-free fetal DNA and to identify variables that affect performance.

*Data Sources.*—Systematic review and meta-analysis with search of PubMed (January 1, 1997-April 17, 2011) to identify English-language human studies reporting primary data. References from review articles were also searched.

*Study Selection and Data Extraction.*—Abstracts were read independently to identify studies reporting primary data suitable for analysis. Covariates included publication year, sample type, DNA amplification methodology, Y chromosome sequence, and gestational age. Data were independently extracted by 2 reviewers.

*Results.*—From 57 selected studies, 80 data sets (representing 3524 male-bearing pregnancies and 3017 female-bearing pregnancies) were analyzed. Overall performance of the test to detect Y chromosome sequences had the following characteristics: sensitivity, 95.4% (95% confidence interval [CI], 94.7%-96.1%) and specificity, 98.6% (95% CI, 98.1%-99.0%); diagnostic odds ratio (OR), 885; positive predictive value, 98.8%; negative predictive value, 94.8%, area under curve (AUC), 0.993 (95% CI, 0.989-0.995), with significant interstudy heterogeneity. DNA methodology and gestational age had the largest effects on test performance. Methodology test characteristics were AUC, 0.988 (95% CI, 0.979-0.993) for polymerase chain reaction (PCR) and AUC, 0.996 (95% CI, 0.993-0.998) for real-time quantitative PCR (RTQ-PCR) ($P = .02$). Gestational age test characteristics were AUC, 0.989 (95% CI, 0.965-0.998) (<7 weeks); AUC, 0.994 (95% CI, 0.987-0.997) (7-12 weeks); AUC, 0.992 (95% CI, 0.983-0.996) (13-20 weeks); and AUC, 0.998 (95% CI, 0.990-0.999) (>20 weeks) ($P = .02$ for comparison of diagnostic ORs across age ranges). RTQ-PCR (sensitivity, 96.0%; specificity, 99.0%) outperformed conventional PCR (sensitivity, 94.0%; specificity, 97.3%). Testing after 20 weeks (sensitivity, 99.0%; specificity, 99.6%) outperformed testing prior to 7 weeks (sensitivity, 74.5%; specificity, 99.1%), testing at 7 through 12 weeks (sensitivity, 94.8%; specificity, 98.9%), and 13 through 20 weeks (sensitivity, 95.5%; specificity, 99.1%).

*Conclusions.*—Despite interstudy variability, performance was high using maternal blood. Sensitivity and specificity for detection of Y chromosome sequences was greatest using RTQ-PCR after 20 weeks' gestation. Tests using urine and tests performed before 7 weeks' gestation were unreliable.

▶ All the world would love a totally safe, noninvasive method to determine fetal sex. The gold standard, of course, for fetal sex determination involves invasive cytogenetic determination usually via chorionic villus sampling or amniocentesis. Fetal sex determination is commonly performed by sonography, which can be applied as early as 11 weeks' gestation. Sex determination is important for X-linked disorders such as adrenal hyperplasia. Unfortunately, sonography is not entirely reliable. Test performance across published series varies significantly. Data suggest that fetal sex cannot be determined by ultrasound examination in 7.5% to 50% of pregnancies at 12 weeks' gestation, a set of statistics that decreases to 3% to 24% at 13 weeks. When performed at 11 weeks, most reports suggest that sex determination will be incorrect as often as 40% of the time, although by 13 weeks, accuracy improves dramatically.

The presence of cell-free circulating Y chromosome DNA sequences in the plasma of pregnant women was first described back in 1997. A number of published reports have validated the initial finding that the Y chromosome sequences can be amplified and used to identify male fetuses simply by taking a sample of blood from a pregnant woman. More recently, companies have begun offering this technology directly to the consumer over the Internet. The tests are marketed for nonmedical use to curious parents-to-be with promises of accuracy running as high as 99% as early as 5 to 7 weeks gestation.

The authors of the report abstracted sought to determine the analytic validity of cell-free fetal DNA testing in the correct identification of fetal sex. The authors simply asked the question: "How reliably can fetal sex be predicted by sex-specific markers in cell-free fetal DNA from a maternal blood or urine sample?" The authors attempted to answer this question by looking at a systematic review of 146 publications that examined the clinical validity of noninvasive prenatal sex determination using cell-free fetal DNA and maternal blood in urine.

So what did the authors find? They observed that any test performed before 7 weeks' gestation was unreliable. Also, tests using urine were unreliable at any gestational age. That said, the overall performance of noninvasive fetal sex determination using maternal blood is high if performed after 7 weeks' gestation. This technology can be useful in clinical settings for early detection for fetuses at risk for sex-linked disorders. Although the sensitivity can be as low as 75% at these very early ages, the sensitivity rises quickly during later stages of pregnancy. Despite the sensitivity problems of this method of determining fetal sex, if a Y chromosome is detected, the specificity is 100%.

This commentary closes with a profound question: How does the human sperm detect ovulated eggs? The answer lies in an unusual ion channel that could aid in the development of a new class of nonhormonal contraception. Progesterone is released by the cumulus cells that surround ovulated eggs. This induces an influx of calcium ions in sperm, increasing their activity and moving them towards the egg. The underlying mechanism seems to be the activation of a pH sensitive calcium channel called CarSper in sperm.[1] One wonders if homing pigeons operate in a similar manner.

**J. A. Stockman III, MD**

*Reference*

1. Editorial comment. The attraction of sperm to ova. *Nature.* 2011;471.

## Trends in selective abortions of girls in India: analysis of nationally representative birth histories from 1990 to 2005 and census data from 1991 to 2011

Jha P, Kesler MA, Kumar R, et al (Univ of Toronto, Ontario, Canada, Post Graduate Inst of Med Res and Education, Chandigarh, India; et al)
*Lancet* 377:1921-1928, 2011

*Background.*—India's 2011 census revealed a growing imbalance between the numbers of girls and boys aged 0—6 years, which we postulate is due to increased prenatal sex determination with subsequent selective abortion of female fetuses. We aimed to establish the trends in sex ratio by birth order from 1990 to 2005 with three nationally representative surveys and to quantify the totals of selective abortions of girls with census cohort data.

*Methods.*—We assessed sex ratios by birth order in 0·25 million births in three rounds of the nationally representative National Family Health Survey covering the period from 1990 to 2005. We estimated totals of selective abortion of girls by assessing the birth cohorts of children aged 0—6 years in the 1991, 2001, and 2011 censuses. Our main statistic was the conditional sex ratio of second-order births after a firstborn girl and we used 3-year rolling weighted averages to test for trends, with differences between trends compared by linear regression.

*Findings.*—The conditional sex ratio for second-order births when the firstborn was a girl fell from 906 per 1000 boys (99% CI 798—1013) in 1990 to 836 (733—939) in 2005; an annual decline of 0·52% (*p* for trend=0·002). Declines were much greater in mothers with 10 or more years of education than in mothers with no education, and in wealthier households compared with poorer households. By contrast, we did not detect any significant declines in the sex ratio for second-order births if the firstborn was a boy, or for firstborns. Between the 2001 and 2011 censuses, more than twice the number of Indian districts (local administrative areas) showed declines in the child sex ratio as districts with no change or increases. After adjusting for excess mortality rates in girls, our estimates of number of selective abortions of girls rose from 0—2·0 million in the 1980s, to 1·2—4·1 million in the 1990s, and to 3·1—6·0 million in the 2000s. Each 1% decline in child sex ratio at ages 0—6 years implied 1·2—3·6 million more selective abortions of girls. Selective abortions of girls totalled about 4·2—12·1 million from 1980—2010, with a greater rate of increase in the 1990s than in the 2000s.

*Interpretation.*—Selective abortion of girls, especially for pregnancies after a firstborn girl, has increased substantially in India. Most of India's population now live in states where selective abortion of girls is common.

▶ This is one of a number of reports coming from India documenting information from the 2011 Indian Census. The latter revealed that 7.1 million fewer girls than boys aged 0 to 6 years were found in the census. This was a notable increase in the gap of 6.0 million fewer girls recorded in the 2001 census and the gap of 4.2 million fewer girls recorded in the 1991 census. The masculine nature of the Indian population, as indicated by the lower than normal sex ratio (defined as female-to-male ratio in India), has been a matter of concern since the first Indian census back in 1871.[1] Almost a century and a half later, the sex ratio in children aged 0 to 6 years in India (915 girls to 1000 boys) is the lowest ratio recorded since data became available in 1961. The steady decline in the ratio is surprising and counterintuitive, in view of India's progress in recent decades in improving the levels of female literacy and increases in income per person. Jha et al present an analysis of trends in sex ratio at birth in India showing that the ratio for second-ordered births, conditional on the firstborn being a girl, fell from 906 per 1000 boys in 1990 to 836 girls per 1000 boys in 2005. On the basis of this finding, the investigators estimate that there would have been between 3.1 and 6.0 million abortions of female fetuses in the past decade alone.

The sex ratio imbalance in children in India was initially attributed to gender discrimination in the allocation of health-related resources within households—indicative of the strong societal norm of a son preference—leading to excess mortality in girls. Recent declines in the child sex ratio, however, are thought now to be driven largely by medical technologies to determine the sex of fetuses, followed by selective abortion of girls. Although the implementation by the PreNatal Diagnostic Techniques Act makes it illegal to identify the sex of a fetus, there is little evidence that the law is accomplishing its goal. Rather, it seems that states with increased availability per person of registered prenatal diagnostic facilities do indeed have lower girl to boy sex ratios than states where this equipment is less available.

The prospects look grim that India can balance its distribution of sexes at birth. The demand for sons among wealthy parents is being satisfied by the medical community through the provision of illegal services of fetal sex-determination and sex-selective abortion. The financial incentives for physicians to undertake this illegal activity seems to be far greater than the penalties associated with breaking the law. It is likely that it is the medical establishment that must be held accountable on moral, social, and legal grounds in India. As a result of the enactment of the law precluding prenatal sex determination in India, only 800 court cases have been brought against doctors, and these have resulted in only 55 convictions.

Interestingly, whereas abortion is highly prevalent in India, a bill has been introduced into the Russian parliament that sharply curbs the availability of abortions in an attempt to reverse that country's chronic depopulation crisis. In a controversial move backed by the Russian Orthodox Church, legislation introduced in 2011 proposed that the country's public health service stop offering abortions altogether, forcing women who want to have an abortion to pay for one at a private clinic. At the time of this writing, the bill had not yet been acted on. One of the most contentious parts of the legislation was the language that a married woman wanting an abortion must obtain the written consent of her husband. Government figures in Russia show that more than 1.5 million abortions are performed in Russia each year, a statistic that the United Nations says means that Russia has more abortions per capita than any other country in the world. The country's population has shrunk by 2.2 million in the past 8 years and stood at roughly 143 million as of 2011, down from 148.5 million in 1995. Experts say that alcohol and drug misuse and the fact that many Russian men die in their 50s are also to blame. Interestingly, Vladimir Putin, the Russian prime minister, has revived the Soviet era practice of giving medals to women who bear many children, and in 2007, he introduced cash payments for women who have 2 children or more. Under the latter scheme, Russian women who have 2 children are eligible for a 1-time payment of approximately $13 000.

**J. A. Stockman III, MD**

*Reference*

1. Natarajan D. *Changes in sex ratio.* New Delhi, India: Census of India; 1972.

## China's facility-based birth strategy and neonatal mortality: a population-based epidemiological study

Feng XL, Guo S, Hipgrave D, et al (Peking Univ, Beijing, China, et al)
*Lancet* 378:1493-1500, 2011

*Background.*—China's success in improving the quality of and access to obstetric care in hospitals offers an opportunity to examine the effect of a large-scale facility-based strategy on neonatal mortality. We aimed to establish this effect by assessing how the institutional strategy of intrapartum care has affected neonatal mortality and its regional inequalities.

*Methods.*—We did a population-based epidemiological study of China's National Maternal and Child Mortality Surveillance System from 1996 to 2008. We used data from 116 surveillance sites in China (37 urban districts and 79 rural counties) to examine neonatal mortality by cause, socioeconomic region, and place of birth, with Poisson regression to calculate relative risks. Rural counties were categorised into types 1–4, with type 4 being the least developed. We report attributable risks and preventable fractions for hospital births versus home births.

*Findings.*—Neonatal mortality decreased by 62% between 1996 and 2008. The rate of neonatal mortality was much lower for hospital births than for home births in all regions, with relative risks (RR) ranging from 0·30 (95% CI 0·22—0·40) in type 2 rural counties, to 0·52 (0·33—0·83) in type 4 counties ($p < 0·0001$). The proportion of neonatal deaths prevented by hospital birth ranged from 70% (95% CI 59·7—77·8) to 48% (16·9—67·3). Babies born in urban hospitals had a low rate of neonatal mortality ($5 \cdot 7$ per 1000 livebirths); but those born in hospitals in type 4 rural counties were almost four times more likely to die than were children born in urban hospitals (RR $3 \cdot 80$, $2 \cdot 53 - 5 \cdot 72$).

*Interpretation.*—Other countries can learn from China's substantial progress in reducing neonatal mortality. The major effect of China's facility-based strategy on neonatal mortality is much greater than that reported for community-based interventions. Our findings will provide a great impetus for countries to increase demand for and quality of facility-based intrapartum care.

▶ Worldwide, it is estimated that neonatal deaths, which occur almost exclusively in low-income and middle-income countries, represent 41% of all deaths in children younger than 5 years. There is a lot all can learn from experiences in China and elsewhere with regard to improvements in neonatal mortality. As in Brazil and Mexico, China has accomplished substantial reductions in mortality rates of children younger than 5 years with socioeconomic development and targeted investments in primary health care, maternal and child health programs, and reproductive health. China's progress is unique because the decline in mortality rates overall is accompanied by a similarly marked reduction in neonatal mortality rates.

Feng et al report empirical, nationally representative data for neonatal mortality rates from the most populous country in the world. The data also expose large and persisting inequities in neonatal mortality across socioeconomic strata and in outcomes between infants born in hospital versus those delivered at home. Using district-leveled data from China's National Maternal and Child Mortality Surveillance System, Feng et al were able to show the apparent effect of China's strategy to promote facility-based deliveries on reduction in neonatal mortality between 1996 and 2008. Being born in hospital is what made the difference, and the difference was a positive one across all diverse socioeconomic strata. It was clear that reductions in neonatal mortality coincided with increasing proportion of births in hospitals. Unfortunately, there was wide variation across socioeconomic strata about the ability to be born in hospital.

An editorial accompanied the Feng et al report.[1] It is noted that concerns have existed about the quality of data from China's National Maternal and Child Mortality Surveillance System. Although the system is a rich source of demographic data, it has been criticized for systematically underreporting births and deaths and for the large variation in the distribution of surveillance sites in the last 2 decades. Inaccurate estimation, for example, of the number of births, might have biased the analysis performed by Feng et al. For example, if home births are less likely to be reported than hospital births, home-birth mortality rates could be seriously inflated because adverse outcomes would be more likely to be reported than satisfactory birthing at home. That said, the data are impressive that China is on the right pathway to improving what previously had been very high neonatal mortality rates.

The data from China document clearly something that we have known for some time in the United States and that is that home delivery is for pizza.

**J. A. Stockman III, MD**

*Reference*

1. Bassani DG, Roth DE. China's progress in neonatal mortality. *Lancet.* 2011;378: 1446-1447.

## A Hemoglobin Variant Associated with Neonatal Cyanosis and Anemia

Crowley MA, Mollan TL, Abdulmalik OY, et al (Case Western Reserve Univ, Cleveland, OH; Rice Univ, Houston, TX; Children's Hosp of Philadelphia, PA; et al)
*N Engl J Med* 364:1837-1843, 2011

Globin-gene mutations are a rare but important cause of cyanosis. We identified a missense mutation in the fetal Gγ-globin gene (*HBG2*) in a father and daughter with transient neonatal cyanosis and anemia. This new mutation modifies the ligand-binding pocket of fetal hemoglobin by means of two mechanisms. First, the relatively large side chain of methionine decreases both the affinity of oxygen for binding to the mutant hemoglobin subunit and the rate at which it does so. Second, the mutant methionine is converted to aspartic acid post-translationally, probably through oxidative mechanisms. The presence of this polar amino acid in the heme pocket is predicted to enhance hemoglobin denaturation, causing anemia.

▶ The infant described in this report has what is known as the *happy blue baby* syndrome. Specifically, a full term infant female weighing 2825 g was born by vaginal delivery to a 20-year-old woman who had been pregnant for the second time. The infant had Apgar scores of 8 at 1 minute and 5 minutes and was described as a "happy blue baby"—that is, cyanotic, but well appearing. Initial hemoglobin oxygen saturation, measured in ambient air with pulse oximetry was 30% to 50%, and the partial pressure of arterial oxygen tension (PaO$_2$) was 107 mm Hg. After intubation and delivery of 100% oxygen, the hemoglobin saturation fluctuated around 85%, and the arterial PaO$_2$ reached 369 mm Hg. The physical examination revealed only cyanosis and moderate hepatomegaly. The infant was extubated with a transition to oxygen delivered by means of nasal cannula. The oxygen saturation remained low at 80% to 90% despite the absence of arterial hypoxemia. The infant had evidence of a moderate anemia. The methemoglobin level was normal, and a review of the red cell smear was unremarkable. Cardiac examination, including echocardiography, was normal. On the first day of life, a hemoglobin electrophoresis performed with cellulose acetate revealed that total hemoglobin consisted of approximately 90% hemoglobin F and 10% hemoglobin A, with no variant hemoglobin bands. The infant received red cell transfusions, which raised her hemoglobin oxygen saturation from approximately 80% to more than 90%. She was discharged home at 6 days of age with oxygen saturations in the range of 90% to 95%. Her clinical course was unremarkable, and by 2 months of age her hemoglobin oxygen saturation was consistently higher than 95%. This infant's family history was positive in her father for transient neonatal cyanosis with a demonstrated hemoglobin oxygen saturation of approximately 80%.

If you have not figured out what was going on with this child, she had a globin gene mutation. This mutation was in the fetal gamma-globin gene (*HBG2*), an abnormality the infant and father shared. This mutation modified the structure of fetal hemoglobin causing a decrease in the affinity of fetal hemoglobin for oxygen, resulting in better oxygen release than would be expected, allowing blood to become readily desaturated as oxygen came off of the hemoglobin easily. This is what caused the cyanosis. Because less hemoglobin was necessary because of the facilitated oxygen delivery, the anemia was expected. As the fetal hemoglobin went away with age, the problem corrected itself.

Fetal hemoglobin contains 2 alpha globins and 2 gamma globins. Mutations in the gamma-globin gene are uncommon, but when the fetal hemoglobin is affected, it may result in neonatal cyanosis. It seems odd and perhaps counter-intuitive that a gene defect would improve oxygen delivery, but when it affects a hemoglobin, such as fetal hemoglobin, which tends to avidly bind oxygen, the reverse effect occurs.

The underlying teaching point here is that when a healthy blue baby appears before you, the likelihood is either that that baby has cyanotic congenital heart disease, a mild methemoglobinemia, or a mutant fetal hemoglobin. Remember the happy blue baby syndrome. If you live long enough, you may see a case.

This commentary closes with an observation having to do with bed placement in neonatal nurseries. In 2005, a Department of Health in England published the document mandating same sex accommodations in hospitals, aiming to ensure the privacy and dignity of all patients during their hospital stays. The intention was that patients of the opposite sex would never room together. By 2010, the British National Health Service began to apply sanctions against hospitals that did not comply with the new requirement. When it came to neonatal nurseries this meant that baby boys' and baby girls' bassinets could not be juxtaposed. Needless to say, most neonatal units did not comply with this mandate as it could be reasonably believed that a newborn baby is unlikely to be aware of nor worried about principles of privacy or dignity.

This is no joke. See the article by Green and Davison.[1]

**J. A. Stockman III, MD**

*Reference*

1. Green M, Davison M. Political correctness: A step too far? *BMJ*. 2011;343:d7451.

---

**Functional Polymorphism in Gamma-Glutamylcarboxylase is a Risk Factor for Severe Neonatal Hemorrhage**
Vanakker OM, De Coen K, Costrop L, et al (Ghent Univ Hosp, Belgium)
*J Pediatr* 159:347-349, 2011

---

A neonate who received vitamin K (VK) supplementation then developed severe late-onset bleeding with abnormal prothrombin time and activated partial thromboplastine time. The bleeding was corrected after intravenous VK. Molecular analysis of the gamma-glutamylcarboxylase gene revealed a heterozygous single nucleotide polymorphism, which decreases carboxylase activity and induces VK-dependent coagulation deficiency.

▶ When I was in training, hemorrhagic disease of the newborn was a fairly straightforward entity, one caused simply by having too little vitamin K on board. At present, hemorrhagic disease of the newborn is classified according to the presentation timing after birth: early (0-24 hours), classic (2-7 days), and late (1-8 weeks). The etiologies of vitamin K deficiency include abnormal maternal vitamin K absorption or medication use that alters maternal vitamin K uptake (early onset), breastfeeding (classic), or malabsorption syndromes (late onset). Also, loss-of-function mutations in genes that encode the vitamin K—cycle key enzymes, gamma-glutamylcarboxylase (GGCX) and VKORC1, can cause a deficiency of the vitamin K—dependent clotting factors. The pathophysiology of neonatal hemorrhage results from a deficient activation of the vitamin K—dependent coagulation factors. After translation, these proteins have essential posttranslational modification in the vitamin K cycle, in which hepatic endoplasmic reticulum GGCX carboxylate glutamate changes into glutamic acid residues. The fully carboxylated coagulation factors are then secreted into the circulation. Vitamin K is an essential cofactor in this carboxylation step.

Vanakker et al describe a newborn with hemorrhagic disease of the newborn period. This was the second child of healthy, nonconsanguineous parents who was born at term after a noncomplicated pregnancy and delivery. The mother had not taken any medication before or during pregnancy. The family history–taking result was negative for any bleeding disorders. Immediately after birth, routine vitamin K prophylaxis was given intramuscularly. Because the mother was breastfeeding, oral supplementation with vitamin K was begun. At 3 weeks of age, the infant was admitted to hospital because of hematemesis resulting from gastrointestinal hemorrhage. The platelet count was normal. The prothrombin time and activated partial thromboplastin times were significantly prolonged. Intravenous vitamin K was administered, and, within 24 hours, the coagulation study results returned to normal. A cranial MRI revealed a large subdural hematoma and several intracerebral hemorrhages. Molecular analyses of the genes that encode the vitamin K—cycle enzymes, GGCX and VKORC1, were performed. Molecular analysis of the VKORC1 gene was normal, whereas the GGCX gene had a known single gene mutation.

In this particular child, although conventional oral vitamin K supplementation was given, this amount of vitamin K is insufficient because of the decreased gamma-carboxylase activity, which leads to inadequate coagulation factor activation and bleeding. High doses of intravenous vitamin K will pass the critical threshold required for adequate protein carboxylation and hence result in normalization of coagulation factors. It turns out that the father was homozygous for the gene defect the child had in the heterozygous state. It is not clear why he never had any bleeding by history taking.

**J. A. Stockman III, MD**

### Risk of Hyperbilirubinemia in Breast-Fed Infants

Chang P-F, Lin Y-C, Liu K, et al (Far Eastern Memorial Hosp, Pan-Chiao, Taipei, Taiwan; et al)
*J Pediatr* 159:561-565, 2011

*Objective.*—To investigate the risk factors for hyperbilirubinemia in infants who are exclusively breast-fed.

*Study Design.*—A prospective study was conducted to investigate the effects of birth body weight, sex, mode of delivery, glucose-6-phosphate dehydrogenase (G6PD) deficiency, variant *UDP-glucuronosyltransferase 1A1 (UGT1A1)* gene, and *hepatic solute carrier organic anion transporter 1B1 (SLCO1B1)* gene on hyperbilirubinemia in neonates who were breast-fed. Hyperbilirubinemia was diagnosed when a full term neonate had a bilirubin level $\geq 15.0$ mg/dL (256.5 $\mu$M) in serum at 3 days old. The polymerase chain reaction-restriction fragment length polymorphism method was used as a means of detecting the known variant sites in the *UGT1A1* and *SLCO1B1* gene.

*Results.*—Of 252 infants born at term who were exclusively breast-fed, 59 (23.4%) had hyperbilirubinemia. The significant risk factors were a variant nucleotide 211 in *UGT1A1* (2.48; 95% CI, 1.29 to 4.76; $P = .006$), G6PD deficiency (12.24; 95% CI, 1.08 to 138.62; $P < .05$), and vaginal delivery (3.55; 95% CI, 1.64 to 7.66; $P < .001$).

*Conclusion.*—Breast-fed neonates who are 211 variants in the *UGT1A1*, G6PD deficiency, and vaginal delivery are at high-risk for hyperbilirubinemia.

▶ All of us know that breast-feeding is associated with a higher risk of neonatal hyperbilirubinemia. This risk varies with certain risk factors. For example, in the report of Chang et al, the incidence of hyperbilirubinemia in breast-fed infants of Asian background is relatively high (23.4%) versus that in Caucasians (5%–12%). This suggests that demographic and genetic factors may play a significant role in the development of hyperbilirubinemia in breast-fed infants.

The etiology of hyperbilirubinemia in breast-fed neonates is not clearly understood. Inadequate breast milk intake can aggravate hyperbilirubinemia by increasing the enterohepatic circulation of bilirubin and subsequent hepatic bilirubin load or dehydration. Breast milk feeding may also act as an external factor for certain variant genotypes, predisposing to the development of hyperbilirubinemia. For example, variation at nucleotide 211 of the *UGT1A1* gene is the most common mutation associated with hyperbilirubinemia in breast-fed infants. This gene affects the handling of bilirubin in the liver. This report from Taiwan shows that variation in the *UGT1A1* gene places infants at significantly higher risk for the development of hyperbilirubinemia. Also, G6PD deficiency strongly correlates with jaundice in the newborn period. This report also found that breast-fed neonates postvaginal delivery had a higher risk for the development of hyperbilirubinemia. Vaginal delivery may be associated with oxytocin usage, vacuum extraction, and cephalohematoma, all of which are known risk factors for hyperbilirubinemia. This relationship with oxytocin exposure was first recognized well over a quarter of a century ago. Oxytocin may have some direct effect on neonatal bilirubin metabolism. In contrast, it appears that cesarean delivery may protect against jaundice. A possible explanation is that infants who are delivered by cesarean delivery tend to receive some supplementation with infant formula, which would perhaps offset the effect of breast milk intake.

If there is a lesson from this report, it is that one should be aware that certain populations are at significantly higher risk for the development of hyperbilirubinemia in the setting of breast-feeding. Infants of Asian background are at greater risk. Those who have an ethnic background that predisposes for a higher probability of having G6PD deficiency are therefore also at greater risk. Whether one can predict all of these risk factors is speculative, but we should at least be aware of the associations.

This commentary closes with a question. You know the origin of the word oxytocin? Oxytocin gets its name from the Greek word for "rapid birth." It was in 1953 that the first hormone from the pituitary was synthesized. It was adrenocorticotropic hormone (ACTH). The second hormone synthesized was oxytocin. Soon after came vasopressin. All were synthesized at virtually the same time.[1]

**J. A. Stockman III, MD**

*Reference*

1. Editorial comment. 'Love' hormone has a dark side. *Science News.* 2011;179.

## A global reference for fetal-weight and birthweight percentiles

Mikolajczyk RT, Zhang J, Betran AP, et al (Bremen Inst for Prevention Res and Social Medicine, Germany; Natl Insts of Health, Bethesda, MD; World Health Organization, Geneva, Switzerland; et al)
*Lancet* 377:1855-1861, 2011

*Background.*—Definition of small for gestational age in various populations worldwide remains a challenge. References based on birthweight are deficient for preterm births, those derived from ultrasound estimates might not be applicable to all populations, and the individualised reference can be too complex to use in developing countries. Our aim was to create a generic reference for fetal weight and birthweight that overcame these deficiencies and could be readily adapted to local populations.

*Methods.*—We used the fetal-weight reference developed by Hadlock and colleagues and the notion of proportionality proposed by Gardosi and colleagues and made the weight reference easily adjustable according to the mean birthweight at 40 weeks of gestation for any local population. For application and validation, we used data from 24 countries in Africa, Latin America, and Asia that participated in the 2004—08 WHO Global Survey on Maternal and Perinatal Health (237 025 births). We compared our reference with that of Hadlock and colleagues (non-customised) and with that of Gardosi and colleagues (individualised). For every reference, the odds ratio (OR) of adverse perinatal outcomes (stillbirths, neonatal deaths, referral to higher-level or special care unit, or Apgar score lower than 7 at 5 min) for infants who were small for gestational age versus those who were not was estimated with multilevel logistic regression.

*Findings.*—OR of adverse outcomes for infants small for gestational age versus those not small for gestational age was 1·59 (95% CI 1·53–1·66) for the non-customised fetal-weight reference compared with 2·87 (2·73–3·01) for our country-specific reference, and 2·84 (2·71–2·99) for the fully individualised reference.

*Interpretation.*—Our generic reference for fetal-weight and birthweight percentiles can be easily adapted to local populations. It has a better ability to predict adverse perinatal outcomes than has the non-customised fetal-weight reference, and is simpler to use than the individualised reference without loss of predictive ability (Fig 2).

► Even in the United States, the definition of small for gestational age is viewed differently by different people. When it comes to the global definition of small for gestational age, you begin to see real problems with uniformity of definitions. References based on birth weight are particularly deficient for preterm births. Often ultrasound measurements are used as references for fetal development, but these are not applicable to all populations. The most popular and widely

| Gestational age* (weeks) | Weight percentiles† for the local population | | | | | | | | | | |
|---|---|---|---|---|---|---|---|---|---|---|---|
| | 99th | 97th | 95th | 90th | 75th | Mean | 25th | 10th | 5th | 3rd | 1st |
| 24 | 820 | 786 | 768 | 741 | 695 | 644 | 593 | 547 | 520 | 502 | 468 |
| 25 | 957 | 918 | 897 | 865 | 812 | 752 | 692 | 639 | 607 | 586 | 547 |
| 26 | 1110 | 1064 | 1040 | 1003 | 941 | 872 | 803 | 741 | 703 | 679 | 634 |
| 27 | 1278 | 1225 | 1198 | 1155 | 1083 | 1004 | 924 | 853 | 810 | 782 | 730 |
| 28 | 1461 | 1401 | 1369 | 1320 | 1238 | 1147 | 1057 | 975 | 926 | 894 | 834 |
| 29 | 1658 | 1590 | 1554 | 1498 | 1405 | 1302 | 1199 | 1106 | 1051 | 1015 | 947 |
| 30 | 1869 | 1792 | 1751 | 1689 | 1584 | 1468 | 1352 | 1247 | 1184 | 1144 | 1067 |
| 31 | 2091 | 2005 | 1960 | 1890 | 1773 | 1643 | 1513 | 1395 | 1325 | 1280 | 1194 |
| 32 | 2324 | 2228 | 2178 | 2100 | 1970 | 1825 | 1681 | 1551 | 1473 | 1422 | 1327 |
| 33 | 2564 | 2459 | 2403 | 2317 | 2173 | 2014 | 1854 | 1711 | 1625 | 1569 | 1464 |
| 34 | 2809 | 2694 | 2632 | 2538 | 2381 | 2206 | 2032 | 1874 | 1780 | 1719 | 1604 |
| 35 | 3056 | 2930 | 2864 | 2761 | 2590 | 2400 | 2210 | 2039 | 1937 | 1870 | 1745 |
| 36 | 3301 | 3165 | 3093 | 2983 | 2798 | 2593 | 2387 | 2203 | 2092 | 2020 | 1885 |
| 37 | 3540 | 3395 | 3318 | 3199 | 3001 | 2781 | 2561 | 2362 | 2244 | 2167 | 2021 |
| 38 | 3770 | 3615 | 3533 | 3407 | 3196 | 2961 | 2727 | 2516 | 2390 | 2308 | 2153 |
| 39 | 3987 | 3823 | 3736 | 3603 | 3380 | 3132 | 2884 | 2660 | 2527 | 2440 | 2276 |
| 40 | 4186 | 4014 | 3923 | 3783 | 3549 | 3288 | 3028 | 2794 | 2653 | 2562 | 2390 |
| 41 | 4365 | 4185 | 4090 | 3944 | 3700 | 3428 | 3157 | 2913 | 2766 | 2671 | 2492 |

**FIGURE 2.**—Selected percentiles of fetal weight and birthweight for a population with the mean birthweight at 40 weeks of gestation of 3288 g in Mexico Data obtained from the calculation sheet for Microsoft Office Excel software (webappendix B). *Gestational age in completed weeks. †Standard deviation of 13·2% of the corresponding mean weight was used for calculation of percentiles. (Reprinted from The Lancet, Mikolajczyk RT, Zhang J, Betran AP, et al. A global reference for fetal-weight and birthweight percentiles. *Lancet.* 2011;377:1855-1861. © 2011, with permission from Elsevier.)

accepted ultrasound-based reference for estimated fetal weight was proposed by Hadlock and colleagues[1] and is as follows:

Fetal weight (g) = exp $(0.578 + 0.332 \times GA - 0.00354 \times GA^2)$

Unfortunately, ultrasound estimates are not applicable in all populations, and the complexity of the individualized reference hinders wide use in developing countries.

Mikolajczyk et al decided to simplify matters by creating straightforward reference tables based on a extensive search of Medline using the terms "definition" and "classification" with "small for gestational age," the aim being to create a generic reference for fetal weight and birthweight that overcomes the many current deficiencies that exist worldwide and that can be readily adapted in local populations. The authors compared the performance of a new global reference with that of the individualized references currently in place in various countries that are part of the World Health Organization and showed that adjustment for ethnicity improves the classification of small for gestational age substantially, whereas addition of more parameters for individualization provides little further improvement against the ethnicity-adjusted reference. Fig 2 is an example of selected percentiles of fetal weight and birth weight for a specific population based on information provided from this report.

While on the topic of population-based data, did you know that 1 in 5 children who die before age 5 years live in India? There are about 2.35 million such deaths in that country each year. Forty-three percent of these deaths occur during the neonatal period, with the remainder occurring after 1 month of age. The 3 main causes of neonatal death are prematurity and low birth weight, accounting for 33% of neonatal deaths, neonatal infections (27%), and birth asphyxia or birth trauma (19%). In the 1- to 59-month age range, there were 2 main causes: pneumonia (28% of deaths) and diarrhea (22% of deaths). Girls had almost a 50% more likely demise in the first 5 years of life. For more on this sad story, see the editorial comment.[2]

In another commentary,[3] it was mentioned that oxytocin was synthesized in 1953. The researcher who synthesized oxytocin received the Nobel Prize 2 years later. The award was given in recognition that this new agent would speed delivery time for women in labor and that the synthesis of other similar molecules promised a new era in hormone treatment. What was not obvious in the 1950s was the role that oxytocin might play in behavior. In more recent decades, researchers have discovered that female virgin rats injected with the hormone will mother rat pups—building nests, licking the pups, and attempting to nurse. Additional work has shown that oxytocin is important in pair bonding among prairie voles, as well as in forming social bonds and in developing trust among humans. Today, oxytocin is more widely known as a "love hormone" than as a labor drug. Recent studies also suggest that studies on oxytocin may lead to yet more treatments, including therapies for social phobia, autism, infertility, and addiction. Who would have believed all this from a drug discovered more than 60 years ago?[4]

**J. A. Stockman III, MD**

*References*

1. Hadlock FP, Harrist RB, Martinez-Poyer J. In utero analysis of fetal growth: a sonographic weight standard. *Radiology*. 1991;181:129-133.

2. Editorial comment. Causes of death in India. *Arch Dis Child.* 2011;96:496.
3. Chang PF, Lin YC, Liu K, Yeh SJ, Ni YH. Risk of hyperbilirubinemia in breast-fed infants. *J Pediatr.* 2011;159:561-565.
4. Quill E. Oxytocin goes from birthing drug to love hormone. *Science News.* January 14, 2012:32.

## Gestational Age at Birth and Mortality in Young Adulthood

Crump C, Sundquist K, Sundquist J, et al (Stanford Univ, CA; Lund Univ, Malmö, Sweden)
*JAMA* 306:1233-1240, 2011

*Context.*—Preterm birth is the leading cause of infant mortality in developed countries, but the association between gestational age at birth and mortality in adulthood remains unknown.

*Objective.*—To examine the association between gestational age at birth and mortality in young adulthood.

*Design, Setting, and Participants.*—National cohort study of 674 820 individuals born as singletons in Sweden in 1973 through 1979 who survived to age 1 year, including 27 979 born preterm (gestational age <37 weeks), followed up to 2008 (ages 29-36 years).

*Main Outcome Measures.*—All-cause and cause-specific mortality.

*Results.*—A total of 7095 deaths occurred in 20.8 million person-years of follow-up. Among individuals still alive at the beginning of each age range, a strong inverse association was found between gestational age at birth and mortality in early childhood (ages 1-5 years: adjusted hazard ratio [aHR] for each additional week of gestation, 0.92; 95% CI, 0.89-0.94; $P < .001$), which disappeared in late childhood (ages 6-12 years: aHR, 0.99; 95% CI, 0.95-1.03; $P = .61$) and adolescence (ages 13-17 years: aHR, 0.99; 95% CI, 0.95-1.03; $P = .64$) and then reappeared in young adulthood (ages 18-36 years: aHR, 0.96; 95% CI, 0.94-0.97; $P < .001$). In young adulthood, mortality rates (per 1000 person-years) by gestational age at birth were 0.94 for 22 to 27 weeks, 0.86 for 28 to 33 weeks, 0.65 for 34 to 36 weeks, 0.46 for 37 to 42 weeks (full-term), and 0.54 for 43 or more weeks. Preterm birth was associated with increased mortality in young adulthood even among individuals born late preterm (34-36 weeks, aHR, 1.31; 95% CI, 1.13-1.50; $P < .001$), relative to those born full-term. In young adulthood, gestational age at birth had the strongest inverse association with mortality from congenital anomalies and respiratory, endocrine, and cardiovascular disorders and was not associated with mortality from neurological disorders, cancer, or injury.

*Conclusion.*—After excluding earlier deaths, low gestational age at birth was independently associated with increased mortality in early childhood and young adulthood.

▶ Obviously, there is a lot written about the long-term effects of being born prematurely. Unfortunately, most of the data in this regard do not tell us about longer-term outcomes into adulthood. We are now just beginning to see data emerge in this regard, particularly because in the last 3 decades, the prevalence of preterm birth (prior to 37 weeks gestation) has increased to more than 12% among newborns in the United States. Advances in neonatal care (widespread use of antenatal corticosteroids, surfactant therapy, and high frequency ventilation) are at least partially responsible for the survival of preterm infants. The result is an increasingly large number of individuals who were born preterm who are now surviving into adulthood. Prior to the publication of the report of Crump et al, no studies to date have reported the specific contribution of gestational age at birth or mortality in adulthood.

Crump et al have conducted a national cohort study performed in Sweden that examines the association between gestational age at birth (independent of fetal growth) and mortality in young adulthood. The investigators examined infants born from 1973 to 1979 as they were followed up into young adulthood for all-cause and specific mortality. During the period 1973 to 1979, the total prevalence of preterm birth in Sweden was 5.0%. The proportion of infants born preterm ( < 37 weeks) who died in the first year of life was 8.6%, including 70.7% of those born at 22 to 27 weeks, 18.4% of those born at 28 to 33 weeks, and 3.1% of those born 34 to 36 weeks, compared with 0.7% of those born full term (37 to 42 weeks) and 1.0% of those born postterm (≥43 weeks).

It was observed that in early childhood as well as young adulthood, preterm birth was associated with increased mortality even among individuals born late preterm (34 to 36 weeks). Mortality rates per 1000 person-years for individuals born late preterm and full term, respectively, were 0.53 and 0.32 in early childhood and 0.65 and 0.46 in adulthood. Adjusted hazard ratios for the association between late preterm (34 to 36 weeks) and mortality were 1.53 in early childhood and 1.31 in young adulthood, relative to infants born at term. The bottom line was that low gestational age at birth was independently associated with increased mortality in young adulthood among individuals born in Sweden in 1973 to 1979. This was true even among those born late preterm.

This report from Sweden is the first study to tell us about the specific contribution of gestational age at birth on mortality in adulthood. The results document the persistent long-term health sequelae of preterm birth. There were multiple causes for this association, mostly related to congenital anomalies, respiratory and endocrine disorders, and cardiovascular disorders in young adulthood. High risk of asthma, hypertension, diabetes, and hypothyroidism was also noted.

Given that the prevalence of preterm birth in the United States exceeds 12% (more than double the prevalence observed in this Swedish report), you can bet that the data would be more dramatic than that reported from Sweden. The results from this report also underscore the need for adequate transition of care from pediatric care providers to adult care providers in the provision of close follow-up for the long-term consequences of being born prematurely.

**J. A. Stockman III, MD**

## A switch toward angiostatic gene expression impairs the angiogenic properties of endothelial progenitor cells in low birth weight preterm infants

Ligi I, Simoncini S, Tellier E, et al (Unité Mixte de Recherche 608, Marseille, France; et al)
*Blood* 118:1699-1709, 2011

Low birth weight (LBW) is associated with increased risk of cardiovascular diseases at adulthood. Nevertheless, the impact of LBW on the endothelium is not clearly established. We investigate whether LBW alters the angiogenic properties of cord blood endothelial colony forming cells (LBW-ECFCs) in 25 preterm neonates compared with 25 term neonates (CT-ECFCs). We observed that LBW decreased the number of colonies formed by ECFCs and delayed the time of appearance of their clonal progeny. LBW dramatically reduced LBW-ECFC capacity to form sprouts and tubes, to migrate and to proliferate in vitro. The angiogenic defect of LBW-ECFCs was confirmed in vivo by their inability to form robust capillary networks in Matrigel plugs injected in *nu/nu* mice. Gene profile analysis of LBW-ECFCs demonstrated an increased expression of antiangiogenic genes. Among them, thrombospondin 1 (*THBS1*) was highly expressed at RNA and protein levels in LBW-ECFCs. Silencing *THBS1* restored the angiogenic properties of LBW-ECFCs by increasing AKT phosphorylation. The imbalance toward an angiostatic state provide a mechanistic link between LBW and the impaired angiogenic properties of ECFCs and allows the identification of THBS1 as a novel player in LBW-ECFC defect, opening new perspectives for novel deprogramming agents.

▶ We challenge anyone reading to quickly speak aloud the title of this article 3 times. Nonetheless, the topic discussed is a very important one. Over the last 20 years or so, multiple epidemiologic studies have found that individuals born with low birth weight (LBW) are predisposed to cardiovascular disease and hypertension. Unfortunately, both the cellular and molecular mechanisms underlying this association have remained poorly understood. Ligi et al now show that endothelial progenitors from LBW infants exhibit striking reductions in their angiogenic properties compared with those infants born with normal birth weight, thus providing for the first time a potential mechanistic link between LBW and adult hypertension.

The proposed model of the mechanistic link between LBW due to preterm birth and adult developmentally programmed hypertension and arterial vascular disease is that endothelial progenitors in cord blood of LBW infants have increased expression levels of antiangiogenic molecules. The angiostatic profile that is created is associated with substantially decreased angiogenic properties, which, if persistent, could explain the vascular abnormalities found in former LBW infants who will experience developmentally programmed hypertension in adulthood. It remains unclear whether and how the premature transition from intrauterine to extrauterine (oxygen-rich) environment affects the angiogenic properties of LBW endothelial progenitors, how long the angiogenic defects, and how interventions during early neonatal life might influence this process.

The importance of this report is that it opens the door to potential novel therapeutic interventions aimed at preventing developmentally programmed hypertension, arterial vascular disease, and perhaps other diseases characterized by abnormal angiogenesis. To learn more about cardiovascular disease and weight at birth, see the excellent commentary on the Ligi et al report by Sola-Visner.[1] Unlike the actual report of Ligi et al, the commentary is in plain English and understandable even by me.

**J. A. Stockman III, MD**

*Reference*

1. Sola-Visner M. Cardiovascular disease and weight ... at birth. *Blood*. 2011;118: 1439-1441.

## Survival Without Disability to Age 5 Years After Neonatal Caffeine Therapy for Apnea of Prematurity

Schmidt B, for the Caffeine for Apnea of Prematurity (CAP) Trial Investigators (McMaster Univ, Hamilton, Canada; et al)
*JAMA* 307:275-282, 2012

*Context.*—Very preterm infants are prone to apnea and have an increased risk of death or disability. Caffeine therapy for apnea of prematurity reduces the rates of cerebral palsy and cognitive delay at 18 months of age.

*Objective.*—To determine whether neonatal caffeine therapy has lasting benefits or newly apparent risks at early school age.

*Design, Setting, and Participants.*—Five-year follow-up from 2005 to 2011 in 31 of 35 academic hospitals in Canada, Australia, Europe, and Israel, where 1932 of 2006 participants (96.3%) had been enrolled in the randomized, placebo-controlled Caffeine for Apnea of Prematurity trial between 1999 and 2004. A total of 1640 children (84.9%) with birth weights of 500 to 1250 g had adequate data for the main outcome at 5 years.

*Main Outcome Measures.*—Combined outcome of death or survival to 5 years with 1 or more of motor impairment (defined as a Gross Motor Function Classification System level of 3 to 5), cognitive impairment (defined as a Full Scale IQ<70), behavior problems, poor general health, deafness, and blindness.

*Results.*—The combined outcome of death or disability was not significantly different for the 833 children assigned to caffeine from that for the 807 children assigned to placebo (21.1% vs 24.8%; odds ratio adjusted for center, 0.82; 95% CI, 0.65-1.03; *P*= .09). The rates of death, motor impairment, behavior problems, poor general health, deafness, and blindness did not differ significantly between the 2 groups. The incidence of cognitive impairment was lower at 5 years than at 18 months and similar in the 2 groups (4.9% vs 5.1%; odds ratio adjusted for center, 0.97; 95% CI, 0.61-1.55; *P*= .89).

*Conclusion.*—Neonatal caffeine therapy was no longer associated with a significantly improved rate of survival without disability in children with very low birth weights who were assessed at 5 years.

▶ There is a rich history going back some time about the use of caffeine as a respiratory stimulant of choice for the treatment of apnea.[1] Schmidt et al now report the results of their 5-year follow-up of infants enrolled in the Caffeine for Apnea of Prematurity (CAP) trial. This report represents the third in a series of patients enrolled from around the world that assesses the long-term effects of caffeine on neurodevelopmental outcome. In the CAP trial, infants with a birth weight of 500 to 1250 g, whose clinicians consider treatment with a methylxanthine during the first 10 days of life, were randomly assigned to receive caffeine or a placebo. The indications for treatment included the need to prevent or treat apnea or to facilitate endotracheal extubation. There was no specific endpoint to treatment, which was based solely on the clinicians' decision that it was no longer needed. Infants who were part of this trial were examined for their neurologic and developmental outcomes at 18 months using the Bayley Scales of Infant Development, which is the gold standard for neurodevelopmental assessment, at least at the time the study was conducted

The primary outcome of the CAP trial was a composite of death before 18 months and cerebral palsy, cognitive delay, severe hearing loss, or bilateral blindness at a corrected age of 18 months to 21 months. One of these outcomes was seen in 40.2% of the caffeine group compared with 46.2% of the placebo group (odds ratio adjusted for center 0.77; 95% confidence limit, 0.64—0.93, $P = .008$). Treatment with caffeine nearly halved the rate of cerebral palsy and resulted in a modest decrease in cognitive delay. Among short-term outcomes, caffeine substantially reduced the rate of bronchopulmonary dysplasia but did not affect the rates of death, brain injury detected by ultrasonography, or necrotizing enterocolitis. These findings were similar to those presented previously in the CAP trial results. When the children were 5 years of age, further neurocognitive assessments were undertaken including the Wechsler Preschool and Primary School Scale of Intelligence III, Child Behavior Checklist and Movement Assessment Battery for Children. In contrast to the earlier results, when the children were 5 years of age, CAP investigators found no effect of caffeine on the primary outcome of death or survival with severe disability, which was defined differently than in the main trial as motor or cognitive impairment, behavior problems, poor general health, deafness, or blindness. Although rates of moderate and severe cognitive impairment declined overall, the improved cognitive outcomes in the caffeine group at 18 months to 21 months relative to the control group were not sustained at 5 years, and rates of death, severe forms of cerebral palsy, behavior problems, poor general health, deafness, and blindness were no different between the groups. The improved motor function observed at 18 months to 21 months of age was sustained at 5 years. Compared with the placebo group, fewer infants treated with caffeine had any cerebral palsy, and affected children had significantly better scores on the Gross Motor Function Classification System (GMFCS) evaluation. The latter results have longer-term implications, because the GMFCS assessments at 6 years to 7 years of age are predictive of function in adult life, according to prior studies.

In a commentary that accompanied this report by Maitre and Stark,[2] it was noted that caffeine's lack of effect on the IQ of preterm infants at school age is not surprising. Although the mental development index assessment at 18 months in the original CAP trials favored the caffeine group, such cognitive scores are not necessarily predictors of school-age intelligence, thus the lack of sustained improvement in the caffeine group at 5 years reflects the poor precision of the tools available to measure cognitive function rather than any likely decline in function.

The bottom line is that although caffeine did not improve all parameters, many of the most significant outcomes from the CAP trial of caffeine were positive. As the commentary notes, all along, neonatologists were using the first safe neuroprotective agent in this vulnerable population.[2]

While on the topic of caffeine, a recent tidbit appeared in *Science News* talking about how much caffeine we get from various products.[3] The caffeine in a serving of espresso can actually vary by a factor of 6 delivering up to 322 mg—more than 6 times the published estimate for a cup of strong coffee. Researchers at the University of Glasgow College of Medical, Veterinary and Life Sciences analyzed 20 commercial espressos and attribute a wide range of observed chemical differences to how the drinks were prepared. It is obvious that consumers, including pregnant women and children and those with liver disease who may unknowingly ingest excess caffeine, are at risk of toxicity. The research obviously was done in Europe where it is not a rare phenomenon for even children to ingest a single espresso and by doing so may be drinking the equivalent of 6 cups of coffee, caffeine-wise.

It should also be noted that research done in rodents shows that a single dose of caffeine does indeed strengthen cell connection in an underappreciated part of the brain, the hippocampus. In the study commented on in *Science News* it was noted that after feeding rats a caffeine dose equivalent to 2 human cups of coffee (2 mg/kg of body weight of caffeine), investigators at the National Institute of Environmental Health Sciences in the Research Triangle Park, North Carolina were able to assess the strength of nerve cell electrical messaging in slices of brain tissue. Nerve cells in hippocampus showed a large burst of electrical activity when researchers stimulated the cells in comparison with control rats who did not imbibe any caffeine. The higher dose of caffeine, the stronger the effect. These strengthened cell connections may have a role in learning, as a main job of the hippocampus is to form spacial memories. It is unclear as yet how this research actually applies to humans. The implications for the newborn are fairly straightforward.[4]

While on the topic of caffeine, more than one medical complication has been associated with coffee. Of course there is tachycardia related to the caffeine in coffee. There is also the possibility of physical burns from spilling hot coffee on one's self. This commentary closes with updated information from scientists who have studied when and why a cup of coffee spills. Although the problem of why coffee spills may seem trivial, it actually brings together a variety of fundamental scientific issues. These include fluid mechanics, the stability of fluid surfaces, interaction between fluids and structures, and the complex biology of walking. Investigators have photographed the complex motions of coffee-filled cups carried by people, investigating the effects of walking speed and variability among individuals. Using frame-by-frame and analysis, the researchers found that after people reached their desired walking speed, motions of a cup consisted of large, regular oscillations caused by walking, as well as smaller, irregular, and more frequent motions caused by fluctuations from stride to stride, and environmental factors such as uneven floors and distractions.[5] It turns out, coffee spilling depends in large part on the natural oscillation frequency of the beverage, that is, the rate at which it prefers to oscillate, much as every pendulum swings at a precise frequency given its length and the gravitational force it experiences. When the frequency of the large, regular motions that a cup of joe experiences is comparable to its natural oscillation frequency, a state of resonance develops: the oscillations reinforce one another, much as pushing on the playground swing at the right point makes it go higher and higher. At this point, the chances of coffee sloshing its way over the edge rise. Once the key relations between coffee motion and human behavior are understood, it might be possible to develop strategies to control spilling such as using a flexible container to act as a sloshing absorber. Theoretically, a series of rings arranged up and down the inner wall of a container might also diminish the liquid oscillations. Maybe someone should make a recommendation in this regard to Starbucks. Would it not be nice to be able to carry a spill-free cup of java without fear of burning yourself?

**J. A. Stockman III, MD**

*References*

1. Henderson-Smart DJ, De Paoli AG. Methylxanthine treatment for apnoea in preterm infants. *Cochrane Database Syst Rev.* 2010;(12):CD000140.
2. Maitre NL, Stark AR. Neuroprotection for premature infants? Another perspective on caffeine. *JAMA.* 2012;307:304-305.
3. Editorial comment. For daily use. *Sci News.* January 14, 2012:4.
4. Sanders L. Coffee delivers jolt deep in brain: caffeine strengthens electrical signals in rats' hippocampus. *Sci News.* December 31, 2011:16.
5. Choi CQ. Fluid dynamics in a cup. *Scientific American.* December 2011.

---

**Pulse oximetry screening for congenital heart defects in newborn infants (PulseOx): a test accuracy study**

Ewer AK, on behalf of the PulseOx Study Group (Univ of Birmingham, UK; et al)
*Lancet* 378:785-794, 2011

---

*Background.*—Screening for congenital heart defects relies on antenatal ultrasonography and postnatal clinical examination; however, life-threatening defects often are not detected. We prospectively assessed the accuracy of pulse oximetry as a screening test for congenital heart defects.

*Methods.*—In six maternity units in the UK, asymptomatic newborn babies (gestation >34 weeks) were screened with pulse oximetry before discharge. Infants who did not achieve predetermined oxygen saturation thresholds underwent echocardiography. All other infants were followed up to 12 months of age by use of regional and national registries and clinical follow-up. The main outcome was the sensitivity and specificity of pulse oximetry for detection of critical congenital heart defects (causing death or requiring invasive intervention before 28 days) or major congenital heart disease (causing death or requiring invasive intervention within 12 months of age).

*Findings.*—20 055 newborn babies were screened and 53 had major congenital heart disease (24 critical), a prevalence of 2·6 per 1000 livebirths. Analyses were done on all babies for whom a pulse oximetry reading was obtained. Sensitivity of pulse oximetry was 75·00% (95% CI 53·29—90·23) for critical cases and 49·06% (35·06—63·16) for all major congenital heart defects. In 35 cases, congenital heart defects were already suspected after antenatal ultrasonography, and exclusion of these reduced the sensitivity to 58·33% (27·67—84·83) for critical cases and 28·57% (14·64—46·30) for all cases of major congenital heart defects. False-positive results were noted for 169 (0·8%) babies (specificity 99·16%, 99·02—99·28), of which six cases were significant, but not major, congenital heart defects, and 40 were other illnesses that required urgent medical intervention.

*Interpretation.*—Pulse oximetry is a safe, feasible test that adds value to existing screening. It identifies cases of critical congenital heart defects that go undetected with antenatal ultrasonography. The early detection of other diseases is an additional advantage.

▶ The report of Ewer et al adds one more piece of information in the debate about universal screening of newborns with pulse oximetry for the detection of some forms of congenital heart disease. If the results of this study were applied to a population of 100 000 babies, roughly 264 would have major congenital heart defects based on known data from the literature. Of these, 130 would be identified by the use of pulse oximetry. About 120 babies would have critical lesions, and 90 of these would be detected by use of pulse oximetry. If an antenatal detection rate of 50% is assumed in identifying babies before birth with congenital heart disease, pulse oximetry could detect an additional 35 cases of critical congenital heart defects. This number, of course, is likely to be higher in areas with lower rates of detection with antenatal ultrasonography. The math also shows that pulse oximetry is also likely to detect 30 cases of significant congenital heart defects and 199 cases of respiratory or infectious illness that might require medical attention. On the other hand, of 100 000 babies, 843 would have an abnormal pulse oximetry but not have critical or serious congenital heart defects (false positives), but only 614 would be completely healthy (ie, no congenital heart defects or other illness). These numbers would vary drastically depending on what cutoffs were used to determine what an acceptable pulse oximetry reading is. For example, if the investigators had used a postductal saturation threshold of less than 95%, the number of false positives would have been reduced by 84, but 3 critical cases (2 with hypoplastic left heart syndrome identified antenatally and 1 with coarctation of the aorta that was not diagnosed antenatally), 1 serious case (truncus arteriosus not suspected antenatally), 2 babies with significant congenital heart defects, and 9 with respiratory disorders would have been missed.

Routine screening with pulse oximetry looks increasingly feasible. Screening tests in the newborn period need not have an extremely high sensitivity to be acceptable. For example, although screening for congenital adrenal hyperplasia has a sensitivity of just 70%, it is widely endorsed. As such, pulse oximetry can be considered to be similar to some other commonly accepted screening strategies. The cost of pulse oximetry has been questioned relative to its benefit, but in one analysis, the cost was estimated to be just $0.99 per infant when screening was done by a technician.[1]

For an excellent review of pulse oximetry in pediatric practice, see the report of Fouzas et al.[2]

This commentary ends with a query. Might there be so many alarms going off at any one time in an intensive care unit that they are ignored? The answer comes from a recent report that documents that up to 94% of alarms are false. The same study found that by introducing a 19-second alarm delay, 67% of the false alarms would be removed.[3]

**J. A. Stockman III, MD**

*References*

1. Grosse SD, Mahle WT, Koppel RI. Cost effectiveness of routine pulse oximetry examination of newborns in the United States [abstract]. Presented at the 30th Annual Meeting of the Society for Medical Decision Making Annual Meeting; October 19, 2008; Philadelphia, PA; E26.
2. Fouzas S, Priftis KN, Anthracopoulos MB. Pulse oximetry in pediatric practice. *Pediatrics.* 2011;128:740-752.
3. Görges M, Markewitz BA, Westenskoro DR. Improving alarm performance in the medical intensive care unit using delays and clinical context. *Anesth Analg.* 2009; 108:1546-1552.

---

**Impact of prenatal evaluation and protocol-based perinatal management on congenital diaphragmatic hernia outcomes**
Lazar DA, Cass DL, Rodriguez MA, et al (Texas Children's Hosp, Houston; et al)
*J Pediatr Surg* 46:808-813, 2011

---

*Background/Purpose.*—Although intuitive, the benefit of prenatal evaluation and multidisciplinary perinatal management for fetuses with congenital diaphragmatic hernia (CDH) is unproven. We compared the outcome of prenatally diagnosed patients with CDH whose perinatal management was by a predefined protocol with those who were diagnosed postnatally and managed by the same team. We hypothesized that patients with CDH undergoing prenatal evaluation with perinatal planning would demonstrate improved outcome.

*Methods.*—Retrospective chart review of all patients with Bochdalek-type CDH at a single institution between 2004 and 2009 was performed.

Patients were stratified by history of perinatal management, and data were analyzed by Fisher's Exact test and Student's *t* test.

*Results.*—Of 116 patients, 71 fetuses presented in the prenatal period and delivered at our facility (PRE), whereas 45 infants were either outborn or postnatally diagnosed (POST). There were more high-risk patients in the PRE group compared with the POST group as indicated by higher rates of liver herniation (63% vs 36%, $P = .03$), need for patch repair (57% vs 27%, $P = .004$), and extracorporeal membrane oxygenation use (35% vs 18%, $P = .05$). Despite differences in risk, there was no difference in 6-month survival between groups (73% vs 73%).

*Conclusions.*—Patients with CDH diagnosed prenatally are a higher risk group. Prenatal evaluation and multidisciplinary perinatal management allows for improved outcome in these patients.

▶ This report contains a tremendous amount of information about the up-to-date management of congenital diaphragmatic hernia with respect to both diagnosis and management. In the current era, the management of congenital diaphragmatic hernia (CDH) has focused on the early and aggressive treatment of pulmonary pathology rather than solely on the repair of the anatomic defect. These techniques have included gentle ventilation, extracorporeal membrane oxygenation (ECMO), and the advanced medical management of pulmonary hypertension. Astonishing results have resulted from such approaches. Survival rates just a generation ago hovered around 50%. Now survival rates have approached or surpassed 90% in many series of care with CDH.

What has not been so clear in terms of management is whether the diagnosis is best made prenatally or whether it does not matter if one does not detect CDH until the child is born. Most analyses have compared current results with those of historical controls or have had insufficient numbers spread out over many years with variations in management; thus, conclusions have not been able to be drawn about the role of prenatal diagnosis. This report from Houston, Texas tells us about the role of prenatal diagnosis. Patients at Texas Children's Fetal Center were divided into those who were diagnosed prenatally and delivered in the major medical center versus those who were diagnosed postnatally and transferred to that medical center. Based on liver position, patch repair, or ECMO use, the experience at Texas Children's Hospital shows that prenatally managed children comprise a higher risk cohort than those postnatally diagnosed. Intuitively, this actually makes sense because severe lesions are more apparent on prenatal imaging and result in the selection of a group of individuals with more severe diaphragmatic hernias for prenatal diagnosis and management. Furthermore, multiple reports have suggested that overall survival is worse for fetuses with prenatally diagnosed CDH compared with those diagnosed at birth or presenting to a neonatal surgical center. Patients who are born at another facility (out born) and transferred to tertiary centers are those who were likely to be more stable enough to survive the immediate resuscitation and stabilization. Some infants (presumably those with more severe disease) do not survive this critical early period and are not reflected in the mortality rates reported by tertiary centers.

The data from Texas Children's Hospital clearly suggest that prenatal evaluation with protocol-based perinatal management may offer a survival advantage for patients with CDH. A recent report from the Department of Surgery at the Hospital for Sick Children in Toronto also shows that in general, out-born delivery is a significant predictor of mortality for infants with antenatally diagnosed CDH.[1] Clearly, if a fetus with CDH is diagnosed prenatally, delivery in a tertiary care center is highly advised.

If you are tired of reading about neonatal-perinatal medicine, look up a rather "spicy" editorial by Isaacs et al.[2] These authors remind us that life is a fatal sexually transmitted disease, but nonetheless, modern medicine can ease your life journey from womb to tomb or (if you are Dutch or Swiss) from youth to euthanasia. Isaacs et al describe 7 ages of man and woman. The first is conception. We are reminded that if you are unable to conceive naturally despite the assistance of modern radiology, modern fetal medicine can do it for you in the privacy of your own womb. It is stated that in vitro fertilization is the only way to populate a nation. Lie down, close your eyes, and medicine will fertilize. Johnson and Johnson will succeed where Masters and Johnson has failed. The second stage is the womb. This is the stage where the modern ultrasonographer is also the family photographer. Can you conceive of anything finer than a silver-framed ultrasound print of your baby, basking in a warm pool of amniotic fluid? Won't your friends and relatives envy the "womb" with a view hanging above one's mantelpiece? Such images of little fetus can be used on Christmas cards to illustrate the fruits of one's labors, past and future. Stage 3 of the 7 stages of man and woman is one's birth. Labor is no more. To preserve one's figure, reduce pain and prevent those pesky prolapse problems; the modern obstetrician's mode of delivery is the vaginal bypass operation, now commonly known as VBO, once quaintly called a cesarean section. The fourth stage of age is childhood. This is the time where all of us learned to not be responsive to the question "are we nearly there yet?" state Isaacs et al. The usual squabbling really is a minor form of ADHD which can be readily managed with babies being weaned directly onto a preservative-free Ritalin-reinforced formula best called: "Peace At Last." The fifth age as one might suspect is adolescence. There is not much to say about adolescence or the adolescent, according to Isaacs et al. This is the time best described as the Neanderthal period punctuated communication-wise by grunts. Males tend to spend the most of their time in the horizontal position while females seem glued to a mobile phone. The sixth age is adulthood and the seventh is old age. Adulthood is a chronic midlife crisis simply bridging adolescence and old age. For many, such a period of life is a gruel of a daily mixture of a 2000-calorie diet, which is also low-fat and alcohol-free, taken with a chaser of statins, beta blockers and antidepressants, all of which may not help one live longer, only wishing one could. As far as old age is concerned, the modern geriatrician no longer describes this as "Olden is Golden," rather with the motto: "Out of the Stone Age and into the Bone Age." This is the age where many opportunities are provided to orthopedic surgeons who gain more experience with joints than a hippie from the 60s. Isaacs et al remind us that the modern geriatrician has just one "get-out" clause, the "Three Strokes and You're Out" rule.

**J. A. Stockman III, MD**

*References*

1. Nasr A, Langer JC. Influence of location of delivery on outcome in neonates with congenital diaphragmatic hernia. *J Pediatr Surg.* 2011;46:814-816.
2. Isaacs D, Isaacs S, Fitzgerald D. The seven ages of man and woman (or "Sex and the CT"). *Arch Dis Child.* 2008;93:1075-1076.

# 15 Nutrition and Metabolism

## Folic Acid Supplements in Pregnancy and Severe Language Delay in Children

Roth C, Magnus P, Schjølberg S, et al (Norwegian Inst of Public Health, Oslo, Norway; et al)
*JAMA* 306:1566-1573, 2011

*Context.*—Prenatal folic acid supplements reduce the risk of neural tube defects and may have beneficial effects on other aspects of neuro-development.

*Objective.*—To examine associations between mothers' use of prenatal folic acid supplements and risk of severe language delay in their children at age 3 years.

*Design, Setting, and Patients.*—The prospective observational Norwegian Mother and Child Cohort Study recruited pregnant women between 1999 and December 2008. Data on children born before 2008 whose mothers returned the 3-year follow-up questionnaire by June 16, 2010, were used. Maternal use of folic acid supplements within the interval from 4 weeks before to 8 weeks after conception was the exposure. Relative risks were approximated by estimating odds ratios (ORs) with 95% CIs in a logistic regression analysis.

*Main Outcome Measure.*—Children's language competency at age 3 years measured by maternal report on a 6-point ordinal language grammar scale. Children with minimal expressive language (only 1-word or unintelligible utterances) were rated as having severe language delay.

*Results.*—Among 38 954 children, 204 (0.5%) had severe language delay. Children whose mothers took no dietary supplements in the specified exposure interval were the reference group (n = 9052 [24.0%], with severe language delay in 81 children [0.9%]). Adjusted ORs for 3 patterns of exposure to maternal dietary supplements were (1) other supplements, but no folic acid (n = 2480 [6.6%], with severe language delay in 22 children [0.9%]; OR, 1.04; 95% CI, 0.62-1.74); (2) folic acid only (n = 7127 [18.9%], with severe language delay in 28 children [0.4%]; OR, 0.55; 95% CI, 0.35-0.86); and (3) folic acid in combination with other supplements (n = 19 005 [50.5%], with severe language delay in 73 children [0.4%]; OR, 0.55; 95% CI, 0.39-0.78).

*Conclusion.*—Among this Norwegian cohort of mothers and children, maternal use of folic acid supplements in early pregnancy was associated with a reduced risk of severe language delay in children at age 3 years.

▶ We have known for years that folic acid supplementation during pregnancy is critical for neural tube development and that inadequate amounts of folic acid in the diet of pregnant women can lead to neural tube defects at a much higher than expected prevalence. What has not been looked at, however, is what the effect is of folic acid on neurologic development subsequent to birth in otherwise normal-appearing children at the time of birth. This is what Roth et al have attempted to address by exploring the Norwegian Mother and Child Cohort Study (NMCCS). They investigated whether maternal use of folic acid supplements would be associated with a reduced risk of severe language delay in offspring. Interestingly, unlike the United States, Norway does not fortify foods with folic acid. Thus, women who do not take supplements of folic acid during pregnancy are much more likely than women in the United States to have inadequate amounts of folic acid in their diet while pregnant.

The NMCCS yielded information on almost 30 children born between 1999 and the end of December 2008. The investigators examined the relationship between severe language delay in children at age 3 years and maternal use of dietary supplements in the period 4 weeks before to 8 weeks after conception. It was observed that maternal use of supplements during this time was associated with a substantially reduced risk of severe language delay in children at age 3 years. The authors found no association, however, between maternal use of folic acid supplements and significant delay in gross motor skills by 3 years of age. No previous observational study has examined the relation of prenatal folic acid supplements to severe language delay in children. The major strength of this study was the prospective design, in which pregnant women were followed from week 17 of pregnancy. Another strength of the study was that it was conducted in a single country (Norway) that does not fortify food with folic acid, allowing an analysis where folic acid supplements would not therefore eclipse dietary sources of folate.

This report does not provide information about the mechanisms through which folic acid supplements have a protective effect on language development. The authors speculate that folic acid supplements may facilitate reversal or compensation of the epigenetic effects of other early prenatal exposures that disrupt neurodevelopment.

This report has profound implications for public policy regarding folic acid supplementation during pregnancy and routine supplementation of folic acid in commonly available foods. It is probably purely by happenstance that people in the United States are perhaps preventing many children from experiencing language delay by the widely available amount of folic acid that is laced into a variety of foods.

While on the topic of vitamins, while it was well recognized that sailors frequently died of scurvy before the mid-1700s, what was not recognized was that after this period, lead poisoning was also a major cause of death in seafarers. Take for example the 6 sealing vessels off the coast of Sweden. In September

1872, these vessels were forced into a bay and then bound in ice, trapping 6 ships and 59 sealers with the prospect of "overwintering" with few provisions. 17 men managed to set off to spend the winter in the Swedish House at Capp Thordsen in Isfjorden. The remainder stayed on their ships and actually survived when the ice broke up and they were able to sail away. The men at Capp Thordsen hunted polar bear and reindeer until the arctic night descended and then relied on stored tinned food that had been abandoned in the Swedish house. There was more than ample food in these tinned cans. Over the next 6 months, one by one these men died, their deaths being attributed to scurvy. In 2009, investigators from Norway braved the permafrost to examine bones of these buried sailors and documented, without question, that all died of lead poisoning. Rusting tin cans were found all about the house and the solder used to seal the cans contained 40% lead. The sailors probably heated their food in the tin cans on their stove, exposing the lead alloy to acid and dissolving the lead into the food. In retrospect, in 1845 another similar series of deaths occurred. It was in that year that Admiral John Franklin set out with 129 men and 2 ships to find the Northwest Passage. They took huge amounts of tinned food. The expedition was equipped for 4 years, but was never heard from again. Final evidence of the disaster came in 1859, when a written account of their ordeal was found in a crumble of stones. The ships had been wrecked by ice, and the men eventually started to walk south, dying as they walked. In the 1980s, a team from Alberta University exhumed 3 sailors buried in permafrost at the expedition's winter quarters and found high concentrations of lead in hair samples. Bones from crew members found scattered along the track showed high concentrations of lead while Inuit bones did not. The conclusion was that the sailors had lead poisoning, leading to their deaths.

By the way, scurvy, caused by lack of vitamin C, was the plague of seafarers until its prevention was discovered in 1753; an intake of lime juice was implemented in the British Navy in 1795. Obviously this is how the British Navy sailor got his name: "Limey."[1]

**J. A. Stockman III, MD**

*Reference*

1. Aasebo U, Kjaer KG. Lead poisoning at the Swedish House. *BMJ.* 2009;339:1404.

---

**Pediatric Vitamin D Deficiency in a Southwestern Luminous Climate**
Szalay EA, Tryon EB, Pleacher MD, et al (Univ of New Mexico School of Medicine, Albuquerque; Univ of New Mexico Carrie Tingley Hosp, Albuquerque)
*J Pediatr Orthop* 31:469-473, 2011

---

*Background.*—Few studies look at vitamin D levels in children living in sunny climates as it is assumed that they receive adequate vitamin D from sun exposure. In light of changing lifestyles of children and studies documenting vitamin D deficiency among children in extreme climates, a study to examine vitamin D levels in healthy children living in a luminous climate was conducted.

*Methods.*—A retrospective chart review of vitamin D levels in healthy children with vague musculoskeletal pain (such as "growing pains") was done. Healthy children, specifically without musculoskeletal pain, were prospectively recruited as controls.

*Results.*—Eighty-eight children, 42 children with "pain" and 46 controls were studied. No statistical difference in vitamin D levels was found between the "pain" group (mean vitamin D level 29.1 ng/mL) and the control group (mean vitamin D level 32.4 ng/mL, $P < 0.52$). Overall, 14% of the entire group had levels < 20 ng/mL, 49% had levels < 30 ng/mL, and 15% had levels > 40 ng/mL.

*Conclusions.*—A consensus has yet to be established as to what an "optimal" vitamin D level is for growing children to develop strong bones for a lifetime. This study demonstrated that 14% of children living in a sunny climate had vitamin D levels below 20 ng/mL, a level universally accepted as insufficient, and 49% were below 30 ng/mL, arguably a "desired" level. A sunny climate does not assure vitamin D sufficiency. Virtually all children should be supplemented, with laboratory follow-up for those at high risk for low bone density/those with insufficiency fractures.

▶ Although the recommended daily dose of 400 IU is considered to be adequate for the prevention of rickets, there is no consensus on what serum vitamin D levels truly optimize bone health in children. The Institute of Medicine and the American Academy of Pediatrics have defined vitamin D deficiency as a serum 25 hydroxy vitamin D level less than 11 ng/mL. Most experts define vitamin D insufficiency as 25 hydroxy vitamin D levels less than 20 ng/mL. In adults, there are adequate data to show evidence of impaired calcium absorption and lower bone density levels at levels less than 32 ng/mL. Just as important, parathyroid hormone levels begin to increase when vitamin D levels decrease to less than 40 ng/mL. Even more modest levels of vitamin D insufficiency are known to produce musculoskeletal pain, but no threshold serum level has been established relative to this relationship.

To prevent vitamin D deficiency and insufficiency, our Maker has given us sunshine. Deficiency of solar exposure is generally not considered to be a problem in the sun-rich American southwest. In that and many other parts of the country, pediatricians concerned about chronic sun exposure commonly recommend regular use of topical sunscreen. Application of topical sunscreen with a sun protection factor (SPF) of 8 effectively prevents vitamin D production by the skin. At the same time parents are more and more frequently using sunscreen on their children, the amount of time that children play outside is diminishing.

Szalay et al, recognizing the changing lifestyles of children and the increasing prevalence of vitamin D deficiency among children with chronic illnesses, decided to look at vitamin D levels in healthy children in a southwest, sunny climate. The latter was chosen because if there is a problem there, there is likely a problem everywhere with vitamin D deficiency or insufficiency. A study was carried out in Albuquerque, New Mexico, which has a latitude of 31° north and a climate offering virtually year-round sunshine and outdoor recreational activities in all seasons. The investigators examined children who had chronic leg pain thought to be "growing pains," having excluded other causes of leg pain such as from inflammatory arthritis and orthopedic disorders including Legg Perthes disease. Forty-two children with complaints of pain and 46 controls were included in the study for a total of 88 children. Most of the children in the "pain" group complained of intermittent pain that had been present for months to years often awakening them at night. All children in this study had normal complete blood counts, antinuclear antibody studies, erythrocyte sedimentation rates, and in most instances a rheumatoid factor or C-reactive protein. The data from this report showed there was no statistical difference in vitamin D levels between the "pain" group (mean 25 hydroxy vitamin D level 29.1 ng/mL) and the control group (mean 25 hydroxy vitamin D level 32.4 ng/mL). Overall serum vitamin D levels ranged from less than 10 to 55 ng/mL. The mean serum vitamin D level for the entire group was 30.8 ng/mL. There was no significant difference in the ethnicity between the study group and controls.

Although there have been several studies suggesting that low levels of vitamin D can result in musculoskeletal pain, the report from Albuquerque did not correlate serum vitamin D levels with vague musculoskeletal pain. This is a study that had a carefully drawn control group, unlike prior studies. What should be noted, however, is despite a latitude of 31° north and a climate offering year-round sunshine, 14% of both study and control children in Albuquerque demonstrated a serum vitamin D level less than 20 ng/mL, a level that can be associated with rachitic changes, and 49% of children had a level less than 30 ng/mL, which is often defined as minimal sufficiency. Only 15% of the group overall had levels greater than 40 ng/mL, a level universally considered to be sufficient for vitamin D.

The bottom line here is that if vitamin D insufficiency and deficiency can occur in Albuquerque, it certainly can occur anywhere. In this study, interestingly, daily multivitamin use had little effect on vitamin D serum levels. Thirteen percent of the control group actually took a multivitamin daily, whereas 57% reported having never taken a vitamin. The average vitamin D levels of children who always took a multivitamin were quite comparable to those who never took a multivitamin. This suggests 400 IU vitamin D a day is insufficient to affect vitamin D levels in these children and that recommendations for 400 IU of vitamin D a day are set at unrealistically low levels for the prevention of osteoporosis and bone fractures. This study suggests that children might best take 1000 IU of vitamin D a day, the equivalent of drinking ten 8-ounce glasses of milk or the ingestion of certain oily fish every day (one serving of salmon, mackerel, sardines contains 300 IU to 500 IU) with several glasses of milk. Obviously this is an unrealistic approach for the prevention of vitamin D deficiency. Fortunately, vendors are now offering child-friendly vitamin D supplements. Vitamin D3 can be purchased in small tablets or capsules. Gummy forms and liquid are also available. Vitamin D3 is preferred, as vitamin D2 has only one-third the potency of vitamin D3.

There clearly are children at greater risk from vitamin D deficiency than others. Some, for example, on seizure medication require dosing of vitamin D in amounts of 4000 to 5000 IU/d, and in this population, monitoring of blood levels does seem warranted. Vitamin D as a fat-soluble vitamin does have the potential for toxicity, although this is rarely seen at serum levels less than 150 ng/mL.

This important report raises a lot of questions about how we have been approaching the prevention of vitamin D insufficiency and deficiency. A lot of attention is being paid these days to vitamin D sufficiency in children and adults. Hopefully we can learn a lot more about how to better prevent the consequences of not taking enough vitamin D or not having enough sun exposure to make our own. As an aside, a recent report has found that infants who are born with vitamin D deficiency appear to have an increased risk of severe lower respiratory infection development compared with infants born with sufficient amounts of vitamin D. Of 156 newborns, the 23% with the lowest vitamin D concentrations in serum had a 6-fold increased risk of respiratory infection compared with the 46% of infants born with the highest vitamin D concentrations.[1]

**J. A. Stockman III, MD**

*Reference*

1. Editorial comment. Low vitamin D infection risk. *JAMA.* 2011;305:2279.

---

### Normal Hemoglobin at the Age of 1 Year Does not Protect Infants From Developing Iron Deficiency Anemia in the Second Year of Life

Moser AM, Urkin J, Shalev H (Ben-Gurion Univ of the Negev, Be'er Sheva, Israel)
*J Pediatr Hematol Oncol* 33:467-469, 2011

---

*Background.*—Iron deficiency anemia (IDA) is the most common hematologic disorder worldwide. Measures to prevent IDA in infants have been successful with questionable sustainability.

*Aim.*—To evaluate the incidence of developing IDA in the second year of life, in infants who were nonanemic at the age of 1 year on routine blood test.

*Methods.*—Blood samples were obtained from 193, 24-month-old toddlers, from 2 large clinics of both main sectors in Southern Israel, comparable for lower economic status. IDA was defined as hemoglobin < 11 gr% and microcytosis as mean corpuscular volume < 70 fL.

*Results.*—IDA was detected in 8 of 118 Bedouins (5 males) and in 10 of 75 Jewish (6 males) infants ($P < 0.01$). The probability of a nonanemic child to develop IDA in the second year of life for the whole study population was 9.3% (18 of 193 infants) and significantly higher in the Jewish population (13.3.0% vs. 6.8%, $P < 0.01$).

*Conclusions.*—Given the difficulty of toddlers to maintain a non-IDA status, and the very low probability of iron overload, our results clearly support the need to continue iron supplementation into the second year.

▶ This report emanates from Israel. There is no reason, however, to believe that the exact same findings would not be seen in the United States. In Israel, a unique governmental network of well-baby clinics is responsible for the routine care and vaccination of all infants up to 3 years of age. As such, most of the caregivers adhere to the Israeli Ministry of Health recommendation to supplement iron during the first year of life. The investigators from Israel have the opportunity to evaluate the incidence of iron deficiency anemia developing in toddlers (beyond age 1), particularly those who were nonanemic at age 12 months when the usual screenings are done for iron deficiency, as is generally true in the United States as well. As per the Israeli Ministry of Health guidelines, iron supplementation prescriptions were discontinued at age 12 months for nonanemic infants. Preterm infants and infants with chronic illness were excluded from the study. The study group consisted of 193 infants. Although all the infants studied were neither anemic nor microcytic at age 12 months, the mean hemoglobin of the infants with iron deficiency anemia decreased at the 24-month test by an average of 0.7 g/dL to 10.6 ± 0.29 g/dL. The mean corpuscular values of infants with iron deficiency at age 2 decreased by an average of 5.1 fL to 67 ± 2.97 fL (range, 64-71 fL). The calculated probability of a nonanemic child developing iron deficiency anemia in the second year of life was 9.3% (18 of 193 infants) and slightly higher in a Jewish population compared with Bedouin toddlers who were also enrolled in this study.

The data from this report underscore recommendations to supplement with iron at least up to 12 months of age and also not to assume that stopping iron at that age sets one up for success with respect to the development of anemia in the second year of life. Iron supplementation for 12 months does not necessarily protect an infant from developing iron deficiency anemia.

The authors of this report suggest that if iron supplementation is discontinued at 1 year (the most common approach used here on our shores), one should be very vigilant about taking careful dietary history on an ongoing basis and perhaps also to screen for iron deficiency at 18 to 24 months of age. The latter recommendation has been one long espoused by Dr Alvin Eden in New York.[1] Folks should be listening to Dr Eden on these points. He is absolutely correct in advocating for screening for iron deficiency during the second year of life.[2]

This commentary closes with mention of data related to the risks of eating red meat, a great source of iron but a problem for other reasons. Further evidence of a link between red meat and poor health has emerged from a large cohort of older US adults. Men and women in the top fifth of red meat intake have a significantly higher risk of death over 10 years than men and women in the bottom fifth (hazard ratio for men 1.31; for women 1.36). The highest risk seems to be related to the intake of processed meats such as bacon, ham, and sausage. The study involved 545 653 adults between the ages of 50 and 71 who completed detailed fit histories dating back to 1995. By 2005, more than 71 000 of these individuals had passed away. These large numbers mean the authors were able to estimate with some precision the exact risks associated with eating red and processed meats for both men and women. The analyses were fully adjusted for other lifestyle factors likely to influence lifespan, such as smoking. These data add to other observational studies that suggest we should all eat less red and processed meats, not least because the increasing consumption of meat in many countries is putting a strain on global supplies of water, energy, and food in general, suggesting that it is far less expensive to grow vegetables and grains as opposed to growing animals for their meat.[3]

**J. A. Stockman III, MD**

*References*

1. Eden AN. Iron deficiency and impaired cognition in toddlers: an underestimated and undertreated problem. *Paediatr Drugs.* 2005;7:347-352.
2. Eden AN, Mir MA. Iron deficiency in 1- to 3-year-old children? A pediatric failure? *Arch Pediatr Adolesc Med.* 1997;151:986-988.
3. Sinha R, Cross AJ, Graubard BI, Leitzmann MF, Schatzkin A. Meat intake and mortality. *Arch Intern Med.* 2009;169:562-571.

## Factors Associated With Exclusive Breastfeeding in the United States

Jones JR, Kogan MD, Singh GK, et al (Maternal and Child Health Bureau, Rockville, MD; et al)
*Pediatrics* 128:1117-1125, 2011

*Objectives.*—To estimate the proportions of US infants who were breastfed exclusively for 6 months, according to characteristics of the mother, child, and household environment, and to compare associations between those characteristics and exclusive breastfeeding with associations between those characteristics and breastfeeding initiation.

*Methods.*—Data were obtained from the 2007 National Survey of Children's Health, a nationally representative, cross-sectional survey. Multivariate logistic regression was used to calculate the adjusted odds ratios for breastfeeding among all infants and for breastfeeding exclusively for 6 months among infants who had initiated breastfeeding. All analyses were limited to children aged 6 months through 5 years for whom breastfeeding data were available (N = 25 197).

*Results.*—Of the nearly 75% of children in the study who had ever been breastfed, 16.8% had been breastfed exclusively for 6 months. Non-Hispanic black children were significantly less likely to have ever been breastfed compared with their non-Hispanic white counterparts (adjusted odds ratio: 0.54 [95% confidence interval: 0.44−0.66]). However, no significant differences in the odds of exclusive breastfeeding according to race were observed. Children with birth weights of <1500 g were most likely to have ever been breastfed and least likely to have been breastfed exclusively. Maternal age was significantly associated with exclusive breastfeeding; however, maternal age was not associated with breastfeeding initiation.

*Conclusions.*—In the United States, the prevalence of exclusive breastfeeding for 6 months remains low among those who initiate breastfeeding. Factors associated with breastfeeding exclusively for 6 months differ from those associated with breastfeeding initiation.

▶ It is about time that an updated report has appeared in the literature about factors associated with exclusive breastfeeding. Exclusive breastfeeding for the first 6 months of life has been strongly recommended by many organizations involved with the care of children, including the American Academy of Pediatrics and its Section on Breastfeeding. Such a recommendation is in place for all infants in whom breastfeeding is not specifically contraindicated. These recommendations are based on numerous well-documented benefits of breastfeeding for both mothers and children, including greater reductions in an infant's risk for specific negative health problems, including gastrointestinal and respiratory infection. Breastfeeding also has monetary benefits. Results of a recent cost analysis indicated that if 90% of US newborns were fed exclusively for the first 6 months of life, direct medical cost would be reduced by approximately $2.2 billion per year.[1]

According to recent estimates from the National Immunization Survey, only 14.1% of children who were born in 2006 were exclusively breastfed for 9 months.[2] In Healthy People 2020, the prevalence target for 6-month exclusive breastfeeding is 20.5%, and the prevalence target for overall breastfeeding initiation was set at 81.9%.[3] Studies have looked at what has affected breastfeeding prevalence. These studies showed disparities according to race, family income, and population density as well as mother's age, educational level, marital status, and body mass index. The report abstracted deals with other characteristics associated with breastfeeding based on information from the 2007 National Survey of Children's Health.

The results of the national survey that was the basis of this report documented that although nearly 75% of US children were breastfed, the vast majority were not breastfed exclusively for 6 months. Non Hispanic black women were less likely than non-Hispanic white women to initiate breastfeeding. This disparity in breastfeeding was suggested to be the result in part from increased comfort with formula feeding among black women, compared with nonblack women, and this initial acceptance of formula feeding is an important consideration for the promotion of both breastfeeding initiation and exclusive breastfeeding for 6 months. No association could be seen, however, between race and the likelihood of having been breastfed exclusively for 6 months if breastfeeding was initially started, suggesting that differences in rates of exclusive breastfeeding between black and white infants are primarily the result of lower rates of breastfeeding initiation among black infants. The report found that maternal mental and emotional health were significantly associated with exclusive breastfeeding for 6 months but not associated with breastfeeding initiation. Postpartum depression increased the odds of early breastfeeding cessation. Mother's age was strongly associated with the likelihood of breastfeeding exclusively for 6 months. Younger mothers are more likely not to breastfeed.

So we learn from this report that despite a substantial increase in the initiation of breastfeeding in the United States over the past quarter century, few US children are breastfed exclusively for the first 6 months of their life. It is clear that the determinants of exclusive breastfeeding for 6 months do differ somewhat from those of breastfeeding initiation. At greatest risk for unsustained breastfeeding is being a young mother, a mother with poor mental or emotional health resources, and being a mother of a very-low—birth weight infant. These groups should be heavily targeted to assist them with achieving a greater probability of sustained breastfeeding for the first 6 months of life.

**J. A. Stockman III, MD**

*References*

1. Bartick M, Reinhold A. The burden of suboptimal breastfeeding in the United States: a pediatric cost analysis. *Pediatrics.* 2010;125:e1048-e1056.

2. Centers for Disease Control and Prevention (CDC). Breastfeeding among US born children 2000–2008, CDC national immunization survey. http://www.CDC.gov/breastfeeding/data/NIS_data. Accessed February 4, 2010.

3. US Department of health and Human Services. Healthy people 2020: maternal, infant and child health: objectives. http://www.healthypeople.gov/2020/topicsobjectives 2020/objectiveslist.aspx?topicid=26. Accessed February 4, 2012.

## Heating-Induced Bacteriological and Biochemical Modifications in Human Donor Milk After Holder Pasteurisation

de Segura AG, Escuder D, Montilla A, et al (Universidad Complutense de Madrid, Spain; Hospital Universitario 12 de Octubre, Madrid, Spain; Instituto de Investigación en Ciencias de la Alimentación, Madrid, Spain)
*J Pediatr Gastroenterol Nutr* 54:197-203, 2012

*Objectives.*—The objectives of the present study were to enumerate and characterize the pathogenic potential of the *Bacillus* population that may survive holder pasteurisation of human milk and to evaluate the nutritional damage of this treatment using the furosine and lactulose indexes.

*Materials and Methods.*—Milk samples from 21 donors were heated at 62.5°C for 30 minutes. Bacterial counts, lactose, glucose, myoinositol, lactulose, and furosine were determined before and after the heat treatment. Some *B cereus* isolates that survived after pasteurisation were evaluated for toxigenic potential.

*Results.*—Nonpasteurised milk samples showed bacterial growth in most of the agar media tested. Bacterial survival after pasteurisation was observed in only 3 samples and, in these cases, the microorganisms isolated belonged to the species *B cereus*. Furosine could not be detected in any of the samples, whereas changes in lactose, glucose, and myoinositol concentrations after holder pasteurisation were not relevant. Lactulose was below the detection limit of the analytical method in nonpasteurised samples, whereas it was found at low levels in 62% of the samples after holder pasteurisation. The lactation period influenced myoinositol content because its concentration was significantly higher in transition milk than in mature or late lactation milk samples.

*Conclusions.*—Holder pasteurisation led to the destruction of bacteria present initially in donor milk samples, except for some *B cereus* that did not display a high virulence potential and did not modify significantly the concentration of the compounds analyzed in the present study.

▶ Hopefully, no one will argue that mother's milk is the first choice for all newborns, including preterm infants, and when it is not available or not sufficient, donor human milk is a valid alternative. Generally speaking, fresh mother's milk is the first choice not only for term infants, but also for preterm infants. In these tiny infants, fresh mother's milk, when administered within 24 hours, does not require routine culturing or heat treatment. Donor human milk does need to be checked microbiologically and should undergo heat treatment and storage procedures. For human milk banks, pasteurization at 62.5°C for 30 minutes is recommended.

This is known as "Holder" pasteurization. Holder pasteurization allows a good compromise between microbiologic safety and nutritional/biological quality of donor human milk. However, pasteurization does affect some of the nutritional and biological properties of human milk and eliminates the beneficial microbiota present that are good to populate an infant's gut.

The report of de Segura et al focuses attention on the effects of pasteurization on the bacteria present in the initial fresh samples of human milk and on potential nutritional damage. The investigators note that pasteurization at 62.5°C for 30 minutes will lead to the loss of beneficial microbiota present in fresh milk and that spore-forming bacteria such as *Bacillus cereus* may survive the heating process. A reassuring observation is that because the counts of such strains in milk samples were low, the presence of toxins in donor milk is improbable. Another reassuring result from the study is that Holder pasteurization does not significantly modify the concentrations of furosine and lactulose, the biochemical indices used to evaluate the potential nutritional damage resulting from heat treatment.

The study of de Segura et al reminds us of the inadequacy of pasteurization methods for donated human milk used today in the majority of human milk banks to make it safe for feeding premature infants. Clearly, different methodologies for treatment should be investigated. Rapid pasteurization at 72°C for 5 or 10 seconds is a method that seems superior to Holder pasteurization achieving a better compromise between microbiologic safety and nutritional and biological quality of human milk. Unfortunately, this method of pasteurization requires a fairly heavy technological investment and is available only at the industrial level. Studies done thus far show that rapid pasteurization retains the protein profile and many of the biological components of donor human milk, including IgA, lactoferrin, and lipase. In addition, the combination of ultrasound and heat (thermoultrasound) is an emerging food preservation technique that retains higher quantities of bioactive components compared with thermopasteurization. Techniques do not yet exist to allow a scale up to large production levels as of this time, however. High-pressure processing is another method that shows promise as an alternative for the pasteurization of human milk, as is Ohmic heating. Ohmic heating is an advanced thermal processing method wherein the food material, which serves as an electric resistor, is heated by passing electricity through it. The electrical energy is dissipated into heat. It results in rapid and uniform heating. Unlike conventional thermal processing, Ohmic heating heats an entire mass of food quickly and uniformly. More studies are necessary to evaluate the theoretical advantages of such new technologies.

To read more about new methods for pasteurization of human milk, see the excellent commentary by Moro and Arslanoglu.[1] Because of the actual limitations of current pasteurization techniques for the heat treatment of human milk, there is a strong need to investigate alternative pasteurization methods that are capable of retaining the bioactivity of a wider range of human milk components with the highest level of microbiologic safety, including protection against spore-forming bacteria.

**J. A. Stockman III, MD**

*Reference*

1. Moro GE, Arslanoglu S. Heat treatment of human milk. *J Pediatr Gastroenterol Nutr.* 2012;54:165-166.

---

## Decrease of Total Subcutaneous Adipose Tissue From Infancy to Childhood
Kaimbacher PS, Dunitz-Scheer M, Wallner-Liebmann SJ, et al (Med Univ Graz, Austria; et al)
*J Pediatr Gastroenterol Nutr* 53:553-560, 2011

---

*Objectives.*—The observation and research of body composition is a topic of present interest. For the assessment of health and variables influencing growth and nutrition, it is of utmost interest to focus on the population of young children.

*Subjects and Methods.*—The measurements of subcutaneous body fat distribution in a sample of clinically healthy children ages 0 to 7 years were examined. The optical device LIPOMETER was applied to measure the thickness of subcutaneous adipose tissue layers (in millimeters) at 15 well-defined body sites. This set of measurement points defines the subcutaneous adipose tissue topography. In the present study, subcutaneous adipose tissue topography was determined in 275 healthy children (128 girls and 147 boys) divided into 3 age groups.

*Results.*—The results of the measurements are presented in 3 levels: total subcutaneous adipose tissue, 4 body regions, and 15 body sites. Our results show a clear physiological decrease in subcutaneous body fat in boys ($-43.8\%$) and girls ($-39.8\%$). One interesting finding was that the decrease occurs mainly in the trunk, abdomen, and lower extremities, whereas the body fat distribution of the upper extremities did not differ. Furthermore, slight subcutaneous adipose tissue topography differences between both sexes were found.

*Conclusions.*—The present study provides basic documentation of subcutaneous adipose tissue topography in healthy children ages 0 to 7 years. An accurate description of subcutaneous adipose tissue topography in healthy subjects could help to characterize various diseases in relation to overnutrition and malnutrition throughout childhood (Fig 1).

▶ Measurement of the fat composition of the human body has been of increasing relevance in the last decade or so, given the emphasis on reducing risk factors for certain diseases, including obesity, metabolic syndrome, various cardiovascular disorders including hyperinsulinemia and hypertension, and atherogenic levels of blood lipids. Kaimbacher et al present data from the first study to thoroughly investigate and highlight the distribution of subcutaneous fat tissue in a quantified way in healthy infants younger than 12 months of age and in children ages 1 to 7 years. The study documents the subcutaneous adipose tissue topography as a reference for characterizing deviations of subcutaneous fat tissue in real live patients with various disorders.

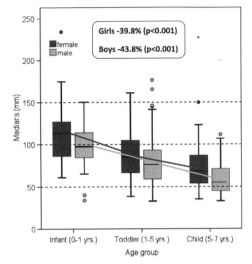

**FIGURE 1.**—Total subcutaneous adipose tissue of 128 girls and 147 boys divided into 3 age groups, showing decreasing medians from infancy to childhood. (Reprinted from Kaimbacher PS, Dunitz-Scheer M, Wallner-Liebmann SJ, et al. Decrease of total subcutaneous adipose tissue from infancy to childhood. *J Pediatr Gastroenterol Nutr.* 2011;53:553-560. © by the AAP.)

This study was reported from Austria and uses a new optical device to determine the fat body composition of the study subjects. The optical device LIPOMETER (European Union patent number 0516251) was used in this report and was developed to generate noninvasive, quick, accurate, and safe measurements of subcutaneous adipose tissue at any given site on the human body. This instrument has been documented to correlate with the gold standard for documenting fat in tissues (computed tomography), showing a correlation coefficient of 0.9863 with the gold standard. The results of the subcutaneous adipose tissue measurements performed in Austria show a clear physiologic decrease in subcutaneous fat from infancy to childhood (Fig 1). The data are supplied with respect to overall subcutaneous adipose tissue and adipose tissue in various body regions and body sites. The decrease in subcutaneous adipose tissue from infancy to childhood was slightly greater in boys (−43.8%) than in girls (−39.4%). This decrease in body fat distribution happens mainly in the trunk, abdomen, and lower extremities, whereas the body fat distribution of the upper extremities does not vary significantly. It is known that small adipocytes, found in great number in subcutaneous adipose tissue, are more insulin sensitive and have higher avidity for uptake by free fatty acids and triglycerides, preventing their deposition in nonadipose tissue. Subcutaneous adipose tissue in the abdominal wall shows the highest rate of uptake of triglycerides and larger free fatty acid release.

If you are at all into nutrition, this report should be read in detail since it provides excellent tabular and graphic information about fat distribution in children. The study is the first to be able to generate basic information of subcutaneous fat tissue topography during infancy and childhood in healthy children.

This commentary ends with some information related to how taxation of sugar-sweetened beverages could be implemented to reduce the number of calories from such beverages that contribute, in part, to obesity in the United States. It should be noted that 33 states already have sales taxes on soft drinks (mean tax 5.2%), but these taxes are too small to affect consumption and the revenues are not earmarked for programs related to health. Consumption of sugar-sweetened beverages has increased throughout the world. Intake in Mexico, for example, doubled within a 7-year period (between 1999 and 2006) in all age groups. Between 1977 and 2002, the per capita intake of caloric beverages doubled in the United States across all age groups. The most recent data from the United States show that children and adults consume about 172 and 175 kcal daily, respectively, per capita from sugar-sweetened beverages. The relationship between consumption of sugar-sweetened beverages and body weight has been examined and documented in many cross-sectional and longitudinal studies. A way of addressing the public health and economic benefits of taxing sugar-sweetened beverages was recently reported in the *New England Journal of Medicine*.[1] The authors of the report propose an excise tax of 1% per ounce of beverages that have any added caloric sweetener. A consumer who drinks a conventional soft drink (20 ounce every day) and switches to a beverage with 0 calories would consume approximately 174 fewer calories a day. The authors of the report recommend a specific excise tax (a tax levied on units such as volume or weight) per ounce or per gram of added sugar as preferable to a sales tax or an ad valorem excise tax (a tax levied as a percentage of price). They note that sales taxes are not desirable since they could encourage the purchase of lower-priced brands resulting in no caloric reduction, or large containers that cost less per ounce. Also, with a sales tax, consumers become aware of the added tax, if at all, only after making a decision to purchase the beverage. Excise taxes could be levied on producers and wholesalers, the cost of which would be passed on to retailers who would then incorporate it into the retail prices and thus the consumers would become aware of the cost at the point of making a purchase. A tax of $0.01 per ounce of beverage would increase the cost of a 20-ounce soft drink by 15% to 20%. The effect on consumption is estimated through research on what is known as "price elasticity" (that is, consumption shifts produced by price). The estimate is that a $0.01 tax per ounce of beverage would cause a decrease in beverage consumption of somewhere between 8% and 10%. It is not recommended that the tax should be applied to noncaloric sweetened drinks. The revenue generated from this type of tax were it a national tax would yield $14.9 billion in the first year alone. Taxes at the state level would generate considerable revenue as well: for example, $139 million in Arkansas, $180 million in Oregon, $221 million in Alabama, $928 million in Florida, $939 million in New York, $1.2 billion in Texas, and $1.8 billion in California.

Obviously there are going to be objections to a national tax on sweetened beverages, the most common argument against it being that the tax is regressive, that is, affecting the poor in our population equally with the wealthy. The analogy, however, that addresses this point is the tobacco tax. Whether you are rich or poor, tobacco is bad for you and in fact smoking-related illness is a greater burden on the less wealthy. Polls over the years of the public support for food and beverage taxes to address obesity have steadily shown favorable responses. In New York, for example, more than 50% of the population supports a soda tax. This percentage rises to 72% if the tax revenue is used to support programs for the prevention of obesity in children and adults as opposed to going into the general coffers of the state.

**J. A. Stockman III, MD**

*Reference*

1. Brownell KD, Farley T, Willett WC, et al. The public health and economic benefits of taxing sugar-sweetened beverages. *N Engl J Med.* 2009;361:1599-1605.

**Fatness leads to inactivity, but inactivity does not lead to fatness: a longitudinal study in children (EarlyBird 45)**
Metcalf BS, Hosking J, Jeffery AN, et al (Peninsula Med School, Plymouth, UK; et al)
*Arch Dis Child* 96:942-947, 2011

*Objective.*—To establish in children whether inactivity is the cause of fatness or fatness the cause of inactivity.

*Design.*—A non-intervention prospective cohort study examining children annually from 7 to 10 years. Baseline versus change to follow-up associations were used to examine the direction of causality.

*Setting.*—Plymouth, England.

*Participants.*—202 children (53% boys, 25% overweight/obese) recruited from 40 Plymouth primary schools as part of the EarlyBird study.

*Main Outcome Measures.*—Physical activity (PA) was measured using Actigraph accelerometers. The children wore the accelerometers for 7 consecutive days at each annual time point. Two components of PA were analysed: the total volume of PA and the time spent at moderate and vigorous intensities. Body fat per cent (BF%) was measured annually by dual energy $x$ ray absorptiometry.

*Results.*—BF% was predictive of changes in PA over the following 3 years, but PA levels were not predictive of subsequent changes in BF% over the same follow-up period. Accordingly, a 10% higher BF% at age 7 years predicted a relative decrease in daily moderate and vigorous intensities of 4 min from age 7 to 10 years (r = 0.17, $p = 0.02$), yet more PA at 7 years did not predict a relative decrease in BF% between 7 and 10 years (r = −0.01, $p = 0.8$).

*Conclusions.*—Physical inactivity appears to be the result of fatness rather than its cause. This reverse causality may explain why attempts to tackle childhood obesity by promoting PA have been largely unsuccessful.

▶ This report smacks of "which is the chicken and which is the egg." Does fatness lead to inactivity, or does inactivity lead to fatness...a burning question that actually has been raised multiple times previously in the literature. It is true that the cause of obesity is multifactorial, resulting from a chronic imbalance between energy intake and energy exposure, but it should be recognized that physical activity accounts for only 25% to 35% of total energy expenditure in children, although this is very important because it is potentially modifiable. The widely held belief that it is inactivity that leads to fatness is the basis for a number of public health initiatives aimed at making children more active. Indeed, although there is overwhelming evidence that physical activity and obesity are linked, observational and experimental data do not always agree. Two large and well-established European observational studies have reported inverse associations between objectively measured physical activity and percent body fat, whereas only 3 of 11 intervention trials have found even a modest impact of physical activity on body composition.[1]

The only way to carefully determine cause and effect is for a longitudinal study to actually contemporaneously measure fatness and activity levels at baseline and then on a regular long-term follow-up basis to investigate the dominant direction of causality. Although such studies have been done in adults, none have been specifically performed in children.

Metcalf et al designed a study that was aimed at using the rule of temporality to elucidate the dominant direction of causality between the objective measures of physical activity and percentage body fat in children. Some 307 healthy children were recruited at school entry (5 years of age) between January 2000 and January 2001 from 54 British primary schools. These youngsters were randomly chosen to ensure a socioeconomic mix representative of the city and of the United Kingdom in general. They participated in what was known as the Early-Bird study. Physical activity was measured objectively on 4 annual occasions throughout the study period using Actigraph accelerometers that were worn for 7 consecutive days (5 school days and 2 weekend days). The Actigraph records the intensity of movement every one-tenth of a second. Actigraphs have been shown to correlate well with free-living measures of energy expenditure in children. Whole body fat, reported as percent body fat, was measured by dual energy x-ray absorptiometry, generally considered to be an excellent criterion method for measuring body composition. Body mass index was measured in the traditional way.

So what is the chicken and what is the egg? Which precedes the other—a decrease in physical activity or a gain in body weight? The answer is physical inactivity is the result rather than the cause of obesity in this study. This reverse causality may explain why physical activity intervention so often failed to prevent excess weight gain in children. The relationship between fatness and physical activity is dominated by the impact of fatness on activity and little or not at all by activity on fatness. Yes, while obesity results from a combination of factors, the principal factor still is too many calories in, which then leads to too few calories out because of physical inactivity. That is quite a snowball effect.

**J. A. Stockman III, MD**

*Reference*

1. Ness AR, Leary SD, Mattocks C, et al. Objectively measured physical activity and fat mass in a large cohort of children. *PLoS Med.* 2007;4:e97.

### Longitudinal analysis of sleep in relation to BMI and body fat in children: the FLAME study

Carter PJ, Taylor BJ, Williams SM, et al (Univ of Otago, Dunedin, New Zealand)
*BMJ* 342:d2712, 2011

*Objectives.*—To determine whether reduced sleep is associated with differences in body composition and the risk of becoming overweight in young children.

*Design.*—Longitudinal study with repeated annual measurements.

*Setting.*—Dunedin, New Zealand.

*Participants.*—244 children recruited from a birth cohort and followed from age 3 to 7.

*Main Outcome Measures.*—Body mass index (BMI), fat mass (kg), and fat free mass (kg) measured with bioelectrical impedance; dual energy x ray absorptiometry; physical activity and sleep duration measured with accelerometry; dietary intake (fruit and vegetables, non-core foods), television viewing, and family factors (maternal BMI and education, birth weight, smoking during pregnancy) measured with questionnaire.

*Results.*—After adjustment for multiple confounders, each additional hour of sleep at ages 3-5 was associated with a reduction in BMI of 0.48 (95% confidence interval 0.01 to 0.96) and a reduced risk of being overweight (BMI ≥ 85th centile) of 0.39 (0.24 to 0.63) at age 7. Further adjustment for BMI at age 3 strengthened these relations. These differences in BMI were explained by differences in fat mass index (−0.43, 0.82 to 0.03) more than by differences in fat free mass index (−0.21, −0.41 to −0.00).

*Conclusions.*—Young children who do not get enough sleep are at increased risk of becoming overweight, even after adjustment for initial weight status and multiple confounding factors. This weight gain is a result of increased fat deposition in both sexes rather than additional accumulation of fat free mass.

▶ This report tells us about the association between reduced sleep time and differences in body composition related to the risk of becoming overweight or obese in young children. Sleep curtailment has been a consistently evolving problem across all age groups. It has been documented that too little sleep is associated with adverse health outcomes, including mortality, stroke, and coronary heart disease in adults.[1] Sleep deprivation also has been found to be associated with type 2 diabetes, hypertension, respiratory disorders, poor self-rated health, and obesity, not only in adults but also in children.[2]

Studies have suspected that short sleep duration may precede the development of overweight or obesity. Most studies, however, have had limitations in that sleep assessment has often been based on parent or self-reports rather than on direct measurements and assessment of body mass index. What Carter et al have done is to report the results of a longitudinal analysis of sleep duration in relation to the development of obesity in 244 children in New Zealand who were followed from age 3 to 7 years. The sleep duration of these children was directly measured using an accelerometer at varying ages and body mass index (BMI), measured yearly. The investigators also looked at yearly measurements of physical activity (as measured by accelerometry), fat mass, and fat-free mass. It was fairly clear that longer sleep duration at age 3 to 5 was associated with a reduction in BMI (0.48 for each extra hour of sleep) and a 61% reduction in the risk of becoming overweight at age 7. This effect was independent of gender, maternal education, BMI, smoking during pregnancy, income, ethnicity, birth weight, and physical activity in some aspects of a child's health. Carter et al concluded that young children with inadequate sleep are at increased risk of overweight as a result of increased fat deposition.

The obvious question raised by this study is how sleep deprivation or short duration of sleep relates to obesity. Is it simply that if you are awake, you are going to have more time to eat? Actually, it has been suggested, mainly through short-lived severe sleep deprivation experiments in young volunteers, that short duration of sleep may cause an increase in energy intake and a reduction in energy exposure through activation of hormonal responses such as reciprocal changes in leptin and ghrelin. Theoretically, this could lead to an increase in appetite, glucose intolerance, and insulin resistance. It could also activate low-grade inflammation and a reduction in energy expenditure mediated by modulation of thyrotropin, cortisol, and noradrenaline. It is also possible that those who are prone to obesity have some other reason to have associated problems with sleep, including hormonal imbalance, anxiety, and so on. It is also possible that sleeping less simply allows more time to eat and engage in other sedentary activities, as exemplified by children and adolescents who stay up late to play on their computer or watch TV while snacking.

In any event, there does appear to be adequate literature to document that short sleep duration or alterations in sleep activity that reduce sleep time are markers for the development of obesity. Unfortunately, as of now there is no intervention tool to interrupt this relationship. Perhaps counting sheep might do the trick.

To read more about the relationship between lack of sleep and obesity, see the excellent editorial on this topic by Cappuccio and Miller.[3]

This commentary closes with a thought or two related to nocturnal feasting and fatness. You may recall that Dr Frank Oski, an internationally known pediatrician, believed that taking one's principal meal in the evening would make one fat. He proffered that one should eat one's principal meal in the morning so that one could metabolize the meal more quickly and efficiently. Eating a principal meal at night when one was sluggish would only put on pounds. For the Oski family, this meant turkey with all the fixings in the morning and oatmeal (perhaps gourmet) for supper. The query is, is there any evidence that nocturnal feasting will make you fatter? The answer is no. A common suggestion to avoid unwanted weight gain has been to avoid eating at night and at first glance, some scientific studies seem to support this. In a study of 83 obese and 94 nonobese women in Sweden, obese women reported eating more meals, and their meals were shifted to the afternoon, evening, or night.[4] However, just because obesity and eating more meals at night are associated, it does not mean that one causes the other. People gain weight because they take in more calories overall than they burn. The obese women were not just night eaters, they were also eating more meals and taking in more calories regardless of when calories were consumed. In fact, other studies have found no link at all between eating at night and weight gain. Swedish men did not show any evidence of weight gain with night-time meals. In a study of 86 obese and 61 normal weight men, there were no differences in the timing of when they ate. Another study of 15 obese people found that the timing of meals did not change the circadian rhythm pattern of energy expenditure. In a study of over 2500 patients, eating at night was not associated with weight gain, but eating more than 3 times a day was. Studies have connected skipping breakfast with gaining more weight, but this is not because breakfast-skippers eat more at night. Breakfast-skippers eat more during the rest of the day. Records of calorie intake suggest that those who eat breakfast maintain healthy weights because their calorie intake is more evenly distributed over the day. In other words, when you eat 3 regular meals, you are not as likely to overeat at any one particular time.

Dr Oski's beliefs about the timing of meals did not serve him very well on one particular occasion. When admitted to an emergency room with chest pain, the physician seeing him mistakenly, for a short time, thought he might have a bowel obstruction. It seems he threw up meatloaf, mashed potatoes, and peas when seen in the emergency room at 8:30 AM, causing the care providers to think that this meal (which had been eaten only an hour before) had been sitting in his stomach overnight. Dr Oski loved to tell this story.

**J. A. Stockman III, MD**

*References*

1. Cappuccio FP, Cooper D, D'Elia L, Strazzullo P, Miller MA. Sleep duration predicts cardiovascular outcomes: a systematic review of meta-analysis of prospective studies. *Eur Heart J Online*. 2011;32:1484-1492.
2. Cappuccio FP, Taggart FM, Kandala N-B, et al. Meta-analysis of short sleep duration and obesity in children and adults. *Sleep*. 2008;31:619-626.
3. Cappuccio FP, Miller MA. Is prolonged lack of sleep associated with obesity? Possibly, and it could have other effects on long-term ill health. *BMJ*. 2011;342:1217-1218.
4. Andersen GS, Stunkard AJ, Sorensen TI, Petersen L, Heitmann BL. Night eating and weight change in middle-aged men and women. *Int J Obes Relat Metab Disord*. 2004;28:1338-1343.

## Effects on Cognitive Performance of Eating Compared with Omitting Breakfast in Elementary Schoolchildren

Kral TVE, Heo M, Whiteford LM, et al (Univ of Pennsylvania School of Nursing and Perelman School of Medicine, Philadelphia; Albert Einstein College of Medicine, Bronx, NY; Univ of Pennsylvania, Philadelphia; et al)
*J Dev Behav Pediatr* 33:9-16, 2012

*Objective.*—The objective of this laboratory-based pilot study was to test the effects of consuming, compared with omitting, breakfast across 6 cognitive domains and on levels of perceived energy and well-being.

*Methods.*—In a crossover design, 21 boys and girls, 8 to 10 years of age, were assessed once a week for 2 weeks. On each test day, subjects performed a series of 8 computerized cognitive performance tasks using the

CogState© software program throughout the morning, but they either consumed or did not consume breakfast. In addition, subjects repeatedly rated their perceived energy level, fatigue, overall well-being, and cheerfulness using a 100-mm Visual Analog Scale.

*Results.*—Results showed no significant main effect of breakfast condition ($p > .17$) or breakfast condition-by-time interaction ($p > .09$) for any of the cognitive performance tasks. On the day when children consumed breakfast, they felt significantly more cheerful ($p = .02$) and indicated to have more energy ($p = .04$) than on the day when they skipped breakfast.

*Conclusion.*—Among children who regularly consume breakfast, skipping breakfast once significantly decreased their perceived level of energy and cheerfulness, but it did not affect their cognitive performance throughout the morning. More experimental studies are needed to assess the effects of different types of breakfast on cognitive performance in children over a prolonged period of time while controlling for familial factors that may affect cognitive performance in children.

▶ Before this report appeared, I was not aware of the magnitude of the issue of elementary school children not eating breakfast. It has been estimated that among 8- to 9-year-old youths, 1 in 5 do not eat breakfast every day.[1] The outcome of not eating breakfast has been looked at in a number of articles over the years. There is a suggestion that not eating breakfast actually leads to becoming overweight. It has also been suggested that omitting breakfast may have detrimental effects on cognitive performance and academic achievement. Why the latter would happen is speculative. Studies have actually looked at the positive effects of breakfast consumption compared with breakfast omission on cognitive performance in children and adolescents, but most of these studies were not well designed or properly controlled.

Kral et al have designed a study to look at the primary outcome of whether eating or omitting breakfast improves cognitive performance in 8- to 10-year-old children across 6 specific cognitive domains. These domains included visual motor function, executive functions/spacial problem solving, psychomotor functions/speed of processing, visual attention/vigilance, visual learning and memory, and attention/working memory. The study also aimed to test the effects of consuming, compared with omitting, breakfast on subjective ratings of perceived energy level, fatigue, overall well-being, and cheerfulness in children. The theory was that on the day when children consumed breakfast they would show improved cognitive performance and would feel more energetic and cheerful and less tired compared with those who omitted breakfast. The study required those who were eating breakfast to eat a specific meal that consisted of 1 of 3 ready-to-eat breakfast cereals along with milk and orange juice. The calorie content of the breakfast was 350 cal. The children were instructed to eat the breakfast at 8:45 AM and consume it entirely. Testing was performed throughout the morning in both the noneating and eating children.

The mean finding of this study indicated that consumption of a cereal-based breakfast, compared with omission of that breakfast, did not significantly affect cognitive performance in an urban (in this case Philadelphia) sample of 8- to

10-year-old children when assessed under controlled laboratory conditions. On the day the child participants did consume breakfast, the youngsters indicated that they were more cheerful and had more energy than on days when they skipped breakfast. None of the 6 cognitive domains were affected by the breakfast manipulation, however. Thus, if one wants their offspring to be cheerful and energized, breakfast it is, but do not expect any miracles in terms of smartness. This report was well designed and hopefully will be the definitive report on this subject. Those who work at Kellogg's and General Mills should read this report in detail. I believe that it would be interesting to repeat this study with some bacon and eggs with a side of fresh toast, butter and marmalade, then see what happens.

This commentary closes within observation having to do with the effects of eating yogurt. Many believe that eating yogurt will in fact change the mix of microbes living in the human intestine. Recent data show that while this is true, the effect is relatively transient. The finding comes from a study of identical twins in which one ate yogurt twice a day for 4 months and the other remained on the infant's original diet. Yogurt enhanced the ability of intestinal bacteria to break down complex carbohydrates found in fruits, vegetables, and other foods. This effect, however, was quite transient. Many use yogurt in an attempt to change the mix of microbes in their intestines to enhance the healthiness of their bowels, but findings now suggest that the benefits of yogurt actually result from a different action and last only a short time.[2]

**J. A. Stockman III, MD**

*References*

1. Miller GD, Forgoc T, Cline T, McBean LD. Breakfast benefits children in the US and aboard. *J Am Coll Nutr.* 1998;17:4-6.
2. Saey T. Yogurt doesn't shift microbes. *Science News.* November 19, 2011:18.

---

**Changes in energy content of lunchtime purchases from fast food restaurants after introduction of calorie labelling: cross sectional customer surveys**
Dumanovsky T, Huang CY, Nonas CA, et al (New York; Pardee RAND Graduate School, Santa Monica, CA; New York City Department of Health and Mental Hygiene; et al)
*BMJ* 343:d4464, 2011

---

*Objective.*—To assess the impact of fast food restaurants adding calorie labelling to menu items on the energy content of individual purchases.

*Design.*—Cross sectional surveys in spring 2007 and spring 2009 (one year before and nine months after full implementation of regulation requiring chain restaurants' menus to contain details of the energy content of all menu items). Setting 168 randomly selected locations of the top 11 fast food chains in New York City during lunchtime hours.

*Participants.*—7309 adult customers interviewed in 2007 and 8489 in 2009.

*Main Outcome Measures.*—Energy content of individual purchases, based on customers' register receipts and on calorie information provided for all items in menus.

*Results.*—For the full sample, mean calories purchased did not change from before to after regulation (828 v 846 kcal, $P = 0.22$), though a modest decrease was shown in a regression model adjusted for restaurant chain, poverty level for the store location, sex of customers, type of purchase, and inflation adjusted cost (847 v 827 kcal, $P = 0.01$). Three major chains, which accounted for 42% of customers surveyed, showed significant reductions in mean energy per purchase (McDonald's 829 v 785 kcal, $P = 0.02$; Au Bon Pain 555 v 475 kcal, $P < 0.001$; KFC 927 v 868 kcal, $P < 0.01$), while mean energy content increased for one chain (Subway 749 v 882 kcal, $P < 0.001$). In the 2009 survey, 15% (1288/8489) of customers reported using the calorie information, and these customers purchased 106 fewer kilocalories than customers who did not see or use the calorie information (757 v 863 kcal, $P < 0.001$).

*Conclusion.*—Although no overall decline in calories purchased was observed for the full sample, several major chains saw significant reductions. After regulation, one in six lunchtime customers used the calorie information provided, and these customers made lower calorie choices.

▶ In response to the obesity epidemic, New York City approved a regulation requiring chain restaurants to show calorie information prominently on all menus and item tags. This regulation became effective March 2008. Dumanovsky et al investigated whether this measure had any effect on consumer choices for lunchtime purchases from fast-food outlets. A comparison was made for information obtained in the spring of 2007 and again in 2009, 1 year before and 9 months after implementation of the regulation. No overall decline in energy content of purchases was observed, but the 15% of customers who actually bothered to read the calorie information reduced the energy content of their lunch by an average of 106 kcal, enough to make a real difference in body weight if sustained.

This report has generated quite a bit of media publicity with decidedly mixed reactions, with some stories claiming it shows the New York City regulation to have been an abject failure, while others have proclaimed it a triumphant success. In a letter to the editor of the *British Medical Journal*, Dr Kathryn Green, a general practitioner in the United Kingdom, wondered how many of the 15% of customers who use the information on calorie content to make healthier choices actually needed to reduce their calorie intake. She suggests that no one wants to live in a nanny state that takes all this too far without evidence of appropriate benefit. While too old to have to worry about being carded for alcohol, Dr Green is concerned that some day in the future she may wind up having to be weighed before being allowed to buy a cake at supermarket checkout.[1] As an aside, it should be noted that in 2011, the French government announced a new tax on sugary soft drinks in a bid to help cut the budget deficit while tackling the country's growing obesity problem. The new tax is projected to raise $170 million for the social security budget. Taxes on tobacco and alcohol were also raised in the enabling legislation.

This commentary closes with an observation. If one compares the calorie counts of 2 McDonald's cheeseburgers, one Big Mac, one Quarter Pounder, a Double Quarter Pounder, and a single serving of an Angus deluxe burger, interestingly, the latter, claiming to have the leanest of meats, has the highest calorie count at 760!

This commentary also closes with an observation from the New York City's Department of Health about the salt content of luncheon meals of New Yorkers. The New York City's Department of Health recently commissioned a survey (with public funds) to find out how much salt New Yorkers were eating at lunch. Researchers stopped people on their way out of 11 fast-food chains, scrutinized their receipts, and calculated the sodium content of full meals from nutritional information on restaurant web sites. The mean sodium content of 6580 lunches was 1.75 g, significantly more than the recommended daily allowance for higher-risk adults (1.5 g), which includes anyone in middle age or beyond, anyone with hypertension, and all African Americans. One in 5 meals gave diners more than the recommended daily allowance for everyone else (2.3 g). Just one in 36 meals met national regulatory standards for a healthy sodium content (0.6 g per meal). Lunches from fried chicken outlets (Kentucky Fried Chicken and Popeye's) were the saltiest. Half of their meals exceeded the higher threshold for daily allowance and 84% exceeded the lower threshold. These statistics did not include the fact that many individuals buying food in fast-food restaurants will add their own salt to the meal for taste purposes. The reason for undertaking the study is that data suggest a 50% cut in dietary salt would help protect individuals from hypertension and heart disease. The math shows an estimated $20 billion annual savings in healthcare cost.[2]

With Mayor Bloomberg's support, New York City has done a lot to modify the commercially available foods in the Big Apple. This spans reducing trans fats in foods supplied by restaurants to now hitting hard on the salt content of food products. Needless to say, in the Big Apple, the philosophy is an apple a day keeps the doctor away.

**J. A. Stockman III, MD**

*References*

1. Green KM. Let them eat cake. *BMJ*. 2011;343:d5366.
2. Dickinson BD, Havas S; Council on Science and Public Health, American Medical Association. Reducing the population burden of cardiovascular disease by reducing sodium intake. *Arch Intern Med*. 2007;167:1460-1468.

---

**Accuracy of Stated Energy Contents of Restaurant Foods**
Urban LE, McCrory MA, Dallal GE, et al (Tufts Univ, Boston, MA; Purdue Univ, West Lafayette, IN; et al)
*JAMA* 306:287-293, 2011

---

*Context.*—National recommendations for the prevention and treatment of obesity emphasize reducing energy intake. Foods purchased in restaurants provide approximately 35% of the daily energy intake in US individuals but the accuracy of the energy contents listed for these foods is unknown.

*Objective.*—To examine the accuracy of stated energy contents of foods purchased in restaurants.

*Design and Setting.*—A validated bomb calorimetry technique was used to measure dietary energy in food from 42 restaurants, comprising 269 total food items and 242 unique foods. The restaurants and foods were randomly selected from quick-serve and sit-down restaurants in Massachusetts, Arkansas, and Indiana between January and June 2010.

*Main Outcome Measure.*—The difference between restaurant-stated and laboratory-measured energy contents, which were corrected for standard metabolizable energy conversion factors.

*Results.*—The absolute stated energy contents were not significantly different from the absolute measured energy contents overall (difference of 10 kcal/portion; 95% confidence interval [CI], −15 to 34 kcal/portion; $P = .52$); however, the stated energy contents of individual foods were variable relative to the measured energy contents. Of the 269 food items, 50 (19%) contained measured energy contents of at least 100 kcal/portion more than the stated energy contents. Of the 10% of foods with the highest excess energy in the initial sampling, 13 of 17 were available for a second sampling. In the first analysis, these foods contained average measured energy contents of 289 kcal/portion (95% CI, 186 to 392 kcal/portion) more than the stated energy contents; in the second analysis, these foods contained average measured energy contents of 258 kcal/portion (95% CI, 154 to 361 kcal/portion) more than the stated energy contents ($P < .001$ for each vs 0 kcal/portion difference). In addition, foods with lower stated energy contents contained higher measured energy contents than stated, while foods with higher stated energy contents contained lower measured energy contents ($P < .001$).

*Conclusions.*—Stated energy contents of restaurant foods were accurate overall. However, there was substantial inaccuracy for some individual foods, with understated energy contents for those with lower energy contents.

▶ With the problem of obesity increasingly rearing its head in the United States, more and more individuals are trying to control their weight or lose weight. The only way to do the latter is by increasing one's energy requirement or decreasing calories in the diet. For those of us who are sedentary, weight control can only be achieved by reducing energy intake. When the total number of calories needed each day to control weight is known and understood, an individual can track caloric intake in an attempt to undercut that number and thereby achieve a net caloric deficit or negative energy balance. Generally, a deficit of 500 calories per day can achieve a 1-pound weight loss per week because a net reduction of 3500 calories is required to lose 1 pound of body weight.

Urban et al have assessed the accuracy of stated energy contents of restaurant foods. They used a special form of calorimetry to assess the actual calorie content of restaurant food, a technique known as bomb calorimetry. The investigators randomly selected low- and high-energy content foods from 7 quick-serve and

7 sit-down chain-type restaurants across 3 states. Foods were ordered, stored, and transported for calorimetry studies. Of 269 foods selected from 42 restaurants, 108 (40%) were found to have measured energy at least 10 kcal/portion higher than the stated amounts. Fifty-two percent were found to have at least 10 kcal/portion lower than the stated amounts, and 19% contained at least 100 kcal/portion higher than the stated amounts. Discrepancies were greater and more frequent in sit-down restaurants that feature foods with lower stated energy contents compared with foods with higher stated energy contents. Desserts, carbohydrates/rich foods, and salads contained significantly more energy content than the stated amounts.

With the passage of the US Patient Protection and Affordable Care Act, labeling of caloric content is mandated in restaurants and by other food vendors with more than 20 locations. Accuracy and standardization of menus, serving sizes, ingredients, and preparation techniques are essential to constituting truth in labeling along with regular monitoring to ensure these standards are being met. Needless to say, in non-chain restaurants, those who prepare the meals probably do not have a great deal of insight into the exact caloric content of what they are making, despite the fact that many patrons would like to know that information.

As an aside, a recent report tells us exactly what the effect is of adding 1 serving per day of certain foods to a person's diet when it comes to weight gain over a period of some years.[1] In a report that involved more than 22 000 men and nearly 100 000 women, it was shown that on average, an individual will gain 3.35 pounds at each 4-year point in time. The effect of adding 1 serving a day of nuts and fruits along with whole grains and vegetables tends to produce a net negative weight gain over a 4-year period of time. On the other hand, having 1 serving a day of unprocessed meats, sugar-sweetened sodas, potato chips, or french fries will increase weight gain anywhere from 1 pound to 3.5 pounds over 4 years (the latter impact is greatest when eating french fries). Although there are no surprises here, it is clear that it not only depends on how much you eat but what you eat when it comes to being overweight.

**J. A. Stockman III, MD**

*Reference*

1. Seppa N. Certain foods pack on the pounds: French fries, soda among biggest causes of weight gain. *Science News.* July 30, 2011:10.

---

## Mild Infantile Hypercalcemia: Diagnostic Tests and Outcomes

Koltin D, Rachmiel M, Wong BYL, et al (The Hosp for Sick Children, Toronto, Ontario, Canada; Assaf Harofeh Med Ctr, Zrifin, Israel; Sunnybrook Health Sciences Centre, Toronto, Ontario, Canada; et al)
*J Pediatr* 159:215-221, 2011

*Objective.*—To assess outcome in a cohort of patients with infantile hypercalcemia followed over 3 years.

*Study Design.*—Patients (n = 32) presenting to the calcium clinic between July 2002 and September 2008 were studied. In addition to tests of calcium phosphate metabolism, serum insulin-like growth factor-1, calcitonin, urine citrate, and *calcium-sensing* receptor gene analysis were obtained.

*Results.*—Mean age at presentation was 6.0 ± 6.3 months. Mean calcium level was 11.4 ± 0.7 mg/dL (2.84 ± 0.17 mmol/L). A recognized cause was found in 14% and a probable cause in 14% of the cohort. Those with nephrocalcinosis (n = 11) had significantly lower mean weight SDS and higher mean calcium levels. The biochemical profile of those in whom no cause could be determined included nonsuppressed parathyroid hormone with either normal or increased $1,25(OH)_2D$. Hypercalcemia resolved in 20 patients. However, in approximately a third, there was persistence in hypercalcemia, hypercalciuria, or nephrocalcinosis.

*Conclusions.*—The addition of $1,25(OH)_2D$ and calcium-sensing receptor mutation analysis to a panel of investigations may improve diagnostic yield. Clinical outcome is overall good, however, one-third need ongoing follow-up.

▶ It has been more than 60 years since Lightwood and Stapleton first described the disorder we now call *infantile hypercalcemia.*[1] In most children, the only manifestation of infantile hypercalcemia is detection when laboratory profiles are done in otherwise asymptomatic infants. In some cases, however, it may present with failure to thrive, poor feeding, irritability, muscle weakness, abdominal pain, constipation, vomiting, and tachycardia, all typical signs of high serum calcium levels. Some infants will suffer more serious consequences, including seizures, diabetes insipidus, and nephrocalcinosis. In the large majority of infants, the hypercalcemia can be predicted to resolve by school age, although there are few reports telling us what happens with these youngsters on the long haul. Since the first description of the disorder by Lightwood and Stapleton, 2 disorders have been identified as causative in a small percentage of children. One is William syndrome, and the other is familial hypocalciuric hypercalcemia (FHH). Increased levels of $1,25(OH)_2D$ and an elevation in serum insulinlike growth factor (IGF)-1 can also result in high calcium levels. Other rare causes include defects in the metabolism of calcitonin and type 1 (distal) renal tubular acidosis. Although such disorders should be looked for in persistent cases of hypercalcemia, more often than not, no etiology is identified, and the infant is designated as having idiopathic infantile hypercalcemia.

The investigators from the Hospital for Sick Children in Toronto, the authors of this report threw their hat into the diagnostic dilemma of infantile hypercalcemia by telling us the extent to which a broad panel of investigations will or will not determine the etiology or suggest a plausible mechanism for the hypercalcemia. The authors also designed a study to tell us the outcomes in a cohort of patients with the disorder.

Koltin et al did a retrospective chart review of all infants referred for hypercalcemia to the Calcium Clinic at the Hospital for Sick Children in Toronto between July 2002 and September 2008. Some 32 infants were identified. History, physical findings, biochemical profiles, genetic screening for William syndrome, and findings on renal ultrasound scan were evaluated. The mean findings were that a specific diagnosis could be made in only 14% of infants with mild infantile hypercalcemia. It was also clear that normocalcemia in parents does not rule out a diagnosis of FHH. Those with nephrocalcinosis at presentation had higher plasma calcium levels and lower weights. Other findings from this report showed a male excess of cases and that renal disease is somewhat unusual at the time of presentation. None of the study subjects had excess vitamin D levels or vitamin D toxicity, but 2 of the infants did appear to have a vitamin D—sensitive form of infantile hypercalcemia. Both responded to reductions in vitamin D in the diet. None of the study subjects in this report had disturbances of IGF-1 or evidence of Bartter syndrome (renal tubular acidosis type 1). None showed evidence of calcitonin problems. Approximately one-third of the cohort had nephrocalcinosis. This problem persisted in the majority but appears to be nonprogressive. The authors suggest that genetic testing for William syndrome is probably not needed in the absence of specific phenotypic features and that parent normocalcemia does not exclude the diagnosis of FHH.

**J. A. Stockman III, MD**

*Reference*

1. Lightwood R, Stapleton T. Idiopathic hypercalcaemia in infants. *Lancet.* 1953; 265:255-256.

## Neonatal screening for lysosomal storage disorders: feasibility and incidence from a nationwide study in Austria

Mechtler TP, Stary S, Metz TF, et al (Med Univ of Vienna, Austria; et al)
*Lancet* 379:335-341, 2012

*Background.*—The interest in neonatal screening for lysosomal storage disorders has increased substantially because of newly developed enzyme replacement therapies, the need for early diagnosis, and technical advances. We tested for Gaucher's disease, Pompe's disease, Fabry's disease, and Niemann-Pick disease types A and B in an anonymous prospective nation wide screening study that included genetic mutation analysis to assess the practicality and appropriateness of including these disorders in neonatal screening panels.

*Methods.*—Specimens from dried blood spots of 34 736 newborn babies were collected consecutively from January, 2010 to July, 2010, as part of the national routine Austrian newborn screening programme. Anonymised samples were analysed for enzyme activities of acid β-glucocerebrosidase, α-galactosidase, α-glucosidase, and acid sphingomyelinase by electrospray ionisation tandem mass spectrometry. Genetic mutation analyses were done in samples with suspected enzyme deficiency.

*Findings.*—All 34 736 samples were analysed successfully by the multiplex screening assay. Low enzyme activities were detected in 38 babies. Mutation analysis confirmed lysosomal storage disorders in 15 of them. The most frequent mutations were found for Fabry's disease (1 per 3859 births), followed by Pompe's disease (1 per 8684), and Gaucher's disease (1 per 17 368). The positive predictive values were 32% (95% CI 16—52),

80% (28–99), and 50% (7–93), respectively. Mutational analysis detected predominantly missense mutations associated with a late-onset phenotype.

*Interpretation.*—The combined overall proportion of infants carrying a mutation for lysosomal storage disorders was higher than expected. Neonatal screening for lysosomal storage disorders is likely to raise challenges for primary health-care providers. Furthermore, the high frequency of late-onset mutations makes lysosomal storage disorders a broad health problem beyond childhood.

▶ Improvements in bone marrow transplantation and the development of recombinant enzyme replacement therapies for children with lysosomal storage disorders have raised the expectation that neonatal screening might enable early treatment before irreversible damage occurs. An example of greatly improved early outcomes has been noted in infants treated soon after birth following identification through the Taiwanese Pompe disease screening program.[1]

Mechtler et al tells about the outcome of neonatal screening in Austria for a group of 4 treatable lysosomal storage disorders. These included Pompe disease, Fabry disease, Gaucher disease, and Niemann-Pick diseases types A and B. The experience in Austria showed a higher-than-expected incidence of these 4 problems (1 per 2315) with a high frequency of mutations that are associated with late onset of symptoms, often in adulthood. The authors correctly speculate that consideration of neonatal screening for this group of disorders now raises many ethical issues given the late onset of symptoms in a significant proportion of patients.

In the United States, dried blood spot screening now includes more than 50 disorders. This is in comparison with just 5 disorders being screened for in the United Kingdom. The rub with some of these screening tests is the increased rate of screening diagnosis compared with the much lower actual clinical onset of disease for many of the disorders.

Many uncertainties remain for clinicians and families confronted by positive results from screening for lysosomal storage disorders. Precise genotype-phenotype correlation is not possible for many of these entities, leaving the treating physician uncertain when counseling a child's family about the implications of the results. Whereas the best possible treatment for mucopolysaccharidosis type 1 is generally accepted to be bone marrow transplantation before the age of 2 years, the appropriate age (or even need) for commencement of enzyme replacement therapy for mild forms of disorders such as for some cases of Fabry disease is a matter of debate, particularly with mutations predicted to have a late-onset phenotype. Even with evidence of efficacy, the very high cost of treatment is likely to be beyond the capacity of health system funding in many countries.

The study design used by Mechtler et al shows the feasibility of screening and establishes frequency of the 5 disorders in question but precluded clinical assessment of neonates identified because the study was anonymous. Future research studies with long-term follow-up, informed consent, and clinical assessment could be considered unethical. Thus, we are left with the dilemma of not knowing what precisely we should be doing with many of the patients who are identified as having lysosomal storage disorders.

**J. A. Stockman III, MD**

*Reference*

1. Chien YH, Lee NC, Thurberg BL, et al. Pompe disease in infants: improving the prognosis by newborn screening and early treatment. *Pediatrics.* 2009;124: e1116-e1125.

**Later-Onset Pompe Disease: Early Detection and Early Treatment Initiation Enabled by Newborn Screening**

Chien Y-H, Lee N-C, Huang H-J, et al (Natl Taiwan Univ Hosp and Nal Taiwan Univ College of Medicine, Taipei; et al)

*J Pediatr* 158:1023-1027, 2011

*Objective.*—To determine whether newborn screening facilitates early detection and thereby early treatment initiation for later-onset Pompe disease.

*Study Design.*—We have conducted a newborn screening program since 2005. Newborns with deficient skin fibroblast acid α-glucosidase activity and two acid α-glucosidase gene mutations but no cardiomyopathy were defined as having later-onset Pompe disease, and their motor development and serum creatine kinase levels were monitored every 3 to 6 months.

*Results.*—Among 344 056 newborns, 13 (1 in 26 466) were found to have later-onset Pompe disease. During a follow-up period of up to 4 years, four patients were treated because of hypotonia, muscle weakness, delayed developmental milestones/motor skills, or elevated creatine kinase levels starting at the ages of 1.5, 14, 34, and 36 months, respectively. Muscle biopsy specimens obtained from the treated patients revealed increased storage of glycogen and lipids.

*Conclusion.*—Newborn screening was found to facilitate the early detection of later-onset Pompe disease. A subsequent symptomatic approach then identifies patients who need early treatment initiation.

▶ Pompe disease is also known as glycogen storage disease type II, glycogenosis II, or acid maltase deficiency. It is a lysosomal storage disorder resulting from a deficiency of the enzyme acid α-glucosidase (GAA). Absence of this enzyme causes the lysosome to accumulate glycogen in all tissues, particularly skeletal muscles. Pompe disease presents in 2 forms. The infantile form occurs very early in life and is usually characterized by the presence of hypertrophic cardiomyopathy. There is a more slowly progressive later-onset form of disease that most commonly has no cardiac manifestations but does result in increasingly profound weakness and ultimately death. The age of diagnosis of the later-onset form can range from anywhere less than 1 year to as late as 78 years. About half of adult patients who have the later-onset form of the disease do report the presence of mild muscular symptoms during childhood. By the time symptoms present, enzyme replacement therapy with GAA is not capable of reversing existing damaged muscle tissue. Chien et al have conducted a large-scale newborn screening program for the early detection and treatment of Pompe disease. These investigators were most interested in detecting the condition in patients very early in life who would have the later-onset form of the disease, allowing for early institution of treatment prior to the development of symptoms. Data from the report show that 1 in 26 466 newborns was found to have later-onset Pompe disease. These patients were followed for up to 4 years. Four individuals were treated because of the development of hypotonia, muscle weakness, delayed developmental milestones/motor skills, or elevated creatine kinase levels starting at ages 1.5, 14, and 36 months. These patients were able to be treated quite promptly with the first onset of symptoms and seem to have done well, validating the usefulness of newborn screening.

While on the topic of orphan enzyme drug replacement, in early spring of 2011, Genzyme announced that it had another batch of its fabrazyme drug, an enzyme replacement therapy used to treat Fabry disease, which failed to meet industry standards for manufacturing procedures. For the second time in less than a year, a group of people with Fabry disease, a rare lysosomal storage disorder, petitioned the US National Institutes of Health to override Genzyme's patent rights and license the intellectual property related to fabrazyme to other drug manufacturers. Such a move is permitted under the Byh-Dole Act of 1980, which gave universities and small businesses that use government funds control of their inventions but enabled funding agencies to "march in" and license patents to third parties when contractors failed to satisfy the health and safety needs of the public. This provision, however, has rarely been tested. Prior to the first fabrazyme petition, the government has only intervened on 3 occasions and in none of these situations has actually granted the petitioner's request when push came to shove. In any event, those with Fabry disease found themselves in 2010 and 2011 not getting the amount of enzyme replacement they needed and also received little help from the federal government via the Byh-Dole Act. Thus far, in no situation has the Byh-Dole Act ever been implemented on behalf of individuals with orphan diseases where pharmaceutical companies have failed to keep the drug supply at adequate levels.

This commentary closes within observation having to do with nutrition. Are you familiar with the term "vitamer"? This is one of several related chemical compounds that act as a vitamin. What is commonly known as vitamin B1—the immune system booster found in pork, legumes, and brewer's yeast—is really 4 different vitamers. In some cases, certain vitamers act as more potent vitamins than others. An international team has discovered a new way to inventory the B1 vitamer content of alcoholic beverages.[1] Studying 204 beers picked from the 2010 Australian International Beer Awards, scientists compared the vitamer counts of lagers, ales, wheat beers, stouts, and porters. Lagers scored lowest, likely because they were pasteurized. So it is that if you want to keep your immune system in tip-top shape, a good stoutly ale will do the trick!

**J. A. Stockman III, MD**

*Reference*

1. Editorial comment. Say what? *Science News*. December 31, 2011:4.

# 16 Oncology

**Associations between Vaccination and Childhood Cancers in Texas Regions**

Pagaoa MA, Okcu MF, Bondy ML, et al (The Univ of Texas School of Public Health, Houston; Baylor College of Medicine, Houston, TX; MD Anderson Cancer Ctr, Houston, TX)

*J Pediatr* 158:996-1002, 2011

*Objectives.* To determine whether children born in Texas regions with higher vaccination coverage had reduced risk of childhood cancer.

*Study Design.*—The Texas Cancer Registry identified 2800 cases diagnosed from 1995 to 2006 who were (1) born in Texas and (2) diagnosed at ages 2 to 17 years. The state birth certificate data were used to identify 11 200 age- and sex-matched control subjects. A multilevel mixed-effects regression model compared vaccination rates among cases and control subjects at the public health region and county level.

*Results.*—Children born in counties with higher hepatitis B vaccine coverage had lower odds of all cancers combined (OR – 0.81, 95% CI: 0.67 to 0.98) and acute lymphoblastic leukemia (ALL) specifically (OR = 0.63, 95% CI: 0.46 to 0.88). A decreased odds for ALL also was associated at the county level with higher rates of the inactivated poliovirus vaccine (OR = 0.67, 95% CI: 0.49 to 0.92) and 4-3-1-3-3 vaccination series (OR = 0.62, 95% CI: 0.44 to 0.87). Children born in public health regions with higher coverage levels of the *Haemophilus influenzae* type b-conjugate vaccine had lower odds of ALL (OR: 0.58; 95% CI: 0.42 to 0.82).

*Conclusions.*—Some common childhood vaccines appear to be protective against ALL at the population level.

▶ With all the antivaccination groups around these days, this report comes none too soon. While based on information that affects only a tiny percentage of the US childhood population, this report of Pagaoa et al does show that children who receive hepatitis B vaccine do have lower overall odds of developing a malignancy. Specifically, the risk of the development of any form of cancer is reduced by 19% and that of acute lymphoblastic leukemia by 27%. These data were derived from an analysis of children born in Texas where regions with higher vaccination coverage clearly showed a reduced risk of the development of childhood cancer. The analysis of a large pool of population-based control subjects resulted in a distribution of potential risk factors and confounding factors that leveled the playing field between vaccinated and unvaccinated children, making the conclusions of the report quite valid. Although the biologic mechanism behind the effect of vaccinations on childhood cancer remains to be determined, the results from this Texas study corroborate findings from previous studies that point to a reduced risk from common vaccines against the development of acute lymphoblastic leukemia. Lots of theories are being examined now to determine exactly what the cause-and-effect relationship is in this regard. Presumably, immunization programs not only reduce the number of infectious diseases in childhood but also contribute to some immunologic defense against the development of certain cancers.

On a somewhat related topic, there is much press these days about shortages of cancer drugs. In certain parts of the United States, vincristine and cytarabine have been in extremely short supply in recent times. Shortages of other drugs, mostly generic, including anesthesia drugs and antibiotics as well as cancer drugs, have tripled over the 5-year period from 2006 through 2011.[1] The US Food and Drug Administration (FDA) has approximately 30 or so cancer drugs on its shortage list in 2010. Many of these cancer drugs are decades old but are still quite effective. The cytarabine shortage has been particularly worrisome because there is no substitute agent for treating acute myeloid leukemia.

It is not entirely clear why the shortages of cancer drugs have only recently appeared. It has been pointed out that nearly all these scarce drugs are generics, which are not particularly profitable. Pharmaceutical companies have little incentive to add back-up capacity to current levels of production. Such shortages rarely happen with brand-name drugs. A bill introduced in 2011 by Senators Amy Klobuchar (D-MN) and Robert Casey (D-PA) was designed in such a way that requires manufacturers to notify the FDA when they have production problems or expect to stop making a drug. This will permit the FDA to work with other companies to ramp up production. Clearly something has to be done. In 2004, the number of new drug shortages identified by the FDA was just 58. By 2010, it increased steadily to 211!

This commentary closes with a bit of history. It is hard to imagine a time when HeLa cells did not exist. Rapidly reproducing and amazingly robust, these cervical cancer cells have become indispensable in modern biomedical research. The cell line is now ubiquitous and has been used in numerable experiments that require human cell culture, having served in the creation of the polio vaccine, the development of leukemia treatments, discoveries in cloning, and gene mapping. Despite the vast amounts of scientific data on HeLa cells, most people know very little about the cell's origin. Obviously they came from a woman, but who was she? HeLa, from the initial letters of the donor's first and last names, provide the clue. Commonly reported as Helen Lane, her actual name was Henrietta Lacks, but just knowing her name does not tell us that she was poor, black, or largely uneducated. It does not tell us how she died in the free ward of Johns Hopkins Hospital in 1951 when she was barely 31 years old, leaving 5 children, nor does it tell us how her cells were taken without her knowledge and without her consent. The Chair of the Department of Pediatrics at Hopkins' Gynecology Department was the one who obtained the cells and offered them to the Head of Tissue Culture Research at Hopkins. It was the latter who was able to culture the cells and discover their amazing capacity for reproduction. All of this was done without permission of the patient or her family. Unfortunately, at the time, it was generally held that physicians could use patients treated in a free ward as research subjects.

If you want to read about the background and life of Henrietta (and her husband Davis), see the book written by Rebecca Skloot.[2] Henrietta died from cervical cancer in 1951. Her DNA continues to live in thousands of laboratories throughout the world.

**J. A. Stockman III, MD**

*References*

1. Kaiser J. Shortages of cancer drugs put patients, trials at risk. *Science*. 2011;332: 523.
2. Skloot R. *The Immortal Life of Henrietta Lacks*. New York, NY: Crown Books; 2010.

---

**Adulthood residential ultraviolet radiation, sun sensitivity, dietary vitamin D, and risk of lymphoid malignancies in the California Teachers Study**

Chang ET, Canchola AJ, Cockburn M, et al (Cancer Prevention Inst of California, Fremont; Univ of Southern California Keck School of Medicine, Los Angeles, CA; et al)
*Blood* 118:1591-1599 2011

To lend clarity to inconsistent prior findings of an inverse association between ultraviolet radiation (UVR) exposure and risk of lymphoid malignancies, we examined the association of prospectively ascertained residential ambient UVR exposure with risk of non-Hodgkin lymphomas (NHLs), multiple myeloma (MM), and classical Hodgkin lymphoma in the California Teachers Study cohort. Among 121 216 eligible women, 629 were diagnosed with NHL, 119 with MM, and 38 with Hodgkin lymphoma between 1995-1996 and 2007. Cox proportional hazards regression was used to estimate incidence rate ratios (RRs) with 95% confidence intervals (CIs). Residential UVR levels within a 20-km radius were associated with reduced risk of overall NHL (RR for highest vs lowest statewide quartile of minimum UVR [$\geq 5100$ vs $< 4915$ W-h/m$^2$], 0.58; 95% CI, 0.42-0.80), especially diffuse large B-cell lymphoma (RR, 0.36; 95% CI, 0.17-0.78) and chronic lymphocytic leukemia/small lymphocytic lymphoma (RR, 0.46; 95% CI, 0.21-1.01), and MM (RR for maximum UVR, 0.57; 95% CI, 0.36-0.90). These associations were not modified by skin sensitivity to sunlight, race/ethnicity, body mass index, or neighborhood socioeconomic status. Dietary vitamin D also was not associated with risk of lymphoid malignancies. These results support a protective effect of routine residential UVR exposure against lymphomagenesis through mechanisms possibly independent of vitamin D.

▶ During the last 10 years or so, there have been several studies that have shown an inverse association between intensity of childhood or adult exposure to ultraviolet radiation and the risk of non-Hodgkin lymphomas (NHLs). The theory has been that ultraviolet light activates vitamin D, which has an antiproliferative and prodifferentiative effect on lymphocytes. One limitation of most existing studies is their retrospective nature. It is important to understand exactly what the role of ultraviolet radiation is in relationship to lymphoid malignancies, as few other modifiable risks have ever been found for NHL. This and related disorders cause more than 36 000 deaths per year in the United States.

Chang et al in a prospective cohort study of 121 216 California women report on an inverse association between ultraviolet radiation exposure and a 40% to 50% reduced risk of developing NHL, particularly diffuse large B-cell lymphoma and chronic lymphocytic leukemia/small lymphocytic lymphoma and multiple myeloma. Using the large prospective California Teachers Study cohort, the authors identified 629 and 119 women who developed NHL and multiple myeloma, respectively, after joining the cohort. The authors examined the association of ambient ultraviolet radiation exposure among these patients in relation to the entire cohort group that served as control. The reduced risk of 40% to 50% of developing NHL in association with high exposure to ultraviolet radiation was independent of race/ethnicity, body mass index, and socioeconomic stature. Thus, the results from this large prospective study suggest that regular routine residential ultraviolet exposure may have a protective effect against lymphoma and multiple myeloma and that this effect may be because of a mechanism that is completely independent of dietary vitamin D. The total and dietary intakes of vitamin D, retinol, and calcium were not associated with alterations in the risk of the malignancies studied.

In a commentary that accompanied this report, it was stated that given the observed lack of a role for vitamin D, the association between ultraviolet radiation exposure and a reduced risk of 40% to 50% of developing NHL and multiple myeloma remains a mystery.[1] It is entirely possible that ultraviolet radiation—mediated induction of regulatory T cells may play a crucial role in the prevention of malignancy. Given that exposure to ultraviolet radiation is an established risk factor for melanoma and nonmelanoma skin cancer, augmenting ultraviolet radiation exposure is unlikely to be an acceptable means of reducing lymphoma risk at a population level. However, this does not mean that the amount of ultraviolet radiation one might normally get from some outdoor activities should be avoided. It should also be noted that there are other ways to induce regulatory T-cell activity, such as with the use of probiotics.[2]

This commentary closes with some thoughts on shift work and the development of cancer. This is particularly relevant not just to patients, but also to US medical trainees who are increasingly subject now to regulatory processes that control their work hours, processes that are leading to more and more shift work. The effect of shift work on cancer, particularly breast cancer, has received interest from the lay media since a panel of the International Agency for Research on Cancer (IARC) declared in 2007 that "shift work that involves circadian disruption is probably carcinogenic to humans."[3] This conclusion was based on evidence from animal studies, with limited evidence from human studies. The evidence is strongest for breast cancer, although the risk of prostate and colorectal cancer may also be increased by shift work. Recently, 38 women with breast cancer who had previously worked night shifts for at least 20 years were compensated by the Danish National Board of Industrial Industries, underscoring the belief, at certain governmental levels, in the theory relating shift work to cancer. Meta-analyses have suggested that the risk of breast cancer is increased by almost 50% in night workers, and by about 70% in flight personnel. The aviation industry in particular has an intense interest in research in this area given the fact that in addition to the theoretical risk of an increased risk of cancer from shift work, there is also an increased risk of cancer from cosmic radiation for many aviation industry employees such as pilots and flight attendants. If there is a relationship, it will be important to see what mechanisms explain the relationship. Some have suspected disruption in melatonin production, which has direct and indirect anticancer effects. Variation in steroid levels can also alter immune function and shift work may result in changes in lifestyle factors such as smoking, diet, alcohol use, or exercise. To read more about the potential link between shift work and cancer, see the report by Fritschl.[4] In a world that is now 24/7, we need to learn more about subjects such as this.

**J. A. Stockman III, MD**

*References*

1. Landgren O. Sun, mother of life, prevents cancer. *Blood.* 2011;118:1431-1432.
2. de Roock S, van Elk M, van Dijk ME, et al. Lactic acid bacteria differ in their ability to induce functional regulatory T cells in humans. *Clin Exp Allergy.* 2010;40: 103-110.
3. Straif K, Baan R, Grosse Y, et al. Carcinogenicity of shift work, painting, and firefighting. *Lancet Oncol.* 2007;8.1065-1066.
4. Fritschl L. Shift work and cancer. Short- and long-term effects provide compelling reasons to act now. *BMJ.* 2009,330:307-308.

---

**Effectiveness of high-dose methotrexate in T-cell lymphoblastic leukemia and advanced-stage lymphoblastic lymphoma: a randomized study by the Children's Oncology Group (POG 9404)**
Asselin BL, Devidas M, Wang C, et al (Univ of Rochester Med Ctr, NY; Univ of Florida, Gainesville; et al)
*Blood* 118:874-883, 2011

---

The Pediatric Oncology Group (POG) phase 3 trial 9404 was designed to determine the effectiveness of high-dose methotrexate (HDM) when added to multi-agent chemotherapy based on the Dana-Farber backbone. Children with T-cell acute lymphoblastic leukemia (T-ALL) or advanced lymphoblastic lymphoma (T-NHL) were randomized at diagnosis to receive/not receive HDM (5 g/m$^2$; as a 24-hour infusion) at weeks 4, 7, 10, and 13. Between 1996 and 2000, 436 patients were enrolled in the methotrexate randomization. Five-year and 10-year event-free survival (EFS) was 80.2% ± 2.8% and 78.1% ± 4.3% for HDM (n = 219) versus 73.6% ± 3.1% and 72.6% ± 5.0% for no HDM (n = 217; $P$ =.17). For T-ALL, 5-year and 10-year EFS was significantly better with HDM (n = 148,

5 years: 79.5% ± 3.4%, 10 years: 77.3% ± 5.3%) versus no HDM (n = 151, 5 years: 67.5% ± 3.9%, 10 years: 66.0% ± 6.6%; $P = .047$). The difference in EFS between HDM and no HDM was not significant for T-NHL patients (n = 71, 5 years: 81.7% ± 4.9%, 10 years: 79.9% ± 7.5% vs n = 66, 5 years: 87.8% ± 4.2%, 10 years: 87.8% ± 6.4%; $P = .38$). The frequency of mucositis was significantly higher in patients treated with HDM ($P = .003$). The results support adding HDM to the treatment of children with T-ALL, but not with NHL, despite the increased risk of mucositis.

▶ Recent nonrandomized studies of childhood T-cell acute lymphoblastic leukemia (T-ALL) report approximately a 70% to 75% 5-year event-free survival. The trial reported by Asselin et al undertaken within the Children's Oncology Group confirms the benefit of high-dose methotrexate in this high-risk group of patients.[1] In this clinical trial, children with newly diagnosed T-ALL or non-Hodgkin lymphoma (NHL) were randomly assigned to receive 4 doses (5 g/m$^2$) of high-dose methotrexate as a 24-hour infusion in the context of a modified intensive Dana-Farber Cancer Institute regimen. The benefits of high-dose methotrexate were substantial enough to warrant early closure of the randomization.

In an editorial that accompanied this report, it was noted that the benefits of high-dose methotrexate being substantial enough to warrant early closure of study randomization was good news. The not-so-good news was that outcome on high-dose methotrexate—treated patients ultimately was no better than that of other forms of T-ALL treatment regimens.[1] It is noted that the report by Asselin et al, while confirming the activity of high-dose methotrexate in newly diagnosed childhood T-ALL, also demonstrates that reductions in the intensity of central nervous system—directed therapy may dilute its therapeutic benefit. How, when, and in what therapeutic context to best supply high-dose methotrexate in this population thus remains unclear. The editorial accompanying this report suggests that "rearranging the deck chairs on the Titanic will not benefit children with T-ALL; it's time to move on to the evaluation of molecularly targeted therapies in this disorder."

This commentary closes with an observation having to do with soy intake and the development of cancer. Soy foods are known to be rich in isoflavones, a major group of phytoestrogens that had been hypothesized to reduce the risk of breast cancer. At the same time, the estrogen-like effect of isoflavones and the potential interaction between these and tamoxifen have led to concerns about soy food consumption among breast cancer patients. Investigators in Shanghai have studied whether diets high in soy in any way affect the outcomes of patients with breast cancer. The bottom line is that among women with breast cancer, soy food consumption is significantly associated with a decreased risk of death and recurrence. The hazard ratio associated with the highest quartile of soy protein intake was just 0.71 for total mortality and 0.68 for recurrence compared with the lowest quartile of intake. It is hard to compare the situation in the United States and China since soy food consumption among US women is substantially lower. Nonetheless, since this report from Shanghai appeared in a very reputable US journal, one can bet that the stock in Archer Daniel's *Midland* (the major US producer of soy products) is on the upswing.[2]

**J. A. Stockman III, MD**

*References*

1. Whitlock JA, Silverman LB. Childhood T-all: it's time to move on. *Blood*. 2011; 118:828-829.
2. Shu XO, Zheng Y, Cai H, et al. Soy food intake and breast cancer survival. *JAMA*. 2009;302:2437-2443.

**Long-term health-related outcomes in survivors of childhood cancer treated with HSCT versus conventional therapy: a report from the Bone Marrow Transplant Survivor Study (BMTSS) and Childhood Cancer Survivor Study (CCSS)**

Armenian SH, Sun C-L, Kawashima T, et al (City of Hope, Duarte, CA; Fred Hutchinson Cancer Res Ctr, Seattle, WA; et al)

*Blood* 118:1413-1420, 2011

HSCT is being increasingly offered as a curative option for children with hematologic malignancies. Although survival has improved, the long-term morbidity ascribed to the HSCT procedure is not known. We compared the risk of chronic health conditions and adverse health among children with cancer treated with HSCT with survivors treated conventionally, as well as with sibling controls. HSCT survivors were drawn from BMTSS (N = 145), whereas conventionally treated survivors (N = 7207) and siblings (N = 4020) were drawn from CCSS. Self-reported chronic conditions were graded with CTCAEv3.0. Fifty-nine percent of HSCT survivors reported $\geq$ 2 conditions, and 25.5% reported severe/life-threatening conditions. HSCT survivors were more likely than sibling controls to have severe/life threatening (relative risk [RR] = 8.1, $P < .01$) and 2 or more (RR = 5.7, $P < .01$) conditions, as well as functional impairment (RR = 7.7, $P < .01$) and activity limitation (RR = 6.3, $P < .01$). More importantly, compared with CCSS survivors, BMTSS survivors demonstrated significantly elevated risks (severe/life-threatening conditions: RR = 3.9, $P < .01$; multiple conditions: RR = 2.6, $P < .01$; functional impairment: RR = 3.5, $P < .01$; activity limitation: RR = 5.8, $P < .01$). Unrelated donor HSCT recipients were at greatest risk. Childhood HSCT survivors carry a significantly greater burden of morbidity not only compared with noncancer populations but also compared with conventionally treated cancer patients, providing evidence for close monitoring of this high-risk population.

▶ Armenian et al have studied the late-term effects of treatment of childhood cancers comparing the consequences of bone marrow transplant with survival afforded by chemotherapy alone. Those who underwent bone marrow transplantation had more long-term chronic health problems, but interestingly there were no differences in the prevalence and severity of chronic health conditions among bone marrow transplant survivors who underwent stem cell transplantation in first remission compared with those with more advanced disease who had had much greater degrees of prior chemotherapy.

The overall goals of the study of Armenian et al were to understand the long-term burden of morbidity associated with hematopoietic stem cell transplantation in childhood; to compare this burden of morbidity with that reported by an unaffected comparison group; and to evaluate the burden of morbidity among hematopoietic stem cell transplantation survivors that was over and above that associated with conventional therapy. It was observed that the burden of chronic health conditions among children treated with hematopoietic stem cell transplantation is high. Some 80% reported at least 1 chronic health condition; 25% had severe/life-threatening conditions; and nearly 60% had 2 or more conditions. In contrast, just 5% of siblings reported severe/life-threatening conditions; 12.4% had 2 or more conditions. Compared with sibling controls, bone marrow transplantation survivors were 2.6 times as likely to report a chronic health condition of any severity. The risk for a severe/life-threatening condition was 8.1-fold increased, and the risk was 5.7-fold increased for having 2 or more conditions. Chronic graft versus host (GVH) disease contributed significantly to the increased risk of adverse health status in most patients. The health status in survivors with resolved chronic GVH disease was equivalent to those who had never been diagnosed with chronic GVH disease. This finding is similar to that previously reported in adult long-term hematopoietic stem cell transplantation survivors.

Among all survivors of cancer, those who have received unrelated hematopoietic stem cell transplants are at greatest risk. Conditioning with total body irradiation and the presence of active chronic GVH disease remain the critical modifiers of chronic health conditions and adverse health status.

**J. A. Stockman III, MD**

---

## High success rate of hematopoietic cell transplantation regardless of donor source in children with very high-risk leukemia

Leung W, Campana D, Yang J, et al (St Jude Children's Res Hosp, Memphis, TN)
*Blood* 118:223-230, 2011

---

We evaluated 190 children with very high-risk leukemia, who underwent allogeneic hematopoietic cell transplantation in 2 sequential treatment eras, to determine whether those treated with contemporary protocols had a high risk of relapse or toxic death, and whether non—HLA-identical transplantations yielded poor outcomes. For the recent cohorts, the 5-year overall survival rates were 65% for the 37 patients with acute lymphoblastic leukemia and 74% for the 46 with acute myeloid leukemia; these rates compared favorably with those of earlier cohorts (28%, n = 57; and 34%, n = 50, respectively). Improvement in the recent cohorts was observed regardless of donor type (sibling, 70% vs 24%;

unrelated, 61% vs 37%; and haploidentical, 88% vs 19%), attributable to less infection (hazard ratio [HR] = 0.12; $P = .005$), regimen-related toxicity (HR = 0.25; $P = .002$), and leukemia-related death (HR = 0.40; $P = .01$). Survival probability was dependent on leukemia status (first remission vs more advanced disease; HR = 0.63; $P = .03$) or minimal residual disease (positive vs negative; HR = 2.10; $P = .01$) at the time of transplantation. We concluded that transplantation has improved over time and should be considered for all children with very high-risk leukemia, regardless of matched donor availability.

▶ There are varying recommendations for the use of allogeneic hematopoietic cell transplantation (HCT) for the management of children with acute myeloid leukemia (AML) and acute lymphoblastic leukemia (ALL). Several studies have shown that survival rates for AML patients treated with HLA-identical sibling HCT are superior to those patients treated with chemotherapy alone, leading to a recommendation in favor of HCT by the American Society for Blood and Marrow Transplantation Evidence-based Review Committee.[1] Also, HCT has been documented to produce higher cure rates in patients with certain cytogenetic abnormalities such as t(9;22) and t(4;11) or who experience induction failure. Additionally, patients with persistent minimal residual disease or relapse while on therapy are also considered candidates for HCT in current protocols.

One of the lingering questions now is whether HCT benefits patients whose leukemia is chemo-resistant to current intensive chemotherapy. Concerns exist about the use of HCT. Toxicity may be excessive because of preexisting organ dysfunction or infections caused by prior intensive chemotherapy. It is also not well known whether there is a significant role for HCT when a matched sibling donor is not available. Some of these issues are addressed in the report of Leung, which evaluates the outcomes and causes of death of 83 patients with very high-risk ALL or high-risk AML who undergo allogeneic HCT after receiving intensive multiagent chemotherapy. The data of these patients were compared with 107 patients who did not receive HCT. The study found that patients who had very high-risk leukemia did have favorable outcomes after HCT. Transplantation-regimen—related death for these patients was much lower than for patients treated with other forms of therapy. The 5-year overall survival for patients with ALL was 65%. It was 74% for those with AML. These are significant improvements over prior studies.

The results published by Leung et al indicate that all patients with very high-risk leukemia should be considered as potential candidates for HCT early in the course of diagnosis or relapse treatment, regardless of the availability of a matched donor or the intensity of prior chemotherapy. This means that such high-risk patients should have HLA typing and a donor search performed as soon as possible with referral to a transplant center. All too often, insurance approval is denied for HCT because of the notion that these patients are not salvageable by this procedure, especially if a sibling donor is not available. The findings from the report of Leung et al contradict this belief and should be a powerful tool for care providers to argue on behalf of their patients if an insurance company balked at payment.

This commentary closes with a comment on a cancer drug regimen. On Christmas Day 2000, Navy, a golden retriever aged 18 months, began a cocktail of celecoxib, tamoxifen, and doxycycline to target blood vessels supplying a tumor on her chest. Her owner, a veterinary student at Tufts University, Boston, was acquainted with the work of angiogenesis pioneer, Judah Folkman at the nearby Children's Hospital, Harvard Medical School. Soon the golden retriever became a golden guinea pig. The treatment was blinded to the patient, who unknowingly polished off the regimen with her dog biscuits. Three months later, Navy was cancer free and the following year a healthy report was published.[2] The excitement around the story led to the drug combination being renamed the Navy protocol, which remains a familiar term in veterinary oncology today.[3]

**J. A. Stockman III, MD**

*References*

1. Oliansky DM, Rizzo JD, Aplan PD, et al. The role of cytotoxic therapy in hematopoietic stem cell transplantation in the therapy of acute myeloid leukemia in children: an evidence-based review. *Biol Blood Marrow Transplant*. 2007;13:1-25.
2. Kirk E. Dog's tale of survival opens door in cancer research. *USA Today*. July 24, 2002.
3. Lane R. A protocol for laboratory retrievers? *Lancet*. 2009;374:2038-2039.

---

**Survival Rates of Children With Acute Lymphoblastic Leukemia Presenting to a Pediatric Rheumatologist in the United States**

Hashkes PJ, Wright BM, Lauer MS, et al (Cleveland Clinic, OH; The Children's Hosp at MCCG, Macon, GA; Lung and Blood Inst, Bethesda, MD; et al)

*J Pediatr Hematol Oncol* 33:424-428, 2011

---

*Background.*—Approximately 30% of pediatric acute lymphoblastic leukemia patients present with musculoskeletal symptoms and are often referred first to a pediatric rheumatologist. We examined the survival and causes of death of these patients presenting to a pediatric rheumatologist and compared the rates with that reported in the hematology-oncology literature.

*Procedure.*—We used the Pediatric Rheumatology Disease Registry, including 49,023 patients from 62 centers, newly diagnosed between 1992 and 2001. Identifiers were matched with the Social Security Death Index censored for March 2005. Deaths were confirmed by death certificates, referring physicians, and medical records. Causes of death were derived by chart review or from the death certificate.

*Results.*—There were 7 deaths of 89 patients (7.9%, 95% confidence interval: 3.9%-15.4%) with acute lymphoblastic leukemia with a 5-year survival rate of 95.5% (88.3 to 98.3) and 10-year survival rate of 89.8% (79.0% to 95.2%). The causes of death were sepsis (bacterial and/or fungal) in 4 (57%) patients, the disease in 2 (29%) and post bone-marrow transplantation in 1 (14%).

*Conclusion.*—The overall survival of patients with acute lymphoblastic leukemia seen first by pediatric rheumatologists is higher than the range reported in the pediatric oncology literature for the same period of diagnosis.

▶ This report contains some important statistics that all of us should become familiar with as pediatric care providers. Musculoskeletal pain is a common symptom in children. Somewhere between 10% and 20% of children of school age will have musculoskeletal pain of some sort. Less than 1% of such children will turn out to have a malignancy, but conversely, 40% of children with malignancy, particularly acute lymphoblastic leukemia (ALL), will have musculoskeletal pain as a presenting symptom. Another 20% will have such symptoms mixed in with other findings consistent with ALL.

All too often, children with musculoskeletal pain and ALL present to either an orthopedist or a rheumatologist, and in such cases the referral is either to rule out structural causes of musculoskeletal pain or to exclude juvenile idiopathic arthritis. Fortunately, well-trained pediatric rheumatologists are more than able to look for the clinical findings and laboratory clues that would trigger a suspicion of malignancy. Nocturnal pain is one such sentinel finding for ALL and often for other types of malignancy. Thus, pain awakening a patient from sleep is not a good finding. In such cases, pediatric rheumatologists know to look carefully at the complete blood count and peripheral blood smear, the lactate dehydrogenase and uric acid levels, as well as x-rays showing the typical bone findings of leukemia (lytic lesions or metaphyseal rarefactions).

The reason it is important for all of us, including our pediatric rheumatology colleagues, to recognize the musculoskeletal findings in ALL relates to the fact that delayed diagnosis can affect survival in an adverse way. Hashkes et al report on just how good pediatric rheumatologists are quickly making a diagnosis of ALL when the latter is a presenting sign of musculoskeletal pain. Using the pediatric rheumatology disease registry, the authors of this report were able to find 89 patients who presented with musculoskeletal pain and who ultimately had a diagnosis of ALL. The survival rate in these patients was 95.5%, and the 10-year survival rate was just under 90%. These survival rates actually are higher than the overall survival rates from the literature of all children presenting with leukemia within similar time frames. These data suggest that such patients may actually have improved survival compared with the general ALL population, a phenomenon that is not easily explained. It should be noted that other studies have also suggested a better-than-average prognosis in children with ALL presenting with bone abnormalities on radiographic study.[1] It would be interesting to see someone put together the data from the pediatric rheumatology disease registry to correlate survivorship with initial prognostic features other than musculoskeletal pain. Such features could include immunophenotyping, genetic markers, and evidence of minimal residual disease after initial induction therapy. These data surely exist in these kids' cancer registry database. It would be an easy undertaking to study this information.

**J. A. Stockman III, MD**

*Reference*

1. Dini G, Taccone A, De Bernardi B, Comelli A, Garrè ML, Gandus S. [Skeletal changes in acute lymphoblastic leukemia in children. Incidence and prognostic significance]. *Radiol Med.* 1983;69:644-649.

---

**Early human cytomegalovirus replication after transplantation is associated with a decreased relapse risk: evidence for a putative virus-versus-leukemia effect in acute myeloid leukemia patients**

Elmaagacli AH, Steckel NK, Koldehoff M, et al (Univ of Duisburg-Essen, Germany)

*Blood* 118:1402-1412, 2011

---

The impact of early human cytomegalovirus (HCMV) replication on leukemic recurrence was evaluated in 266 consecutive adult (median age, 47 years; range, 18-73 years) acute myeloid leukemia patients, who underwent allogeneic stem cell transplantation (alloSCT) from 10 of 10 high-resolution human leukocyte Ag-identical unrelated (n = 148) or sibling (n = 118) donors. A total of 63% of patients (n = 167) were at risk for HCMV reactivation by patient and donor pretransplantation HCMV serostatus. In 77 patients, first HCMV replication as detected by pp65-antigenemia assay developed at a median of 46 days (range, 25-108 days) after alloSCT. Taking all relevant competing risk factors into account, the cumulative incidence of hematologic relapse at 10 years after alloSCT was 42% (95% confidence interval [CI], 35%-51%) in patients without opposed to 9% (95% CI, 4%-19%) in patients with early pp65-antigenemia ($P < .0001$). A substantial and independent reduction of the relapse risk associated with early HCMV replication was confirmed by multivariate analysis using time-dependent covariate functions for grades II to IV acute and chronic graft-versus-host disease, and pp65-antigenemia (hazard ratio = 0.2; 95% CI, 0.1-0.4, $P < .0001$). This is the first report that demonstrates an independent and substantial reduction of the leukemic relapse risk after early replicative HCMV infection in a homogeneous population of adult acute myeloid leukemia patients.

▶ Most believe that cytomegalovirus (CMV) is a bad actor in patients with leukemia, including those who have had stem cell transplantation. Not quite, so say Elmaagacli et al. These investigators have found an unexpected favorable association of a low rate of leukemic relapse in acute myeloid leukemia patients who reactivate CMV in the first few weeks following stem cell transplantation. Analyzing 266 consecutive patients with acute myeloblastic leukemia (AML) who received stem cell transplants from HLA-identical relatives or unrelated donors between 1997 and 2009, the authors found an unusual association between early CMV reactivation and transplantation outcome. Seventy-seven patients developing their first CMV antigenemia at a median of 6 weeks after transplantation were found to have a remarkably low risk of leukemic relapse

(9% at 10 years after transplant compared with a 42% risk in patients not reactivating CMV). Furthermore, they found that, far from being a risk for increased transplant-related mortality, the occurrence of CMV reactivation was not deleterious for survival.

In the past, CMV reactivation seemed to imply immunodeficiency and breakdown of immunosurveillance against residual leukemia. Normally, one would think that the detection of virus early after transplantation might be expected to be associated with an increased risk of relapse. The findings from Germany, therefore, fly in the face of established perceptions. Needless to say, unexpected findings merit special scrutiny if they are to be believed, and in this report the authors have gone to extensive lengths to support their conclusions. Elmaagacli et al propose several explanations for their findings. First, myeloid cells are a reservoir for CMV. It is possible that viral reactivation in AML blasts makes them a target for subsequent attack by virus-specific cytotoxic T cells. Alternatively, CMV reactivation in AML cells may up-regulate leukocyte fixation antigen-3 expression and enhance natural killer cell cytotoxicity against the leukemic cells. Also, the virus could have a direct cytotoxic effect on AML cells: a virus-versus-leukemia effect. Of these various possibilities, the hypothesis that CMV renders the leukemia a target for immune attack seems the most likely.

The data from this report do in fact seem quite solid. It is interesting when bad viruses actually turn out to be the good ones.

**J. A. Stockman III, MD**

## A Home-based Maintenance Therapy Program for Acute Lymphoblastic Leukemia—Practical and Safe?

Phillips B, Richards M, Boys R, et al (St James's Hosp, Leeds, UK)
*J Pediatr Hematol Oncol* 33:433-436, 2011

The maintenance phase of treatment for childhood acute lymphoblastic leukemia is characterized by daily oral chemotherapy dose-adjusted on the basis of toxicity, monitored by regular (1 to 2 weekly) blood counts. A traditional approach is undertaking this at out-patient clinics. A home maintenance program was commenced to reduce visits to hospital and associated family disruption. The program organizes blood tests arranged to be taken at or near the patients' home. The results are examined by a pharmacist and specialist nurse; changes in therapy are communicated by telephone call and written confirmation. Hospital attendance is reduced to monthly visits. To assess the program, tablet counting and before-and-after audits of parental satisfaction were undertaken. Results of the first 2 years are presented. Preliminary analysis to identify predictors of nonadherence was performed. Fifty families were included in the evaluation. There were no critical incidents. Poor adherence rates in the initial 3-month period (overall 24%) improved after increased support and advice were offered to 78%. Increasing age was correlated with good adherence ($r = 0.37$, $P = 0.02$).

Partnership status of the child's caretakers was strongly associated with adherence (14% of poor adhering patients had caretakers in stable partnerships, compared with 87% of good adhering patients, $P < 0.01$).

▶ This report comes from Great Britain. The authors of the report decided to assess safety and parent satisfaction with a home maintenance program for care of children with acute lymphoblastic leukemia (ALL). In the United States, the more traditional approach has been to bring children with ALL back to the primary cancer treatment center to undertake periodic blood testing, physical examination, physician review, and modification of therapy as needed. Given the overall survivorship of children with ALL these days, this can amount to a fair commitment time-wise and logistically for a family. What Phillips et al have done is to design a regional oncology program covering a population base of approximately 3.7 million people. The oncology center represented in the report sees about 35 newly diagnosed acute leukemia patients each year. The center provides support for shared care by partner district general hospitals. It is the latter, often in one's own hometown, that provides the maintenance therapy. There is a continuous dialogue between the cancer center and the regional programs. The authors of this report found that the home-based maintenance program was reliable, safe, and preferred by families compared with the oncology-center approach. Adherence to the therapy regimen was excellent.

In the United States, we see this type of program described largely in rural parts of the country. It is hard to say whether most oncology programs would be willing to accept the data from Great Britain. Parents, however, seem to like the results. As an aside, a recent report from Copenhagen tells us that the periodic courses of steroid therapy children with ALL receive can produce adrenal insufficiency such that during times of stress, these youngsters are at significant risk for an adrenal crisis.[1] The authors suggest that as adrenal insufficiency is frequent in children treated for ALL, and because they often experience infections or other stressors, adrenal status should be assessed and steroid substitution therapy given during stressful episodes in those who are demonstrated to have adrenal insufficiency.

**J. A. Stockman III, MD**

*Reference*

1. Vestergaard TR, Juul A, Lausten-Thomsen U, et al. Duration of adrenal insufficiency during treatment for childhood acute lymphoblastic leukemia. *J Pediatr Hematol Oncol.* 2011;33:442-449.

**Bone mineral density in adult survivors of childhood acute leukemia: impact of hematopoietic stem cell transplantation and other treatment modalities**

Le Meignen M, Auquier P, Barlogis V, et al (Hosp L'Archet II, Nice, France; Hôpital Nord, Marseille, France; Children's Hosp of La Timone, Marseille, France; et al)

*Blood* 118:1481-1489, 2011

Femoral and lumbar bone mineral densities (BMDs) were measured in 159 adults enrolled in the Leucémies de l'Enfant et de l'Adolescent program, a French prospective multicentric cohort of childhood leukemia survivors. BMDs were expressed as Z-scores, and multivariate linear regression analyses were used to construct association models with potential risk factors. Mean age at evaluation and follow-up was 23 and 14.7 years, respectively. In the whole cohort, mean femoral Z-score was $-0.19 \pm 0.08$. Two factors were associated with lower femoral BMD transplantation ($-0.49 \pm 0.15$ vs $0.04 \pm 0.10$ in the chemotherapy group; $P = .006$) and female sex ($-0.34 \pm 0.10$ vs $-0.03 \pm 0.13$; $P = .03$). Among patients who received a transplant, the only significant risk factor was hypogonadism ($-0.88 \pm 0.16$ vs $-0.10 \pm 0.23$; $P = .04$). A slight reduction in lumbar BMD (mean Z-score, $-0.37 \pm 0.08$) was detected in the whole cohort without difference between the transplantation and chemotherapy groups. Among patients who received a transplant, younger age at transplantation was correlated with a low lumbar BMD ($P = .03$). We conclude that adults who had received only chemotherapy for childhood leukemia have a slight reduction in their lumbar BMD and a normal femoral BMD. Patients who received a transplant with gonadal deficiency have a reduced femoral BMD which might increase the fracture risk later in life.

▶ It is well known that childhood acute leukemia (ALL)-affected youngsters have a much increased likelihood of having reduced bone mineral density (BMD). The cause of this relates to a number of different factors. This could be because of the disease process itself, the use of steroids, intensive chemotherapy, abnormalities of endocrine function that control bone metabolism, immunosuppressive agents used as part of stem cell transplantation, poor nutrition, and decreased physical activity. What is not known is whether survivors of childhood ALL maintain low BMD long after the end of treatment. Le Meignen et al designed a study to determine the long-term effects of abnormalities in BMD in childhood survivors of ALL by looking at 159 adults who fell into the latter category. The study was carried out in France. It was a prospective study. Adult survivors were examined at a median age of 23 years, some 14.7 years after disease diagnosis and treatment.

This report showed that most survivors of childhood ALL do not sustain significant long-term impairment of BMD. That is not to say, however, that all subjects fared well. There was a subset of patients that had lower-than-expected BMD for age. This appeared to be related to specific aspects of their treatment and its consequences. The use of chemotherapy alone did not correlate with long-term reductions in BMD. The study did not detect a more pronounced BMD involvement in patients with ALL who received steroids or methotrexate, which are known to cause an osteopathy. Patients who underwent hematopoietic stem cell transplantation were a different kettle of fish, however. In addition to the intensity of the conditioning programs these patients received, immunosuppressive agents used after hematopoietic stem cell transplantation appeared to have accelerated bone loss. A younger age at transplantation correlated with a lower BMD.

These findings highlight the significance of bone mass measurements in the survivor group who underwent hematopoietic stem cell transplantation. Bone mineral assessment should be part of the routine long-term follow-up of these patients, particularly if related to gonadal failure. These patients should avoid smoking, limit intake of caffeine and carbonated beverages, and assure themselves of adequate intakes of calcium and vitamin D. They should also engage in weight-bearing exercise programs for the remainder of their lives.

Needless to say, BMD problems may turn out to be a significant long-term complication for survivors of ALL who have undergone hematopoietic stem cell transplantation. The data from this report represent only 15 years of follow-up. One would like to see 25 years and 50 years of follow-up to know exactly how well these youngsters will do into adulthood.

**J. A. Stockman III, MD**

---

## Prevalence and risk factors of the metabolic syndrome in adult survivors of childhood leukemia

Oudin C, Simeoni M-C, Sirvent N, et al (Hôpital de la Timone Enfants, Marseille, France; Hôpital de la Timone, Marseille, France; CHU l'Archet, Nice, France; et al)
*Blood* 117:4442-4448, 2011

---

We evaluate the prevalence and risk factors of the metabolic syndrome (MS) in young adults surviving childhood leukemia. During the years 2007 to 2008, assessment of MS was proposed to all adults included in the Leucémie de l'Enfant et de l'Adolescent program, a French prospective multicentric cohort of leukemia survivors. Among 220 eligible patients, 184 (83.6%) had complete evaluation. Median age at evaluation and follow-up duration were 21.2 and 15.4 years. Overall prevalence of MS was 9.2% (95% confidence interval, 5.5-14.4). There was no association of MS with sex, age at diagnosis, leukemia subtype, steroid therapy, and central nervous system irradiation. Patients were stratified according to 4 therapeutic modalities: chemotherapy alone (n = 97), chemotherapy and central nervous system irradiation (n = 27), hematopoietic stem cell transplantation (HSCT) without (n = 17) or with (n = 43) total body irradiation (TBI). MS occurred in 5.2%, 11.1%, 5.9%, and 18.6% of them, respectively. The higher risk observed in the HSCT-TBI group was significant in univariate and in multivariate analysis (odds ratio [OR] = 3.9, $P = .03$). HSCT with TBI was associated with a higher rate of hypertriglyceridemia (OR = 4.5, $P = .004$), low level of high-density lipoprotein cholesterol

(OR = 2.5, *P* =.02), and elevated fasting glucose (OR = 6.1, *P* =.04) So, TBI is a major risk factor for MS. Further studies are warranted to explain this feature.

▶ Currently it is estimated that there are more than 50 000 survivors of childhood acute lymphocytic leukemia (ALL) in the United States. These numbers continue to increase every day. Although ALL survivors are generally at lower risk of developing long-term sequelae of therapy compared with survivors of other cancer diagnoses (notably Hodgkin lymphoma, brain tumors, and sarcomas), this group has a particular predisposition for metabolic derangements. A number of studies have demonstrated an increased prevalence of the metabolic syndrome (MS) and its various components, including central obesity, hypertension, impaired glucose metabolism, and dyslipidemia. Those particularly vulnerable to the development of MS are patients with ALL who have had cranial radiation and hematopoietic stem-cell transplantation (HSCT).

In the study of Oudin et al, 18.6% of survivors of ALL who had a combination of HSCT and total body irradiation met the criteria for MS. Obesity was the highest prevalence manifestation of MS in this patient population. In those undergoing cranial irradiation, it is thought that obesity is in part the result of radiation-induced growth hormone insufficiency and leptin insensitivity. Even survivors treated without radiation (most children with ALL today) can be at increased risk for obesity as a consequence of cancer therapy. Steroid therapy may lead to physical inactivity secondary to myopathy, osteonecrosis, and reduced bone mineral density. Vincristine-induced peripheral neuropathy may further limit physical activity. In addition, unhealthy lifestyles, such as poor diet and increased sedentary time, may develop during treatment protocols that last over a number of years.

The result of the problems associated with MS in childhood survivors of ALL is an increased risk of cardiovascular disease. Data to date suggest that ALL survivors are 4.2 times more likely than the general population to die of heart disease.[1] They are also 6.4 times as likely to suffer a late-occurring stroke. Consequently, all survivors of ALL, particularly those exposed to cranial radiation therapy, HSCT, or total body radiation, must have regular follow-up care that is adapted to address the metabolic and cardiovascular risks that arise from their prior therapy. All too often, however, these children enter adulthood and do not have a receptor piece in the adult health care provider community that provides these comprehensive services.

It is a shame to win the battle with childhood cancer only to lose the long-term battle of life because of poor provision of health care.

**J. A. Stockman III, MD**

*Reference*

1. Armstrong GT, Liu Q, Yasui Y, et al. Late mortality among 5-year survivors of childhood cancer: a summary from the Childhood Cancer Survivor Study. *J Clin Oncol.* 2009;27:2328-2338.

## Cardiovascular Hospitalizations and Mortality Among Recipients of Hematopoietic Stem Cell Transplantation

Chow EJ, Mueller BA, Baker KS, et al (Fred Hutchinson Cancer Res Ctr, Seattle, WA; Seattle Children's Hosp, WA; Univ of Washington, Seattle; et al)
*Ann Intern Med* 155:21-32, 2011

*Background.*—Hematopoietic stem cell transplantation (HSCT) is increasingly used to treat multiple malignant and nonmalignant conditions. The risk for cardiovascular disease after the procedure has not been well-described.

*Objective.*—To compare rates and hazards of cardiovascular-related hospitalization and death among persons who were still alive at least 2 years after HSCT with those in a population-based sample.

*Design.*—Retrospective cohort study.

*Setting.*—Comprehensive cancer center.

*Patients.*—1491 patients who had survived 2 years or longer after HSCT received between 1985 and 2006, and frequency-matched persons who were randomly selected from drivers' license files in the state of Washington.

*Measurements.*—Cardiovascular hospitalizations and death, as determined from statewide hospital discharge records and death registries in Washington.

*Results.*—Compared with the general population, transplant recipients experienced increased cardiovascular death (adjusted incidence rate difference, 3.6 per 1000 person-years [95% CI, 1.7 to 5.5]). Recipients also had an increased cumulative incidence of ischemic heart disease, cardiomyopathy or heart failure, stroke, vascular diseases, and rhythm disorders and an increased incidence of related conditions that predispose toward more serious cardiovascular disease (hypertension, renal disease, dyslipidemia, and diabetes). No consistent differences in hazards were observed after total-body irradiation or receipt of an allogeneic versus an autologous graft, aside from an increased rate of hypertension among recipients of allogeneic grafts. Disease relapse after transplantation was associated with an increased hazard of cardiovascular death (hazard ratio, 2.3 [CI, 1.1 to 4.8]).

*Limitation.*—All patients received HSCT at a single institution, and no information was available on pretransplantation treatment and lifestyle factors that may influence risk for cardiovascular disease.

*Conclusion.*—Increased rates of cardiovascular disease should be taken into account when caring for patients who have received HSCT. Future efforts should be directed toward improved screening and controlling of factors that predispose toward cardiovascular disease.

▶ At the time this report appeared, more than 60 000 individuals worldwide had received either allogeneic or autologous hematopoietic stem-cell transplantation (HSCT). That is an annual figure. HSCT is most commonly used as part of the management of hematologic cancer but is also used for other types of cancer and an increasing number of nonmalignant conditions. While graft-versus-host disease and recurrent cancer are the most common problems post-HSCT, investigators have increasingly recognized that HSCT recipients are also at great risk for the longer-term cardiovascular morbidity and mortality complications of the procedure. Patients who receive HSCT are at greater risk for dyslipidemia, hypertension, and diabetes, which in turn increase the risk for nonfatal and fatal cardiovascular disease in people who were previously diagnosed with a malignancy. Unfortunately, until the report of Chow et al appeared, we had limited information about the probable risks of such complications in adults who have survived a childhood malignancy.

Chow et al examined the experience at the Fred Hutchinson Cancer Research Center in Seattle. The center is a National Cancer Institute—designated comprehensive cancer center and the only accredited institution that performs both allogeneic and autologous HSCTs in the state of Washington. The researchers followed up with almost 1500 patients who survived 2 years or longer after HSCT that had been performed between 1985 and 2006. Approximately one-fourth of the patients were diagnosed in childhood. It was clear that rates of cardiovascular morbidity and mortality were significantly increased in patients who had received HSCT compared with the general population. These rates were increased the most in individuals younger than 60 years of age at the time of treatment. They were also more significantly increased among those who already had multiple cardiovascular risk factors (hypertension, diabetes, dyslipidemia, and renal disease). The risk of cardiovascular death was increased by almost 4-fold in HSCT recipients compared with normal controls.

The findings of this report emphasize the need for clinicians to be especially aware of late cardiovascular effects in HSCT recipients. Unfortunately, the latter often are cured of their basic underlying disease, and the index of suspicion of long-term complications may be lower. Screening programs need to be in place to detect the long-term consequences of HSCT. Handoffs from pediatric to adult care providers must have clear guidelines for each patient in this regard.

**J. A. Stockman III, MD**

---

## Long-term Risks of Subsequent Primary Neoplasms Among Survivors of Childhood Cancer

Reulen RC, for the British Childhood Cancer Survivor Study Steering Group (Univ of Birmingham, Edgbaston, UK; et al)
*JAMA* 305:2311-2319, 2011

---

*Context.*—Survivors of childhood cancer are at excess risk of developing subsequent primary neoplasms but the long-term risks are uncertain.

*Objectives.*—To investigate long-term risks of subsequent primary neoplasms in survivors of childhood cancer, to identify the types that contribute most to long-term excess risk, and to identify subgroups of survivors at substantially increased risk of particular subsequent primary neoplasms that may require specific interventions.

*Design, Setting, and Participants.*—British Childhood Cancer Survivor Study—a population-based cohort of 17 981 5-year survivors of childhood cancer diagnosed with cancer at younger than 15 years between 1940 and 1991 in Great Britain, followed up through December 2006.

*Main Outcome Measures.*—Standardized incidence ratios (SIRs), absolute excess risks (AERs), and cumulative incidence of subsequent primary neoplasms.

*Results.*—After a median follow-up time of 24.3 years (mean=25.6 years), 1354 subsequent primary neoplasms were ascertained; the most frequently observed being central nervous system (n=344), nonmelanoma skin cancer (n=278), digestive (n=105), genitourinary (n=100), breast (n=97), and bone (n=94). The overall SIR was 4 times more than expected (SIR, 3.9; 95% confidence interval [CI], 3.6-4.2; AER, 16.8 per 10 000 person-years). The AER at older than 40 years was highest for digestive and genitourinary subsequent primary neoplasms (AER, 5.9 [95% CI, 2.5-9.3]; and AER, 6.0 [95% CI, 2.3-9.6] per 10 000 person-years, respectively); 36% of the total AER was attributable to these 2 subsequent primary neoplasm sites. The cumulative incidence of colorectal cancer for survivors treated with direct abdominopelvic irradiation was 1.4% (95% CI, 0.7%-2.6%) by age 50 years, comparable with the 1.2% risk in individuals with at least 2 first-degree relatives affected by colorectal cancer.

*Conclusion.*—Among a cohort of British childhood cancer survivors, the greatest excess risk associated with subsequent primary neoplasms at older than 40 years was for digestive and genitourinary neoplasms (Table 4).

▶ It is well known that if a child survives a cancer, he or she may grow up to be an adult with a significantly higher risk of the development of a secondary malignancy. Survivors of childhood cancer have about a 3- to 6-fold increased risk of developing a subsequent primary neoplasm. Unfortunately, there is not much information about the specific long-term risk associated with this, thus the importance of the report of Reulen et al.

Reulen et al have investigated the long-term risk of the subsequent development of a primary neoplasm in survivors of childhood leukemia. Their study was part of the British Childhood Cancer Survivor Study. The latter has followed almost 20 000 5-year survivors of childhood cancer for an average of at least 25 years. The study certainly has important findings including the recognition of an increased risk of the development of colorectal cancer, the latter occurring at a rate comparable to that seen in individuals with a strong family history of this cancer. Another important finding of this study is that childhood cancer survivors remain at risk for developing subsequent primary neoplasms even beyond 40 years of age. Among survivors younger than 20 years, bone cancer and glioma account for more than 50% of overall late-occurring primary neoplasms. In contrast, digestive and genitourinary subsequent primary neoplasms are low among survivors younger than 20 years but increase substantially with age older than 40 years. This risk multiplies significantly if a youngster has received direct irradiation of the abdomen or pelvis. The highest risk for the development of a genitourinary secondary neoplasm is seen in patients with inherited forms of retinoblastoma, suggesting that this excess risk is at least partially attributable to genetic predisposition.

Given the excesses observed among those older than 40 years of age, the data from this report clearly indicate that survivors of childhood cancer should be

TABLE 4.—Absolute Excess Risk for Digestive, Genitourinary, Breast, and Respiratory Subsequent Primary Neoplasms in Survivors Older Than 40 Years by Type of Childhood Cancer

| Type of Childhood Cancer | Digestive | | Genitourinary | | Breast | | Respiratory | |
|---|---|---|---|---|---|---|---|---|
| | No. Obs/Exp | AER (95% CI)[a] | No. Obs/Exp | AER (95% CI)[a] | No. Obs/Exp | AER (95% CI)[a] | No. Obs/Exp | AER (95% CI)[a] |
| Central nervous system | 9/5.1 | 3.6 (−1.8 to 9.0) | 13/6.6 | 5.9 (−0.6 to 12.4) | 7/9.0 | −1.8 (−6.6 to 3.0) | 3/3.3 | −0.2 (−3.4 to 2.9) |
| Leukemia | 0/0.3 | −2.8[b] | 1/0.5 | 4.0 (−11.8 to 19.7) | 0/0.9 | −7.3[b] | 0/0.2 | −1.4[b] |
| Hodgkin lymphoma | 7/1.7 | 15.1 (0.3 to 29.9) | 3/2.0 | 2.9 (−6.8 to 12.6) | 11/1.7 | 26.4 (7.9 to 44.9) | 7/1.1 | 16.9 (2.1 to 31.7) |
| Non-Hodgkin lymphoma | 4/1.3 | 11.5 (−5.0 to 28.1) | 5/1.5 | 14.7 (−3.8 to 33.3) | 1/1.5 | −2.0 (−10.3 to 6.3) | 2/0.8 | 5.0 (−6.7 to 16.7) |
| Neuroblastoma | 0/0.4 | −3.9[b] | 1/0.5 | 4.3 (−14.1 to 22.7) | 1/0.7 | 2.7 (−15.7 to 21.2) | 0/0.2 | −2.3[b] |
| Heritable retinoblastoma | 3/0.6 | 15.4 (−6.6 to 37.4) | 8/0.8 | 46.5 (10.5 to 82.5) | 3/1.3 | 10.7 (−11.3 to 32.8) | 5/0.4 | 30.0 (1.5 to 58.4) |
| Nonheritable retinoblastoma | 1/0.9 | 0.4 (−9.6 to 10.3) | 1/1.2 | −1.1 (−11.1 to 8.8) | 3/1.7 | 6.7 (−10.5 to 24.0) | 0/0.6 | −3.0[b] |
| Wilms tumor | 5/0.8 | 20.7 (−0.7 to 42.1) | 0/1.0 | −5.1[b] | 1/1.7 | −3.5 (−13.1 to 6.0) | 0/0.4 | −2.2[b] |
| Bone tumor | 1/1.0 | −0.1 (−10.1 to 9.8) | 1/1.4 | −1.9 (−11.8 to 8.0) | 4/1.9 | 10.8 (−9.1 to 30.7) | 1/0.7 | 1.7 (−8.3 to 11.6) |
| Soft tissue sarcoma | 2/1.6 | 1.1 (−7.2 to 9.4) | 6/2.1 | 11.8 (−2.6 to 26.3) | 2/2.5 | −1.6 (−9.9 to 6.8) | 1/1.0 | −0.1 (−6.0 to 5.8) |
| Other | 4/2.0 | 4.6 (−4.3 to 13.5) | 2/2.8 | −1.7 (−8.0 to 4.5) | 3/5.2 | −4.9 (−12.6 to 2.8) | 1/1.2 | −0.5 (−5.0 to 3.9) |

*Abbreviations:* AER, absolute excess risk; CI, confidence interval; Exp, expected; Obs, observed.
[a] AER per 10 000 person-years; CIs should be interpreted cautiously if based on fewer than 5 observed events.
[b] CI could not be calculated because observed number of events is zero.

encouraged to participate in existing general population screening programs. These should include breast, cervical, and bowel cancer screening. Table 4 shows those who would be at highest risk for the development of later-occurring neoplasms.

This commentary closes with an interesting observation having to do with fingerprints. In the United States, it is increasingly common to see one finger-printed when checking in on certain air flights. Recently, a patient who had been receiving capecitabine, an antimetabolite drug, to prevent recurrence of his nasopharyngeal cancer was detained by immigration officials because his fingerprints had mysteriously disappeared.[1] The drug is known to cause chronic inflammation of the palms and soles that can over time eradicate fingerprints. Oncologists are now warning patients to carry a letter with them when they travel that explains they are not a security risk.

**J. A. Stockman III, MD**

*Reference*

1. Wong M, Choo SP, Tan EH. Travel warning with capecitabine. *Ann Oncol.* 2009; 20:1281.

---

### Lung nodules in pediatric oncology patients: a prediction rule for when to biopsy

Murrell Z, Dickie B, Dasgupta R (Cincinnati Children's Hosp Med Ctr, OH)
*J Pediatr Surg* 46:833-837, 2011

---

*Purpose.*—The purpose of the study was to develop a prediction rule regarding the factors that most accurately predict the diagnosis of a malignancy in a lung nodule in the pediatric oncology patient.

*Methods.*—A retrospective review of pediatric oncology patients that underwent lung nodule resection between 1998 and 2007 was performed. Multivariable logistic regression was used to create a prediction rule.

*Results.*—Fifty pediatric oncology patients underwent 21 thoracotomies and 48 thoracoscopies to resect discrete lung nodules seen on computed tomographic scans during workup for metastasis or routine surveillance. The mean nodule size was 10.43 ± 7.08 mm. The most significant predictors of malignancy in a nodule were peripheral location (odds ratio [OR], 9.1); size between 5 and 10 mm (OR, 2.78); location within the right lower lobe (OR, 2.43); and patients with osteosarcoma (OR, 10.8), Ewing sarcoma (OR, 3.05), or hepatocellular carcinoma (OR, 2.38).

*Conclusions.*—Lesions that are between 5 and 10 mm in size and peripherally located in patients with osteosarcoma, Ewing sarcoma, or hepatocellular carcinoma are most likely to be malignant. Use of a prediction rule can help guide clinical practice by determining which patients should undergo surgical resection of lung nodules and which patients may be closely observed with continued radiologic studies.

▶ The lung is a frequent metastatic site in children who have solid tumor malignancies. All too often with routine chest x-ray surveillance or magnetic resonance imaging/computed tomography scanning, a nodule is detected, and the conundrum then is whether that nodule is likely to be benign or malignant. The challenge for the multidisciplinary collaborative efforts of the radiologist, oncologist, and surgeon is how to best identify the benign or malignant nature of these pulmonary nodules. Primary solid tumors of childhood, such as osteosarcoma, Ewing sarcoma, hepatoblastoma, and rhabdomyosarcoma, commonly spread at the lungs.

The authors of this report have given us good information about which pulmonary nodules are more likely to be benign or malignant in children who have been diagnosed with a primary cancer. Without question, to determine the disease status of the lesion, histologic assessment is definitive. The authors remind us that benign lesions have been reported in 15% to 45% of patients with a known tumor undergoing surgery for suspected thoracic nodules. In the authors' experience, 33% of biopsies turned out to be benign. The authors showed that if a nodule is between 5 mm and 10 mm in size and peripherally located in patients with osteosarcoma, Ewing sarcoma, and hepatocellular carcinoma, the lesions are overwhelmingly likely to be malignant. Using this size and location as a predictive rule, the authors were able to demonstrate a benign biopsy rate that can be as low as 12%.

Obviously, the goal is to decrease the number of biopsies in children who may have benign lesions. While there is no golden rule as yet for this, the authors of this report do provide us with useful information about the predictability of both size and location of nodules.

While on the topic of cancers, recently a 36-year-old arc welder presented with a persistent nodular lesion overlying his left nasal alar. Excisional biopsy confirmed a basal cell carcinoma with evidence of severe solar damage in the surrounding skin. The patient strongly denied exposure to sun. He was, however, an arc welder. It is known that arc welding produces considerable amounts of ultraviolet radiation. Presumably the latter was the cause of his skin cancer. Remember the phenomenon of arc welder's basal cell carcinoma.[1]

**J. A. Stockman III, MD**

*Reference*

1. Vhatt YM, Nigam A, Sissons MCJ. Arc welder's basal cell carcinoma. *BMJ.* 2010; 341:227.

---

### KIT as a Therapeutic Target in Metastatic Melanoma

Carvajal RD, Antonescu CR, Wolchok JD, et al (Memorial Sloan-Kettering Cancer Ctr, NY; et al)
*JAMA* 305:2327-2334, 2011

---

*Context.*—Some melanomas arising from acral, mucosal, and chronically sun-damaged sites harbor activating mutations and amplification of the type III transmembrane receptor tyrosine kinase KIT. We explored the effects of KIT inhibition using imatinib mesylate in this molecular subset of disease.

*Objective.*—To assess clinical effects of imatinib mesylate in patients with melanoma harboring *KIT* alterations.

*Design, Setting, and Patients.*—A single-group, open-label, phase 2 trial at 1 community and 5 academic oncology centers in the United States of 295 patients with melanoma screened for the presence of *KIT* mutations and amplification between April 23, 2007, and April 16, 2010. A total of 51 cases with such alterations were identified and 28 of these patients were treated who had advanced unresectable melanoma arising from acral, mucosal, and chronically sun-damaged sites.

*Intervention.*—Imatinib mesylate, 400 mg orally twice daily.

*Main Outcome Measures.*—Radiographic response, with secondary end points including time to progression, overall survival, and correlation of molecular alterations and clinical response.

*Results.*—Two complete responses lasting 94 (ongoing) and 95 weeks, 2 durable partial responses lasting 53 and 89 (ongoing) weeks, and 2 transient partial responses lasting 12 and 18 weeks among the 25 evaluable patients were observed. The overall durable response rate was 16% (95% confidence interval [CI], 2%-30%), with a median time to progression of 12 weeks (interquartile range [IQR], 6-18 weeks; 95% CI, 11-18 weeks), and a median overall survival of 46.3 weeks (IQR, 28 weeks-not achieved; 95% CI, 28 weeks-not achieved). Response rate was better in cases with mutations affecting recurrent hotspots or with a mutant to wild-type allelic ratio of more than 1 (40% vs 0%, $P = .05$), indicating positive selection for the mutated allele.

*Conclusions.*—Among patients with advanced melanoma harboring *KIT* alterations, treatment with imatinib mesylate results in significant clinical responses in a subset of patients. Responses may be limited to tumors harboring *KIT* alterations of proven functional relevance.

*Trial Registration.*—clinicaltrials.gov Identifier: NCT00470470.

▶ Melanoma remains a major cause of morbidity in both adults and children with approximately 70 000 invasive melanomas diagnosed each year, resulting in almost 10 000 deaths related to metastatic disease. Melanoma comprises several subtypes. The most common melanoma subtype in the United States arises from nonchronically sun-damaged skin and often harbors activating mutations in *BRAF*. Melanoma arising from mucosal, acral, and chronically sun-damaged sites infrequently have *BRAF* mutations but not commonly have amplifications or activating mutations of *KIT*. The latter produce a protein (KIT) that mediates cancer cell growth, proliferation, invasion, metastases, and inhibition of apoptosis. The importance of *KIT* and normal melanocyte development is well established, but its role in the development of cancer is less well known. *KIT* is an established therapeutic target in cancers with activating mutations of *KIT*, such as gastrointestinal stromal tumors. Given the preclinical activity of a drug that inhibits *KIT*, Carvajal et al have studied the effects of imatinib mesylate, a *KIT* inhibitor, in 295 patients with melanoma. In a small but significant subset of patients with advanced melanoma harboring *KIT* alterations, substantial responses were noted.

The results of this report are significant and give great promise to new agents that are being developed that specifically inhibit the functional aspects of onco-genes related to the development of melanoma. While on the topic of melanoma, it should be commented that evidence from recent randomized control trials has demonstrated that regular sunscreen use prevents cutaneous squamous cell carci-noma, and recent data suggest that the regular use of sunscreen can help prevent melanoma. A study of Green et al from subtropical regions of Australia that included 1621 adults randomized to regular or discretionary sunscreen use (which included no use at all) demonstrated a reduced incidence of new primary melanomas over a 10-year period.[1] Because exposure to ultraviolet radiation is the only known modifiable cause of melanoma, the report of Green et al is a poten-tial "game changer" for the primary prevention of melanoma. Without question, patients at high risk for skin cancer because of phenotypic characteristics (fair skin, freckling, and tendency to sunburn) who live in or visit sunny climates or who have a family history of melanoma should routinely and thoroughly apply sunscreen before going outside. In the United States, this recommendation is particularly relevant for those who reside in locations with relatively high levels of ambient ultraviolet radiation, such as Arizona, California, and Florida, and for those living in temperate climates who often vacation in sunny places during the winter and experience seasonal variations in ambient ultraviolet light.

To read more about sunscreen use, see the excellent commentary on this topic by Robinson and Bigby.[2] These authors remind us how important it is to instruct both adults and children on the proper use of sunscreens. For adults, 2 coats or about 1 full teaspoon of sunscreen should be applied to each body part before going outside: head, neck and ears; front of trunk; back of trunk; each arm, dorsum of hand, and shoulder; and each lower leg, upper leg, and dorsum of the foot. The leg needs to be divided into upper and lower segments with each getting 1 teaspoon. One can figure that children probably need close to this amount of protection as well, obviously depending on size.

This commentary ends with a description of a high-tech methodology that might assist in the management and/or cure of certain forms of cancer. Two tiny electronic lights embedded in a small flexible bandage may in fact provide a new way to zap tumor cells in people with skin cancer. The technology, emerging from two British companies, harnesses a type of light source known as "organic" light-emitting diodes (OLEDs). OLEDs are made from semiconducting organic polymers that can convert electrical energy into light and already form the basis for the displays in certain cellular phones and MP3 players. One of their main advantages is that, unlike conventional LEDs, OLEDs can be printed onto a wide range of materials, making them an ideal light source for light-emitting bandages. These can be embedded in flexible plastic strips and pads. These light-emitting bandages are designed to be used in conjunction with photodynamic therapy, in which patients with skin cancer receive an anticancer drug that is activated by red light. Currently such technology is usually used in medical center settings and can be painful because of the heat generated locally. The new technology, however, offers a convenient way for people to treat themselves at home. The idea is for patients to rub a cream containing the anticancer drug into the area of skin cancer and then attach the pad or strip for several hours. This allows the OLEDs to emit red light at levels that do not generate excessive heat, but that are still capable of activating the drug to selectively kill cancer cells. One of the interesting aspects of OLEDs is that they can be custom produced to create an exact outline of a cancer to be treated. Clinical trials are now underway to determine the effectiveness of such an approach.[3]

**J. A. Stockman III, MD**

*References*

1. Green AC, Williams GM, Logan V, Strutton GM. Reduced melanoma after regular sunscreen use: randomized trial follow-up. *J Clin Oncol.* 2011;29:257-263.
2. Robinson JK, Bigby M. Prevention of melanoma with regular sunscreen use. *JAMA.* 2011;306:302-303.
3. Evans J. High-tech bandages lighten the load of light therapy. *Nat Med.* 2009;15: 713.

## Cancer Risks Associated With Germline Mutations in *MLH1*, *MSH2*, and *MSH6* Genes in Lynch Syndrome

Bonadona V, for the French Cancer Genetics Network (Université Lyon 1, France; et al)
*JAMA* 305:2304-2310, 2011

*Context.*—Providing accurate estimates of cancer risks is a major challenge in the clinical management of Lynch syndrome.

*Objective.*—To estimate the age-specific cumulative risks of developing various tumors using a large series of families with mutations of the *MLH1*, *MSH2*, and *MSH6* genes.

*Design, Setting, and Participants.*—Families with Lynch syndrome enrolled between January 1, 2006, and December 31, 2009, from 40 French cancer genetics clinics participating in the ERISCAM (Estimation des Risques de Cancer chez les porteurs de mutation des gènes MMR) study; 537 families with segregating mutated genes (248 with *MLH1*; 256 with *MSH2*; and 33 with *MSH6*) were analyzed.

*Main Outcome Measure.*—Age-specific cumulative cancer risks estimated using the genotype restricted likelihood (GRL) method accounting for ascertainment bias.

*Results.*—Significant differences in estimated cumulative cancer risk were found between the 3 mutated genes ($P = .01$). The estimated cumulative risks of colorectal cancer by age 70 years were 41% (95% confidence intervals [CI], 25%-70%) for *MLH1* mutation carriers, 48% (95% CI, 30%-77%) for *MSH2*, and 12% (95% CI, 8%-22%) for *MSH6*. For endometrial cancer, corresponding risks were 54% (95% CI, 20%-80%), 21% (95% CI, 8%-77%), and 16% (95% CI, 8%-32%). For ovarian cancer, they were 20% (95% CI, 1%-65%), 24% (95% CI, 3%-52%), and 1% (95% CI, 0%-3%). The estimated cumulative risks by age 40 years did not exceed 2% (95% CI, 0%-7%) for endometrial cancer nor 1% (95% CI, 0%-3%) for ovarian cancer, irrespective of the gene. The estimated lifetime risks for other tumor types did not exceed 3% with any of the gene mutations.

*Conclusions.*—*MSH6* mutations are associated with markedly lower cancer risks than *MLH1* or *MSH2* mutations. Lifetime ovarian and endometrial cancer risks associated with *MLH1* or *MSH2* mutations were high but do not increase appreciably until after the age of 40 years.

▶ Lynch syndrome affects children as well as adults. It is an autosomal dominant multicancer disorder and is the most common form of hereditary colorectal cancer. It has a prevalence in the general population of 0.9% and accounts also for approximately 2.3% of all endometrial cancers. All too often, patients with Lynch syndrome are unrecognized because family history is not fully assessed and patients most commonly have few or no colorectal polyps, as opposed to the more easily identifiable polyposis syndromes. Patients with Lynch syndrome present with cancer at a relatively young age, and they are at higher risk of developing more than 1 type of cancer. The most common extracolonic tumors derive from the endometrium, stomach, ovary, small bowel, and urinary tract.

Bonadona et al report estimates of cancer risk for carriers of mutations in the most common Lynch-causing genes. The study includes the largest number of families reported so far with age-specific cumulative estimates of cancer risk. The authors find wide variation in the development of specific forms of cancer in those with Lynch syndrome, depending on the specific Lynch causing genes that a patient might happen to have. For example, the risk of development of colorectal cancer in those carrying a Lynch syndrome gene varies from as low as 12% to as high as 50%. The results of this study help clarify what type of specific cancer a particular patient with Lynch syndrome might have the greatest risk of developing, helping us to focus surveillance more intensively in specific circumstances. It should be noted that while endometrial, ovarian, stomach, small bowel, and urinary tract cancers tend to develop beyond adolescence, colorectal cancer can affect those in their teens. Surveillance for the latter with regular colonoscopy is critical.

This commentary closes with a question about cancer risk. You are seeing a woman who has recently become pregnant. She is starting early to interview potential pediatricians. She is a business woman who flies a great deal. For the next 6 months she anticipates flying from New York City to Japan approximately every 3 weeks. She has read about the risk to the fetus of such long-distance hauls. She wants to know the real "skinny" on cosmic radiation and the dangers to both herself and her future offspring. How would you answer? The answer comes from a recent report that summarizes such risks.[1] This review reminds us that cosmic radiation comes from outside the solar system and from particles released during solar flares. Intensity of radiation depends on the year (due to solar cycles), altitude, latitude, and length of exposure. Because many types of cancer can be linked to cosmic radiation—especially breast cancer, skin cancer, and melanoma—effects of radiation on flight crews and frequent air travelers are indeed of concern. In 1991, the International Commission on Radiological Protection (ICRP) declared cosmic radiation an occupational risk for flight crews, which led to exposure monitoring and guidelines to reduce crew annual exposure to 20 mSv, which is more than double the exposure of most crews. Ground-radiation exposure is generally considered something that should be restricted to 1 mSv per year in the general population, but air-travel—related cosmic-radiation exposure does not have a specific limit. There is a solar-radiation alert system that monitors high-particle intensity from sudden episodes of solar radiation. The FAA issues a solar-radiation advisory to air carriers via a National Oceanic and Atmospheric Administration weather wire service when solar flares might cause increased radiation at commercial-aircraft altitudes. Unfortunately, no studies have been done to assess the health consequences of cosmic-radiation exposure during travel in the general population other than among flight crews. Even the most frequent air travelers are unlikely to be at risk—except for the pregnant woman since her fetus is exposed to the same radiation dose as the mother. The ICRP recommends a radiation limit of 1 mSv during the whole pregnancy, whereas the National Council on Radiation Protection and Measurements recommends a monthly limit of 0.5 mSv. These recommendations limit pregnant crew members and frequent air travelers, because flying roughly 15 long-haul trips, for example, can expose a fetus to more than 1 mSv. To avoid a risk to a fetus, the FAA recommends that pregnant crew members be reassigned to short, low-altitude, low-latitude flights and also request that employers of a pregnant crew member schedule her flights so that she remains clearly under the 1-mSv limit.

So the answer to this woman's query is pretty straightforward. Since she would be flying many long-haul (greater than 8 hours) flights at high latitudes, she would do best by taking a desk job while she is pregnant. Please note that pregnant women and air travelers in general can access the solar-radiation alert system online before traveling and change flight days accordingly.

**J. A. Stockman III, MD**

*Reference*

1. Silverman D, Gendreau M. Medical issues associated with commercial flights. *Lancet.* 2009;373:2067-2077.

---

## Strategies to Identify the Lynch Syndrome Among Patients With Colorectal Cancer: A Cost-Effectiveness Analysis

Ladabaum U, Wang G, Terdiman J, et al (Stanford Univ School of Medicine, CA; Univ of California, San Francisco; Baylor Univ Med Ctr, Dallas, TX; et al)
*Ann Intern Med* 155:69-79, 2011

---

*Background.*—Testing has been advocated for all persons with newly diagnosed colorectal cancer to identify families with the Lynch syndrome, an autosomal dominant cancer-predisposition syndrome that is a paradigm for personalized medicine.

*Objective.*—To estimate the effectiveness and cost-effectiveness of strategies to identify the Lynch syndrome, with attention to sex, age at screening, and differential effects for probands and relatives.

*Design.*—Markov model that incorporated risk for colorectal, endometrial, and ovarian cancers.

*Data Sources.*—Published literature.

*Target Population.*—All persons with newly diagnosed colorectal cancer and their relatives.

*Time Horizon.*—Lifetime.

*Perspective.*—Third-party payer.

*Intervention.*—Strategies based on clinical criteria, prediction algorithms, tumor testing, or up-front germline mutation testing, followed by tailored screening and risk-reducing surgery.

*Outcome Measures.*—Life-years, cancer cases and deaths, costs, and incremental cost-effectiveness ratios.

*Results of Base-Case Analysis.*—The benefit of all strategies accrued primarily to relatives with a mutation associated with the Lynch syndrome, particularly women, whose life expectancy could increase by approximately 4 years with hysterectomy and salpingo-oophorectomy and adherence to colorectal cancer screening recommendations. At current rates of germline testing, screening, and prophylactic surgery, the strategies reduced deaths from colorectal cancer by 7% to 42% and deaths from endometrial and ovarian cancer by 1% to 6%. Among tumor-testing strategies, immunohistochemistry followed by *BRAF* mutation testing was preferred, with an incremental cost-effectiveness ratio of $36 200 per life year gained.

*Results of Sensitivity Analysis.*—The number of relatives tested per proband was a critical determinant of both effectiveness and cost-effectiveness, with testing of 3 to 4 relatives required for most strategies to meet a threshold of $50 000 per life-year gained. Immunohistochemistry followed by *BRAF* mutation testing was preferred in 59% of iterations in probabilistic sensitivity analysis at a threshold of $100 000 per life-year gained. Screening for the Lynch syndrome with immunohistochemistry followed by *BRAF* mutation testing only up to age 70 years cost $44 000 per incremental life-year gained compared with screening only up to age 60 years, and screening without an upper age limit cost $88 700 per incremental life-year gained compared with screening only up to age 70 years.

*Limitation.*—Other types of cancer, uncertain family pedigrees, and genetic variants of unknown significance were not considered.

*Conclusion.*—Widespread colorectal tumor testing to identify families with the Lynch syndrome could yield substantial benefits at acceptable costs, particularly for women with a mutation associated with the Lynch syndrome who begin regular screening and have risk-reducing surgery. The cost-effectiveness of such testing depends on the participation rate among relatives at risk for the Lynch syndrome.

▶ This report tells us a great deal about Lynch syndrome and the cancer manifestations of those who carry 1 or more of the gene defects related to Lynch syndrome. This report from Stanford University, Baylor University, and Memorial Sloan-Kettering Cancer Center in New York reminds us how important it is to identify families with Lynch syndrome. This is true since distinctive features of the Lynch syndrome are seldom apparent in affected individuals until the diagnosis of cancer is made. Thus, the syndrome is usually suspected on the basis of a strong family history of colorectal cancer and other types of cancer.

Ladabaum et al used a modeling analysis to examine the medical and cost-effectiveness of each of the potential approaches currently possible to diagnose the Lynch syndrome in patients with colorectal cancer. Performing tumor testing in all colorectal cancer patients or proceeding directly to genetic testing regardless of family risk was also examined. The study found that proceeding directly to genetic testing starting at age 20 to 30 years in patients with a 5% or higher risk (regardless of whether the index case had cancer) was both medically effective and cost-effective compared with the usual practice of immunohistochemistry tumor testing of all patients initially presenting with colorectal cancer.

To read more about the Lynch syndrome and who should have genetic testing, see the excellent editorial on this topic by Burt.[1]

**J. A. Stockman III, MD**

*Reference*

1. Burt RW. Who should have genetic testing for the Lynch syndrome? *Ann Intern Med.* 2011;155:127-128.

---

### Use of mobile phones and risk of brain tumours: update of Danish cohort study

Frei P, Poulsen AH, Johansen C, et al (Danish Cancer Society, Copenhagen, Denmark; et al)
*BMJ* 343:d6387, 2011

---

*Objective.*—To investigate the risk of tumours in the central nervous system among Danish mobile phone subscribers.

*Design.*—Nationwide cohort study.

*Setting.*—Denmark.

*Participants.*—All Danes aged ≥30 and born in Denmark after 1925, subdivided into subscribers and non-subscribers of mobile phones before 1995.

*Main Outcome Measures.*—Risk of tumours of the central nervous system, identified from the complete Danish Cancer Register. Sex specific incidence rate ratios estimated with log linear Poisson regression models adjusted for age, calendar period, education, and disposable income.

*Results.*—358 403 subscription holders accrued 3.8 million person years. In the follow-up period 1990-2007, there were 10 729 cases of tumours of the central nervous system. The risk of such tumours was close to unity for both men and women. When restricted to individuals with the longest mobile phone use—that is, ≥13 years of subscription—the incidence rate ratio was 1.03 (95% confidence interval 0.83 to 1.27) in men and 0.91 (0.41 to 2.04) in women. Among those with subscriptions of ≥10 years, ratios were 1.04 (0.85 to 1.26) in men and 1.04 (0.56 to 1.95) in women for glioma and 0.90 (0.57 to 1.42) in men and 0.93 (0.46 to 1.87) in women for meningioma. There was no indication of dose-response relation either by years since first subscription for a mobile phone or by anatomical location of the tumour—that is, in regions of the brain closest to where the handset is usually held to the head.

*Conclusions.*—In this update of a large nationwide cohort study of mobile phone use, there were no increased risks of tumours of the central nervous system, providing little evidence for a causal association.

▶ This report found no evidence that the risk of brain tumors was increased in 358 403 Danish mobile phone subscribers. These findings were also true when the data from this report were restricted to people who have been subscribing to mobile telephone use for more than 10 years, when gliomas and meningiomas were analyzed separately, and when tumors in the anatomic regions closest to the handset were analyzed. It should be noted that 1 weakness of the report was that having a mobile phone subscription is not equivalent to using a mobile phone, and conversely some mobile phone users will be nonsubscribers. The resulting misclassification could dilute any association between mobile phone use and cancer risk, and this is important for a negative study such as reported by Frei et al. However, for long-term users, this misclassification would have only a small effect in that long-term users who did not hold personal subscriptions would make up a tiny portion of the group overall.

In an editorial that accompanied this report, Ahlbom and Feychting state that the results of the Frei et al report are largely reassuring.[1] They conclude "continued monitoring of health registers and prospective cohorts is warranted, but more case control or other studies with built-in selection and recall bias are not needed."

While on the topic of things having to do with hearing, add exposure to second-hand smoke to the list of things that can cause hearing loss in teens. Data from 1 533 nonsmokers age 12 years to 19 years showed that teens with the highest blood levels of cotinine, a biomarker for exposure to secondhand smoke, have the greatest degree of hearing loss. A growing body of literature suggests that exposure to cigarette smoke can lead to sensory impairment in nonsmokers.[2] Also, please note that the Centers for Disease Control and Prevention recently noted that prior military service is associated with a higher prevalence of hearing loss independent of other factors related to age. Military service can entail harmful exposure to high-intensity noise from firearms, explosives, jet engines, and machinery during combat operations and training and in the course of general job duties. Such noise-induced hearing loss is a permanent disability. Across all age groups, veterans are more than twice as likely to suffer hearing loss compared with their nonveteran colleagues matched for age.[3]

This commentary closes with some discussion about a new form of radiation and its potential hazard. This has to do with the use of full-body scanners at airports. Full-body scanners or whole-body scanners are generally classified into two types: millimeter radiowave or backscatter technologies. Millimeter radiowave systems scan travelers by bombarding them with radiowaves and collecting the reflected radiowaves via antennae to generate an image. This technology does not use x-rays. In contrast, backscatter systems use low-intensity x-rays to scan the body. The x-rays do not penetrate the body; instead they bounce off the skin and are then captured by detectors to create images. These x-rays are useful for detecting objects hidden under clothing and taped on the body, but not for detecting objects hidden inside the body. For the latter purpose, only transmission x-ray systems can be used and the amount of radiation would be prohibitive. A typical backscatter scan takes about 8 to 15 seconds to perform and provides 2 images: front and back. For the past few years, full-body scanners have been used as screening devices at a number of airports. Several important concerns exist regarding full-body scanners: biological risk to travelers and concerns about privacy, the longevity of images, and the stability of scanners. In this context, it is recommended that the radiation doses from backscatter systems should not exceed 0.1 uSv, and the doses measured have been reported to be between 0.05 uSv and 0.1 uSv per scan.[4] Based on this, a person would have to undergo 1000 to 2000 backscatter scans before receiving a dose equivalent to a medical chest x-ray (100 uSv). The dose of radiation from a single backscatter scan is equivalent to that received from less than 30 minutes of background irradiation and to 10 minutes of average air travel where exposure to cosmic radiation occurs. A person would have to undergo 100 to 200 backscatter scans before receiving a dose equivalent to one day of natural background irradiation that all of us are exposed to. The Nuclear Regulatory Commission in the United States recommends an annual limit on radiation doses to the public of 1000 uSv and 250 uSv a year from any single source or practice. To exceed 250 uSv a year at a dose of 0.1 or 0.05 uSv per scan, a traveler would need to have 2500 to 5000 scans, which is highly unlikely in one year.

The bottom line is that propriety and embarrassment aside, current calculations indicate that backscatter systems are safe for general use, even in infants and children, pregnant women, and people with genetically based hypersensitivity to radiation such as those with Fanconi anemia. When considered in the context of a potential increase in security, most believe that the benefits outweigh the potential for harm, but that is for society to ultimately decide.[5]

**J. A. Stockman III, MD**

*References*

1. Ahlbom A, Feychting M. Mobile phones and brain tumors: evidence is reassuring, but continued monitoring of health registers and prospective cohorts is still warranted. *BMJ*. 2005;343:914-915.
2. Kuehn BM. Author Insights: Secondhand Smoke Exposure Linked to Hearing Loss in Teens. http://newsatjama.jama.com/2011/07/18/author-insight-secondhand-smoke-exposure-linked-to-hearing-loss-in-teens/. Accessed August 2, 2012.
3. Centers for Disease Control and Prevention (CDC). Severe hearing impairment among military veterans—United States, 2010. *MMWR Morb Mortal Wkly Rep*. 2011;60:955-958.
4. National Council on Radiation Protection and Measurements. Commentary No. 16 — Screening of humans for security purposes using ionizing radiation scanning systems. 2003. www.ncrppublications.org/commentary/16. Accessed August 2, 2012.
5. Mahesh M. The use of full body scanners at airports. Medical risk is negligible but concerns about privacy remain. *BMJ*. 2010;340:490-491.

# 17 Ophthalmology

An Evidence-Based Approach to Physician Etiquette in Pediatric Ophthalmology
Reddy AK, Coats DK, Yen KG (Texas Children's Hosp, Houston)
*J Pediatr Ophthalmol Strabismus* 48:336-339, 2011

*Purpose.*—Little objective evidence exists to guide physician etiquette in pediatric ophthalmology. This article describes the preferences of families visiting a pediatric ophthalmology clinic for the first time.

*Methods.*—Review of 149 questionnaires completed by the families of patients visiting a pediatric ophthalmology clinic in a tertiary care center. The Fisher exact and chi-square tests were used to compare subpopulations.

*Results.*—Most respondents preferred that their physician wear a white coat. Men preferred a handshake to a verbal greeting ($P = .0264$) and professional to business casual attire for both male and female physicians ($P = .01$, both). African-American parents were more likely to prefer being addressed by surname than other races ($P = .008$). No statistically significant differences were found comparing the preferences of parents with an advanced education (bachelor and graduate degrees) to those without.

*Conclusion.*—Pediatric ophthalmologists may wish to consider wearing white coats and business casual attire in clinic and addressing parents informally as "mom" or "dad" or by their first name, although etiquette should ultimately be determined on an individual patient basis.

▶ While this tidy little report refers to how parents view physician etiquette involving pediatric ophthalmologists, the information provided probably applies to all medical professionals. Parents or guardians of children visiting the Texas Children's Hospital Pediatric Ophthalmology Clinic for the first time were asked to complete a questionnaire regarding their preferences on physician attire, the way they were greeted, and provider gender. More than 200 surveys were distributed to families. The average age of the children being seen by the pediatric ophthalmologist was 4.5 years. Of those responding, 75.8% felt the way they were greeted by their physician affected their trust and confidence in him or her. The majority of parents (91.9%) expressed no preference with regard to the gender of their physician, but 7.4% preferred a female physician and 0.7% (a single patient's family) preferred a male physician. Of the 11 parents who preferred their child be examined by a female physician, 91.0% were female. Informal greetings such as "mom" or "dad" were popular. Only 40.9% of respondents reported that the way their physician dressed affected their trust and confidence in him or her. Although 67.8% of respondents had no preference with regard to the attire of their male physician, 22.1% preferred their male physician to dress in business casual attire. No preference with regard to the attire of their female physicians was indicated by 65.5% of respondents, and 22.3% preferred their female physician to dress in business attire. A total of 57.7% of respondents preferred their physician wear a white coat while examining their child. Four respondents (2.7%) expressed a preference for male physicians to wear scrubs; 5.4% expressed a preference for female physicians to wear scrubs. Men were more likely than women to prefer a handshake to a verbal greeting for their children. No statistically significant differences were found comparing the preferences of parents with advanced education to those without.

Based on the results of these findings, it is suggested that care providers may wish to consider wearing white coats and business casual attire in clinic, greeting parents and children with a handshake (especially if the parent accompanying the child is male), and addressing parents informally as "mom" or "dad" or by their first name. Again, it is difficult to be absolutely sure about extrapolation of these data to other types of health care providers. The wearing of white coats has recently come under a fair amount of scrutiny.[1,2] While white coats are traditionally worn to communicate a level of professionalism, it has been argued that they should be abandoned in patient-centered practices because they make the wearer appear more authoritative and less compassionate with the suggestion that the effect of wearing a white coat is strong enough to cause significant physiologic changes, at least in adults (ie, white coat hypertension) and induce anxiety in children, although this has been debated.

Please note that this report and many that have preceded it have surveyed families seeing a physician for the first time. One wonders after one has established a relationship with a family whether it is at all important what one wears (within the boundaries of common sense).

This commentary closes with an observation having to do with Dr Conan Doyle. Bet you were not aware of Dr Doyle's specialty area. He in fact was an ophthalmologist. In 1881, Conan Doyle was struggling to build an ophthalmic practice in two rented rooms, one to be a consulting room and the other a waiting room, close to Harley Street. He later wrote that both proved to be waiting rooms, so much so that he had time to prepare and submit for publication his first successful Sherlock Holmes stories, collected in *The Adventures of Sherlock Holmes*. This was in 1891, a year in which he developed influenza and was sick for a fair amount of time, the cost of the illness essentially bankrupting him. It was in this same month that Conan Doyle decided to terminate his medical practice and sold his eye instruments for just 6 pounds and 10 shillings. To read more about Arthur Conan Doyle, see the book by Lellenberg Stashower and Folley: *Arthur Conan Doyle: A Life in Letters* (published by Harper Press, 2007).

**J. A. Stockman III, MD**

*References*

1. Parker-Pope T. Do you really want to see your doctor's elbows? *New York Times.* http://well.blogs.newyorktimes.com/2008/09/08. September 8, 2008.
2. Jones A. Bare below the elbows: a brief history of surgeon attire and infection. *BJU Int.* 2008;102:665-666.

## Pediatric Ocular Injuries From Airsoft Toy Guns

Shazly TA, Al-Hussaini AK (Massachusetts Eye and Ear Infirmary/Harvard Med School, Boston; Assiut Univ Hosp, Egypt)
*J Pediatr Ophthalmol Strabismus* 49:54-57, 2012

*Purpose.*—To report ocular injuries caused by airsoft guns in children.

*Methods.*—A retrospective chart review of pediatric patients who sustained ocular injuries related to airsoft guns between November 2005 and December 2007. Place of trauma, presenting symptoms and signs, surgical interventions performed, and final visual outcome were reviewed.

*Results.*—Thirty-two patients with a mean age of 8.8 ± 4.0 years (range: 1.5 to 18 years) were examined; 28 were boys (87.5%). Presenting visual acuity ranged from hand motions to 20/20 and could not be assessed in 2 patients. Hyphema was a common finding that was present in 24 cases, corneal abrasions were present in 10 cases, and raised intraocular pressure was present in 7 cases. Seven patients presented with traumatic cataract, and two had iridodialysis. Immediate surgical intervention was performed in 7 patients and 7 patients were scheduled for elective surgery. The patients presented after an average of 1.9 ± 1.9 days (range: 4 hours to 6 days) after the injury. Average follow-up was 18 days (range: 7 days to 5 months). Final visual acuity was 20/200 or worse in 5 patients, 20/40 or better in 23 patients, and could not be assessed in 2 cases.

*Conclusion.*—Airsoft guns can cause a variety of serious injuries, sometimes necessitating operative intervention. The long-term morbidity from some of these injuries is significant. Airsoft guns are capable of inflicting serious and permanent ocular damage.

▶ Trauma to the eye remains one of the most significant causes of visual loss in children. This report from the Boston Children's Hospital reminds us that airsoft toy guns can be a significant cause of ocular trauma in children. Airsoft guns are found in many consumer stores these days. The Consumer Product Safety Commission has estimated that nonpowder weapon injuries result in more than 20 000 visits to emergency departments in the United States. Airsoft guns are nonpowder firearms in which a plastic pellet is propelled by compressed gas. The gas may be compressed by a powerful spring or by the repetitive pumping of air into a gas chamber. Air guns also can expel copper-plated BBs, small plastic balls measuring 6 mm in diameter, and paintball gelatin balls, usually measuring 11 mm in diameter. Most airsoft guns are restricted to firing plastic pellets. When compared with ocular injuries caused by paintball pistols, this series did not include any cases with corneal/corneoscleral ruptures or retinal breaks. Although airsoft guns are similar in operation and muzzle velocity (300—400 feet/second) to paintball guns, airsoft guns use lighter-weight projectiles. The difference in momentum of the projectiles may explain the more severe ocular comorbidities caused by paintball guns.

If a parent buys an airsoft gun for their child, it is imperative they understand that protective eyewear use is mandatory to guard against ocular injuries. Airsoft guns are a weapon and not a toy. Until stricter control is exercised over the sale and design of these weapons, the role of the pediatrician, emergency physician, and surgeon in educating families cannot be overemphasized. Parents must be instructed about the potential for serious injury with airsoft gun use by children and inadequately trained adults.

While on the topic of things having to do with the eye, research performed at the Scheie Eye Institute at the University of Pennsylvania has shown that gene therapy can cure retinitis pigmentosa in dogs. While there is a distinct similarity between humans and dogs in terms of eye anatomy, physiology, and disease characteristics, the positive response to the forms of gene therapy used to treat retinitis pigmentosa in dogs raises hope for a clear path to human therapy.[1]

This commentary closes with a question. You own a pet tarantula that you keep in a terrarium. From time to time, you have to clean the terrarium. Why should you use eye protection? The answer to this question comes from a description of a 29-year-old man who developed a red watery and photophobic eye. He failed treatment with topical antibiotics and a slitlamp examination was performed where multiple corneal subepithelial infiltrates were visible as well as scattered white spots. These findings were thought to be consistent with a viral keratoconjunctivitis. A second examination with higher magnification, however, showed hair-like projections in the center of each of the corneal infiltrates. These were noted at varying depths within the cornea. Some had migrated through the innermost endothelial layer producing mild anterior chamber inflammation. A dilated fundal examination was carried out which showed one small focus of retinitis in association with a hair-like projection. When these findings were described to the patient, he immediately recalled an incident that preceded the onset of his symptoms a couple of weeks earlier. He had been cleaning the glass tank of his pet, a Chilean Rose tarantula. While his attention was focused on a stubborn stain, he sensed movement in the terrarium. He turned his head and found that the tarantula, which was in close proximity, had released a "mist" of hairs, which hit his face and eyes. The patient's ophthalmologist attempted removal of the corneal hairs under an operating microscope, but they proved to be too fine to be removed even with micro-forceps. Treatment was instituted with topical steroids with significant, but not complete improvement. The patient now wears eye protection before handling the tarantula.

It should be note that the Chilean Rose tarantula *(Grammostola rosea)* has urticating hairs over the posterior surface of his body. As a defense mechanism against potential predators, the tarantula will rub his hind legs against his abdomen to dislodge these hairs into the air. Multiple barbs allow the hairs to migrate through ocular tissue as well as other surfaces. The inflammatory reaction that results in the eye is called ophthalmia nodosa, a broad diagnostic category covering the response of the eye to insect or vegetable material. A few other cases of ophthalmia nodosa secondary to tarantula hairs have been reported. Long-term topical steroid treatment is the only effective management for this clinical presentation. While the condition is rare, if you happen to keep a tarantula around the house, wear eye protection or otherwise you might get a case of Spiderman's eye.[2]

**J. A. Stockman III, MD**

*References*

1. Stratton K. Penn vet professor Gustavo D. Aguirre receives grant from foundation fighting blindness. *Penn News*. September 20, 2011. http://www.upenn.edu/pennnews/news/penn-vet-professor-gustavo-d-aguirre-vmd-phd-receives-grant-foundation-fighting-blindness. Accessed August 2, 2012
2. Norris JH, Carrim ZI, Morrell AJ. Spiderman's eye. *Lancet*. 2010;375:92.

---

**Self correction of refractive error among young people in rural China: results of cross sectional investigation**
Zhang M, Zhang R, He M, et al (Joint Shantou Int Eye Centre, Shantou, People's Republic of China; Sun Yat Sen Univ, Yuexiu, Guangzhou, China; et al)
*BMJ* 343:d4767, 2011

---

*Objective.*—To compare outcomes between adjustable spectacles and conventional methods for refraction in young people.

*Design.*—Cross sectional study.

*Setting.*—Rural southern China.

*Participants.*—648 young people aged 12-18 (mean 14.9 (SD 0.98)), with uncorrected visual acuity ≤ 6/12 in either eye.

*Interventions.*—All participants underwent self refraction without cycloplegia (paralysis of near focusing ability with topical eye drops), automated refraction without cycloplegia, and subjective refraction by an ophthalmologist with cycloplegia.

*Main Outcome Measures.*—Uncorrected and corrected vision, improvement of vision (lines on a chart), and refractive error.

*Results.*—Among the participants, 59% (384) were girls, 44% (288) wore spectacles, and 61% (393/648) had 2.00 dioptres or more of myopia in the right eye. All completed self refraction. The proportion with visual acuity ≥ 6/7.5 in the better eye was 5.2% (95% confidence interval 3.6% to 6.9%) for uncorrected vision, 30.2% (25.7% to 34.8%) for currently worn spectacles, 96.9% (95.5% to 98.3%) for self refraction, 98.4% (97.4% to 99.5%) for automated refraction, and 99.1% (98.3% to 99.9%) for subjective refraction ($P = 0.033$ for self refraction v automated refraction, $P = 0.001$ for self refraction v subjective refraction). Improvements over uncorrected vision in the better eye with self refraction and subjective refraction were within one line on the eye chart in 98% of participants. In logistic regression models, failure to achieve maximum recorded visual acuity of 6/7.5 in right eyes with self refraction was associated with greater absolute value of myopia/hyperopia ($P < 0.001$), greater astigmatism ($P = 0.001$), and not having previously worn spectacles ($P = 0.002$), but not age or sex. Significant inaccuracies in power (≥ 1.00 dioptre) were less common in right eyes with self refraction than with automated refraction (5% v 11%, $P < 0.001$).

*Conclusions.*—Though visual acuity was slightly worse with self refraction than automated or subjective refraction, acuity was excellent in nearly all these young people with inadequately corrected refractive error at baseline. Inaccurate power was less common with self refraction than automated refraction. Self refraction could decrease the requirement for scarce trained personnel, expensive devices, and cycloplegia in children's vision programmes in rural China.

▶ Testing eyesight just is not feasible or affordable in many parts of the world. It is estimated that more than 150 million individuals worldwide are visually impaired simply for lack of eyeglasses. To address this, Dr Josh Silver several years ago invented the Adspecs adjustable spectacles, the 2 fluid-filled lenses that can be deformed by attached pumps until the wearer can clearly see letters on a vision chart and thus determine what corrective lens they need. Investigators in China studied 648 school students age 12 to 18 years who had uncorrected visual acuity ≤6/12 in either eye. Although the Adspecs did not perform as well as automated refraction with expensive devices, they did allow 97% of participants to achieve visual acuity within an excellent range to permit normal visual function in a classroom.

Adspecs cost approximately $20 and have adjustable mechanisms with fluid-filled lenses that increase the volume to change the refraction of the lens. This is done with a small syringe that either adds or withdraws fluid. Once the correct refraction is found, the amount of fluid is locked down and the syringe is withdrawn. One could then use the Adspecs as regular glasses, but as the authors of this report note, at $20 they are still too expensive for average use. The solution then comes from ready-made glasses, available off the shelf that match the prescription needed. Such glasses can cost as little as $1.60. To learn more about this revolutionary and innovative approach to solving visual problems, see: www.bmj.com/site/video/innovations.xhtml.

While on the topic of things related to vision, an interesting tidbit appeared recently in the *British Medical Journal* concerning James Joyce. Of many numerous biographies about James Joyce and his life, virtually all have commented on his nearsightedness, or myopia. Joyce is known to have had bad vision and to have had a cataract removed once. Photographs of him wearing glasses showed very thick convex lenses that appeared to make his blue eyes quite large. It is curious why so many writers found Joyce's eye problems interesting, but they were dead wrong when it came to the correct diagnosis of his refractive error, which was hyperopia. In 1932 a prescription for his lens correction was written by his ophthalmologist, Dr Alfred Vogt. That prescription was recently found. The prescription for both lenses showed a refractive power of +17 diopters. Thus is that the preeminent author of the 20th century, James Joyce, wrote his most famous novel, Ulysses, from afar![1]

**J. A. Stockman III, MD**

*Reference*

1. Ascaso F, Veize JL. Was James Joyce myopic or hyperopic? *BMJ*. 2011;344:1295.

**Surgical Management of Adult Onset Age-Related Distance Esotropia**
Mittelman D (Rush Univ Med Ctr and Advocate Lutheran General Children's
Hosp, Chicago, IL)
*J Pediatr Ophthalmol Strabismus* 48:214-216, 2011

*Purpose.*—To study the effects of bilateral medial rectus recession for
the management of adult onset age-related distance esotropia.

*Methods.*—Ten patients with adult onset age-related distance esotropia
measuring 14 prism diopters or greater underwent bilateral medial rectus
recession to eliminate the need for prism glasses.

*Results.*—In all but one case, the diplopia completely resolved postoper-
atively, with a median residual deviation of 1 prism diopter esophoria for
distance and 2 prism diopters exophoria at near.

*Conclusion.*—Bilateral medial rectus recession is a useful technique for
the management of adult onset age-related distance esotropia.

► If you are not familiar with adult-onset age-related distance esotropia, it is
a syndrome characterized by esotropia greater at distance than near fixation,
occurring in individuals older than 60 years. The etiology of this condition is
unknown, but is likely to be due to involutional changes within the orbit, most
notably sagging and inferior displacement of the lateral rectus muscle and/or its
pulley. The most common associated symptom is horizontal diplopia. In most
cases, the double vision can be readily managed with prism glasses. More severely
affected individuals have to have management of the strabismus with surgery. So
why do we mention this condition? It is included simply to indicate that children
are not the only ones affected with strabismus. There is an adult-onset form of this
as well.

**J. A. Stockman III, MD**

**Lenticular Abnormalities in Children**
Khokhar S, Agarwal I, Kumar G, et al (AIIMS, New Delhi, India)
*J Pediatr Ophthalmol Strabismus* 49:32-37, 2012

*Purpose.*—To study the lenticular problems in children presenting at an
apex institute.

*Methods.*—Retrospective analysis of records (<14 years) of new lens
clinic cases was done.

*Results.*—Of 1,047 children, 687 were males. Mean age at presentation
was 6.35 ± 4.13 years. Developmental cataract was seen in 45.6% and
posttraumatic cataract in 29.7% of patients. Other abnormalities were
cataract with retinal detachment, persistent hyperplastic primary vitreous,
subluxated lens, micro/spherophakia, cataract secondary to uveitis, intraocular lens complications, cataract with choroidal coloboma, and visual
axis opacification.

TABLE 1.—Analysis of Subtypes

| Code | Frequency | Male (%) | Bilateral (%) | Age (Y)[a] |
|---|---|---|---|---|
| 1: Developmental cataract | 477 (45.6%) | 63.7 | 44 | 4.53 ± 3.92 |
| 2: Posttraumatic cataract | 311 (29.7%) | 69.1 | 4 | 7.73 ± 3.53 |
| 3: Cataract with retinal detachment | 18 (1.7%) | 61.1 | 33.3 | 8.95 ± 4.16 |
| 4: Persistent hyperplastic primary vitreous | 13 (1.2%) | 46.2 | 20 | 4.61 ± 3.53 |
| 5: Subluxated/dislocated lens | 62 (5.9%) | 69.4 | 54 | 9.36 ± 3.56 |
| 6: Cataract with uveitis | 37 (3.5%) | 67.6 | 38 | 7.79 ± 3.31 |
| 7: Micro/spherophakia | 16 (1.5%) | 56.3 | 94 | 6.56 ± 4.52 |
| 8: Complications of cataract surgery | 31 (3.0%) | 74.2 | 29 | 8.07 ± 3.73 |
| 9: Choroidal coloboma | 12 (1.1%) | 33.3 | 60 | 8.5 ± 4.16 |
| 10: Visual axis opacification | 70 (6.7%) | 67.1 | 61 | 7.58 ± 3.51 |

[a]Values given as mean ± standard deviation.

*Conclusion.*—Developmental and posttraumatic cataracts were the most common abnormalities. Delayed presentation is of concern (Table 1).

▶ This article reminds us that some 1.4 million children younger than 15 years are blind worldwide. Most of this blindness (estimated to be 80%) is avoidable. About three-quarters of blind children in the world live in developing countries in Africa and Asia. Lens abnormalities are among the most important causes of childhood blindness. The human lens, which begins to develop around the fourth week of intrauterine life, reacts very easily to any insult by losing its clarity and developing opacity. This will manifest as a congenital cataract at birth and later as a developmental cataract. There are many other causes of cataract formation as well.

This report from New Delhi, India, attempts to establish the different causes of lens abnormalities and how these cases present in childhood. A table illustrates the various subtypes of lens abnormalities that can lead to cataract formation. The information in the table represents data derived from 1047 children. Developmental cataract was the most common diagnosis (45.6%) in this study. Congenital cataracts were usually present at birth, but not always. Posttraumatic cataract was the second largest group (29.7%). The mean age of this group was 7.73 ± 3.53 years. In all, 70% of traumatic cataracts occurred in boys. Only 4% of such cases were bilateral.

This report represents the largest documented series of cataracts in children. As the study demonstrates, given proper and timely care, many lenticular problems can be addressed and rehabilitated.

**J. A. Stockman III, MD**

## Embryonic stem cell trials for macular degeneration: a preliminary report

Schwartz SD, Hubschman J-P, Heilwell G, et al (Univ of California, Los Angeles; et al)
*Lancet* 379:713-720, 2012

---

*Background.*—It has been 13 years since the discovery of human embryonic stem cells (hESCs). Our report provides the first description of hESC-derived cells transplanted into human patients.

*Methods.*—We started two prospective clinical studies to establish the safety and tolerability of subretinal transplantation of hESC-derived retinal pigment epithelium (RPE) in patients with Stargardt's macular dystrophy and dry age-related macular degeneration—the leading cause of blindness in the developed world. Preoperative and postoperative ophthalmic examinations included visual acuity, fluorescein angiography, optical coherence tomography, and visual field testing. These studies are registered with ClinicalTrials.gov, numbers NCT01345006 and NCT01344993.

*Findings.*—Controlled hESC differentiation resulted in greater than 99% pure RPE. The cells displayed typical RPE behaviour and integrated into the host RPE layer forming mature quiescent monolayers after transplantation in animals. The stage of differentiation substantially affected attachment and survival of the cells in vitro after clinical formulation. Lightly pigmented cells attached and spread in a substantially greater proportion (>90%) than more darkly pigmented cells after culture. After surgery, structural evidence confirmed cells had attached and continued to persist during our study. We did not identify signs of hyperproliferation, abnormal growth, or immune mediated transplant rejection in either patient during the first 4 months. Although there is little agreement between investigators on visual endpoints in patients with low vision, it is encouraging that during the observation period neither patient lost vision. Best corrected visual acuity improved from hand motions to 20/800 (and improved from 0 to 5 letters on the Early Treatment Diabetic Retinopathy Study [ETDRS] visual acuity chart) in the study eye of the patient with Stargardt's macular dystrophy, and vision also seemed to improve in the patient with dry age-related macular degeneration (from 21 ETDRS letters to 28).

*Interpretation.*—The hESC-derived RPE cells showed no signs of hyperproliferation, tumorigenicity, ectopic tissue formation, or apparent rejection after 4 months. The future therapeutic goal will be to treat patients earlier in the disease processes, potentially increasing the likelihood of photoreceptor and central visual rescue.

▶ In 1998 investigators first suggested that human embryonic stem cells could be a promising source of replacement cells for regenerative medicine applications. It has been a long road since then in demonstrating the clinical applicability of this form of therapy. For a number of reasons, disorders that affect the eye and other immunoprivileged sites will probably be the first targets of study for stem cell—based therapy in humans. It is well established that the subretinal space is protected by a blood—ocular barrier and is characterized by antigen-specific inhibition of both the cellular and humeral immune responses. For this reason, certain forms of eye disease represent this target.

In the retina, degeneration of the retinal pigment epithelium results in photoreceptor loss in many site-threatening disorders, including dry, age-related ocular degeneration and an entity called Stargardt macular degeneration. These conditions are the leading causes of blindness in the developing world. Although currently untreatable, there is evidence from animal models that transplantation with the retinal pigment epithelium using stem cells can prevent loss of vision. Retinal pigment epithelium maintains that health of photoreceptors by recycling photopigments and metabolizing vitamin A. Transplantation of intact sheets and suspensions of primary retinal pigment epithelium have been previously attempted in people with mixed results, both in terms of graft survival and improvement in vision. Theoretically there are advantages to the use of stem cells as an alternative source of replacement tissue. However, stem cells must be free of pathogens, possess the appropriate characteristics of the differentiated cell, and be free of undifferentiated cells. They also must be extensively tested in animals for absence of teratoma, migration of cells into other organs, and other untoward effects.

The goal of this study was to assess the safety and tolerability of stem cell—derived retinal pigment epithelium cells in the management of macular degeneration. The report is a preliminary one, describing the experience with 2 patients. Through a complicated process, using existing embryonic cell lines, the investigators injected specialized stem cells subretinally into 2 patients with macular degeneration. Mild immunosuppression with tacrolimus was used. In follow-up, there was anatomical evidence of survival of the graft. The investigators were able to clinically detect increased pigmentation at the level of the retinal pigment epithelium. Functional improvements in vision were observed.

The findings from this study suggest that transplanted stem cells might be useful in the management of certain forms of ocular disease. In the 2 patients evaluated, the stem cells seemed to have been transplanted into the eye without abnormal proliferation, teratoma formation, graft rejection, or other untoward pathological reactions or safety problems. Needless to say, continued follow-up is necessary as well as significantly larger clinical trials to document whether this form of innovative therapy is worthwhile.

This commentary closes with a clinical conundrum. An 18-year-old boy in your practice is being seen for severe abdominal pain. The history is complicated by the fact that this teenager binge drinks. In fact, he has been drinking hard liquor for the past several days. He has 2 physical findings of importance. One is that his abdomen is diffusely tender and slightly swollen. The other is that the eye exam shows cotton-wool spots and intraretinal hemorrhages surrounding a normal optic disc. These findings alone should be sufficient for you to order very specific laboratory studies. You suspect what diagnosis? If you suspect that this patient has pancreatitis you would be correct. One complication of pancreatitis is what is known as Purtscher retinopathy.[1] This can be associated with the sudden onset of blindness. Purtscher retinopathy is caused by microembolization of retinal and parietal arterioles by fat emboli and is characterized by retinal ischemia and hemorrhages. Characteristic retinal findings of Purtscher retinopathy include multiple cotton-wool spots that surround the optic nerve. Purtscher retinopathy itself was first described in 1912 as a syndrome of sudden blindness associated with severe head trauma. Patients had findings of multiple white retinal patches and retinal hemorrhages that were associated with severe vision loss. Since its original description, Purtscher retinopathy has been associated with traumatic injury, primarily blunt thoracic trauma and head trauma, and numerous nontraumatic diseases. Purtscher-like retinopathy is seen in other diverse conditions, including acute pancreatitis; fat embolization; amniotic fluid embolization; preeclampsia; hemolysis, and low platelets (HELLP) syndrome; and vasculitic diseases, such as lupus.

**J. A. Stockman III, MD**

*Reference*

1. Mayer C, Khoramnia R. Purtscher-like retinopathy caused by acute pancreatitis. *Lancet.* 2011;378:1653.

---

### Childhood optic neuritis clinical features and outcome

Absoud M, Cummins C, Desai N, et al (Birmingham Children's Hosp, UK; Great Ormond Street Hosp, London, UK; et al)
*Arch Dis Child* 96:860-862, 2011

---

*Aim.*—To describe clinical features and outcome of a series of children with first-episode optic neuritis investigated in three paediatric neurology centres.

*Methods.*—Databases were searched to identify children (<16 years) with optic neuritis and life table analysis was used.

*Results.*—44 children (female/male ratio 1.8) median age 10.9 years were followed up for median 1 year. Optic neuritis was unilateral in 43%. Maximal visual deficit was severe (<6/60) in 77%, with full recovery in 70%. Cumulative probability of developing MS (11/44) or NMO (3/44) at 2 years was 0.45. Relapsing optic neuritis was a strong predictor for development of MS or NMO. A positive MRI (>1 brain T2 hyperintense lesion) was a strong predictor for development of MS.

*Discussion.*—Childhood optic neuritis is associated with severe visual deficit with good recovery. An initial abnormal MRI brain scan or relapsing optic neuritis should alert the clinician to MS or NMO diagnosis.

▶ This important report tells us a lot about optic neuritis occurring in childhood. All pediatricians should be familiar with the presentation and natural course of optic neuritis even though it is a fairly rare disorder. It is an important entity because, if not properly treated, it can lead to blindness.

The report of Absoud et al provides information from a multicenter study of children with optic neuritis. It is clear that acute optic neuritis in children differs from the typical adult form. Bilateral disease is more common in children, as is severe loss of visual acuity. We see that the average age of presentation is

10 years to 11 years with a female predominance of almost 2 to 1. As in adults, the condition is predictive of the subsequent risk of multiple sclerosis. Optic neuritis may also represent the first attack of Devic neuromyelitis optica. The latter is an inflammatory, demyelinating condition in which clinical disease is referable to the optic nerves and spinal cord without involvement of the remaining central nervous system white matter. Devic disease is associated with a high mortality rate in adults (30%), but the same process may have milder manifestations in children. In Devic disorder, a serum antibody that targets the aquaporin 4 molecule has been identified. As far as multiple sclerosis is concerned, the latter has been diagnosed in 13% of children within 10 years after a first episode of optic neuritis and in 19% within 20 years. Some studies have reported even higher frequencies of the development of multiple sclerosis. In the series from Great Britain, a positive magnetic resonance image (MRI) of the brain/spinal cord showing demyelination at the presentation of optic neuritis is the strongest predictor for the development of multiple sclerosis. In this series, only 1 patient with a normal MRI ultimately developed multiple sclerosis.

The value of steroid treatment and other therapies on the recovery of visual function and on the subsequent risk of multiple sclerosis in children with optic neuritis has not been established by randomized trials. These therapies are applied on the basis of adult data. Generally speaking, intravenous methylprednisolone is generally recommended if visual loss is unilateral and severe or if it is bilateral. Some will also use interferon if an abnormal MRI is present, but again there are little data to either support or reject this form of therapy.

The bottom line here is that childhood optic neuritis is nothing to sneeze at with the risk of development of multiple sclerosis or Devic disorder being high. The tipoff to the 2 latter entities is an abnormal MRI brain scan.

**J. A. Stockman III, MD**

---

### Measurement of Intraocular Pressure With Pressure Phosphene Tonometry in Children

Fan DSP, Chiu TYH, Congdon N, et al (The Chinese Univ of Hong Kong, Kowloon, People's Republic of China; Prince of Wales Hosp, Hong Kong, People's Republic of China)
J Pediatr Ophthalmol Strabismus 48:167-173, 2011

---

*Purpose.*—To study the accuracy and acceptability of intraocular pressure (IOP) measurement by the pressure phosphene tonometer, non-contact tonometer, and Goldmann tonometer in children.

*Methods.*—Fifty children (5 to 14 years old) participated in this prospective comparative study. IOP was measured with the pressure phosphene tonometer, non-contact tonometer, and Goldmann tonometer by three different examiners who were masked to the results. The children were also asked to grade the degree of discomfort from 0 to 5 (0 = no discomfort; 5 = most discomfort).

*Results.*—The mean IOPs measured by the Goldmann tonometer, pressure phosphene tonometer, and non-contact tonometer were 15.9 mm Hg (standard deviation [SD]: = 5.5 mm Hg; range: 10 to 36 mm Hg), 16.0 mm Hg (SD: 2.9 mm Hg; range: 12 to 25 mm Hg), and 15.7 mm Hg (SD = 5.1 mm Hg; range: 8 to 32 mm Hg), respectively ($P = .722$). The mean difference between pressure phosphene tonometer and Goldmann tonometer readings was 2.9 mm Hg and that between non-contact tonometer and Goldmann tonometer readings was 2.1 mm Hg. The 95% confidence interval of the mean difference between pressure phosphene tonometer and Goldmann tonometer readings was −1.07 and 1.19, and that between non-contact tonometer and Goldmann tonometer readings was −1.07 and 0.53. The mean discomfort ratings for the pressure phosphene tonometer, non-contact tonometer, and Goldmann tonometer were 0.6, 2.0, and 2.3, respectively ($P < .001$).

*Conclusion.*—Although the pressure phosphene tonometer was less accurate than the non-contact tonometer compared with Goldmann tonometer, it gave a reasonably close estimate and had a high specificity of raised IOP. In addition, measurement by the pressure phosphene tonometer is most acceptable to children. The pressure phosphene tonometer can be considered as an alternative method of IOP measurement in children.

▶ It is difficult to imagine any adult being happy with someone, even an ophthalmologist, coming near their eye with an instrument. Normal avoidance reflexes take over when this happens. Imagine the situation, however, if you were just a tiny tike and the same thing is taking place with an eye doctor attempting to measure ocular pressure. Indeed, accurate, simple and noninvasive measurement of intraocular pressure (IOP) in children remains a major challenge in pediatric ophthalmology. There have been instruments designed for this purpose such as the Goldmann Tonometer and the electronic Tono-Pen XL. Both still require the placement of an instrument directly onto the cornea using topical anesthetics. It is not uncommon for a child to struggle and resist the measurement of IOP in such circumstances. Unfortunately, vigorous resistance may produce a Valsalva effect, thereby causing an increase in systemic venous pressure that can transiently increase IOP. The bottom line is that neither of the 2 instruments described for use in children are particularly effective in an uncooperative patient. So what might work? The noncontact pulse air tonometer could offer a descent alternative for IOP measurement in children, but there are some disadvantages associated with the use of this type of equipment. It is not portable, and the reliability of noncontact pulse air tonometry in children is not based on solid literature.

What Fan et al have done is to show us the potential benefits of a new form of tonometry called pressure phosphene tonometry. This is a psychophysical technique to evaluate IOP based on the entopic phenomenon of pressure phosphene. The word *phosphene* comes from the Greek, meaning "to show a light." Phosphene is the sensation of light elicited by a nonphotic stimuli. Technically, according to something known as Imbert-Fick's law, when the globe of the eye is deformed, which occurs in the application of a force over a given area, the perception of a phosphene occurs and can be related to pressure. It is applied through the eyelid, and no direct eyeball contact or topical anesthesia is required. Although there are controversies in the application of pressure phosphene tonometry, previous data have shown that when used by a professional, it can produce accurate IOP measurements comparable to that of the Goldmann Tonometer.

The authors of this report aimed to evaluate the potential use of pressure phosphene tonometry in pediatric patients by investigating the accuracy of the pressure phosphene tonometer compared with the Goldman Tonometer and noncontact pulse air tonometer in children, assessing the sensitivity and specificity in detecting an elevated IOP as well as the applicability and acceptance of its use in children. Some 100 eyes in children ranging from 5 to 14 years were evaluated using the pressure phosphene tonometer (Proview Eye Pressure Monitor; Bausch & Lomb, Tampa, FL). You will have to read this report in detail to understand exactly how the technology is applied. The bottom line is that although the Goldmann Tonometer remains the gold standard of IOP measurement in all ages, it may not be all that applicable to children because of discomfort and avoidance. The noncontact pulse air tonometer seems to have better accuracy than the pressure phosphene tonometer. However, with clear instructions and proper guidance, the pressure phosphene tonometer can be considered in selected children. Although the average pediatrician will not be performing this, it is nice to know that technologies exist to measure IOP in children. Again, a complete reading of this article is necessary to understand the physics involved, along with the pros and cons of each of the techniques that ophthalmologists may apply for the detection of increased IOP.

While on the topic of things having to do with the eye, is it possible that the coughing associated with pertussis might be a cause of retinal hemorrhages? Recently a prospective study of children aged 15 days to 2 years was undertaken to determine whether pertussis infection and its associated cough would cause retinal hemorrhages.[1] In 35 children confirmed to have pertussis, no patient was found to have retinal hemorrhages. Statistical analysis of this study showed that the chance of pertussis causing retinal hemorrhage was less than 1 in 100. Thus, if you see a coughing child and suspect pertussis but also find on physical examination the presence of retinal hemorrhages, think nonaccidental trauma.

**J. A. Stockman III, MD**

*Reference*

1. Curcoy AI, Trenchs V, Morales M, Serra A, Pou J. Is pertussis in infants a potential cause of retinal hemorrhages? *Arch Dis Child*. 2012;97:239-240.

### Manifestations of Ocular Fundus in Children With Febrile Seizures

Guo H, Lan Y, Wang M, et al (Second Affiliated Hosp of Sun Yat-sen Univ, People's Republic of China)

*J Pediatr Ophthalmol Strabismus* 48:182-186, 2011

*Purpose.*—To study the potential incidence of retinopathy in children with febrile seizures.

*Methods.*—Thirty-four children with febrile seizures, aged 3 months to 9 years and admitted from January 2000 to June 2008, were retrospectively analyzed. All cases received fundus examination within 24 hours after admission and the incidence of retinopathy was calculated.

*Results.*—None of the subjects was found to have retinal hemorrhages. Therefore, using Hanley's Rule of Three, the upper limit of 95% confidence interval of retinal hemorrhages following febrile seizures in children is less than 10%.

*Conclusion.*—The incidence of retinal hemorrhages in children with febrile seizures is lower than 10%. If retinal hemorrhages are found in children with febrile seizures, other causes need to be considered (Table 1).

▶ Trauma, cardiopulmonary resuscitation, vomiting, seizures, and coughing can theoretically cause forceful contraction of the thoracoabdominal muscles, resulting in a sudden increase in intrathoracic pressure and subsequently an increase in cranial and retinal venous pressure. These sudden transient changes in pressures may cause cerebral and retinal hemorrhages. What Guo et al have done is to inform us about whether retinal hemorrhages can be expected in children who have experienced febrile seizures. This report is extremely important to the practice of general pediatrics and to those who provide expert testimony in the area of child abuse.

What these investigators have done is examine the records of all children with a diagnosis of febrile seizures who were admitted to a hospital in the People's Republic of China. The classification of febrile seizures was made according to the following definitions. Simple seizures were self-limiting and of short

TABLE 1.—Diagnosis of Children With Retinopathy

| Retinal Manifestation | Diagnosis | No. of Children (N = 34) |
|---|---|---|
| Mild bilateral retinal edema | Severe pneumonia with systemic inflammatory response syndrome, type I respiratory failure, and heart failure; upper gastrointestinal hemorrhage; febrile seizures (simple) | 1 (2.9%) |
| Bilateral retinas showed signs of ischemia and became pale | Case 1: febrile seizures (complex), acute bronchitis, and microcytic hypochromic anemia; Case 2: bronchial pneumonia, febrile seizures (simple), congenital heart disease, and anemia | 2 (5.9%) |
| Mild bilateral retinal veins congestion | Febrile seizures (simple) and acute upper respiratory tract infection | 2 (5.9%) |

duration (less than 15 minutes), had tonic-clonic features, had no reoccurrence within the next 24 hours, and had no postictal pathology. Complex seizures were of longer duration (greater than 15 minutes), might present as a series of seizures with limited time interval, could have new events recurring within the next 24 hours, and could include focal seizures with clonic and/or tonic movements, with loss of muscle tone, beginning on one side of the body with or without secondary generalization, and/or with eye deviation to one side, or seizure activity followed by transient unilateral paralysis (lasting minutes to hours, occasionally days). Only children with simple febrile seizures (not complex) were evaluated with funduscopic examination by a trained ophthalmologist using direct ophthalmoscopy. The procedure included dilation of pupils with permission from parents and care providers if the pupil size was inadequate to allow a full examination.

Of 261 children with febrile seizures, 35 underwent a full fundus examination by an ophthalmologist using direct ophthalmoscopy. Pupils were dilated if necessary to enable a full examination. Five children were found to have mild retinopathy (Table 1). In no case was a retinal hemorrhage found.

We should all be aware of the conclusions of this report. Retinal hemorrhages rarely, if at all, occur as a result of febrile seizures. The finding of retinal hemorrhages in a child after a seizure should trigger an extensive search for other causes.

This commentary closes with a question. Why do drive-up ATM keypads have Braille dots? The answer is simple, because it is cheaper to make the same machine for both drive-up and walk-up locations.

**J. A. Stockman III, MD**

# 18 Respiratory Tract

---

**Main Air Pollutants and Myocardial Infarction: A Systematic Review and Meta-analysis**

Mustafić H, Jabre P, Caussin C, et al (Univ Paris Descartes, France; Marie Lannelongue Hosp, Le Plessis Robinson, France; et al)

*JAMA* 307:713-721, 2012

---

*Context.*—Short-term exposure to high levels of air pollution may trigger myocardial infarction (MI), but this association remains unclear.

*Objective.* To assess and quantify the association between short-term exposure to major air pollutants (ozone, carbon monoxide, nitrogen dioxide, sulfur dioxide, and particulate matter $\leq 10$ μm [$PM_{10}$] and $\leq 2.5$ μm [$PM_{2.5}$] in diameter) on MI risk.

*Data Sources.*—EMBASE, Ovid MEDLINE in-process and other nonindexed citations, and Ovid MEDLINE (between 1948 and November 28, 2011), and EBM Reviews—Cochrane Central Register of Controlled Trials and EBM Reviews—Cochrane Database of Systematic Reviews (between 2005 and November 28, 2011) were searched for a combination of keywords related to the type of exposure (air pollution, ozone, carbon monoxide, nitrogen dioxide, sulfur dioxide, $PM_{10}$, and $PM_{2.5}$) and to the type of outcome (MI, heart attack, acute coronary syndrome).

*Study Selection.*—Two independent reviewers selected studies of any study design and in any language, using original data and investigating the association between short-term exposure (for up to 7 days) to 1 or more air pollutants and subsequent MI risk. Selection was performed from abstracts and titles and pursued by reviewing the full text of potentially eligible studies.

*Data Extraction.*—Descriptive and quantitative information was extracted from each selected study. Using a random effects model, relative risks (RRs) and 95% CIs were calculated for each increment of 10 μg/m$^3$ in pollutant concentration, with the exception of carbon monoxide, for which an increase of 1 mg/m$^3$ was considered.

*Data Synthesis.*—After a detailed screening of 117 studies, 34 studies were identified. All the main air pollutants, with the exception of ozone, were significantly associated with an increase in MI risk (carbon monoxide: 1.048; 95% CI, 1.026-1.070; nitrogen dioxide: 1.011; 95% CI, 1.006-1.016; sulfur dioxide: 1.010; 95% CI, 1.003-1.017; $PM_{10}$: 1.006; 95% CI, 1.002-1.009; and $PM_{2.5}$: 1.025; 95% CI, 1.015-1.036). For ozone, the RR was 1.003 (95% CI, 0.997-1.010; $P = .36$). Subgroup analyses provided results comparable with those of the overall analyses. Population attributable fractions ranged between 0.6% and 4.5%, depending on the air pollutant.

*Conclusion.*—All the main air pollutants, with the exception of ozone, were significantly associated with a near-term increase in MI risk.

▶ So much has been written about air pollution over the past 50 years that it is hard to figure out where to start this commentary. The rise in solid or liquid pollutants suspended in the air includes nitrates, ozone, and sulfates emitted from road traffic, construction, and industry, all found to adversely affect health in both the long and short term. The effect of air pollution is pervasive. There are studies linking air pollution with stroke and heart attacks, including research published in 2011 in the *Lancet* that showed air pollution to be a trigger of myocardial infarction and that this effect was of a similar magnitude to that of physical exertion, alcohol, and coffee.

Mustafić et al recognized that a comprehensive and systematic meta-analysis of studies investigating the association of short-term exposure to air pollutants with myocardial infarction risk had not been performed. These investigators systematically reviewed associations between air pollutants and risk of myocardial infarction and quantified these associations. They reviewed all the literature related to this topic between 1948 and 2011. The data obtained from the study did demonstrate a significant association between all analyzed pollutants, with the exception of ozone, and myocardial infarction risk The magnitude of the association between air pollution and myocardial infarction is relatively small compared with the risks associated with factors such as smoking, hypertension, or diabetes mellitus that increase risk from 2-fold to 3-fold.

This report is important for pediatricians to understand. At greatest risk from air pollution are the young and the disabled. Even short-term exposure to air pollution can have its consequences. Although the relative risks reported here are somewhat low, they are not negligible because the majority of the population is exposed to air pollution all the time in industrialized countries. Further research is certainly needed to determine whether effective interventions that improve air quality would be associated with a decrease in the risk of myocardial infarction over one's lifetime.

This commentary closes with an observation about how powerful certain industries are that generate pollution. Recently, it was noted that at least 4 medical journals were warned by an attorney to hold off distributing data they had under review related to pollution from diesel exhaust fumes. The admonition—which concerns a large US study of the effects of diesel exhaust on miners' lungs—came from an attorney in Washington, DC, who is a lobbyist for the Mining Awareness Resource Group, a mining industry coalition. Editors at 2 United Kingdom—based publications, *Occupational and Environmental Medicine* and the *Annals of Occupational Hygiene*, say they and others received a letter advising them against "publication or other distribution" of the diesel exhaust data in the miners study until the data have been more thoroughly vetted by this attorney's clients.[1]

So much for freedom of speech.

**J. A. Stockman III, MD**

Reference

1. Kean S. Journals warned to keep a tight lid on diesel exposure data. *Science*. February 12. http://news.sciencemag.org/scienceinsider/2012/02/journals-warned-to-keep-a-tight.html. Accessed August 8, 2012.

---

**A Randomized Trial of Nicotine-Replacement Therapy Patches in Pregnancy**
Coleman T, Pregnancy (SNAP) Trial Team (Univ of Nottingham, UK)
*N Engl J Med* 366:808-818, 2012

---

*Background.*—Nicotine-replacement therapy is effective for smoking cessation outside pregnancy and its use is widely recommended during pregnancy. We investigated the efficacy and safety of nicotine patches during pregnancy.

*Methods.*—We recruited participants from seven hospitals in England who were 16 to 50 years of age with pregnancies of 12 to 24 weeks' gestation and who smoked five or more cigarettes per day. Participants received behavioral cessation support and were randomly assigned to 8 weeks of treatment with active nicotine patches (15 mg per 16 hours) or matched placebo patches. The primary outcome was abstinence from the date of smoking cessation until delivery, as validated by measurement of exhaled carbon monoxide or salivary cotinine. Safety was assessed by monitoring for adverse pregnancy and birth outcomes.

*Results.*—Of 1050 participants, 521 were randomly assigned to nicotine-replacement therapy and 529 to placebo. There was no significant difference in the rate of abstinence from the quit date until delivery between the nicotine-replacement and placebo groups (9.4% and 7.6%, respectively; unadjusted odds ratio with nicotine-replacement therapy, 1.26; 95% confidence interval, 0.82 to 1.96), although the rate was higher at 1 month in the nicotine-replacement group than in the placebo group (21.3% vs. 11.7%). Compliance was low; only 7.2% of women assigned to nicotine-replacement therapy and 2.8% assigned to placebo used patches for more than 1 month. Rates of adverse pregnancy and birth outcomes were similar in the two groups.

*Conclusions.*—Adding a nicotine patch (15 mg per 16 hours) to behavioral cessation support for women who smoked during pregnancy did not significantly increase the rate of abstinence from smoking until delivery or the risk of adverse pregnancy or birth outcomes. However, low compliance rates substantially limited the assessment of safety. (Funded by the National Institute for Health Research Health Technology Assessment Programme; Current Controlled Trials number, ISRCTN07249128.)

▶ There is no question that smoking at any time of life is a hazard to one's health. Smoking while pregnant is a hazard not just to the individual who smokes but also to the unborn baby. Despite the hazards of smoking while pregnant, 10% to 12% of pregnant women in the United States and 6% to 18% of pregnant women in high-income countries smoke, making cigarette smoking a major modifiable cause of adverse pregnancy outcomes in high-income countries. Traditionally, behavioral counseling has been the therapy of choice for pregnant smokers, increasing quit rates in this population by 6% to 10% over usual care. Other than counseling, however, it is not clear how best to treat pregnant smokers. Nicotine-replacement therapy does increase the rate at which smokers quit smoking among nonpregnant smokers, but its efficacy during pregnancy has not been well examined.

The authors report the results of a controlled trial of nicotine-replacement patches in pregnant women. Pregnant smokers were randomly assigned to receive behavioral counseling and either a standard course of nicotine patches (at a dose of 15 mg per 16 hours a day) or a visually identical placebo. The study treatment was administered for 4 weeks, followed by an additional 4 weeks of treatment that was contingent on biochemical evidence of smoking abstinence. Although smoking cessation rates at 1 month were higher in the nicotine-replacement group than in the placebo group, prolonged cessation rates were similar in the nicotine-replacement and placebo groups (9.4% and 7.6%, respectively). Overall adherence to therapy was low; only 7.2% of women in the nicotine-replacement group and 2.8% of those in the placebo group used the treatment for more than 4 weeks.

The finding that nicotine-replacement therapy does not improve long-term quit rates is disappointing, to say the least. With the demonstrated low adherence rates in placebo-controlled trials of nicotine-replacement therapy in pregnant smokers, it is difficult for any care provider to counsel patients regarding whether such treatment would be efficacious or safe if used as directed. In this study, the higher abstinence rate at 1 month in the nicotine-replacement group than in the placebo group (21.3% vs 11.7%) indicates the efficacy of the medication. However, most women who quit smoking for a short time did not use the patch for more than 4 weeks.

In a commentary that accompanied this report, Oncken[1] asked the question whether participants stopped the study treatment before or after a smoking relapse, since the former would suggest that future trials should focus on adherence to therapy, whereas the latter would suggest that the medication is not efficacious for smoking cessation. Elucidating the reasons for the low adherence among pregnant smokers in this and other trials would also increase our understanding of the potential usefulness of nicotine-replacement therapy for smoking cessation during pregnancy and would inform the design of future pharmacotherapy trials. Fortunately, adverse events did not appear to be a major factor in the low adherence to therapy in the current study.

A few other comments seem relevant. The clearance of nicotine is accelerated during pregnancy, and it has been suggested that to optimize efficacy, higher doses of nicotine-replacement therapy may be needed in pregnant smokers. Given that nicotine is a teratogen in animals, it would be important, particularly in any study using higher doses, to monitor the overall exposure to nicotine in order to ensure that exposure during the use of nicotine-replacement therapy does not exceed baseline exposure. Pending more data on the efficacy and safety of nicotine-replacement therapy during pregnancy, it seems clear that this form of treatment cannot be recommended with any level of clinical certainty at the present time. Thus we are left with only behavioral therapy with all of its warts and failures.

This commentary concludes with a few remarks about less toxic cigarette use. Manufacturers are currently promoting less toxic cigarettes these days, meaning lower nicotine content cigarettes. It has been suggested, however, that such cigarettes may actually backfire, in the sense, of leading to an increase in lung cancer. Of the excess deaths caused by smoking, about 29% have been caused by heart disease and stroke and about 16% by lung cancer, with the rest mostly due to assorted other kinds of cancers. Many people think of lung cancer as the chief culprit because lung cancer is a relatively rare disease in the absence of smoking, whereas heart disease is quite common. Nonsmokers get lung cancer at about one-fortieth the rate of smokers, whereas heart disease and stroke are major causes of death in both smokers and nonsmokers. Studies have shown that nicotine addicts smoke until they inhale enough nicotine to satisfy their craving. This means that if one switches to low-nicotine cigarettes, the addicted individual will likely smoke more cigarettes in the long run. This in turn means that they will be subjected to more of the "tars" (cancer-causing ingredients of the smoke) in their attempts to get their usual dosage of nicotine (the ingredient responsible for heart disease and stroke). In the end, smokers of low-nicotine cigarettes will remain at the same risk for heart disease and stroke, but increase their chances of developing cancer—or so say some investigators.[2]

**J. A. Stockman III, MD**

*References*

1. Oncken C. Nicotine replacement for smoking cessation during pregnancy. *N Engl J Med.* 2012;366:846-847.
2. Deutsch M. Less toxic cigarette use may backfire. *Science.* 2009;325:944.

## Parental Smoking and Vascular Damage in Their 5-year-old Children

Geerts CC, Bots ML, van der Ent CK, et al (Univ Med Ctr Utrecht, The Netherlands)
*Pediatrics* 129:45-54, 2012

*Background.*—The relation between smoke exposure in early life, the prenatal period in particular, and the vascular development of young children is largely unknown.

*Methods.*—Data from the birth cohort participating in the WHISTLER-Cardio study were used to relate the smoking of parents during pregnancy to subsequent vascular properties in their children. In 259 participating children who turned 5 years of age, parental smoking data were updated and children's carotid artery intima-media thickness (CIMT) and arterial wall distensibility were measured by using ultrasonography.

*Results.*—Children of mothers who had smoked throughout pregnancy had 18.8 μm thicker CIMT (95% confidence interval [CI] 1.1, 36.5, $P = .04$) and 15% lower distensibility (95% CI −0.3, −0.02, $P = .02$)

after adjustment for child's age, maternal age, gender, and breastfeeding. The associations were not found in children of mothers who had not smoked in pregnancy but had smoked thereafter. The associations were strongest if both parents had smoked during pregnancy, with 27.7 $\mu$m thicker CIMT (95% CI 0.2, 55.3) and 21% lower distensibility (95% CI $-0.4$, $-0.03$).

*Conclusion.*—Exposure of children to parental tobacco smoke during pregnancy affects their arterial structure and function in early life.

▶ The evidence is overwhelmingly clear that secondhand smoke is not good for children. This report from the Netherlands documents that mothers who smoke during pregnancy expose their babies to the ultimate form of secondhand smoke, and this has profound consequences for the vasculature of the unborn child when such children are studied later at 5 years of age. The report is the first to show the effect of smoking during pregnancy on the vasculature of children and the fact that smoking during pregnancy appears to be a terrible habit at a critical period for such damage to occur.

Over time, fewer and fewer adults are now smoking. However, data show that about half of children have biochemical evidence of exposure to second-hand smoke.[1] The American Academy of Pediatrics has partnered with organizations around the world to improve efforts in tobacco control as they relate to children. Many of these efforts involve supporting policies that will protect children from exposure to secondhand smoke, including smoke-free laws to promote clean air in places where children spend their time, such as outdoor areas, public spaces, and public housing. It is clear that it is never too late to try to protect children from secondhand smoke. A recent report by Rosen et al analyzes a systematic review and meta-analysis to quantify the effects of interventions that encourage parents to stop smoking.[2] It was determined that interventions to achieve cessation among parents for the sake of their children do in fact work and can help protect vulnerable children from harm due to tobacco smoke exposure. Unfortunately, however, most parents do not quit, and additional strategies to protect children are badly needed.

The preceding commentary closed with some remarks about low-nicotine cigarettes.[3] This commentary closes with some reflections on electronic cigarettes. The results of a US Food and Drug Administration (FDA) analysis of widely marketed electronic cigarette products suggest these devices may contain some of the same toxic or carcinogenic compounds as traditional cigarettes. Electronic cigarettes, or E-cigarettes, or battery-powered devices vaporize nicotine, flavoring, and/or chemicals into an inhalable vapor. Chemical analyses of several samples of products by FDA scientists detected tobacco-associated chemicals that may be harmful to humans, including known human carcinogens. One cigarette type also contained 1% ethylene glycol, a toxic chemical. Additionally, investigators found varying levels of nicotine. Electronic cigarettes are marketed for a range of uses, including as a cessation aid and as an alternative to cigarettes in smoke-free zones. It should be noted that the FDA has detained or refused numerous shipments of E-cigarettes at US borders because the agency classifies these as an unapproved drug or drug administration device. However, these products do continue to be available to US consumers as of this writing via online sales and at mall kiosks.

If you want to read more about E-cigarettes, see the article by Kuehn.[4]

**J. A. Stockman III, MD**

*References*

1. Centers for Disease Control and Prevention (CDC). Vital signs: nonsmokers' exposure to secondhand smoke — United States, 1999-2008. *MMWR Morb Mortal Wkly Rep.* 2010;59:1141-1146.
2. Rosen LJ, Noach MB, Winickoff JP, Hovell MF. Parental smoking cessation to protect young children: a systematic review and meta-analysis. *Pediatrics.* 2012; 129:141-152.
3. Coleman T, Cooper S, Thornton JG, et al. A randomized trial of nicotine-replacement therapy patches in pregnancy. *N Engl J Med.* 2012;366:808-818.
4. Kuehn BM. FDA: Electronic cigarettes may be risky. *JAMA.* 2009;302:937.

### The tumor necrosis factor family member LIGHT is a target for asthmatic airway remodeling

Doherty TA, Soroosh P, Khorram N, et al (La Jolla Inst for Allergy and Immunology, CA; Univ of California—San Diego (UCSD), La Jolla; et al)
*Nat Med* 17:596-603, 2011

Individuals with chronic asthma show a progressive decline in lung function that is thought to be due to structural remodeling of the airways characterized by subepithelial fibrosis and smooth muscle hyperplasia. Here we show that the tumor necrosis factor (TNF) family member LIGHT is expressed on lung inflammatory cells after allergen exposure. Pharmacological inhibition of LIGHT using a fusion protein between the IgG Fc domain and lymphotoxin β receptor (LTβR) reduces lung fibrosis, smooth muscle hyperplasia and airway hyperresponsiveness in mouse models of chronic asthma, despite having little effect on airway eosinophilia. LIGHT-deficient mice also show a similar impairment in fibrosis and smooth muscle accumulation. Blockade of LIGHT suppresses expression of lung transforming growth factor-β (TGF-β) and interleukin-13 (IL-13), cytokines implicated in remodeling in humans, whereas exogenous administration of LIGHT to the airways induces fibrosis and smooth muscle hyperplasia. Thus, LIGHT may be targeted to prevent asthma-related airway remodeling.

▶ This is another report describing a mechanism associated with airway remodeling in patients with asthma. Unfortunately, over time, those affected with reactive airway disease develop thickening and increasing rigidity of their airways. This results in part from accumulation of extracellular matrix protein, such as collagen and thickening of smooth muscle. Current therapies for asthma are beneficial in controlling symptoms and airway inflammation but have little effect on lung remodeling. Thus far, anti-inflammatory therapy with corticosteroids seems to have no effect on levels of subepithelial fibrosis, suggesting that the mechanisms that regulate remodeling may be distinct from those that induce eosinophilia or other aspects of inflammation.

Doherty et al have identified the tumor necrosis factor (TNF) family ligand LIGHT (lymphotoxin-related inducible ligand) that competes for glycoprotein D binding to herpesvirus entry mediator on T cells (also known as TNFSF14) as a crucial regulator of airway remodeling in mouse models of chronic asthma. They show that blockade or absence of LIGHT induces subepithelial fibrosis, smooth muscle hypertrophy and hyperplasia, and airway hyper-responsiveness after allergen challenge, but does not affect airway eosinophilia. These results suggest that LIGHT could be targeted to treat airway remodeling in asthma. This is noteworthy because there are currently no drugs specifically available that target the mechanisms of asthmatic lung remodeling. If LIGHT is to be developed as a treatment for asthma-related remodeling, future research should focus on determining whether anti-LIGHT therapeutics can slow or reverse the progression of established airway disease. We may very well be at the dawn of new management strategies for an age-old disease!

This commentary closes with some observations on avian and alligator airways. Bet you were not aware that the lungs of birds move air in only one direction during inspiration and exhalation through most of the tubular gas-exchanging bronchi (parabronchi), whereas in the lungs of mammals and presumably other vertebrates, air moves tidally into and out of gas-exchange structures, which in essence are cul-de-sacs. This unidirectional flow in birds purportedly depends on bellows like ventilation by air sacs and may have evolved to meet the high aerobic demands of sustained flight. The anatomical similarity with the avian lung has led investigators to hypothesize that airflow might also be unidirectional in crocodilians. Indeed, studies of airflow in the American alligator show that it is extremely bird-like. This suggests that this pattern of respiration dates back to the dinosaurs of the Triassic period. For what it is worth, unidirectional airflow in both bird and the alligator facilitates extraordinary extraction of oxygen under conditions of hypoxia.

If you want to learn more about the extraordinary tidbit of unidirectional airflow in the lungs of both birds and alligators, read the report of Farmer and Sanders.[1]

**J. A. Stockman III, MD**

*Reference*

1. Farmer CG, Sanders K. Unidirectional airflow in the lungs of alligators. *Science*. 2010;327:338-339.

---

**Effect of Bronchoconstriction on Airway Remodeling in Asthma**
Grainge CL, Lau LCK, Ward JA, et al (Univ of Southampton School of Medicine, UK)
*N Engl J Med* 364:2006-2015, 2011

---

*Background.*—Asthma is characterized pathologically by structural changes in the airway, termed airway remodeling. These changes are associated with worse long-term clinical outcomes and have been attributed to eosinophilic inflammation. In vitro studies indicate, however, that the compressive mechanical forces that arise during bronchoconstriction may induce remodeling independently of inflammation. We evaluated the influence of repeated experimentally induced bronchoconstriction on airway structural changes in patients with asthma.

*Methods.*—We randomly assigned 48 subjects with asthma to one of four inhalation challenge protocols involving a series of three challenges with one type of inhaled agent presented at 48-hour intervals. The two active challenges were with either a dust-mite allergen (which causes bronchoconstriction and eosinophilic inflammation) or methacholine (which causes bronchoconstriction without eosinophilic inflammation); the two control challenges (neither of which causes bronchoconstriction) were either saline alone or albuterol followed by methacholine (to control for nonbronchoconstrictor effects of methacholine). Bronchial-biopsy specimens were obtained before and 4 days after completion of the challenges.

*Results.*—Allergen and methacholine immediately induced similar levels of bronchoconstriction. Eosinophilic inflammation of the airways increased only in the allergen group, whereas both the allergen and the methacholine groups had significant airway remodeling not seen in the two control groups. Subepithelial collagen-band thickness increased by a median of 2.17 $\mu$m in the allergen group (interquartile range [IQR], 0.70 to 3.67) and 1.94 $\mu$m in the methacholine group (IQR, 0.37 to 3.24) ($P < 0.001$ for the comparison of the two challenge groups with the two control groups); periodic acid–Schiff staining of epithelium (mucus glands) also increased, by a median of 2.17 percentage points in the allergen group (IQR, 1.03 to 4.77) and 2.13 percentage points in the methacholine group (IQR, 1.14 to 7.96) ($P = 0.003$ for the comparison with controls). There were no significant differences between the allergen and methacholine groups.

*Conclusions.*—Bronchoconstriction without additional inflammation induces airway remodeling in patients with asthma. These findings have potential implications for management.

▶ This report, dealing with how the airways remodel themselves in patients with asthma, definitely has implications for the care of children and adolescents, even though the target range of the study participants barely overlapped the teen years. We would likely see identical findings in the older childhood age group with reactive airway disease for whom we provide care.

Asthma is known to be accompanied by changes in the structure and composition of the airway walls, collectively termed *airway remodeling*. The key features of airway remodeling include increased numbers of mucous-secreting epithelial cells, thickening of the subepithelial collagen layer, and increases in vascularity and smooth muscle mass around the airways. There seems to be no argument that airway remodeling contributes to the decline in lung function and the development of fixed airway obstruction present in some patients with chronic persistent asthma, particularly as the patient grows older. Evidence does indicate that aspects of airway remodeling can be detected early in life, with the implication that remodeling may contribute prominently to both early-onset and persistent airway dysfunction.

Although the main culprit responsible for airway remodeling in asthma has been suspected to result from inflammation, the authors of this report suggest another possibility. Their investigation demonstrates selected aspects of airway remodeling that can be promoted simply by the episodic administration of an inhaled bronchoconstrictor, methacholine. They suggest that physical forces are involved with the remodeling process, not just inflammation. Using a prospective, randomized, controlled study design, the authors measured indices of airway remodeling in 4 groups of subjects with mild atopic asthma. Subjects were studied at baseline and after exposure to inhaled allergen, methacholine, saline, or methacholine after pretreatment with the bronchodilator albuterol. Allergen exposure caused both bronchoconstriction and eosinophilic inflammation as assessed by means of biopsy and bronchoalveolar-lavage fluid examination, whereas methacholine challenge led to bronchoconstriction without changes in eosinophils or other airway leukocytes. Both exposures were titrated to produce similar levels of immediate airway narrowing, as indicated by falls in forced inspiratory volume in 1 second. The methacholine and allergen challenges strikingly promoted marked and indistinguishable changes from baseline in measures of airway remodeling, including subepithelial collagen thickness, epithelial mucous staining, epithelial proliferation, and increased expression of transforming growth factor beta. In the group pretreated with albuterol before methacholine challenge, airway narrowing in response to methacholine was prevented. These data strongly support a direct role for the physical forces of bronchoconstriction in promoting the measured indices of airway remodeling.

The bottom line from this report is that it is not only inflammation that can permanently change the airways of patients with asthma. Airway smooth muscle contraction on a repetitive basis, absent inflammation, is capable of producing fixed damage to the airways. This study offers a tentative and compelling rationale for further investigation of whether strategies specifically aimed at preventing bronchoconstriction might positively affect airway remodeling, and, by extension, airway function. The failure of inhaled steroids alone to modify the natural history of lung-function changes in asthma underscores the need for continued innovation and exploration for agents that are specifically capable of preventing bronchoconstriction.

To read more about the physical forces and airway remodeling in asthma, see the excellent commentary by Tschumperlin.[1]

This commentary closes with an observation having to do with reactive airway disease. The 2011 IG Nobel award in medicine was given to Simon Rietveld of the University of Amsterdam, the Netherlands. The award was given for discovering the symptoms of asthma can be treated with a roller coaster ride. Presumably the effect was most dramatic on the down sloping of the roller coaster, although this was not pointed out in the article. Also, the age of the patients in this report was not described. Presumably all were over 42 inches tall as that is the requirement for roller coaster riding in Disney World and presumably elsewhere.[2]

**J. A. Stockman III, MD**

*Reference*

1. Tschumperlin DJ. Physical forces and airway remodeling in asthma. *N Engl J Med.* 2011;364:2058-2059.
2. Rietveld S, van Beest I. Roller coaster asthma. *Behav Res Ther.* 2006;45:977-987.

---

**A Hemodynamic Study of Pulmonary Hypertension in Sickle Cell Disease**
Parent F, Bachir D, Inamo J, et al (Université Paris-Sud, Clamart, France; Hôpital Henri Mondor, France; Hôpital La Meynard, France; et al)
*N Engl J Med* 365:44-53, 2011

---

*Background.*—The prevalence and characteristics of pulmonary hypertension in adults with sickle cell disease have not been clearly established.

*Methods.*—In this prospective study, we evaluated 398 outpatients with sickle cell disease (mean age, 34 years) at referral centers in France. All patients underwent Doppler echocardiography, with measurement of tricuspid-valve regurgitant jet velocity. Right heart catheterization was performed in 96 patients in whom pulmonary hypertension was suspected on the basis of a tricuspid regurgitant jet velocity of at least 2.5 m per second. Pulmonary hypertension was defined as a mean pulmonary arterial pressure of at least 25 mm Hg.

*Results.*—The prevalence of a tricuspid regurgitant jet velocity of at least 2.5 m per second was 27%. In contrast, the prevalence of pulmonary hypertension as confirmed on catheterization was 6%. The positive predictive value of echocardiography for the detection of pulmonary hypertension was 25%. Among the 24 patients with confirmed pulmonary hypertension, the pulmonary-capillary wedge pressure was 15 mm Hg or less (indicating precapillary pulmonary hypertension) in 11 patients. Patients with confirmed pulmonary hypertension were older and had poorer functional capacity and higher levels of N-terminal pro—brain natriuretic peptide than other patients. In contrast, patients who had a tricuspid regurgitant jet velocity of at least 2.5 m per second without pulmonary hypertension and patients with a tricuspid regurgitant jet velocity of less than 2.5 m per second had similar clinical characteristics.

*Conclusions.*—In this study of adults with sickle cell disease, the prevalence of pulmonary hypertension as confirmed on right heart catheterization was 6%. Echocardiographic evaluation alone had a low positive predictive value for pulmonary hypertension. (Funded by the French Ministry of Health and Assistance Publique—Hôpitaux de Paris; Clinical Trials.gov number, NCT00434902.)

▶ Sickle cell disease affects 80 000 to 100 000 Americans and is considered a global health burden. The pathophysiology of sickle cell disease is initiated by polymerization of the deoxy sickle hemoglobin, which results in sickling of red blood cells and hemolytic anemia. This reduces red cell lifespan to an average of just 16 days. The deformed red cells adhere to endothelium and cause a cascade of secondary pathologies, including adhesion of other cell types, vaso-occlusion, inflammation, vascular remodeling, and widespread organ damage. Anemia contributes to cardiomegaly and exercise intolerance. More recently reported has been a high prevalence of pulmonary hypertension, particularly pulmonary arterial hypertension. Pulmonary arterial hypertension in the case of a patient with sickle cell disease is characterized by the presence of precapillary pulmonary hypertension in the absence of left-sided heart disease, lung disease, or chronic thromboembolism. In studies involving adults, the prevalence of pulmonary hypertension associated with sickle cell disease runs as high as 30%.

What Parent et al have done is study the prevalence of pulmonary hypertension as assessed by right-sided heart catheterization in young adults and older adults with sickle cell disease in whom pulmonary hypertension was suspected on the basis of echocardiography. The data from this report have significant applicability to our understanding of the evolution of this complication in childhood. The study found that the prevalence of pulmonary hypertension on the basis of echocardiography ran 27%, but when confirmed by right-side heart catheterization, the prevalence was just 6%. The annual rate of death in those with pulmonary hypertension was about 2%, significantly lower than that observed in other reports. The bottom line is that echocardiographic evaluation alone seems to have a low positive predictive value for pulmonary hypertension. Echocardiography, however, is the screening test of choice because of its ease of application. Unfortunately, the optimal diagnostic procedure is right-side heart catheterization, a little too much to use unless there is a very good reason to want to be certain about whether pulmonary hypertension is present.

While on the topic of sickle cell disease, Meiler et al[1] now report that pomalidomide, an immunomodulatory drug, will stimulate fetal hemoglobin production in a mouse model of sickle cell disease and does so without the toxic side effects seen with hydroxyurea, the most commonly used drug to increase fetal hemoglobin production in humans with sickle cell disease. This is a highly encouraging development for a serious disease with only 1 approved therapeutic agent.

This commentary closes with a few facts having to do with high-altitude flying and its effects on the respiratory and cardiovascular systems in humans. Although commercial air flights usually cruise at altitudes of 7010 to 12 498 m above sea level, the passenger cabin is pressurized only to an altitude of 1524 to 2438 m. Most regulatory governmental agencies require the cabin altitude not to exceed 2438 m. Most healthy individuals tolerate this cabin pressure. Studies, however, of adult volunteers simulating a 20-hour flight showed that the frequency of reported complaints associated with acute mountain sickness (fatigue, headache, lightheadedness, and nausea) increased with increasing altitude and peaked at 2438 m, with the most symptoms becoming apparent after 3 hours to 9 hours of exposure. Long-haul aircraft such as the Airbus 380 and Boeing 777 LR are now capable of extending flight times to as much as 18 to 20 h. Thus, you can see what the problem is. Cabin pressurization at 2438 m reduces the atmospheric pressure of the cabin, resulting in a concomitant decrease of arterial oxygen saturation ($PaO_2$) from 95 Hg to 60 mm Hg at the maximum cabin altitude of 2438 m. In healthy passengers these pressures lead to a 3% to 4% decrease in systemic oxyhemoglobin saturation, which is still well within the flat portion of the oxyhemoglobin dissociation curve. However, many passengers (adults and/or children) with preexisting cardiac, pulmonary and hematologic conditions may have a reduced baseline $PaO_2$, so reduced cabin pressure leads to further reduction in oxygen saturation, which lowers further with increasing flight times. It is known that about 1 in 5 passengers with chronic obstructive pulmonary disease will have at least mild respiratory distress during a routine flight.

Current guidelines suggest that oxygen supplementation is recommended for passengers with either a resting oxygen saturation of 92% or lower ($PaO_2 \leq 67$ mm Hg) or if the expected in-flight $PaO_2$ is less than 50 mm Hg to 55 mm Hg.

One final comment about air flight and gases in the body. Gas in body cavities is also affected by cabin pressure. According to Boyle's Law, the volume that a gas occupies is inversely proportional to the surrounding pressure. Thus, at the low cabin pressures associated with cruising altitudes, gas in the body cavities expands by 30%. For healthy passengers this expansion can result in minor abdominal cramping and barotrauma to the ears in certain circumstances. However, passengers who have undergone recent surgical procedures are at increased risk of problems related to gas expansion, and many anecdotal reports, including those of bowel perforation and wound dehiscence, have been published. These are usually the result of patients who have had intraperitoneal gas instilled for laparoscopic procedures or who have recently undergone colonoscopy with air having been put into the bowel. Guidelines recommend delaying air travel for 14 days after major surgical procedures. Individuals who have experienced bowel obstruction or diverticulitis are advised to wait 7 days to 10 days before air travel. Please note that passengers who scuba dive also have an increased risk of decompression sickness if they fly too soon after diving. A divers' alert network recommends a 12-hour interval between diving and air travel for divers who make a dive per day without decompression. Divers who participate in several dives a day, or who dive requiring decompression, should wait 24 hours before air travel. Last, recognize that gas expansion also affects medical devices such as pneumatic splints, feeding tubes, urinary catheters, and cuffed endotracheal or tracheostomy tubes. Gas expansion concerns with these devices can be eliminated by installation of water rather than air during air travel.

To learn more about gases and medical issues related to flying, see the excellent summary by Silverman and Gendreau.[2]

**J. A. Stockman III, MD**

*References*

1. Meiler SE, Wade M, Kutlar F, et al. Pomalidomide augments fetal hemoglobin production without the myelosuppressive effects of hydroxyurea in transgenic sickle cell mice. *Blood.* 2011;118:1109-1112.
2. Silverman D, Gendreau M. Medical issues associated with commercial flights. *Lancet.* 2009;373:2067-2077.

### Effect of Bronchoalveolar Lavage–Directed Therapy on *Pseudomonas aeruginosa* Infection and Structural Lung Injury in Children with Cystic Fibrosis: A Randomized Trial

Wainwright CE, for the ACFBAL Study Investigators (Univ of Queensland, Brisbane, Australia; et al)

*JAMA* 306:163-171, 2011

*Context.*—Early pulmonary infection in children with cystic fibrosis leads to increased morbidity and mortality. Despite wide use of oropharyngeal cultures to identify pulmonary infection, concerns remain over their diagnostic accuracy. While bronchoalveolar lavage (BAL) is an alternative diagnostic tool, evidence for its clinical benefit is lacking.

*Objective.*—To determine if BAL-directed therapy for pulmonary exacerbations during the first 5 years of life provides better outcomes than current standard practice relying on clinical features and oropharyngeal cultures.

*Design, Setting, and Participants.*—The Australasian Cystic Fibrosis Bronchoalveolar Lavage (ACFBAL) randomized controlled trial, recruiting infants diagnosed with cystic fibrosis through newborn screening programs in 8 Australasian cystic fibrosis centers. Recruitment occurred between June 1, 1999, and April 30, 2005, with the study ending on December 31, 2009.

*Interventions.*—BAL-directed (n = 84) or standard (n = 86) therapy until age 5 years. The BAL-directed therapy group underwent BAL before age 6 months when well, when hospitalized for pulmonary exacerbations, if *Pseudomonas aeruginosa* was detected in oropharyngeal specimens, and after *P. aeruginosa* eradication therapy. Treatment was prescribed according to BAL or oropharyngeal culture results.

*Main Outcome Measures.*—Primary outcomes at age 5 years were prevalence of *P. aeruginosa* on BAL cultures and total cystic fibrosis computed tomography (CF-CT) score (as a percentage of the maximum score) on high-resolution chest CT scan.

*Results.*—Of 267 infants diagnosed with cystic fibrosis following newborn screening, 170 were enrolled and randomized, and 157 completed the study. At age 5 years, 8 of 79 children (10%) in the BAL-directed therapy group and 9 of 76 (12%) in the standard therapy group had *P. aeruginosa* in final BAL cultures (risk difference, −1.7% [95% confidence interval, −11.6% to 8.1%]; $P = .73$). Mean total CF-CT scores for the BAL-directed therapy and standard therapy groups were 3.0% and 2.8%, respectively (mean difference, 0.19% [95% confidence interval, −0.94% to 1.33%]; $P = .74$).

*Conclusion.*—Among infants diagnosed with cystic fibrosis, BAL-directed therapy did not result in a lower prevalence of P. aeruginosa infection or lower total CF-CT score when compared with standard therapy at age 5 years.

▶ This is one of the most important articles that have appeared in the recent literature with respect to the treatment of patients with cystic fibrosis. One of the difficult encounters physicians have in caring for such patients is making a correct diagnosis of the organism that may be causing a pulmonary exacerbation.

Bronchoalveolar lavage (BAL) has rapidly become the diagnostic tool of choice to identify culprit organisms. Prior to the introduction of BAL, oropharyngeal cultures were widely used, particularly in nonexpectorating patients. These types of cultures have limited sensitivity and variable specificity for predicting the presence of lower airway pathogens. There have been longitudinal BAL-based studies. These studies have documented that by 5 years of age, 30% of patients are already colonized with *Pseudomonas aeruginosa*. By adulthood, 80% of patients with cystic fibrosis are colonized with this organism. While *P aeruginosa* may be easily treated early in its established course, once firmly established in the lungs, *P aeruginosa* infection is rarely eliminated, leading to lung injury with deteriorated pulmonary function and increased treatment requirement. For this reason, early detection and treatment seems to offer the greatest opportunity for preventing or delaying chronic *P aeruginosa* infection.

Investigators with the Australasian Cystic Fibrosis Bronchoalveolar Lavage Trial established a protocol whereby all newly diagnosed patients with cystic fibrosis (detected on newborn screening) would have BAL-directed therapy for pulmonary exacerbations in their first 5 years of life. They investigated whether this approach would reduce the establishment of *P aeruginosa* infection and structural lung injury by 5 years of age compared with standard management based on clinical features and oropharyngeal culture results. In this randomized controlled trial, BAL directed therapy did not reduce structural lung abnormalities seen on high-resolution chest computed tomography (CT) scans or prevalence of *P aeruginosa* infection at 5 years of age when compared with standard treatment. The trial interestingly found an unexpectedly low prevalence of *P aeruginosa* infection, which limited its statistical power for the primary outcome. At 5 years of age, only one child met the clinical criteria for chronic *P aeruginosa* infection.

It should be noted that compared with children receiving standard therapy, BAL-directed therapy was associated with reduced length of stay for non–*P aeruginosa* respiratory-related hospital admissions, which may partially offset the increased health care cost associated with the procedure itself. Despite children in this study having excellent nutritional and clinical status and relatively normal lung function and having received aggressive treatment of infection, many still had mild structural changes on high-resolution chest scans, with 57% showing signs of bronchiectasis and 45% demonstrating air trapping. Air trapping may in fact be a very sensitive marker of early lung disease.

The importance of this report is that it is the first large multicenter, randomized controlled trial in young children with cystic fibrosis using carefully designed CT scores as a primary outcome measure. High-resolution chest CT scans do provide a sensitive direct measure of structural lung damage caused by cystic fibrosis, especially bronchiectasis, the most important component of cystic fibrosis lung disease associated with increased morbidity and early mortality. Spirometry is unable to detect these early changes. As valuable as high-resolution chest CT scans are, their use needs to be balanced by the potential risk associated with increased radiation exposure over one's lifetime. The study does tell us that BAL-directed therapy provides no clinical, microbiologic, or radiographic advantage and does lead to an increased risk of predominantly mild adverse events as a direct result of bronchoscopy as well as disadvantages such as the need to fast prior to the procedure, exposure to anesthesia, and potential perioperative anxiety. BAL is still, however, a very useful research tool in young patients with cystic fibrosis who are unable to bring up sputum. BAL is probably best reserved for young children whose conditions are deteriorating despite parenteral antibiotic therapy. In such circumstances, unusual or antibiotic-resistant pathogens are much more likely to be found.

**J. A. Stockman III, MD**

## A CFTR Potentiator in Patients with Cystic Fibrosis and the *G551D* Mutation

Ramsey BW, for the VX08-770-102 Study Group (Seattle Children's Hosp and Univ of Washington School of Medicine; et al)
*N Engl J Med* 365:1663-1672, 2011

*Background.*—Increasing the activity of defective cystic fibrosis transmembrane conductance regulator (CFTR) protein is a potential treatment for cystic fibrosis.

*Methods.*—We conducted a randomized, double-blind, placebo-controlled trial to evaluate ivacaftor (VX-770), a CFTR potentiator, in subjects 12 years of age or older with cystic fibrosis and at least one *G551D-CFTR* mutation. Subjects were randomly assigned to receive 150 mg of ivacaftor every 12 hours (84 subjects, of whom 83 received at least one dose) or placebo (83, of whom 78 received at least one dose) for 48 weeks. The primary end point was the estimated mean change from baseline through week 24 in the percent of predicted forced expiratory volume in 1 second ($FEV_1$).

*Results.*—The change from baseline through week 24 in the percent of predicted $FEV_1$ was greater by 10.6 percentage points in the ivacaftor group than in the placebo group ($P < 0.001$). Effects on pulmonary function were noted by 2 weeks, and a significant treatment effect was maintained through week 48. Subjects receiving ivacaftor were 55% less likely to have a pulmonary exacerbation than were patients receiving placebo, through week 48 ($P < 0.001$). In addition, through week 48, subjects in the ivacaftor group scored 8.6 points higher than did subjects in the placebo group on the respiratory-symptoms domain of the Cystic Fibrosis Questionnaire—revised instrument (a 100-point scale, with higher numbers indicating a lower effect of symptoms on the patient's quality of life) ($P < 0.001$). By 48 weeks, patients treated with ivacaftor had gained, on average, 2.7 kg more weight than had patients receiving placebo ($P < 0.001$). The change from baseline through week 48 in the concentration of sweat chloride, a measure of CFTR activity, with ivacaftor as compared with placebo was −48.1 mmol per liter ($P < 0.001$). The incidence of adverse events was similar with ivacaftor and placebo, with a lower proportion of serious adverse events with ivacaftor than with placebo (24% vs. 42%).

*Conclusions.*—Ivacaftor was associated with improvements in lung function at 2 weeks that were sustained through 48 weeks. Substantial improvements were also observed in the risk of pulmonary exacerbations, patient-reported respiratory symptoms, weight, and concentration of sweat chloride. (Funded by Vertex Pharmaceuticals and others; VX08-770-102 ClinicalTrials.gov number, NCT00909532.)

▶ The gene for cystic fibrosis was discovered back in 1989. This gene regulates the cystic fibrosis membrane conductance regulator (CFTR) protein, an epithelial ion channel protein contributing to the regulation of absorption and secretion of salt and water in various tissues, including the lung, sweat glands, pancreas, and gastrointestinal tract. Cystic fibrosis is caused by mutations in the CFTR that affect the quantity of protein that reaches the cell's surface or that affects the function of CFTR channels at the cell's surface.

Ramsey et al report on a relatively new agent, ivacaftor (VX770), an investigational, orally bioavailable agent that is designed to increase the time for which activated CFTR channels at the cell's surface remain open. Thus the drug is called a potentiator. Specifically, ivacaftor has been shown to augment the chloride transport activity of 551D-CFTR protein. It should be noted that just 4% to 5% of patients with cystic fibrosis have the G551D mutation on at least 1 allele. More than 90% of patients with cystic fibrosis in the United States have the most common mutant form of CFTR, delta F508-CFTR. In vitro, ivacaftor stimulates activity in delta F508-CFTR, but to a much lesser extent than it does in G551D. It is not clear whether such a level of stimulation is sufficient to produce any clinical benefit in patients with this most common form of mutation.

While there is not yet a magic bullet to deal with cystic fibrosis in most patients, the findings of Ramsey et al document a remarkable degree of improvement in affected patients with one of the lesser genetic forms of the disorder. Daily administration of oral ivacaftor for almost a year was not associated with greater safety risks than were observed with placebo. Side effects were minimal. Thus, the findings from this report represent an important milestone in the development of treatments designed to improve CFTR protein function as a means of addressing the underlying cause of cystic fibrosis and, as the authors of this report note, begin to fulfill the promise ushered in with the discovery of the CFTR gene more than 20 years ago.

**J. A. Stockman III, MD**

---

### Increasing Severity of Pectus Excavatum is Associated with Reduced Pulmonary Function

Lawson ML, Mellins RB, Paulson JF, et al (Kennesaw State Univ, GA; Morgan Stanley Children's Hosp of New York-Presbyterian at Columbia Univ Med Ctr; Eastern Virginia Med School, Norfolk, VA; et al)
*J Pediatr* 159:256-261, 2011

---

*Objective.*—To determine whether pulmonary function decreases as a function of severity of pectus excavatum, and whether reduced function is restrictive or obstructive in nature in a large multicenter study.

*Study Design.*—We evaluated preoperative spirometry data in 310 patients and lung volumes in 218 patients aged 6 to 21 years at 11 North American centers. We modeled the impact of the severity of deformity (based on the Haller index) on pulmonary function.

*Results.*—The percentages of patients with abnormal forced vital capacity (FVC), forced expiratory volume in 1 second ($FEV_1$), forced expiratory flow from 25% exhalation to 75% exhalation, and total lung capacity findings increased with increasing Haller index score. Less than 2% of patients demonstrated an obstructive pattern ($FEV_1/FVC$ <67%), and 14.5% demonstrated a restrictive pattern (FVC and $FEV_1$ <80% predicted; $FEV_1/FVC$ >80%). Patients with a Haller index of 7 are >4 times more likely to have an FVC of ≤80% than those with a Haller index of 4, and are also 4 times more likely to exhibit a restrictive pulmonary pattern.

*Conclusions.*—Among patients presenting for surgical repair of pectus excavatum, those with more severe deformities have a much higher likelihood of decreased pulmonary function with a restrictive pulmonary pattern.

▶ Most patients with pectus excavatum will have some minor loss of pulmonary function. This is usually in the range of 80% to 85% of normal average values for the overall population. Such minimal depressions and pulmonary function do not cause symptoms at rest but could at varying levels of significant exercise. To date, no studies have calculated the projected decrease in pulmonary function with the actual depth of chest wall depression in those with pectus excavatum. Lawson et al examined lung function in a large multicenter study, hypothesizing that the severity of chest wall depression could be used to accurately predict the amount of decreased pulmonary function that one would expect in affected individuals.

The investigation of Lawson et al involved 326 patients across 11 North American pediatric medical centers. A full battery of pulmonary function tests was performed. The magnitude of the pectus deformity was determined calculating a Haller index. One needs a computed tomography scan to do this. The index is calculated as the inner transverse thoracic diameter divided by the anterior posterior distance between the anterior thoracic wall and the spine at the narrowest point. The study did show that there was a strong correlation between the depth of chest wall depression and alterations in pulmonary function. Also, the effect on pulmonary function is primarily lung restriction, not airway obstruction. The correlation between the Haller index and the degree of pulmonary dysfunction was not absolute.

For more than 60 years, medical reports have consistently referred to symptomatic complaints related to pectus excavatum. Symptoms have included limited exercise ability, easy fatigability, and a subjective sense of inability to breathe easily. This report provides evidence that pulmonary function is related to the depth of the depression in a causal way and may explain why repairing the defect can result in improved pulmonary function and better exercise tolerance. The study does not assess the additional possibility that impaired right ventricular function from external pressure of the deformed chest wall could interfere with cardiac output and cardiopulmonary function. This study provides no specific indications for surgical correction of pectus excavatum. This remains a clinical decision. Altered pulmonary function is just one of several factors to be considered.

This commentary closes with an observation regarding Vicks VapoRub. Just how safe is this product for use in children? Most of us know that Vicks VapoRub (Proctor & Gamble, Cincinnati, Ohio) is frequently used to relieve symptoms of cold and congestion. Its active ingredients are camphor (4.8%), menthol (2.7%), and eucalyptus oil (91.2%). These aromatics provide the sensation of increased nasal air flow, but in fact studies have documented no improvement in airflow or decrease in nasal resistance with the use of Vicks VapoRub. It is not recommended for direct application in the nostril and is not recommended for children younger than 2 years of age, although this advice is not infrequently ignored by parents or in fact may not be known by parents to be a potential issue. Recently, an 18-month-old previously healthy girl was brought to an emergency room in significant respiratory distress. She had had a relatively minor upper respiratory tract infection as she had been in the care of her grandparents, who spontaneously stated that Vicks VapoRub had been placed under the child's nostrils, following which the respiratory distress rapidly evolved over the course of half an hour. The child had developed severe wheezing and intercostal retractions. Her initial pulse oximetry saturation was just 66% in room air. She had to be admitted to the hospital and was treated with high-dose steroids and bronchodilators, which improved her oxygen saturations, and she eventually recovered.

The physicians caring for this youngster decided to do an experiment using ferrets, exposing ferrets to Vicks VapoRub. Ferrets have an airway anatomy and cellular composition that is similar to humans and other carnivores and have been used in the past to study airway inflammation and mucus secretion.[1] The ferrets were exposed to Vicks VapoRub and clearly showed increases in mucin secretion as well as lung inflammation in the pulmonary airways. It is obvious that Vicks VapoRub, at least in tiny folks, can possibly make you feel better before it is capable of doing you in.

By way of background, Lunsford Richardson II and John Farris first compounded Vicks VapoRub in 1891 in Greensboro, North Carolina, soon after buying the local W.C. Porter Drug Store. They introduced this product onto the market in 1905 with the name Vicks Magic Croup Salve. The flu epidemic of 1918 was a boon to Vicks VapoRub with sales rising from $900 000 to $2.9 million in just 12 months. Proctor & Gamble has since marketed Vicks VapoRub as "the only thing more powerful than a mother's touch." It is thought that Vicks VapoRub works by the menthol in it activating trigeminal cold receptors, which through a series of reactions causes the brain to recognize what is going on as a cooling sensation and perceives it to be due to increased airflow across the nostrils despite an actual decrease in air flow. In the human nasal cavity, menthol actually increases nasal resistance within one minute and the increased resistance can persist for several hours.

Needless to say, it is not nice of Vicks VapoRub to fool Mother Nature, nor the human brain, into perceiving something that is not there.

**J. A. Stockman III, MD**

*Reference*

1. Abanses JC, Arima S, Rubin BK. Vicks VapoRub induces mucin secretion, decreases ciliary beat frequency, and increases tracheal mucus transport in the ferret trachea. *Chest.* 2009;135:143-148.

# 19 Therapeutics and Toxicology

**Antibiotic Prescribing in Ambulatory Pediatrics in the United States**
Hersh AL, Shapiro DJ, Pavia AT, et al (Univ of Utah, Salt Lake City; Univ of California, San Francisco; et al)
*Pediatrics* 128:1053-1061, 2011

*Background.*—Antibiotics are commonly prescribed for children with conditions for which they provide no benefit, including viral respiratory infections. Broad-spectrum antibiotic use is increasing, which adds unnecessary cost and promotes the development of antibiotic resistance.

*Objective.*—To provide a nationally representative analysis of antibiotic prescribing in ambulatory pediatrics according to antibiotic classes and diagnostic categories and identify factors associated with broad-spectrum antibiotic prescribing.

*Patients and Methods.*—We used the National Ambulatory and National Hospital Ambulatory Medical Care surveys from 2006 to 2008, which are nationally representative samples of ambulatory care visits in the United States. We estimated the percentage of visits for patients younger than 18 years for whom antibiotics were prescribed according to antibiotic classes, those considered broad-spectrum, and diagnostic categories. We used multivariable logistic regression to identify demographic and clinical factors that were independently associated with broad-spectrum antibiotic prescribing.

*Results.*—Antibiotics were prescribed during 21% of pediatric ambulatory visits; 50% were broad-spectrum, most commonly macrolides. Respiratory conditions accounted for >70% of visits in which both antibiotics and broad-spectrum antibiotics were prescribed. Twenty-three percent of the visits in which antibiotics were prescribed were for respiratory conditions for which antibiotics are not clearly indicated, which accounts for >10 million visits annually. Factors independently associated with broad-spectrum antibiotic prescribing included respiratory conditions for which antibiotics are not indicated, younger patients, visits in the South, and private insurance.

*Conclusions.*—Broad-spectrum antibiotic prescribing in ambulatory pediatrics is extremely common and frequently inappropriate. These findings can inform the development and implementation of antibiotic stewardship efforts in ambulatory care toward the most important geographic regions, diagnostic conditions, and patient populations (Table 1).

▶ It is hard to deny that misuse of antibiotics is a major problem in the US pediatric care. Studies have shown that more than 150 million ambulatory visits annually result in an antibiotic prescription, including more than 30 million prescriptions dispensed for children.[1] The Centers for Disease Control and Prevention (CDC) initiated major efforts in the 1990s to raise awareness about inappropriate antibiotic prescribing. The CDC's initiatives seem to have had some traction because the overall rate of antibiotic prescribing in ambulatory settings has been declining. When one looks carefully, however, at specific types of antibiotics, the prescribing of broad-spectrum agents, particularly macrolides, has increased substantially during the last decade. This antibiotic overuse drives up cost and the numbers of adverse events and influences the development of antibiotic-resistant infections.

Hersh et al have looked at the problem of antibiotic overprescribing, addressing 2 objectives. The authors sought to describe the overall use of antibiotics in ambulatory pediatric settings according to antibiotic classes with a particular focus on estimating the tendency for physicians to prescribe antibiotics for certain diagnoses. They also sought to identify factors associated with broad-spectrum antibiotic prescribing during ambulatory care visits.

The authors analyzed data from the National Ambulatory Medical Care Survey and the National Hospital Ambulatory Medical Care Survey between the periods 2006 and 2009. Between 2006 and 2008, the investigators documented that antibiotics were prescribed in an estimated 49 million ambulatory pediatric visits annually, which represents 21% of all ambulatory visits for children. To say this differently, 1 visit out of 5 will result in an antibiotic being prescribed in a pediatrician's office. Half of the time these antibiotics will be broad-spectrum

TABLE 1.—Antibiotic-Prescribing Patterns Across Diagnostic Conditions

| Condition | Across-Condition Contribution to Antibiotic Prescribing, % |
|---|---|
| Respiratory | 72.3 |
| ARTIs for which antibiotics are indicated | 48.9 |
| ARTIs for which antibiotics are not indicated | 13.1 |
| Other respiratory conditions for which antibiotics are not definitely indicated | 10.3 |
| Other | 27.7 |
| Skin/cutaneous/mucosal | 11.9 |
| Urinary tract infections[a] | 2.0 |
| Gastrointestinal infections | 0.3 |
| Miscellaneous infections | 1.9 |
| Other | 11.6 |
| Total | 100[a] |

Data indicate the percentage that each condition contributed to overall antibiotic prescribing on the basis of an estimated total of 43.9 million visits in which antibiotics were prescribed. This total does not include 2036 sampled visits excluded in which a concomitant infection appeared as a secondary or tertiary diagnosis. See Appendix for ICD-9-CM codes specified by each condition.
[a]Excludes nitrofurantoin.

antibiotics. The most commonly prescribed antibiotic classes include narrow-spectrum penicillins (38% of visits in which antibiotics were prescribed) and macrolides (20%). Quinolones, tetracyclines, lincomycin derivatives, and sulfon-amides were prescribed relatively infrequently, together accounting for less than 11% of visits in which antibiotics were prescribed. Macrolides clearly were the most commonly prescribed broad-spectrum antibiotics. Of the various conditions for which antibiotic prescribing was initiated, more than 70% were related to respiratory disorders. An antibiotic was prescribed during 48.4% of visits in which a respiratory condition was the primary diagnosis. Twenty-three percent of the visits in which antibiotics were prescribed were for respiratory conditions for which antibiotics are clearly not indicated. Table 1 shows the pattern of anti-biotic prescribing by diagnostic classification.

The conclusion of this report is fairly obvious. The overuse of broad-spectrum antibiotics remains quite problematic because many of these agents are prescribed unnecessarily, have high cost, and do in fact promote bacterial resis-tance. Antibiotic stewardship programs have been shown to be effective in inter ventions for improving antibiotic prescribing patterns in hospital settings (see the report that follows) including reducing overall use of broad-spectrum antibiotics. Unfortunately, there is no such equivalent stewardship program for office-based practice, and the "big brotherism" that could be associated with such ambulatory monitoring would likely to be found to be unacceptable. What we need is a quality improvement program to promote a reduction in antibiotic use that most, if not all pediatricians, could participate in on a voluntary basis.

This commentary ends with a query. Just how safe is it to use a spoon as a dosing instrument for liquid medicines? The answer is that the spoon has been identified as a major cause of dosing error in pediatric poisonings.[2] Indeed, the US Food and Drug administration recommends against using kitchen uten-sils to dose liquid medicines. Despite this, most individuals still use spoons when pouring medicine for themselves and their families. These dosing errors remain relatively minor when using kitchen teaspoons, but they increase fairly signifi-cantly when using various sizes of larger spoons. If the size of a spoon leads to suspect that it holds more or less than 5 ml (a true teaspoon), a person may compensate by over- or underdosing. In fact, investigators have examined this phenomenon during the flu season of 2009 by asking 195 university students to dose 5 ml of cold medicine into a teaspoon (5 ml, 2.7 × 4 cm), a medium-size tablespoon (15 ml, 4 × 6 cm), and a larger spoon (45 ml, 6 × 9 cm). Partic-ipants were asked to pour exactly one teaspoon (5 ml); next they were asked to pour the same 5-ml dose into each of the remaining two spoons in a randomized order. After each of these two pours, the participants were asked to indicate how confident they were that they had poured 5 ml. The investigators then measured the actual volume of the medicine poured. It was observe that although the capacity of the spoons was never a constraint, participants dosed 8.4% less than prescribed into the medium-sized spoon and 11.6% more into the larger spoon. Participants stated an above-average confidence that their pouring tech-nique was accurate, when indeed it was not. Needless to say that whereas the clinical implications of an underdosing of 8% or an overdosing of 12% would likely be minimal, the dosing error, if compounded with multiple dosings over a day or several days, could be quite significant. To read more about this, see the report of Wansink and van Ittersum.[3]

On a similar theme, here is a tidbit for you. Although one would expect more experienced pourers to be more accurate with the volumes they dispense, this is not always necessarily so. It has been shown that confident veteran bartenders pour 28% more liquor into short, wide glasses than into tall slender glasses of the same volume.[4] A "proud" bartender would never use a shot glass to do the measuring, right?

**J. A. Stockman III, MD**

*References*

1. McCaig LF, Besser RE, Hughes JM. Trends in antimicrobial prescribing rates for children and adolescents. *JAMA*. 2002;287:3096-3102.
2. Litovits T. Implications of dispensing cups in dosing errors and pediatric poisonings: a report from the Association of Poison Control Centers. *Ann Pharmacother*. 1992; 26:917-918.
3. Wansink B, van Ittersum K. Spoons systematically biased dosing of liquid medicine. *Ann Intern Med*. 2010;152:66-67.
4. Wansink B, van Ittersum K. Shape of glass and amount of alcohol poured. Comparative study of effective practice and concentration. *BMJ*. 2005;331:152-154.

### Benefits of a Pediatric Antimicrobial Stewardship Program at a Children's Hospital

Di Pentima MC, Chan S, Hossain J (Vanderbilt Univ, Nashville, TN; Alfred I. duPont Hosp for Children, Wilmington, DE; Nemours Biomedical Res, Wilmington, DE)
*Pediatrics* 128:1062-1070, 2011

*Objective.*—To prospectively evaluate the effect of a comprehensive antimicrobial stewardship program on antimicrobial use, physician interventions, patient outcomes, and rates of antimicrobial resistance.

*Methods.*—Active surveillance of antimicrobial use with intervention and real-time feedback to providers and reinforcement of prior authorization for selected antimicrobials were introduced at a pediatric teaching hospital. Antimicrobial-use indications were incorporated as a mandatory field in the computerized information system. An automated report of antimicrobials prescribed, doses, patient demographics, and microbiology data was generated and reviewed by an infectious-disease pharmacist and a pediatric infectious-disease physician. Antimicrobial use, expressed as the number of doses administered per 1000 patient-days, was measured 3 years before and after the implementation of the program.

*Results.*—Total antimicrobial use peaked at 3089 doses administered per 1000 patient-days per year in 2003–2004 before implementation of the program and steadily decreased to 1904 doses administered per 1000 patient-days per year during the postintervention period. Targeted-antimicrobial use declined from 1250 to 988 doses administered per 1000 patient-days per year. Nontargeted-antimicrobial use declined from

1839 to 916 doses administered per 1000 patient-days per year. Rates of antimicrobial resistance to broad-spectrum antimicrobials among the most common Gram-negative bacilli remained low and stable over time.

*Conclusions.*—The successful implementation of antimicrobial stewardship strategies had a significant impact on reducing targeted- and nontargeted-antimicrobial use, improving quality of care of hospitalized children and preventing emergence of resistance.

▶ This article by Di Pentima et al. deals with antibiotic oversubscribing in the office setting, hospital antibiotic prescribing, and the role of antimicrobial stewardship programs within children's hospitals. Antimicrobial stewardship programs were introduced in the 1980s and have been pivotal in reducing unnecessary antibiotic use. Five years ago, the Infectious Disease Society of America, in collaboration with other professional organizations, released guidelines to assist in the implementation of multidisciplinary antimicrobial stewardship programs. Although many institutions have picked up on these practices, few children's hospitals have actually implemented comprehensive stewardship programs in comparison with their adult institution counterparts. Complete data about the extent of antimicrobial use in pediatric hospitals before and after the introduction of such programs have been sparse, thus the value of this report evaluating the effects of such programs on antibiotic use, physician intervention, patient outcomes, and rates of antimicrobial resistance. This report is the first publication that thoroughly describes the impact of antibiotic stewardship programs in a children's hospital.

This report emanates from the Alfred I. duPont Hospital for Children, which approved the implementation of an inpatient stewardship program beginning in 2004. The stewardship program team included a full-time doctoral-level clinical pharmacist with postdoctoral training in infectious diseases and a physician director who was a board-certified pediatric infectious disease practitioner. The antibiotic stewardship program used 2 strategies: prospective audit with intervention and feedback to all prescribers and enforcement of prior authorization for selected antimicrobials. A figure shows the trends of antimicrobial use 3 years before and 3 years after institution of the stewardship program. Total antimicrobial use peaked in 2003 to 2004 and decreased steadily over the next 3 years. Total antimicrobial use decreased by 38% despite a 7% increase in the acuity of patient care. Furthermore, targeted antimicrobials that required prior authorization (36%) had a more significant decline when compared with nonrestricted antimicrobials. Over time, the rates of noncompliance with antimicrobial stewardship recommendations decreased by more than 50%. A 92% rate of compliance with antimicrobial recommendations was higher than rates previously reported by other investigators.

While it is true that this study was reported out of a single children's hospital (the Nemours Children's Hospital in Wilmington, Delaware), it is likely that similar success could be seen in any other children's hospital that does not have such a program already underway. The successful experience at the Nemours Children's Hospital should encourage other pediatric centers to pursue similar programs.

**J. A. Stockman III, MD**

**566** / Pediatrics

### The Growing Impact of Pediatric Pharmaceutical Poisoning
Bond GR, Woodward RW, Ho M (Cincinnati Children's Hosp Med Ctr, OH)
*J Pediatr* 160:265-270, 2012

*Objective.*—To understand which medications, under which circumstances, are responsible for the noted increase in pediatric medication poisonings, resource use, and morbidity.

*Study Design.*—Patient records from 2001-2008 were obtained from the National Poison Data System of the American Association of Poison Control Centers for children aged ≤5 years evaluated in a health care facility following exposure to a potentially toxic dose of a pharmaceutical agent. Pharmaceutical agents were classified as over-the-counter or prescription and by functional category. Exposures were classified as child self-ingested the medication or as therapeutic error. For the 8-year period, emergency visits, admissions, significant injuries, and trends in these events were calculated for each substance category.

*Results.*—We evaluated 453 559 children for ingestion of a single pharmaceutical product. Child self-exposure was responsible for 95% of visits. Child self-exposure to prescription products dominated the health care impact with 248 023 of the visits (55%), 41 847 admissions (76%), and 18 191 significant injuries (71%). The greatest resource use and morbidity followed self-ingestion of prescription products, particularly opioids, sedative-hypnotics, and cardiovascular agents.

*Conclusions.*—Prevention efforts have proved to be inadequate in the face of rising availability of prescription medications, particularly more dangerous medications (Fig 2).

▶ I was not aware that emergency department visits by young children for medication poisonings now exceed those for motor vehicle occupant injuries. This is despite tamper-proof medicine bottles and a widespread awareness of the problem of medication poisonings in youngsters. Bond et al undertook

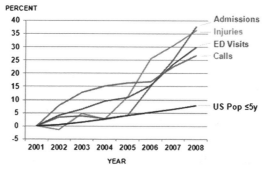

FIGURE 2.—Pediatric poisoning trends vs population change from 2001 baseline. Visual display shows actual values, see text for linear trend changes. US population data are from http://webappa.cdc.gov/sasweb/ncipc/nfirates2001.html; all other data relate to poisoning data from NPDS as defined in text. (Reprinted from Journal of Pediatrics, Bond GR, Woodward RW, Ho M. The growing impact of pediatric pharmaceutical poisoning. *J Pediatr.* 2012;160:265-270. Copyright 2012 with permission from Elsevier.)

a study to explore all electronic medical records related to the National Poison Data System, the electronic database of all calls to member poison centers of the American Association of Poison Control Centers. These centers provide service to every citizen of the United States. Data from every poison control center call are recorded electronically, in real time, and in a standardized format. Bond et al examined the records of children 5 years and younger whose call type was unintentional exposure to a pharmaceutical agent that involved presenting to a health care facility during the period 2001 to 2008. Combination agents such as antihistamines/decongestant cough and cold products were considered a single product in the analysis of the data.

In this series, more than half a million children 5 years of age or younger were exposed to pharmaceuticals over an 8-year period. Child self-exposure to prescription products represented the largest category of ingestions with more than half of the poisonings falling into this category as well as 76% of admissions. Fig 2 shows the overall trend from baseline for exposures with very significant increases in such exposures during the 8-year period, despite a relatively modest increase in the US population of youngsters 5 years and under.

The data from this report are alarming and show that the greatest increase in medication exposure resulting in emergency department visits is from prescription pharmaceuticals, particularly opioid analgesics, sedative hypnotics (benzodiazepines, muscle relaxants, and sleep aids) and cardiovascular medications. Therapeutic errors by parents at home represented a relatively small component of the problem and did not seem to increase over time. These data indicate that "poison-proofing" efforts, while important, are insufficient strategies to deal with the magnitude of the problem observed.

The most likely explanation for the observations found in this report is the increase in the number of medications in the environment of small children. In a recent survey, 50% of adults are now taking at least 1 prescription medication, and 7% of adults are taking 5 or more medications at any one time.[1] The 24% increase in the number of visits following self-ingestion is best explained by more medication being available in the home or by less-effective home prevention. It is possible that some types of medication previously less available in the environment of young children have become more available. As obesity and the metabolic syndrome have increased in prevalence and have affected younger adults, more homes of small children may have antihypertensive and antidiabetic medicines prescribed for parents or siblings. Teen and preteen prescriptions for attention-deficit/hyperactivity disorder have increased as well.

The only conclusion one can reach is that the problem of pediatric medication poisoning is getting worse, not better, and existing preventive efforts have proven to be inadequate. Educational efforts are important but are unlikely to make a significant improvement by themselves. We must readdress home storage of all medications and repackaging of medications (particularly grandparents' medications and "pill minders"). Storage devices and child-resistant closures need to improve even more. Blister packs should be used for more drugs.

This commentary closes with a remark about medications and their use by those who are colorblind. For most of us, color is one good way we often use to differentiate certain medications from one another. In fact, as one ages and vision may decline, color may be the major differentiator as opposed to the difficulties some have in reading print on labels. Unfortunately, 8% of men and 0.4% of women have impaired color vision, of whom half are unable to recognize the main colors used in color coding. In a survey of 100 people with impaired color vision, 2% reported that they had confused their medication because they had mistaken the color of tablets. A pink-colored tablet appears blue to a color-blind individual and a green tablet appears gray. It is thought that doctors and pharmacists should only use color to instruct patients on how to identify tablets if they know that patient has normal color vision. People with red-green color deficiency can recognize yellow, blue, gray, and white. Perhaps manufacturers should incorporate this information into guidelines about the use of color for tablet identification.[2]

**J. A. Stockman III, MD**

*Reference*

1. Kaufman DW, Kelly JP, Rosenberg L, Anderson TE, Mitchell AA. Recent patterns of medication use in the ambulatory adult population of the United States: the Slone survey. *JAMA.* 2002;287:337-344.
2. Cole BL, Harris RW. Caution: colored medication and the colorblind. *Lancet.* 2009;374:720.

---

**Impact of CYP2C19 variant genotypes on clinical efficacy of antiplatelet treatment with clopidogrel: systematic review and meta-analysis**
Bauer T, Bouman HJ, van Werkum JW, et al (Univ Hosp of Cologne, Germany; Univ Maastricht, Netherlands; et al)
*BMJ* 343:d4588, 2011

---

*Objective.*—To evaluate the accumulated information from genetic association studies investigating the impact of variants of the cytochrome P450 (CYP) 2C19 genotype on the clinical efficacy of clopidogrel.

*Design.*—Systematic review and meta-analysis with a structured search algorithm and prespecified eligibility criteria for retrieval of relevant studies; dominant genetic model assumptions and quantitative methods for calculating summary effect estimates from study level odds ratios; systematic assessment of bias within and between studies; and grading of the cumulative evidence by consensus criteria.

*Data sources.*—Medline, Embase, the Cochrane Library, online databases, contents pages and bibliographies of general medical, cardiovascular, pharmacological, and genetic journals.

*Eligibility Criteria for Selecting Studies.*—Original full length reports assessing the cumulative incidence of major adverse cardiovascular events or stent thrombosis over a follow-up period of at least a month in association with carrier status for the loss of function or gain of function CYP2C19 allele in adult patients with coronary artery disease and a clinical presentation of acute coronary syndrome or stable angina pectoris who were taking clopidogrel.

*Results.*—15 studies met the inclusion criteria. The random effects summary odds ratio for stent thrombosis in carriers of at least one CYP2C19 loss of function allele versus non-carriers combining nine studies was 1.77 (95% confidence interval 1.31 to 2.40; $P < 0.001$). This nominally significant odds ratio was subject to considerable bias across the studies (small study effect bias and replication diversity). The adjustment for these quality modifiers tended to abolish the association. The corresponding random effects summary odds ratio of major adverse cardiovascular events for 12 studies combined was 1.11 (0.89 to 1.39; $P = 0.36$). The random effects summary odds ratio of stent thrombosis in carriers versus non-carriers of at least one CYP2C19*17 gain of function allele for three studies combined was 0.99 (0.60 to 1.62; $P = 0.96$), and the corresponding odds ratio of major adverse cardiovascular events in five studies was 0.93 (0.75 to 1.14; $P = 0.48$). The overall quality of epidemiological evidence was graded as low, which excludes reliable clinical assessments.

*Conclusions.*—Accumulated information from genetic association studies does not indicate a substantial or consistent influence of CYP2C19 gene polymorphisms on the clinical efficacy of clopidogrel. The current evidence does not support the use of individualised antiplatelet regimens guided by CYP2C19 genotype.

▶ Clopidogrel is an antiplatelet agent used as an antithrombotic agent in both children and adults. Although much more commonly prescribed in adults to prevent atherothrombotic events, it is occasionally used in children when it is desirable to inhibit platelet adhesion to vascular endothelium, such as when there are prosthetic materials that have been placed within the vasculature. Also, patients with abnormal heart valves commonly are prescribed antiplatelet agents to prevent clots from forming. This report by Bauer et al is included mainly to show how far along we have come in integrating information from the human genome project into clinical practice.

Variation in the human genome has long been considered to contribute to individual differences in disease susceptibility and drug response. Bauer and colleagues report on a systematic review and meta-analysis of studies examining the association of variation in the CYP2C19 and atherothrombotic events during treatment with clopidogrel. The sequence of the human genome is now known, as are the positions of several million nucleotides that differ most commonly from one person to the next. Laboratory techniques currently permit rapid, cost-effective genotyping of single nucleotide polymorphisms in the genomes of many thousands of people to gain insight into gene regions that influence disease-related biomarkers, susceptibility to common diseases, and the response to widely prescribed drugs. By the end of 2011, nearly 1000 such genome-wide association studies had reported findings. These studies have yielded valuable early insights into disease pathogenesis that will yield future dividends in the form of new treatment. Unfortunately, the genetic variants that have been studied so far have too weak an effect to be predictive of certain outcomes. What one would like for each person is a personalized medical profile that can influence decisions regarding disease status and the treatment.

In their systematic review and meta-analysis, Bauer et al evaluated the strength of evidence on the association between the variation in the CYP2C19 gene and atherothrombotic events during treatment with clopidogrel. Clopidogrel, a widely prescribed, now off-patent, antiplatelet agent (originally licensed at Plavix), requires metabolism for its activation. Several hepatic cytochrome enzymes contribute to this activation, including CYP2C19. There is an emerging view that people who carry reduced activity CYP2C19 are less well protected from cardiovascular events during clopidogrel treatment and that a genotype-based test could help inform decisions on the dose of this drug necessary to prevent thrombosis and whether to opt for newer and more expensive antiplatelet agents such as prasugrel or ticagrelor, both drugs that are on patent and are less dependent on metabolism for their activation.

Bauer et al answered the question of whether variants of the cytochrome P450 (CYP) 2C19 genotype influence the clinical efficiency of clopidogrel. Their careful analysis of the literature does not support a substantial or consistent influence of the CYP2C19 gene polymorphisms on the incidence of major adverse cardiovascular events. The problems identified by Bauer et al may not be unique to the CYP2C19 genotyping and clopidogrel response. All of us need to be careful about gene-disease associations, cancer biomarker studies, and genetic tests as predictors of disease and of indicators of variation in drug metabolism. This is not to say that these associations may not be present, just that they need to be very carefully understood. Currently, the Food and Drug Administration has issued a boxed warning on clopidogrel that tells clinicians about reduced effectiveness in patients who are poor metabolizers of Plavix and that tests are available to identify gene differences that could help inform clinicians. It is entirely possible that this boxed warning itself is not entirely accurate.

In the next few years, we will be learning a great deal more about the interactions between various genotypes and drugs. It's personalized medicine. Stay tuned.

This commentary closes with a quiz. See what you would do with the following case scenario: A young adult male presents to the emergency room after awakening from a nap. He has numbness around his mouth, tingling in his hands, and slight dyspnea. This is in Juneau, Alaska. At the same time you are seeing this patient, 2 of his friends arrive in the emergency room. Both have similar symptoms to the first patient. One is severely ill, requiring intubation. All 3 individuals shared a meal of boiled, noncommercially harvested mussels. Your diagnosis? If you diagnosis paralytic shellfish poisoning, you would have been absolutely correct. Recently reported from the Centers for Disease Control and Prevention were a series of patients, all from southeast Alaska, with paralytic shellfish poisoning. The signs and symptoms in these patients ranged from mild, short-lived paresthesias of the mouth or extremities to severe, life-threatening paralysis. Paralytic shellfish poisoning results from ingestion of saxitoxins, toxins produced by marine dinoflagellate algae that accumulate in bivalve mollusks such as clams, cockles, and mussels. It should be noted that in 2011, 21 cases of paralytic shellfish poisoning were identified in southeast Alaska during the months of May and June.[1] These numbers represent a considerable increase in the numbers normally expected. All care providers should be aware of this problem, which is not restricted to the shore-lines of Alaska.

**J. A. Stockman III, MD**

*Reference*

1. Centers for Disease Control and Prevention (CDC). Paralytic shellfish poison-ing—Southeast Alaska, May—June 2011. *MMWR Morb Mortal Wkly Rep.* 2011;60:1554-1556.

## ADHD Drugs and Serious Cardiovascular Events in Children and Young Adults

Cooper WO, Habel LA, Sox CM, et al (Vanderbilt University, Nashville, TN; Kaiser Permanente Northern California, Oakland, CA; Boston Univ School of Medicine, MA; et al)
*N Engl J Med* 365:1896-1904, 2011

*Background.*—Adverse-event reports from North America have raised concern that the use of drugs for attention deficit—hyperactivity disorder (ADHD) increases the risk of serious cardiovascular events.

*Methods.*—We conducted a retrospective cohort study with automated data from four health plans (Tennessee Medicaid, Washington State Medicaid, Kaiser Permanente California, and OptumInsight Epidemiology), with 1,200,438 children and young adults between the ages of 2 and 24 years and 2,579,104 person-years of follow-up, including 373,667 person-years of current use of ADHD drugs. We identified serious cardiovascular events (sudden cardiac death, acute myocardial infarction, and stroke) from health-plan data and vital records, with end points validated by medical-record review. We estimated the relative risk of end points among current users, as compared with nonusers, with hazard ratios from Cox regression models.

*Results.*—Cohort members had 81 serious cardiovascular events (3.1 per 100,000 person-years). Current users of ADHD drugs were not at increased risk for serious cardiovascular events (adjusted hazard ratio, 0.75; 95% confidence interval [CI], 0.31 to 1.85). Risk was not increased for any of the individual end points, or for current users as compared with former users (adjusted hazard ratio, 0.70; 95% CI, 0.29 to 1.72). Alterna-tive analyses addressing several study assumptions also showed no signif-icant association between the use of an ADHD drug and the risk of a study end point.

*Conclusions.*—This large study showed no evidence that current use of an ADHD drug was associated with an increased risk of serious cardiovas-cular events, although the upper limit of the 95% confidence interval indi-cated that a doubling of the risk could not be ruled out. However, the absolute magnitude of such an increased risk would be low. (Funded by the Agency for Healthcare Research and Quality and the Food and Drug Administration.)

▶ Reports of adverse events from Canada and the United States that have included cases of sudden death, myocardial infarction, and stroke in conjunction with the use of drugs used to manage attention-deficit/hyperactivity disorder (ADHD) have raised concern about the safety of these drugs. The lay press has written much about this in the past couple of years. ADHD medications, such as amphetamines, atomoxetine, and methylphenidate, are taken by as many as 3 million youngsters aged 4 to 17 years in the United States. In addition to the afore-mentioned risk, these drugs do cause a slight increase in systolic and diastolic blood pressures (on average, 1-4 mm Hg) and heart rate (on average, 3-8 beats per minute). Public awareness about their use and the ubiquity with which they are dispensed have raised concerns about their safety. This is why the report of Cooper et al is so important because earlier studies of the relationship between cardiovascular events and the use of ADHD drugs have been largely inconclusive.

Cooper et al have used data from 4 large geographically and demographically diverse US health care plans to conduct a retrospective cohort study of the use of ADHD drugs and the risk of serious cardiovascular events in children and young adults. The investigators obtained data from computerized health records of 4 health plans that together annually covered 22.4 million people during this study period. These plans included Tennessee Medicaid, Washington State Medicaid, Kaiser Permanente California (Northern and Southern Regions), and OptumInsight Epidemiology (National Private Insurance Health-Plan data). The study examined the use of ADHD management drugs (dexmethylphenidate, dextroamphetamines, and amphetamine salts, atomoxetine, or pemoline). Patient data included those as young as 2 years to those aged up to 24 years. The primary end point of the study was a serious cardiovascular event defined as sudden cardiac death, myocardial infarction, or stroke. Sudden cardiac death was defined as a sudden, pulseless condition or collapse consistent with a ventricular tachy-arrhythmia occurring in a community setting and including both fatal and resus-citated cardiac arrest. The study cohort included 1 200 438 children and young adults. The mean age of those included in this report was 11.1 years. The mean length at follow-up for this cohort was 2.1 years.

Data from this report showed that a total of 81 cohort members had a serious cardiovascular event for a rate of 3.1 per 100 000 person-years. This included 31 sudden cardiac deaths, 9 acute myocardial infarctions, and 39 strokes. As compared with nonusers, the adjusted rate of serious cardiovascular events did not differ significantly among current users of ADHD drugs (hazard ratio, 0.75). Even if former ADHD medication users were included among those with cardio-vascular events, there was still no statistical association with drug use. The study by Cooper et al concluded that in their study involving children and young adults with 2.5 million person-years of follow-up, there were just 3.1 serious cardiovas-cular events per 100 000 person-years and that the absolute magnitude of any increased risk must be low. The data from this report are perfectly in line with those that appeared a few months later that were published in *Pediatrics*. Schelle-man et al[1] also performed a large cohort study using data from 2 administrative databases that included 241 417 children aged 3 to 17 years. These investigators found no statistically significant difference between ADHD medication users and nonusers with respect to sudden death or ventricular arrhythmias. The same was true of myocardial infarctions and stroke. The conclusion also was that the rate of cardiovascular events in exposed children must be very low.

**J. A. Stockman III, MD**

*Reference*

1. Schelleman H, Bilker WB, Strom BL, et al. Cardiovascular events and death in children exposed and unexposed to ADHD agents. *Pediatrics.* 2011;127:1102-1110.

---

**Ciprofloxacin safety in paediatrics: a systematic review**
Adefurin A, Sammons H, Jacqz-Aigrain E, et al (Derbyshire Children's Hosp, Derby, UK; Hôpital Robert Debré, Paris, France)
*Arch Dis Child* 96:874-880, 2011

---

*Objective.*—To determine the safety of ciprofloxacin in paediatric patients in relation to arthropathy, any other adverse events (AEs) and drug interactions.

*Methods.*—A systematic search of MEDLINE, EMBASE, CINAHL, CENTRAL and bibliographies of relevant articles was carried out for all published articles, regardless of design, that involved the use of ciprofloxacin in any paediatric age group ≤17 years. Only articles that reported on safety were included.

*Results.*—105 articles met the inclusion criteria and involved 16 184 paediatric patients. There were 1065 reported AEs (risk 7%, 95% CI 3.2% to 14.0%). The most frequent AEs were musculoskeletal AEs, abnormal liver function tests, nausea, changes in white blood cell counts and vomiting. There were six drug interactions (with aminophylline (4) and methotrexate (2)). The only drug related death occurred in a neonate who had an anaphylactic reaction. 258 musculoskeletal events occurred in 232 paediatric patients (risk 1.6%, 95% CI 0.9% to 2.6%). Arthralgia accounted for 50% of these. The age of occurrence of arthropathy ranged from 7 months to 17 years (median 10 years). All cases of arthropathy resolved or improved with management. One prospective controlled study estimated the risk of arthropathy as 9.3 (OR 95% CI 1.2 to 195). Pooled safety data of controlled trials in this review estimated the risk of arthropathy as 1.57 (OR 95% CI 1.26 to 1.97).

*Conclusion.*—Musculoskeletal AEs occur due to ciprofloxacin use. However, these musculoskeletal events are reversible with management. It is recommended that further prospective controlled studies should be carried out to evaluate the safety of ciprofloxacin, with particular focus on the risk of arthropathy.

▶ Ciprofloxacin, a commonly used broad-spectrum antibiotic, was introduced back in 1987 as a second-generation fluoroquinolone. The first quinolone discovered was nalidixic acid in 1962. It was discovered as a by-product of antimalarial research. Nalidixic acid is infrequently used these days. Its use is limited because of its narrow spectrum of antibacterial activity, low serum levels, and toxicity issues. Fluorination of the quinolone nucleus at position 6 has resulted in the introduction of second and third as well as fourth generations of fluoroquinolones.

Fluoroquinolones as a whole, including ciprofloxacin, may cause an arthropathy in young weight-bearing joints in animal studies. Cartilage damage caused by quinolones was first reported in juvenile animals (Beagle dogs aged 4-12 months) in 1977.[1] These findings have also been demonstrated in mice, rats, and rabbits. The occurrence of arthropathy in children, however, has been somewhat uncertain and thus the value of the report by Adefurin et al.

Adefurin et al have undertaken a systematic review, pulling together all safety data about the use of ciprofloxacin in pediatrics, with a critical look at the occurrence of arthropathy. The authors found 105 articles that were highly relevant to this subject. The data reported are the first pooled information that reports suspected adverse events due to ciprofloxacin use in pediatric patients. Even though this drug is generally contraindicated for use in pediatrics, the review identified more than 16 000 children who had received this particular antimicrobial. The review confirms that musculoskeletal toxicity is the most frequently reported adverse event following the use of ciprofloxacin. There is, however, a wide range of toxicity that has been reported, and it is important to recognize that, like all anti-infective agents, ciprofloxacin can be associated with a wide variety of adverse events. Based on the information from the review, it can be estimated that there will be 1 musculoskeletal adverse event in every 62.5 patients and a 57% increased risk of arthropathy in patients exposed to ciprofloxacin. These musculoskeletal adverse events appear to be reversible with management.

This review suggests that arthralgia is the most common symptom of arthropathy (50%) in pediatric patients, affecting mostly the knee joint. Tendon or joint disorders and reduced movement also account for a significant proportion of arthropathy cases (19% and 15%, respectively). Tendon disorders, including tendon rupture, are possibilities in the pediatric age population. The authors of this report say that the concern about arthropathy in pediatric patients is appropriate. This risk, however, is relatively low and reversible with management. Obviously the risk of ciprofloxacin-induced arthropathy needs to be considered in relation to the benefits of using ciprofloxacin in children with acute infection.

Although this report identified 389 newborns that were exposed to this antimicrobial, the data are insufficient to say whether ciprofloxacin is problematic when used at this very young age. The role of ciprofloxacin in pediatric and neonatal sepsis can only be clarified by further prospective studies evaluating both the benefit and the risk of toxicity. Such studies should be highly focused on the risk of arthropathy.

**J. A. Stockman III, MD**

*Reference*

1. Ingham B, Brentnall DW, Dale EA, et al. Arthropathy induced by antibacterial fused N-alkyl-4-pyridone-3-carboxylic acids. *Toxicol Lett.* 1977;6:21-26.

## Mycoestrogen Pollution of Italian Infant Food

Meucci V, Soldani G, Razzuoli E, et al (Univ of Pisa, Italy)
*J Pediatr* 159:278-283, 2011

*Objective.*—To determine the concentrations of zearalenone and its metabolites in the leading brands of infant formula milks and meat-based infant foods commonly marketed in Italy, and to assess their repercussion in the provisional tolerable daily intakes of these estrogenic mycotoxins.

*Study Design.*—A total of 185 cow's milk-based infant formulas and 44 samples of meat-based infant foods samples were analyzed. The analysis of mycotoxins was performed by immunoaffinity column clean-up and high-pressure liquid chromatography with fluorescence detection.

*Results.*—Zearalenone was detected in 17 (9%) milk samples (maximum 0.76 μg/L). The α-zearalenol was detected in 49 (26%) milk samples (maximum 12.91 μg/L). The β-zearalenol was detected in 53 (28%) milk samples (maximum 73.24 μg/L). The α-zearalanol and β-zearalanol were not detected in milk samples. Although α-zearalenol was detected in 12 (27%) meat samples (maximum 30.50 μg/kg), only one meat-based sample was contaminated by α zearalanol (950 μg/kg). Zearalenone, β-zearalenol, and β-zearalanol were not detected in meat samples.

*Conclusions.*—This study shows the presence of mycoestrogens in infant (milk-based and meat-based) food, and this is likely to have great implications for subsequent generations, suggesting the need to perform occurrence surveys in this type of food.

▶ In recent times we have heard a lot about problems with the way formulas and infant foods are manufactured. There was a report from Italy of the contamination of infant formula by aflatoxin M1 and ochratoxin A.[1] Although this problem did not occur on the shores of the United States, it does exemplify problems that can arise in the production of what would otherwise be considered a safe food product. Also of concern is the potential for contamination of commercial infant food itself, particularly with respect to zearalenone and its metabolites. Zearalenone is a nonsteroidal mycotoxin produced by *Fusarium* sp on grain. This mycotoxin exhibits estrogenic and anabolic properties in several animal species, including humans. Contamination of food by zearalenone is caused either by direct contamination of grains and fruits or by the carryover of mycotoxins and their metabolites in animal tissues, milk, and eggs after intake of contaminated foodstuffs. The harmful effects of zearalenone are increased through its derivatives and metabolites, which have a remarkable ability to mimic estrogen, acting as an estrogen receptor agonist.

Meucci et al designed a study to determine the concentrations of zearalenone and its metabolites in leading brands of infant formulas (all marketed in Italy, not in the United States). They also determined the level of mycotoxins that contaminate meat-based baby foods. The investigators studied many infant formulas based on cow's milk and also investigated meat-based infant foods. Zearalenone was detected in 9% of milk samples. A derivative of zearalenone was detected in 26% of milk samples. The study clearly documented the presence of mycoestrogens in infant formula produced in Italy. With respect to meat-based food samples, this is the first report showing the presence of zearalenone metabolites. The presence of mycoestrogens in food is likely to have greater implications for infants and young children than for adults. Presumably, mycotoxins result from the ingestion by cattle of feed containing mycoestrogens.

All of us should be aware that since 1969 a derivative of zearalenone, alpha zearalenol, has been widely adopted as a growth stimulant in the United States to improve the fattening rates of cattle. Its use has been banned in the European Union since 1985, along with hormones including estradiol, progesterone, testosterone, trenbolone acetate, and melengestrol acetate. There is also a European ban on imported meat and meat products derived from cattle given these hormones other than for veterinary reasons.

The bottom line here is that it would be interesting to see the studies that have been performed in Italy reproduced in the United States in order to determine the magnitude of a problem, if any exists, with the infant food supply.

This commentary closes with a mention about the therapeutic value of *B serrata*. *B serrata* refers to *Boswellia serrata*, better known as frankincense. Recall Matthew 2:10-11:

> *When they saw the star, they rejoiced exceedingly with great joy. And going into the house they saw the child with Mary, his mother, and they fell down and worshiped him. Then opening their treasures, they offered him gifts, gold and frankincense and myrrh.*

What was being offered by the Three Wise Men were the resin frankincense as well as myrrh, offerings hardly for the purposes of religious ceremony, rather for the medicinal properties of these resins. Frankincense in particular has a long history of use—for example, in religious ceremonies and for perfume production—and its medicinal properties have been appreciated for millennia. Only recently, however, has a systematic review of the medicinal value of frankincense been published.[2] This review suggests that *Boswellia* extracts may show some promise in treating asthma, rheumatoid arthritis, Crohn disease, knee osteoarthritis, and colitis, given the antiinflammatory properties of *Boswellia* extracts. The same systematic review also noted that adverse effects of *B serrata* were minor and not judged to be related to the treatment for which the resin was being used. Before jumping on the frankincense bandwagon, it should be noted that the evidence presented from the systematic review, while encouraging, was not totally convincing. Not enough large randomized clinical trials have been published for any one condition to recommend the use of frankincense to treat disease. The pharmacokinetics and optimal dose of *B serrata* extracts are largely unknown. Usually 600 mg to 3000 mg gum resin per day or equivalence thereof are recommended for oral intake. Dozens of *B serrata* preparations for oral intake are commercially available and frequently found in health food stores. The majority are not regulated as medicine, but sold as food supplements. Fortunately, the safety profile of *B serrata* seems quite good. In the clinical trials undertaken to date, no serious, long-term, or irreversible adverse effects have been noted. Other data indicate that mild adverse effects such as nausea, acid reflux, and gastrointestinal upset may occasionally occur. No evidence of drug interaction with other pharmaceuticals has been noted.

There actually is a lot of street noise about the use of frankincense these days. Currently more than one million web sites exist on "frankincense" and half a million on "*Boswellia.*" The majority fail to offer reliable information on its medicinal uses. The systematic review ends with some interesting words of potential wisdom: "Absence of evidence is not the same as evidence of absence," which is particularly relevant in herbal medicine, where pharmacovigilance is often less than optimal.

**J. A. Stockman III, MD**

*References*

1. Meucci V, Razzuoli E, Soldani G, Massart F. Mycotoxin detection in infant formula milks in Italy. *Food Addit Contam Part A Chem Anal Control Expo Risk Assess.* 2010;27:64-71.
2. Ernst E. Frankincense: a systematic review. *BMJ.* 2008;337:1439-1441.

## Impact of Early-Life Bisphenol A Exposure on Behavior and Executive Function in Children

Braun JM, Kalkbrenner AE, Calafat AM, et al (Harvard Univ, Boston, MA; Univ of North Carolina, Chapel Hill; Natl Ctr for Environmental Health, Atlanta, GA; et al)
*Pediatrics* 128:873-882, 2011

*Objectives.*—To estimate the impact of gestational and childhood bisphenol A (BPA) exposures on behavior and executive function at 3 years of age and to determine whether child gender modified those associations.

*Methods.*—We used a prospective birth cohort of 244 mothers and their 3-year-old children from the greater Cincinnati, Ohio, area. We characterized gestational and childhood BPA exposures by using the mean BPA concentrations in maternal (16 and 26 weeks of gestation and birth) and child (1, 2, and 3 years of age) urine samples, respectively. Behavior and executive function were measured by using the Behavior Assessment System for Children 2 (BASC-2) and the Behavior Rating Inventory of Executive Function-Preschool (BRIEF-P).

*Results.*—BPA was detected in >97% of the gestational (median: 2.0 μg/L) and childhood (median: 4.1 μg/L) urine samples. With adjustment for confounders, each 10-fold increase in gestational BPA concentrations was associated with more anxious and depressed behavior on the BASC-2 and poorer emotional control and inhibition on the BRIEF-P. The magnitude of the gestational BPA associations differed according to child gender; BASC-2 and BRIEF-P scores increased 9 to 12 points among girls, but changes were null or negative among boys. Associations between childhood BPA exposure and neurobehavior were largely null and not modified by child gender.

*Conclusions.*—In this study, gestational BPA exposure affected behavioral and emotional regulation domains at 3 years of age, especially among girls. Clinicians may advise concerned patients to reduce their exposure to certain consumer products, but the benefits of such reductions are unclear.

▶ There has been a great deal written in recent years about the consequences of exposure to bisphenol A (BPA). BPA is found in a number of consumer products ranging from dental sealants, food-beverage containers and linings, medical equipment, and thermal receipts. There is no way currently to avoid some BPA exposure. It is known that BPA can disrupt the endocrine system. Experimental studies in animals indicate that gestational exposure to BPA will influence normal neurodevelopment, affecting sexually dimorphic behavior such as aggression, anxiety, exploration, and spatial memory.[1] The issue is whether any behavioral outcomes reported in nonhuman species translate into the human situation. The authors of this report have noted previously that gestational BPA exposure is associated with increased hyperactivity and aggression scores for 2-year-old girls in a prospective birth cohort from Cincinnati, Ohio.[2] Interestingly, this earlier study did not document persistence of continued development past early childhood and was unable to examine the relationship between BPA exposure and executive function, which is a set of processes involved with inhibiting behavior, modulating emotions, and shifting between activities.

To examine the void that currently exists in our understanding of the impact of BPA exposure early in life, Braun et al carried out studies specifically designed to see whether executive functioning was altered by early BPA exposure as a child matured. Behavior and executive functions were measured by using the Behavior Assessment System for Children 2 (BASC2) and the Behavior Rating Inventory of Executive Function in Preschool (BRIEF-P). In this report, almost 250 mothers and their children were followed in the greater Cincinnati area. Maternal urine samples were collected twice during pregnancy for BPA concentration determination. Children's spot urine samples were collected at 1, 2, and 3 years of age. These samples were taken over a 5-year period from 2004 to 2009. The offspring were then followed for several years to determine any impact of BPA exposure and later changes in childhood behavior and executive function.

Only 3% of mothers showed no detectable BPA in their urine during pregnancy. It was clear that each 10-fold increase in gestational BPA concentrations was associated with more anxious and depressed behavior and poorer emotional control and inhibition in the offspring by 3 years of age. These findings are quite consistent with numerous studies demonstrating altered neurobehavior among BPA-exposed animals. The study also suggested that girls are significantly more sensitive to gestational BPA exposure than are boys. This is an intriguing finding. Perhaps girls are just nicer to begin with, and the fall from grace resulting from BPA seems more dramatic. Just a theory.

This commentary begins to close with some information provided in a letter to the editor of *JAMA* in November 2007. Investigators from the Harvard School of Public Health and the National Center for Environmental Health looked at the impact of eating canned soup on BPA urinary levels in a group of volunteer student and faculty at the Harvard School of Public Health. Using a randomized, single-blinded, 2 × crossover design, for a 5-day period, one study group consumed a 12-ounce serving of fresh soup prepared from fresh materials without canned ingredients daily between 12:15 PM and 2:00 PM. The other group consumed a 12-ounce serving of canned soup (Progresso brand) for the same schedule. After a 2-day washout, treatment assignments were reversed. Urinary samples showed BPA detected in 77% of samples after fresh soup consumption and 100% of samples after canned soup consumption. The difference in actual BPA levels, however, was dramatic. Consumption of 1 serving of canned soup daily over 5 days was associated with a more than 100 000-fold increase in urinary BPA amounts. The absolute urinary BPA concentrations observed following canned soup consumption are among the most extreme reported in nonoccupational settings.[3]

Please note that only 1 brand of canned soup was evaluated as part of this study. It is known that BPA has been found in many canned foods where it is present as a by-product of interior epoxy coatings used to prevent corrosion. It just might be safer eating a can of Campbell's from the 1930s than one from 2012.

Here is a toxicologic "whodunit." In October 8, 1587, Francesco I de'Medici, Grand Duke of Tuscany, and his bride, Bianca Cappello, died of an illness that at the time was attributed to malaria. They were sick for just 11 days before their demise. There were rumors, however, at the time that the two had been murdered by Francesco's brother, Cardinal Ferdinando. Apparently, Ferdinando had a very good motive to kill his brother and the woman that Francesco had loved and then married after the death of his first wife, the Grand Duchess Giovanna of Austria. Ferdinando was at risk of being excluded from the succession if Francesco's illegitimate son, Don Antonio, was to inherit the title of Grand Duke or, even worse, if Bianca, who was no longer able to have children, was to falsify the birth of the heir. The symptoms reported by doctors attending Francesco included nausea and violent vomiting as initial symptoms; cold sweats, repeated requests for cold drinks because of terrible dryness and constant gastric burning; the persistence of violent and convulsive vomiting; aggressive and delirious restlessness; and apparent improvement 4 to 5 days after the onset of illness, followed by the sudden return of symptoms. Much less is known about Bianca's illness, though her doctors reported that she had been struck by a disease very similar in nature to that of her husband. Given the fact that these symptoms are quite different than those of typical malarial infection, what is your hypothesis as to the toxicologic cause of death?

If you answered arsenic poisoning, you would be correct. Investigators from the University of Pisa with authorization from the Director of the Medici Chapels in Florence had the opportunity to collect biological material from the grave of Francesco I as well as from Francesco I's wife, both buried in a crypt in the church of Santa Maria. Multiple samples taken from Francesco I showed clearcut evidence of arsenic poisoning of an acute nature (hair samples showed no evidence of arsenic, whereas tissue samples did). Francesco I did not live long enough to have arsenic showing up in his hair. Thus it is that modern science documented the murders of two of the most important Medicis.[4]

**J. A. Stockman III, MD**

*References*

1. Palanza P, Gioiosa L, vom Saal FS, Parmigiani S. Effects of developmental exposure to bisphenol A on brain and behavior in mice. *Environ Res.* 2008;108: 150-157.
2. Braun JM, Yolton K, Dietrich KN, et al. Prenatal bisphenol A exposure and early childhood behavior. *Environ Health Perspect.* 2009;117:1945-1952.
3. Carwile JL, Ye X, Zhou X, Calafat AM, Michels KB. Canned soup consumption and urinary bisphenol A: a randomized crossover trial. *JAMA.* 2011;306:2218-2220.
4. Mari F, Polettini A, Lippi D, Bertol E. Mysterious death of Francesco I de'Medici and Bianca Cappello: an arsenic murder? *BMJ.* 2006;333:1299-1301.

# Article Index

## Chapter 1: Adolescent Medicine

## Chapter 2: Allergy and Dermatology

## Chapter 3: Blood

## Chapter 4: Child Development/Behavior

## Chapter 5: Dentistry and Otolaryngology (ENT)

## Chapter 6: Endocrinology

## Chapter 7: Gastroenterology

## Chapter 8: Genitourinary Tract

## Chapter 9: Heart and Blood Vessels

## Chapter 10: Infectious Diseases and Immunology

## Chapter 11: Miscellaneous

## Chapter 12: Musculoskeletal

## Chapter 13: Neurology and Psychiatry

## Chapter 14: Newborn

## Chapter 15: Nutrition and Metabolism

## Chapter 16: Oncology

## Chapter 17: Ophthalmology

## Chapter 18: Respiratory Tract

## Chapter 19: Therapeutics and Toxicology

# Author Index

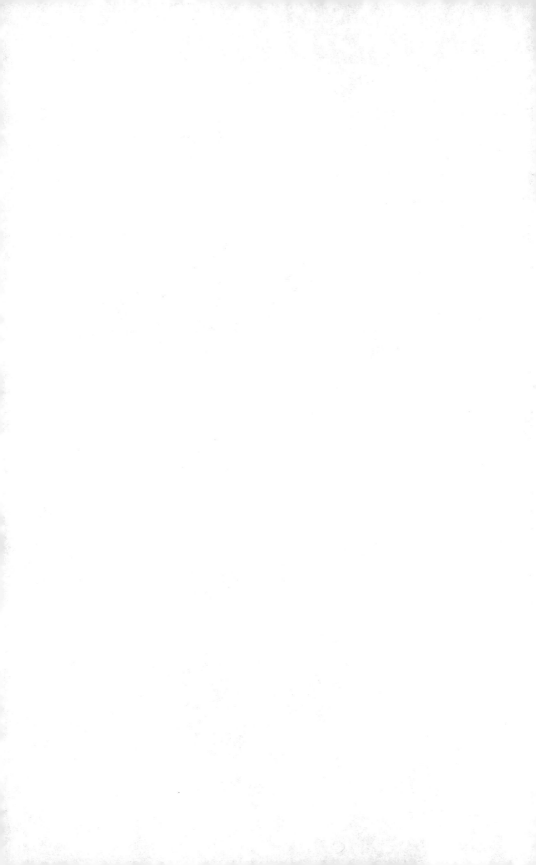

Edwards Brothers Malloy
Ann Arbor MI. USA
June 7, 2013